CLINICIAN'S POCKET REFERENCE

The Scut Monkey Book
1979–2004

Celebrating 25 years of providing medical students, residents, practicing physicians, and health care providers with the essential and up-to-date information for excellence in basic patient care

EDITED BY

LEONARD G. GOMELLA, MD, FACS

The Bernard W. Godwin, Jr., Professor
And Chairman
Department of Urology
Jefferson Medical College
Thomas Jefferson University
Philadelphia, Pennsylvania

STEVEN A. HAIST, MD, MS, FACP

Professor of Medicine
Division of General Internal Medicine
Department of Internal Medicine
University of Kentucky Medical Center
Lexington, Kentucky

Based on a program originally developed
at the University of Kentucky College
of Medicine Lexington, Kentucky
WWW.THESCUTMONKEY.COM

McGraw-Hill
MEDICAL PUBLISHING DIVISION

New York   Chicago   San Francisco   Lisbon   London
Madrid   Mexico City   Milan   New Delhi   San Juan
Seoul   Singapore   Sydney   Toronto

The McGraw-Hill Companies

Clinician's Pocket Reference, 10th Edition

1234567890 DOC/DOC 09876543
ISBN: 0-07-140255-1
ISSN: 1041-1348

Notice

Medicine is an ever-changing science. As new research and clinical experience broaden our knowledge, changes in treatment and drug therapy are required. The authors and the publisher of this work have checked with sources believed to be reliable in their efforts to provide information that is complete and generally in accord with the standards accepted at the time of publication. However, in view of the possibility of human error or changes in medical sciences, neither the editors nor the publisher nor any other party who has been involved in the preparation or publication of this work warrants that the information contained herein is in every respect accurate or complete, and they disclaim all responsibility for any errors or omissions or for the results obtained from use of the information contained in this work. Readers are encouraged to confirm the information contained herein with other sources. For example and in particular, readers are advised to check the product information sheet included in the package of each drug they plan to administer to be certain that the information contained in this work is accurate and that changes have not been made in the recommended dose or in the contraindications for administration. This recommendation is of particular importance in connection with new or infrequently used drugs.

The book was set in Times Roman by Pine Tree Composition, Inc.
The editors were Janet Foltin, Harriet Lebowitz, and Karen G. Edmonson.
The production supervisor was Catherine H. Saggese.
The text designer was Marsha Cohen/Parallelogram Graphics.
The cover designer was Mary McKeon.
The illustration manager was Charissa Baker.
The indexer was Pamela J. Edwards.
R. R. Donnelley was printer and binder.

This book is printed on acid-free paper.

INTERNATIONAL EDITION ISBN: 0-07-121968-4

To Tricia, Mom, Dad, Leonard, Patrick, Andrew, Michael and Aunt Lucy

To Meg, Sarah and Will

"We don't drive the trucks, we only load them."
Nick Pavona, MD
UKMC Class of 1980

CONTENTS

PREFACE

For the last 25 years, students, residents, practicing physicians, nurses and other allied health professionals have turned to the "Scut Monkey Book" for learning the essential information on basic patient care. The *Clinician's Pocket Reference* is based on a University of Kentucky manual entitled *So You Want to Be a Scut Monkey: Medical Student's and House Officer's Clinical Handbook.* The "Scut Monkey" program at the University of Kentucky College of Medicine was first held in the summer of 1979 and was developed by the Class of 1980 to help ease the sometimes frustrating transition from the preclinical to the clinical years of medical school. Based on detailed surveys from the University of Kentucky and 44 other medical schools, the essential information and skills that students should be familiar with at the start of their clinical years was developed.

The "Scut Monkey" program was developed around this core and consisted of a simple reference manual and a series of workshops conducted at the start of the third year. Held originally as a pilot program for the University of Kentucky College of Medicine Class of 1981, the program has become an annual event. Each new fourth-year class has the responsibility of orienting the new third-year students in basic skills. The program is successful because it was developed and taught *by students for other students.* Over the years, students have been the main source of feedback for the book, perhaps another secret to its enduring success. Information on the "Scut Monkey" orientation program is available from Dr. Todd Cheever, Assistant Dean for Academic Affairs at the University of Kentucky College of Medicine in Lexington.

Over the last nine editions and 25 years, the book has been continually updated to reflect the dynamic changes in medical care. Because of the demand for the information in this book, it is now on a two-year revision cycle to keep the information as up to date as possible. An attempt is made to cover the most frequently asked basic management questions that are normally found in many different sources such as procedure manuals, laboratory manuals, drug references, and critical care manuals, to name a few. This book is not meant as a substitute for specialty-specific reference manuals; the core information presented is the essential foundation for the new medical student or health care provider in training.

The book is designed to represent a cross section of medical practices around the country, and over the years, contributors from dozens of medical centers have had input. The *Clinician's Pocket Reference* has been translated into several languages with the much requested electronic media version in development. The "Scut Monkey" was honored to have been asked by Warner Brothers, the producers of the TV show "ER", to be one of the prop books used on their series. The companion manual, the *Clinician's Pocket Drug Reference,* has been very successful and is entering its third edition this year.

We would like to express special thanks to our wives and families for their long-term support of the "Scut Monkey" project. Linda Davoli, our extraordinary copy editor, knows just how to communicate information to busy readers. Janet Foltin, Janene Matragrano Oransky, Harriet Lebowitz, and the team at Mc-Graw-Hill are valued in moving the book forward and assisting in developing the electronic "Scut Monkey." A special thanks to our assistant Conchita Ballard who always keeps things organized.

A word of gratitude to the administration of the University of Kentucky College of Medicine: Drs. Kay Clawson, Terry Leigh, and Roy Jarecky, and the then very young faculty member Dr. Richard Braen, who took a chance and supported a group of third-year medical students who wanted to try something a "little bit different" way back in 1978. Thanks also to the hundreds of past contributors, Dr. Michael Olding, one of the project's cofounders, and readers who have helped to establish the "Scut Monkey Book" as one of the most useful references for students and residents worldwide. Every medical student at the University of Kentucky College of Medicine for the last 25 years has received a courtesy copy of this book as a small token of our appreciation for the University's dedication to producing outstanding and caring physicians who serve patients in the Commonwealth and beyond.

We're always grateful for your comments and suggestions because they allow us to keep the book up to date and useful, an effort that would be impossible if it were not for the ongoing interest of our readers. We hope this book will not only help you learn some of the basics of the art and science of medicine but also allow you to care for your patients in the best way possible.

Lastly (for those of you paying close attention and who actually read the preface of a book!), in honor of our 25th anniversary and his 25th birthday, the Scut Monkey has been given a fresh new look, his third makeover in 25 years. Let us know what you think.

Leonard G. Gomella, MD
Philadelphia, Pennsylvania
Leonard.Gomella@Jefferson.edu

Steven A. Haist, MD
Lexington, Kentucky
sahaist@uky.edu

ABBREVIATIONS

The following are common abbreviations used in medical records and in this edition

÷: divided dose
↓: decrease(d), reduce, downward
×: times for multiplication sign
↑: increase(d), upward (as in titrate upward)
/: per
+/-: with or without
+: with
<: less than, younger than
>: more than, older than
≅: approximately equal to
AAA: abdominal aortic aneurysm
AaDO$_2$: difference in partial pressures of oxygen in mixed alveolar gas and mixed arterial blood
A-a gradient: alveolar-to-arterial gradient
AAI: ankle—arm index
AAS: acute abdominal series
AB: antibody, abortion, antibiotic
A&B: apnea and bradycardia
ABD: abdomen
ABG: arterial blood gas
A/B index: ankle—brachial index
ABMT: autologous bone marrow transplantation
ac: before eating (*ante cibum*), assist controlled
ACCP: American College of Chest Physicians
ACE: angiotensin-converting enzyme
Ach-ase: acetylcholinesterase
ACLS: Advanced Cardiac Life Support
ACP: American College of Physicians
ACS: acute coronary syndrome, American Cancer Society, American College of Surgeons
ACTH: adrenocorticotropic hormone
A.D.C. VAAN DIML: mnemonic for Admit, Diagnosis, Condition, Vitals, Activity, Allergies, Nursing procedures, Diet, Ins and outs, Medications, Labs
A.D.C. VAN DISSL: mnemonic for Admit, Diagnosis, Condition, Vitals, Activity, Nursing procedures, Diet, Ins and outs, Specific drugs, Symptomatic drugs, Labs
ADH: antidiuretic hormone
ADHD: attention-deficit hyperactivity disorder
ad lib: as much as needed (*ad libitum*)
AED: automatic external defibrillator
AEIOU TIPS: mnemonic for Alcohol, Encephalopathy, Insulin, Opiates, Uremia, Trauma, Infection, Psychiatric, Syncope (diagnosis of coma)
AF: afebrile, aortofemoral, atrial fibrillation
AFB: acid-fast bacilli
AFP: alpha-fetoprotein
A/G: albumin/globulin ratio
AHA: American Heart Association
AHF: antihemophilic factor
AI: aortic insufficiency
AIDS: acquired immunodeficiency syndrome
AJCC: American Joint Committee on Cancer
AKA: above-the-knee amputation
ALAT: alanine aminotransferase
ALL: acute lymphocytic leukemia
ALS: amyotrophic lateral sclerosis
ALT: alanine aminotransferase
AM: morning
amb: ambulate
AMI: acute myocardial infarction
AML: acute myelocytic leukemia, acute myelogenous leukemia
AMMoL: acute monocytic leukemia
amp: ampule
AMP: adenosine monophosphate
ANA: antinuclear antibody
ANC: absolute neutrophil count
ANCA: antineutrophil cytoplasmic antibody
ANLL: acute nonlymphoblastic leukemia
ANS: autonomic nervous system
AOB: alcohol on breath
AP: anteroposterior, abdominal—perineal

APAP: acetaminophen
APL: acute promyelocytic leukemia
aPPT: activated partial thromboplastin time
APSAC: anisoylated plasminogen streptokinase activator complex
APUD: amine precursor uptake (and) decarboxylation
Ara-C: cytarabine
ARD: antibiotic removal device
ARDS: adult respiratory distress syndrome
ARF: acute renal failure
AS: aortic stenosis
ASA: American Society of Anesthesiologists
ASAP: as soon as possible
ASAT: aspartate aminotransferase
ASCVD: atherosclerotic cardiovascular disease
ASD: atrial septal defect
ASHD: atherosclerotic heart disease
ASO: antistreptolysin O
AST: aspartate aminotransferase
ATG: antithymocyte globulin
ATN: acute tubular necrosis
ATP: adenosine triphosphate
AUC: area under the curve
AV: atrioventricular
A-V: arteriovenous
A-Vo$_2$: arteriovenous oxygen
B I&II: Billroth I and II
BACOD: bleomycin, doxorubicin (Adriamycin), cyclophosphamide, vincristine (Oncovin), dexamethasone
BACOP: bleomycin, doxorubicin (Adriamycin), cyclophosphamide, vincristine (Oncovin), prednisone
BBB: bundle branch block
BC: bone conduction
BCAA: branched-chain amino acid
BCG: bacille Calmette-Guérin
BE: barium enema
BEE: basal energy expenditure
bid: twice a day (*bis in die*)
bili: bilirubin
BKA: below-the-knee amputation
BM: bone marrow, bowel movement
BMR: basal metabolic rate
BMT: bone marrow transplantation
BOM: bilateral otitis media
BP: blood pressure
BPH: benign prostatic hypertrophy
bpm: beats per minute
BR: bed rest
BRBPR: bright red blood per rectum
BRP: bathroom privileges
bs, BS: bowel sounds, breath sounds
BSA: body surface area
BS&O: bilateral salpingo-oophorectomy

BUN: blood urea nitrogen
BW: body weight
Bx: biopsy
c: with (*cum*)
Ca: calcium
CA: cancer
CAA: crystalline amino acid
CABG: coronary artery bypass graft
CAD: coronary artery disease
CAF: cyclophosphamide, doxorubicin (Adriamycin), 5-fluorouracil
CALGB: Cancer and Leukemia Group B
cAMP: cyclic adenosine monophosphate
Cao$_2$: arterial oxygen content
caps: capsule(s)
CAT: computed axial tomography
CBC: complete blood count
CBG: capillary blood gas
CC: chief complaint
CCI: corrected count increment (platelets)
CCO: continuous cardiac output
CCO$_2$: capillary oxygen content
CCU: clean-catch urine, cardiac care unit
CCV: critical closing volume
CD: continuous dose
CDC: Centers for Disease Control and Prevention
CEA: carcinoembryonic antigen
CEP/CIEP: counterimmunoelectrophoresis
CF: cystic fibrosis
CFU: colony-forming unit(s)
CGL: chronic granulocytic leukemia
CH$_{50}$: (total serum) hemolytic complement
CHD: coronary heart disease
CHF: congestive heart failure
CHO: carbohydrate
CHOP: cyclophosphamide, doxorubicin, vincristine (Oncovin), prednisone
CI: cardiac index
CIE: counterimmunoelectrophoresis
CIS: carcinoma in situ
CK: creatine phosphokinase
CKI: cyclin-dependent kinase inhibitor
CK-MB: isoenzyme of creatine kinase with muscle and brain subunits
Cl: chlorine
CLL: chronic lymphocytic leukemia
cm: centimeter
CML: chronic myelogenous leukemia
CMV: cytomegalovirus
CN: cranial nerve
CNS: central nervous system
CO: cardiac output
C/O: complaining of
COAD: chronic obstructive airway disease
COLD: chronic obstructive lung disease
COMT: catechol-*O*-methyltransferase
conc: concentrate

cont inf: continuous infusion
COPD: chronic obstructive pulmonary disease
COX-2: cyclooxygenase-2
CP: chest pain, cerebral palsy
CPAP: continuous positive airway pressure
CPK: creatinine phosphokinase
CPP: central precocious puberty
CPR: cardiopulmonary resuscitation
CR: controlled release
CrCl: creatine clearance
CREST: calcinosis cutis, Raynaud's disease, esophageal dysmotility, syndactyly, telangiectasia
CRF: chronic renal failure
CRH: corticotropin-releasing hormone
CRP: C-reactive protein
C&S: culture and sensitivity
CSF: cerebrospinal fluid, colony-stimulating factor
C-spine: cervical spine
CT: computed tomography
CVA: cerebrovascular accident, costovertebral angle
CVAT: costovertebral angle tenderness
CVH: common variable hypogammaglobulinemia
Cvo$_2$: oxygen content of mixed venous blood
CVP: central venous pressure
CXR: chest x-ray
d: day
D$_5$LR: 5% dextrose in lactated Ringer's solution
D$_5$W: 5% dextrose in water
DAG: diacylglycerol
DAP: diastolic pulmonary artery pressure
DAT: diet as tolerated
DAW: dispense as written
DC: discontinue, discharge, direct current
D&C: dilation and curettage
ddI: dideoxyinosine
DDx: differential diagnosis
DEA: United States Drug Enforcement Administration
DES: diethylstilbestrol
DEXA: dual-energy x-ray absorptiometer
DFA: direct fluorescent antibody
DHEA: dehydroepiandrosterone
DHEAS: dehydroepiandrosterone sulfate
DI: diabetes insipidus
DIC: disseminated intravascular coagulation
DIP: distal interphalangeal joint
DIT: diiodotyrosine
DJD: degenerative joint disease
DKA: diabetic ketoacidosis
dL: deciliter
DM: diabetes mellitus
DMSA: dimercaptosuccinic acid

DNA: deoxyribonucleic acid
DNP: deoxyribonucleic protein
DNR: do not resuscitate
DOA: dead on arrival
DOCA: deoxycorticosterone acetate
DOE: dyspnea on exertion
DOPA: dihydroxyphenylalanine
DP: dorsalis pedis
2,3-DPG: 2,3-diphosphoglycerate
DPL: diagnostic peritoneal lavage
DPT: diphtheria, pertussis, tetanus
DR: delayed release
DRG: diagnosis-related group
DS: double strength
DSA: digital subtraction angiography
DTPA: diethylenetriamine-pentaacetic acid
DTR: deep tendon reflex
DVT: deep venous thrombosis
Dx: diagnosis
EAA: essential amino acid
EBL: estimated blood loss
EBV: Epstein—Barr virus
EC: enteric-coated
ECG: electrocardiogram
ECOG: Eastern Cooperative Oncology Group
ECT: electroconvulsive therapy
EDC: estimated date of confinement
EDTA: ethylenediamine tetraacetic acid
EDVI: end-diastolic volume index
EFAD: essential fatty acid deficiency
EIA: enzyme immunoassay
ELISA: enzyme-linked immunosorbent assay
EMD: electromechanical dissociation
EMG: electromyelogram
EMS: emergency medical system, eosinophilia-myalgia syndrome
EMV: eyes, motor, verbal response (Glasgow Coma Scale)
ENA: extractable nuclear antigen
ENT: ear, nose, and throat
eod: every other day
EOM: extraocular muscle
EPO: erythropoietin
EPSP: excitatory postsynaptic potential
ER: endoplasmic reticulum, emergency room, extended release
ERCP: endoscopic retrograde cholangiopancreatography
ERV: expiratory reserve volume
ESR: erythrocyte sedimentation rate
ESRD: end-stage renal disease
ET: endotracheal
ETOH: ethanol
ETT: endotracheal tube
EUA: examination under anesthesia
ExU: excretory urogram
Fab: antigen-binding fragment

FANA: fluorescent antinuclear antibody

FBS: fasting blood sugar

Fe: iron

FEV_1: forced expiratory volume in 1 s

FFP: fresh frozen plasma

FHR: fetal heart rate

FIGO: Fédération Internationale de Gynécologie et d'Obstétrique

FiO_2: fraction of inspired oxygen

FRC: functional residual capacity

FSH: follicle-stimulating hormone

FSP: fibrin split product

ft: foot

FTA-ABS: fluorescent treponemal antibody-absorbed

FTT: failure to thrive

FU: follow-up

5-FU: fluorouracil

FUO: fever of unknown origin

FVC: forced vital capacity

Fx: fracture

g: gram

G: gravida

GABA: γ-aminobutyric acid

GAD: glutamic acid decarboxylase

GC: gonorrhea (gonococcus)

G-CSF: granulocyte colony-stimulating factor

GDP: guanosine diphosphate

GERD: gastroesophageal reflux disease

GETT: general by endotracheal tube (anesthesia)

GFR: glomerular filtration rate

GGT: γ-glutamyltransferase

GH: growth hormone

GHIH: growth hormone-inhibiting hormone

GI: gastrointestinal

GM-CSF: granulocyte-macrophage colony-stimulating factor

GNID: gram-negative intracellular diplococci

GnRH: gonadotropin-releasing hormone

GOG: Gynecologic Oncology Group

G6PD: glucose-6-phosphate dehydrogenase

gr: grain

GSW: gunshot wound

gt, gtt: drop, drops (*gutta*)

GTP: guanosine triphosphate

GTT: glucose tolerance test

GU: genitourinary

GVHD: graft-versus-host disease

GXT: graded exercise tolerance (cardiac stress test)

HA: headache

HAA: hepatitis B surface antigen (hepatitis-associated antigen)

HAV: hepatitis A virus

HBcAb: hepatitis B core antibody

HBeAg: hepatitis B e antigen

HBP: high blood pressure

HBsAg: hepatitis B surface antigen

HBV: hepatitis B virus

HCG: human chorionic gonadotropin

HCL: hairy cell leukemia

HCT: hematocrit

HCTZ: hydrochlorothiazide

HCV: hepatitis C virus

HDL: high-density lipoprotein

HEENT: head, eyes, ears, nose, and throat

HFV: high-frequency ventilation

Hgb: hemoglobin

[Hgb]: hemoglobin concentration

H/H: hemoglobin/hematocrit, Henderson—Hasselbalch equation

HIAA: 5-hydroxyindoleacetic acid

HIDA: hepatic 2,6-dimethyliminodiacetic acid

HIV: human immunodeficiency virus

HJR: hepatojugular reflex

HLA: histocompatibility locus antigen

HOB: head of bed

H&P: history and physical examination

hpf: high-power field

HPI: history of the present illness

HPLC: high-pressure liquid chromatography

HPV: human papilloma virus

HR: heart rate

hs: at bedtime (*hora somni*)

HSG: hysterosalpingogram

HSM: hepatosplenomegaly

HSV: herpes simplex virus

$5-HT_3$: 5-hydroxytryptamine

HTLV-III: human T-lymphotropic virus, type III (AIDS agent, HIV)

HTN: hypertension

HUS: hemolytic uremic syndrome

Hx: history

IC: inspiratory capacity

ICN: intensive care nursery

ICS: intercostal space

ICSH: interstitial cell-stimulating hormone

ICU: intensive care unit

ID: identification, infectious disease

I&D: incision and drainage

IDDM: insulin-dependent diabetes mellitus

Ig: immunoglobulin

IgG1κ: immunoglobulin G1 kappa

IHSS: idiopathic hypertrophic subaortic stenosis

IL: interleukin

IM: intramuscular

IMV: intermittent mandatory ventilation

in.: inch

INF: intravenous nutritional fluid

INH: isoniazid

inhal: inhalation
inj: injection
INR: international normalized ratio
I&O: intake and output
IP$_3$: inositol triphosphate
IPPB: intermittent positive pressure breathing
IPSP: inhibitory postsynaptic potential
iPTH: parathyroid hormone by radioimmunoassay
IR: inversion recovery
IRBBB: incomplete right bundle branch block
IRDM: insulin-resistant diabetes mellitus
IRV: inspiratory reserve volume
ISA: intrinsic sympathomimetic activity
IT: intrathecal
ITP: idiopathic thrombocytopenic purpura
IV: intravenous
IVC: intravenous cholangiogram
IVP: intravenous pyelogram
JVD: jugular venous distention
K: potassium
katal: unit of enzyme activity
kg: kilogram
KOR: keep open rate
17-KSG: 17-ketogenic steroids
KUB: kidneys, ureters, bladder
KVO: keep vein open
L: left, liter
LAD: left axis deviation, left anterior descending
LAE: left atrial enlargement
LAHB: left anterior hemiblock
LAP: left atrial pressure, leukocyte alkaline phosphatase
LBBB: left bundle branch block
LDH: lactate dehydrogenase
LDL: low-density lipoprotein
LE: lupus erythematosus
LH: luteinizing hormone
LHRH: luteinizing hormone releasing hormone
LIH: left inguinal hernia
liq: liquid
LLL: left lower lobe
LLSB: left lower sternal border
LMP: last menstrual period
LNMP: last normal menstrual period
LOC: loss of consciousness, level of consciousness
LP: lumbar puncture
lpf: low-power field
LPN: licensed practical nurse
LSB: left sternal border
LSD: lysergic acid diethylamide
LUL: left upper lobe
LUQ: left upper quadrant
LV: left ventricle
LVD: left ventricular dysfunction

LVEDP: left ventricular end-diastolic pressure
LVH: left ventricular hypertrophy
m: meter
MAC: *Mycobacterium avium* complex
MACE: methotrexate, doxorubicin (Adriamycin), cyclophosphamide, epipodophyllotoxin
MAG$_3$: mercaptoacetyltriglycine
MAMC: midarm muscle circumference
MAO: monoamine oxidase
MAOI: monoamine oxidase inhibitor
MAP: mean arterial pressure
MAST: military/medical antishock trousers
MAT: multifocal atrial tachycardia
max: maximum
MBC: minimum bactericidal concentration
MBT: maternal blood type
MCH: mean cell hemoglobin
MCHC: mean cell hemoglobin concentration
MCT: medium-chain triglycerides
MCTD: mixed connective tissue disease
MCV: mean cell volume
MEN: multiple endocrine neoplasia
mEq: milliequivalent
MESNA: 2-mercaptoethane sulfonate sodium
met-dose: metered-dose
mg: milligram
Mg: magnesium
MHA-TP: microhemagglutination-*Treponema pallidum*
MHC: major histocompatibility complex
MI: myocardial infarction, mitral insufficiency
MIBG: metaiodobenzyl-guanidine
MIC: minimum inhibitory concentration
min: minute, minimum
MIT: monoiodotyrosine
mL: milliliter
MLE: midline episiotomy
mm: millimeter
MMEF: maximal midexpiratory flow
mm Hg: millimeters of mercury
mmol: millimole
MMR: measles, mumps, rubella
mon: month
mol: mole
MOPP: mechlorethamine, vincristine (Oncovin), procarbazine, prednisone
6-MP: mercaptopurine
MPF: M phase-promoting factor
MPGN: membrano-proliferative glomerulonephritis
MPTP: analog of meperidine (used by drug addicts)
MRI: magnetic resonance imaging

mRNA: messenger ribonucleic acid

MRS: magnetic resonance spectroscopy

MRSA: methicillin-resistant *Staphylococcus aureus*

MS: mitral stenosis, morphine sulfate, multiple sclerosis

MSBOS: maximal surgical blood order schedule

MSH: melanocyte-stimulating hormone

MTT: monotetrazolium

MTX: methotrexate

MUGA: multigated (image) acquisition (analysis)

μm: micrometer

MVA: motor vehicle accident

MVI: multivitamin injection

MVV: maximum voluntary ventilation

MyG: myasthenia gravis

Na: sodium

NAACP: mnemonic for *N*eoplasm, *A*llergy, *A*ddison's disease, *C*ollagen-vascular disease, *P*arasites (causes of eosinophilia)

NAD: no active disease

Na$^+$/K$^+$-ATPase: sodium/potassium adenosine triphosphate

NAPA: *N*-acetylated procainamide, *N*-acetylparaaminophenol

NAS: no added sodium

NAVEL: mnemonic for *N*erve, *A*rtery, *V*ein, *E*mpty space, *L*ymphatic

NCV: nerve conduction velocity

NE: norepinephrine

neb: nebulizer

NED: no evidence of recurrent disease

ng: nanogram

NG: nasogastric

NIDDM: non-insulin-dependent diabetes mellitus

NK: natural killer

NKA: no known allergies

NKDA: no known drug allergy

nmol: nanomole

NMR: nuclear magnetic resonance

NPC: nuclear pore complex

NPO: nothing by mouth (*nil per os*)

NRM: no regular medicines

NS: normal saline

NSAID: nonsteroidal antiinflammatory drug

NSILA: nonsuppressible insulin-like activity

NSR: normal sinus rhythm

NT: nasotracheal

NTG: nitroglycerin

OB: obstetrics

OCD: obsessive-compulsive disorder

OCG: oral cholecystogram

7-OCHS: 17-hydroxycorticosteroids

OD: overdose, right eye (*oculus dexter*)

oint: ointment

OM: otitis media

OOB: out of bed

ophth: ophthalmic

OPV: oral polio vaccine

OR: operating room

OS: opening snap, left eye (*oculus sinister*)

OTC: over-the-counter (medications)

OU: both eyes

p: para

PA: posteroanterior, pulmonary artery

PAC: premature atrial contraction

PAD: diastolic pulmonary artery pressure/personal automatic defibrillator

PAF: paroxysmal atrial fibrillation

PAL: periarterial lymphatic (sheath)

Pao$_2$: peripheral arterial oxygen content

PAo$_2$: alveolar oxygen

PAOP: pulmonary artery occlusion pressure

PAP: pulmonary artery pressure, prostatic acid phosphatase

PAS: systolic pulmonary artery pressure

PASG: pneumatic antishock garment

PAT: paroxysmal atrial tachycardia

PBM: pharmacy benefit manager

pc: after eating (*post cibum*)

PCA: patient-controlled analgesia

PCI: percutaneous coronary intervention

PCKD: polycystic kidney disease

PCN: percutaneous nephrostomy

pCO$_2$: partial pressure of carbon dioxide

PCP: *Pneumocystis carinii* pneumonia, phencyclidine

PCR: polymerase chain reaction

PCWP: pulmonary capillary wedge pressure

PDA: patent ductus arteriosus

PDGF: platelet-derived growth factor

PDR: *Physicians' Desk Reference*

PDS: polydioxanone

PE: pulmonary embolus, physical examination, pleural effusion

PEA: pulseless electrical activity

PEEP: positive end-expiratory pressure

PEG: polyethylene glycol, percutaneous gastrostomy

PERRLA: pupils equal, round, reactive to light and accommodation

PERRLADC: pupils equal, round, reactive to light and accommodation directly and consensually

PET: positron emission tomography

PFT: pulmonary function test

pg: picogram

PGE$_1$: prostaglandin E1

PI: pulmonic insufficiency (disease), principle investigator

PICC: peripherally inserted central catheter

PID: pelvic inflammatory disease
PIE: pulmonary infiltrates with eosinophilia
PIH: prolactin-inhibiting hormone
PKU: phenylketonuria
PMDD: premenstrual dysphoric disorder
PMH: past medical history
PMI: point of maximal impulse
PMNL: polymorphonuclear leukocyte (neutrophil)
PND: paroxysmal nocturnal dyspnea
PNS: peripheral nervous system
PO: by mouth (*per os*)
pO$_2$: partial pressure of oxygen
POD: postoperative day
postop: postoperative, after surgery
PP: pulsus paradoxus, postprandial
PPD: purified protein derivative
P&PD: percussion and postural drainage
PPN: partial parenteral nutrition
PR: by rectum
PRA: plasma renin activity
PRBC: packed red blood cells
preop: preoperative, before surgery
PRG: pregnancy
PRK: photorefractive keratectomy
PRN: as often as needed (*pro re nata*)
PS: pulmonic stenosis, partial saturation
PSA: prostate-specific antigen
PSV: pressure support ventilation
PSVT: paroxysmal supraventricular tachycardia
Pt: patient
PT: prothrombin time, physical therapy, posterior tibial
PTCA: percutaneous transluminal coronary angioplasty
PTH: parathyroid hormone
PTHC: percutaneous transhepatic cholangiogram
PTT: partial thromboplastin time
PTU: propylthiouracil
PTX: pneumothorax
PUD: peptic ulcer disease
PVC: premature ventricular contraction
PVD: peripheral vascular disease
PVR: peripheral vascular resistance
PWP: pulmonary wedge pressure
PZI: protamine zinc insulin
q: every (*quaque*)
Q: mathematical symbol for flow
qd: every day
qh: every hour
q{_}h: every {_} hours
qhs: every hour of sleep (bedtime)
qid: four times a day (*quater in die*)
QNS: quantity not sufficient
qod: every other day

Qs: volume of blood (portion of cardiac output) shunted past nonventilated alveoli
Qs/Qt: shunt fraction
Qt: total cardiac output
R: right
RA: rheumatoid arthritis, right atrium
RAD: right axis deviation
RAE: right atrial enlargement
RAP: right atrial pressure
RBBB: right bundle branch block
RBC: red blood cell (erythrocyte)
RBP: retinol-binding protein
RCC: renal cell carcinoma
RDA: recommended dietary allowance
RDS: respiratory distress syndrome (of newborn)
RDW: red cell distribution width
REF: right ventricular ejection fraction
REM: rapid eye movement
RER: rough endoplasmic reticulum
%RH: percentage of relative humidity
RIA: radioimmunoassay
RIH: right inguinal hernia
RIND: reversible ischemic neurologic deficit
RL: Ringer's lactate
RLL: right lower lobe
RLQ: right lower quadrant
RME: resting metabolic expenditure
RML: right middle lobe
RMSF: Rocky Mountain spotted fever
RNA: ribonucleic acid
RNase: ribonuclease
R/O: rule out
ROM: range of motion
ROS: review of systems
RPG: retrograde pyelogram
RPR: rapid plasma reagin
rRNA: ribosomal ribonucleic acid
RRR: regular rate and rhythm
RSV: respiratory syncytial virus
RT: rubella titer, respiratory therapy, radiation therapy
RTA: renal tubular acidosis
RTC: return to clinic
RTOG: Radiation Therapy Oncology Group
RU: resin uptake
RUG: retrograde urethrogram
RUL: right upper lobe
RUQ: right upper quadrant
RV: residual volume
RVEDVI: right ventricular end-diastolic volume index
RVH: right ventricular hypertrophy
Rx: treatment
s: without (*sine*), second
SA: sinoatrial
S&A: sugar and acetone

SAA: synthetic amino acid
SaO_2: arterial oxygen saturation
SBE: subacute bacterial endocarditis
SBFT: small bowel follow-through
SBS: short bowel syndrome
SCr: serum creatinine
segs: segmented cells
SEM: systolic ejection murmur
SER: smooth endoplasmic reticulum
SG: Swan—Ganz
SGA: small for gestational age
SGGT: serum gamma-glutamyl transpeptidase
SGOT: serum glutamic-oxaloacetic transaminase
SGPT: serum glutamic-pyruvic transaminase
SI: Système International
SIADH: syndrome of inappropriate antidiuretic hormone
sig: write on label (*signa*)
SIMV: synchronous intermittent mandatory ventilation
SIRS: systemic inflammatory response syndrome
SKSD: streptokinase-streptodornase
SL: sublingual
SLE: systemic lupus erythematosus
SMA: sequential multiple analysis
SMO: slips made out
SMX: sulfamethoxazole
SOAP: mnemonic for *S*ubjective, *O*bjective, *A*ssessment, *P*lan
SOB: shortness of breath
SOC: signed on chart
soln: solution
SPAG: small-particle aerosol generator
S/P: status post
SPECT: single-photon emission computed tomography
SQ: subcutaneous
SR: sustained release
SRP: single recognition particle
SRS-A: slow-reacting substance of anaphylaxis
SSKI: saturated solution of potassium iodide
SSRI: selective serotonin reuptake inhibitor
stat: immediately (*statim*)
STD: sexually transmitted disease
supp: suppository
susp: suspension
SVD: spontaneous vaginal delivery
Svo_2: mixed venous blood oxygen saturation
SVR: systemic vascular resistance
SVT: supraventricular tachycardia
SWOG: Southwest Oncology Group
Sx: symptoms

T: one, TT: two, etc.
T_3: triiodothyronine
T_3 RU: triiodothyronine resin uptake
T_4: thyroxine
tabs: tablet(s)
TAH: total abdominal hysterectomy
TB: tuberculosis
TBG: thyroxine-binding globulin, total blood gas
TBLC: term birth, living child
T&C: type and cross-match
TC&DB: turn, cough, and deep breathe
TCF: triceps skin fold
TCP: transcutaneous pacer
Td: tetanus-diphtheria toxoid
TD: transdermal
TEE: transesophageal echocardiography
TENS: transcutaneous electrical stimulation
TFT: thyroid function test
6-TG: 6-thioguanine
T&H: type and hold
TIA: transient ischemic attack
TIBC: total iron-binding capacity
tid: three times a day (*ter in die*)
TIG: tetanus immune globulin
TKO: to keep open
TLC: total lung capacity
TMJ: temporal mandibular joint
TMP: trimethoprim
TMP-SMX: trimethoprim-sulfamethoxazole
TNFα: tumor necrosis factor alpha
TNM: tumor-nodes-metastases
TNTC: too numerous to count
TO: telephone order
TOPV: trivalent oral polio vaccine
TORCH: toxoplasma, rubella, cytomegalovirus, herpes virus (*O* = other [syphilis])
TPA: tissue plasminogen activator
TPN: total peripheral resistance, total parenteral nutrition
TRH: thyrotropin-releasing hormone
T&S: type and screen
TSH: thyroid-stimulating hormone
TT: thrombin time
TTE: transthoracic echocardiography
TTP: thrombotic thrombocytopenic purpura
TU: tuberculin units
TUR: transurethral resection
TURBT: TUR bladder tumors
TURP: TUR prostate
TV: tidal volume
TVH: total vaginal hysterectomy
Tx: treatment, transplant, transfer
type 2 DM: type 2 diabetes mellitus, non-insulin-dependent diabetes mellitus
U: units

UA: urinalysis
UAC: uric acid: umbilical artery catheter
ud: as directed (*ut dictum*)
UDS: urodynamic studies
UGI: upper gastrointestinal
ULN: upper limit of normal
UPEP: urine protein electrophoresis
URI: upper respiratory infection
US: ultrasonography
USP: United States Pharmacopeia
UTI: urinary infection
UUN: urinary urea nitrogen
V: volt
VAMP: vincristine, doxorubicin (Adri-
    amycin), methylprednisolone
VAP: ventilator associated pneumonia
VC: vital capacity
VCUG: voiding cystourethrogram
VDRL: Venereal Disease Research Labo-
    ratory
VF: ventricular fibrillation
VLDL: very low density lipoprotein

VMA: vanillylmandelic acid
VO: voice order
VP-16: etoposide
V/Q: ventilation—perfusion
VSS: vital signs stable
VT: ventricular tachycardia
W: watt
WB: whole blood
WBC: white blood cell, white blood cell
    count
WD: well developed
WF: white female
wk: week
WM: white male
WN: well nourished
wnl: within normal limits
WPW: Wolff—Parkinson—White
XRT: x-ray therapy
y: year
YO: years old
ZE: Zollinger—Ellison

"SO YOU WANT TO BE A SCUT MONKEY": AN INTRODUCTION TO CLINICAL MEDICINE*

The transition from the preclinical years to the clinical years of medical school is often a difficult one. Understanding the new responsibilities and a set of ground rules can ease this transition. What follows is a brief introduction to clinical medicine for the new clinical clerk.

THE HIERARCHY

Most services can be expected to have at least one of each of the following physicians on the team.

The Intern

In some programs, the intern is known euphemistically as the first-year resident. This person has the day-to-day responsibilities of patient care. This duty, combined with a total lack of seniority, usually serves to keep the intern in the hospital more than the other members of the team and may limit his or her teaching of medical students. Any question concerning details in the evaluation of the patient, for example, whether Mrs. Pavona gets a complete blood count this morning or this evening, is usually referred first to the intern.

The Resident

The resident is a member of the house staff who has completed at least 1 year of postgraduate medical education. The most senior resident is typically in charge of the overall conduct of the service and is the person you might ask a question such as "What might cause Mrs. Pavona's white blood cell count to be 142,000?" You might also ask your resident for an appropriate reference on the subject or perhaps to arrange a brief conference on the topic for everyone on the service. A surgical service typically has a chief resident, a doctor in the last year of residency who usually runs the service. On medical services the chief resident is usually an appointee of the chairman of medicine and primarily has administrative responsibilities with limited ward duties.

The Attending Physician

The attending physician is also called simply "The Attending," and on nonsurgical services, "the attending." (*Note:* Before we get any more letters, yes this is a joke!) This physician has completed postgraduate education and is now a mem-

---

* Based on a concept by and adapted from Epstein A, Frye T (eds.): *So You Want to Be a Toad.* College of Medicine, Ohio State University, Columbus, OH.

ber of the teaching faculty. He or she is usually already boarded in a specialty or may be newly trained and "board eligible." The attending is morally and legally responsible for the care of all patients whose charts are marked with the attending's name. All major therapeutic decisions made about the care of these patients are ultimately passed by the attending. In addition, this person is responsible for teaching and evaluating house staff and medical students. This is the member of the team you might ask, "Why are we treating Mrs. Pavona with busulfan?"

The Fellow

Fellows are physicians who have completed their postgraduate education and elected to do extra study in one special field, such as nephrology, high-risk obstetrics, or surgical oncology. They may or may not be active members of the team and may not be obligated to teach medical students, but usually they are happy to answer any questions you may ask. You might ask this person to help you read Mrs. Pavona's bone marrow smear.

Physician Extenders

Nurse practitioners and physician assistants are being incorporated into the health care system including academic medical centers. Their responsibilities vary by service, hospital, and state regulation. Remember that they are critical members of the team and excellent resources for both the students and patients.

TEAMWORK

The medical student, in addition to being a member of the medical team, must interact with members of the professional team of nurses, dietitians, pharmacists, social workers, PA's, nurse practitioners, and all others who provide direct care for the patient. Good working relations with this group of professionals can make your work go more smoothly; bad relations with them can make your rotation miserable.

Nurses are generally good-tempered, but overworked in most systems. Like most human beings, they respond very favorably to polite treatment. Leaving a mess in a patient's room after the performance of a floor procedure, standing by idly while a 98-lb licensed practical nurse struggles to move a 350-lb patient onto the chair scale, and obviously listening to three ringing telephones while room call lights flash are acts guaranteed not to please. Do not let anyone talk you into being an acting nurse's aide or ward secretary but try to help when you can.

You will occasionally meet a staff member who is having a bad day, and you will be able to do little about it. Returning hostility is unwarranted at these times, and it is best to avoid confrontations except when necessary for the care of the patient.

When faced with ordering a diet for your first sick patient, you might be confronted with the inadequacy of your education in nutrition. Fortunately for your patient, dietitians are available. Never hesitate to call one.

In matters concerning drug interactions, side effects, individualization of dosages, alteration of drug dosages in disease, and equivalence of different brands of the same drug, it never hurts to call the pharmacist. Most medical centers have a pharmacy resident or PharmD candidates who follow every patient on a floor or service and who will gladly answer any questions you have on medications. The pharmacist or pharmacy resident can very often provide pertinent articles on a requested subject.

YOUR HEALTH AND A WORD ON "AGGRESSIVENESS"

In your months of curing disease both day and night, it becomes easy to ignore your own right to keep yourself healthy. There are numerous bad examples of medical and surgical interns who sleep 3 hours a night and get most of their meals from vending machines. Newly mandated "80-hour" work rules will likely make this scenario a thing of the past. Do not let anyone talk you into believing that you are not entitled to decent meals and sleep, even if the 80-hour rule does not apply to students (yet!). If you offer yourself as a sacrifice, it will be a rare rotation on which you will not become one. On the other hand, try to extend yourself when the need arises; the house staff will appreciate it and because they may have significant input into your grade, it may reflect itself in an outstanding grade on the rotation.

You may have the misfortune someday of reading an evaluation that says a student was not "aggressive enough." This is an enigmatic notion to everyone. Does it mean that the student refused to attempt to start an intravenous line after eight previous failures? Does it mean that the student was not consistently the first to shout out the answer over the mumblings of fellow students on rounds? Whatever constitutes "aggressiveness" must be a dubious virtue at best.

A more appropriate virtue might be **assertiveness in obtaining your education.** Ask **good** questions, have the house staff show you procedures and review your chartwork, read about your patient's illness, review the surgery basics before going to the OR, participate actively in your patient's care, and take an interest in other patients on the service. This approach avoids the need for victimizing your patients and comrades that the definition of *aggression* suggests.

ROUNDS

Rounds are meetings of all members of the service for discussing the care of the patient. These occur daily and are of three kinds.

Morning Rounds

Also known as "work rounds," these take place anywhere from 6:00 to 9:00 AM on most services and are attended by residents, interns, and students. This is the time for discussing what happened to the patient during the night, the progress of the patient's evaluation or therapy or both, the laboratory and radiologic tests to be ordered for the patient, and, last but not least, talking with and evaluating the patient. Know about your patient's most recent laboratory reports and progress—this is a chance for you to look good.

Ideally, differences of opinion and any glaring omissions in patient care are politely discussed and resolved here. Writing new orders, filling out consultations, and making any necessary telephone calls are best done right after morning rounds.

Attending Rounds

These vary greatly depending on the service and on the nature of the attending physician. The same people who gathered for morning rounds will be here, with the addition of the attending. At this meeting, the patients are often seen again (especially on the surgical services); significant new laboratory, radiographic, and physical findings are described (often by the student caring for the patient); and new patients are formally presented to the attending (again, often by the medical student).

The most important priority for the student on attending rounds is to **know the patient.** Be prepared to concisely tell the attending what has happened to the patient. Also be ready to give a brief presentation on the patient's illness, especially if it is unusual. The attending will probably not be interested in minor details that do not affect therapeutic decisions. Additionally, the attending will probably not wish to hear a litany of normal laboratory values, only the pertinent ones, such as Mrs. Pavona's platelets are still 350,000/{m}L in spite of her bone marrow disease. You do not have to tell everything you know on rounds, but you must be prepared to do so.

Open disputes among house staff and students are bad form on attending rounds. For this reason, the unwritten rule is that any differences of opinion not previously discussed shall not be initially raised in the presence of the attending.

Check-out or Evening Rounds

Formal evening rounds on which the patients are seen by the entire team a second time are typically done only on surgical services and pediatrics. Other services, such as medicine, often will have check-out with the resident on call for the service that evening (sometimes called "card rounds"). Expect to convene sometime between 3:00 and 7:00 PM on most days.

All new data are presented by the person who collected them (often the student). Orders are again written, laboratory work desired for early the next day is requested, and those on call compile a "scut list" of work to be done that night and a list of patients who need close supervision.

BEDSIDE ROUNDS

Basically, these are the same as any other rounds except that tact is at a premium. The first consideration at the bedside must be for the patient. If no one else on the team says "Good morning" and asks how the patient is feeling, do it yourself; this is not a presumptuous act on your part. Keep this encounter brief and then explain that you will be talking about the patient for a while. If handled in this fashion, the patient will often feel flattered by the attention and will listen to you with interest.

Certain points in a hallway presentation are omitted in the patient's room. The patient's race and sex are usually apparent to all and do not warrant inclusion in your first sentence.

The patient must *never* be called by the name of the disease, eg, Mrs. Pavona is not "a 45-year-old CML (chronic myelogenous leukemia)" but "a 45-year-old *with* CML." The patient's general appearance need not be reiterated. Descriptions of evidence of disease must not be prefaced by words such as *outstanding* or *beautiful.* Mrs. Pavona's massive spleen is not beautiful to her, and it should not be to the physician or student either.

At the bedside, keep both feet on the floor. A foot up on a bed or chair conveys impatience and disinterest to the patient and other members of the team. It is poor form to carry beverages or food into the patient's room.

Although you will probably never be asked to examine a patient during bedside rounds, it is still worthwhile to know how to do so considerately. Bedside examinations are often done by the attending at the time of the initial presentation or by one member of a surgical service on postoperative rounds. First, warn the patient that you are about to examine the wound or affected part. Ask the patient to uncover whatever needs to be exposed rather than boldly removing the patient's clothes yourself. If the patient is unable to do so alone, you may do it, but remember to explain what you are doing. Remove only as much clothing as is necessary and then promptly cover the patient again. In a ward room, remember to pull the curtain.

Bedside rounds in the intensive care unit call for as much consideration as they do in any other room. That still, naked soul on the bed might not be as "out of it" as the resident (or anyone else) might believe and may be hearing every word you say. Again, exercise discretion in discussing the patient's illness, plan, prognosis, and personal character as it relates to the disease.

Remember that the patient information you are entrusted with as a health care provider is confidential. There is a time and place to discuss this sensitive information and public areas such as elevators or cafeterias are not the appropriate location for these discussions.

READING

Time for reading is at a premium on many services, and it is therefore important to use that time effectively. Unless you can remember everything you learned in the first 20 months of medical school, you will probably want to review the basic facts about the disease that brought your patient into the hospital. These facts are most often found in the same core texts that got you through the preclinical years. Unless specifically directed to do so, avoid the temptation to log on to MEDLINE to find all the latest articles on a disease you have not read about for the last 7 months; you do not have the time.

The appropriate time to head for the MEDLINE is when a therapeutic dilemma arises and only the most recent literature will adequately advise the team. You may wish to obtain some direction from the attending, the fellow, or the resident before plunging on line or into the library on your only Friday night off call this month. Ask the residents or fellow students for the pocket manuals or PDA downloads that they found most useful for a given rotation.

THE WRITTEN HISTORY AND PHYSICAL

Much has been written on how to obtain a useful medical history and perform a thorough physical examination, and there is little to add here. Three things worth emphasizing are your own physical findings, your impression, and your own differential diagnosis.

Trust and record your own physical findings, even if other examiners have written things different from those you found. You just may be right, and, if not, you have learned something from it. Avoid the temptation to copy another examiner's findings as your own when you are unable to do the examination yourself. Still, it would be an unusually cruel resident who would make you give Mrs. Pavona her fourth rectal examination of the day, and in this circumstance you may write "rectal per resident." *Do not do this routinely just to avoid performing a complete physical examination. Check with the resident first.*

Although not always emphasized in physical diagnosis, your clinical impression is probably the most important part of your write-up. Reasoned interpretation of the medical history and physical examination is what separates physicians from the computers touted by the tabloids as their successors. Judgment is learned only by boldly stating your case, even if you are wrong more often than not.

The differential diagnosis, that is, your impression, should include only those entities that you consider when evaluating your patient. Avoid including every possible cause of your patient's ailments. List only those that you are seriously considering, and include in your plan what you intend to do to exclude each one. Save the exhaustive list for the time your attending asks for all the causes of a symptom, syndrome, or abnormal laboratory value.

THE PRESENTATION

The object of the presentation is to *briefly* and *concisely* (usually in a few minutes) describe your patient's reason for being in the hospital to all members of the team who do not know the patient and the story. Unlike the write-up, which contains all the data you obtained, the presentation may include only the pertinent positive and negative evidence of a disease and its course in the patient. It is hard to get a feel for what is pertinent until you have seen and done a few presentations yourself.

Practice is important. Try never to read from your write-up, as this often produces dull and lengthy presentations. Most attendings will allow you to carry note cards, but this method can also lead to trouble unless content is carefully edited. Presentations are given in the same order as a write-up: identification, chief complaint, history of the present illness, past medical history, family history, psychosocial history, review of systems, physical examination, laboratory and x-ray data, clinical impression, and plan. Only pertinent positives and negatives from the review of systems should be given. These and truly relevant items from other parts of the interview often can be added to the history of the present illness. Finally, the length and content of the presentation vary greatly according to the wishes of the attending and the resident, but you will learn quickly what they do and do not want.

RESPONSIBILITY

Your responsibilities as a student should be clearly defined on the first day of a rotation by either the attending or the resident. Ideally, this enumeration of your duties should also include a list of what you might expect concerning teaching, floor skills, presentations, and all the other things you are paying many thousand dollars a year to learn.

On some services, you may feel like a glorified unit secretary (clinical rotations are called "clerkships" for good reason!), and you will not be far from wrong. This is *not* what you are going into hock for. The scut work should be divided among the house staff and students.

You will frequently be expected to call for a certain piece of laboratory data or to go review an x-ray with the radiologist. You may then mutter under your breath, "Why waste my time? The report will be on the chart in a day or two!" You will feel less annoyed in this situation if you consider that every piece of data ordered is vital to the care of your patient.

Outpatient clinic experiences are incorporated into many rotations today. The same basic rules and skill set necessary for inpatient care can be easily transferred to the outpatient setting. The student's responsibility, again, may be summarized in three words: **know your patient.** The whole service relies to a great extent on a well-informed presentation by the student. The better informed you are, the more time left for education and the better your evaluation will be. A major part of becoming a physician is learning responsibility.

ORDERS

Orders are the physician's instructions to the nursing and other members of the professional staff on the care of the patient. These may include the frequency of vital signs, medications, respiratory care, laboratory and x-ray studies, and nearly anything else that you can imagine.

There are many formats for writing concise admission, transfer, and postoperative orders. Some rotations may have a precisely fixed set of routine orders, but others will leave you and the intern to your own devices. It is important in each case to avoid omitting instructions critical to the care of the patient. Although you will be confronted with a variety of lists and mnemonics, ultimately it is helpful to devise your own system and commit it to memory. Why memorize? Because when you are an intern and it is 3:30 AM, you may overlook something if you try to think it out. One system for writing admission or transfer orders uses the mnemonic "A.D.C. Vaan Dissl" and is discussed in Chapter 2.

The word *stat* is the abbreviation for the Latin word *statim,* which means "immediately." When added to any order, it puts the requested study in front of all the routine work waiting to be done. Ideally, this order is reserved for the truly urgent situation, but in practice it is often inappropriately used. Most of the blame for this situation rests with physicians who either fail to plan ahead or order stat lab results when routine studies would do.

Student orders usually require a cosignature from a physician, although at some institutions students are allowed to order routine laboratory studies. Do not ask a nurse or pharmacist to act on an unsigned student order; it is **illegal** for them to do so.

The intern is usually responsible for most orders. The amount of interest shown by the resident and the attending varies greatly, but ideally you will review the orders on routinely admitted patients with the intern. Have the intern show you how to write some orders on a few patients, then take the initiative and write the orders yourself and review them with the intern. Even if your center uses computerized orders, follow along with the intern or resident entering them.

THE DAY

The events of the day and the effective use of time are two of the most distressing enigmas encountered in making the transition from preclinical to clinical education. For example, there are no typical days on surgical services because the operating room schedule prohibits making rounds at a regularly scheduled time every day. The following are suggestions that will help on any service.

1. Schedule special studies early in the day. The free time after work rounds is usually ideal for this. Also, call consultants early in the morning. Often, they can see your patient on the same day or at least early the next day.
2. Try to take care of all your business in the radiology department in one trip unless a given problem requires viewing a film promptly. Do *not* make as many separate trips as you have patients.
3. Make a point of knowing when certain services become unavailable, for example, electrocardiograms, contrast-study scheduling, and blood drawing. Be sure to get these procedures done while it is still possible to do so.

4. Make a daily work or "scut"* list, and write down laboratory results as soon as you obtain them. Few people can keep all the daily data in their heads without making errors.

5. Try to arrange your travels around the hospital efficiently. If you have patients to see on four different floors, try to take care of all their needs, such as, drawing blood, removing sutures, writing progress notes, and calling for consultations, in one trip.

6. Strive to work thoroughly but quickly. If you do not try to get work done early, you never will (this is not to say that you will succeed even if you do try). There is no sin in leaving at 5:00 PM or earlier if your obligations are *completed* and the supervising resident has dismissed you.

A PARTING SHOT

The clinical years are when all the years of premed study in college and the first 2 years of medical school suddenly come together. Trying to tell you adequately about being a clinical clerk is similar to trying to make someone into a swimmer on dry land. The terms to describe new clinical clerks may vary at different medical centers ("scut monkey," "scut boy," "scut dog," "torpedoes"). These euphemistic expressions describing the new clinical clerk acknowledge that the transition, a sort of rite of passage, into the next phase of physician training has occurred.

We hope that this "So You Want to Be a Scut Monkey" introduction and the information contained in this book will give you a good start as you enter the "hands-on" phase of becoming a successful and respected physician.

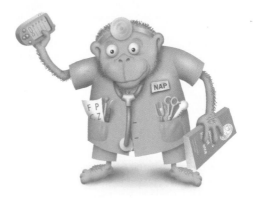

---

* Although the origin of how the word *scut* entered the medical jargon is obscure, we like to think it represents an acronym for "some common unfinished task" or "some clinically useful training."

HISTORY AND PHYSICAL EXAMINATION

HISTORY AND PHYSICAL EXAMINATION

An example of a complete H&P write-up can be found on page 20. The details provided and length of the written H&P can vary with the particular problem and with the service to which the patient is admitted.

History

Identification: Name, age, sex, referring physician, and the informant (eg, patient, relative, old chart) and the informant's reliability.

Chief Complaint: State, in patient's own words, the current problem.

History of the Present Illness (HPI): Defines the present illness by quality; quantity; setting; anatomic location and radiation; time course, including when it began; whether the complaint is progressing, regressing, or steady; of constant or intermittent frequency; and aggravating, alleviating, and associated factors. The information should be in chronologic order, including diagnostic tests done prior to admission. Related history, including previous treatment for the problem, risk factors, and pertinent negatives should be included. Also include any family history and psychosocial history pertinent to the chief complaint. Any other significant ongoing problems should be included in the HPI in a separate section or paragraph. For instance, if a patient with poorly controlled diabetes mellitus comes to the emergency room because of chest pain, the HPI would first include information regarding the chest pain followed by a detailed history of the diabetes mellitus. If the diabetes mellitus was well controlled or diet-controlled, the history of the diabetes mellitus may be placed in the past medical history.

Past Medical History (PMH): Current medications, including OTC medications, vitamins, and herbals; allergies (drugs and other—include how allergies are manifested); surgeries; hospitalizations; blood transfusions, include when and how many units and the type of blood product; trauma; stable current and past medical problems unrelated to the HPI. Specific illnesses to inquire about for adults include diabetes mellitus; HTN; MI;, stroke; PUD; asthma; emphysema; thyroid, liver, and kidney disease; bleeding disorders; cancer; TB; hepatitis; and STDs. Also inquire about routine health maintenance. This category depends on the age and sex of the patient but could include last Pap smear and pelvic exam; breast exam; whether the patient does self breast examination; date of last mammogram; diphtheria/tetanus immunization; pneumococcal, influenza, and hepatitis B vaccines; stool samples for occult blood; sigmoidoscopy or colonoscopy; cholesterol; HDL cholesterol; functioning smoke alarms on each floor at home; and use of seat belts. **Pediatric patients:** Include prenatal and birth history, feedings, food intolerance, immunization history, hot water heater temperature setting, and use of bicycle helmets.

Family History: Age, status (alive, dead) of blood relatives and medical problems for any blood relatives (inquiry about cancer, especially breast, colon, and prostate; TB, asthma; MI; HTN; thyroid disease; kidney disease; PUD; DM; bleeding disorders; glaucoma, macular degeneration, depression, and alcohol or substance abuse). Can be written out or use a family tree.

Psychosocial (Social) History: Stressors (financial, significant relationships, work or school, health) and support (family, friends, significant other, clergy); lifestyle risk factors (alcohol, drugs, tobacco, and caffeine use; diet; exercise; and exposure to environmental agents; and sexual practices); patient profile (may include marital status and children, sexual orientation; present and past employment; financial support and insurance; education; religion; hobbies; beliefs; living conditions); for veterans, include military service history. **Pediatric patients:** Include grade in school, sleep, and play habits.

Review of Systems (ROS)

General. Weight loss, weight gain, fatigue, weakness, appetite, fever, chills, night sweats

Skin. Rashes, pruritus, bruising, dryness, skin cancer or other lesions

Head. Trauma, headache, tenderness, dizziness, syncope

Eyes. Vision, changes in the visual field, glasses, last prescription change, photophobia, blurring, diplopia, spots or floaters, inflammation, discharge, dry eyes, excessive tearing, history of cataracts or glaucoma

Ears. Hearing changes, tinnitus, pain, discharge, vertigo, history of ear infections

Nose. Sinus problems, epistaxis, obstruction, polyps, changes in or loss of sense of smell

Throat. Bleeding gums; dental history (last checkup, etc); ulcerations or other lesions on tongue, gums, buccal mucosa

Respiratory. Chest pain; dyspnea; cough; amount and color of sputum; hemoptysis; history of pneumonia, influenza and pneumococcal vaccinations and positive PPD

Cardiovascular. Chest pain, orthopnea, trepopnea, dyspnea on exertion, PND, murmurs, claudication, peripheral edema, palpitations

Gastrointestinal. Dysphagia, heartburn, N/V/D, hematemesis, indigestion, abdominal pain, constipation, melena (hematochezia), hemorrhoids, change in stool shape and color, jaundice, fatty food intolerance

Gynecologic. Gravida/para/abortions; age at menarche; last menstrual period (frequency, duration, flow); dysmenorrhea; spotting; menopause; contraceptive method; sexual history, including history of venereal disease, frequency of intercourse, number of partners, sexual orientation and satisfaction, and dyspareunia

Genitourinary. Frequency, urgency, hesitancy; dysuria; hematuria; polyuria; nocturia; incontinence; venereal disease; discharge; sterility; impotence; polyuria; polydipsia; change in urinary stream; and sexual history, including frequency of intercourse, number of partners, sexual orientation and satisfaction, and history of STD's.

Endocrine. Polyuria, polydipsia, polyphagia, temperature intolerance, glycosuria, hormone therapy, changes in hair or skin texture

Musculoskeletal. Arthralgias, arthritis, trauma, joint swelling, redness, tenderness, limitations in ROM, back pain, musculoskeletal trauma, gout

Peripheral Vascular. Varicose veins, intermittent claudication, history of thrombophlebitis

Hematology. Anemia, bleeding tendency, easy bruising, lymphadenopathy

Neuropsychiatric. Syncope; seizures; weakness; coordination problems; alterations in sensations, memory, mood, sleep pattern, anhedonia, loss of energy, decreased ability to concentrate, change in weight or appetite, family history of depression or suicide; emotional disturbances; drug and alcohol problems

Physical Examination

General: Mood, stage of development, race, and sex. State if patient is in any distress or is assuming an unusual position, such as, sitting up leaning forward (position often seen in patients with acute exacerbation of COPD or pericarditis). Note if patient appears markedly older or younger than stated age

Vital Signs: Temperature (note if oral, rectal, axillary or ear), pulse, respirations, BP (may include right arm, left arm, lying, sitting, standing), height, weight and BMI. BP and heart rate supine and after standing 1 min should always be included if volume depletion (GI bleeding, pancreatitis, diarrhea, or vomiting) or autonomic insufficiency is suspected, especially if the patient reports dizziness, or syncope.

Skin: Rashes, eruptions, scars, tattoos, moles, hair pattern (See pages 13–15 for definitions of dermatologic lesions.)

Lymph Nodes: Location (head and neck, supraclavicular, epitrochlear, axillary, inguinal), size, tenderness, motility, consistency

Head, Eyes, Ears, Nose, and Throat (HEENT)

Head. Size and shape, tenderness, trauma, bruits. **Pediatric patients:** Fontanels, suture lines

Eyes. Conjunctiva; sclera; lids; position of eyes in orbits; pupil size, shape, reactivity; extraocular muscle movements; visual acuity (eg, 20/20); visual fields; fundi (disc color, size, margins, cupping, spontaneous venous pulsations, hemorrhages, exudates, A-V ratio, nicking)

Ears. Test hearing, tenderness, discharge, external canal, tympanic membrane (intact, dull or shiny, bulging, motility, fluid or blood, injected)

Nose. Symmetry; palpate over frontal, maxillary, and ethmoid sinuses; inspect for obstruction, lesions, exudate, inflammation. **Pediatric patients:** Nasal flaring, grunting

Throat. Lips, teeth, gums, tongue, pharynx (lesions, erythema, exudate, tonsillar size, presence of crypts)

Neck: ROM, tenderness, JVD, lymph nodes, thyroid examination, location of larynx, carotid bruits, HJR. JVD should be reported in relationship to the number of centimeters above or below the sternal angle, such as "1 cm above the sternal angle," rather than "no JVD."

Chest: Configuration and symmetry of movement with respiration; intercostal retractions; palpation for tenderness, fremitus, and chest wall expansion; percussion (include diaphragmatic excursion); breath sounds; adventitious sounds (rales, rhonchi, wheezes, rubs). If indicated: vocal fremitus, whispered pectoriloquy, egophony (found with consolidation)

Heart: Rate, inspection, and palpation of precordium for point of maximal impulse and thrill; auscultation at the apex, LLSB, and right and left second intercostal spaces with diaphragm and apex and LLSB with the bell. (For a description of S_1 and S_2 and where best to hear the heart sounds, see, legend for Figure 1–1.).

Breast: Inspection for nipple discharge, inversion, excoriations and fissures, and skin dimpling or flattening of the contour; palpation for masses, tenderness; gynecomastia in males

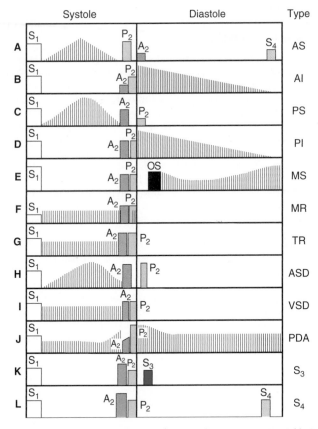

FIGURE 1-1. Graphic representation of common heart murmurs. See Table 1–2 for abbreviations and descriptions. Height of box indicates intensity of heart sound and hatched lines indicate pattern of murmur. S_1: Occurs at beginning of systole; is the closure of the mitral (M_1) and tricuspid (T_1) valves. Normally, you only hear T_1 at the LLSB. S_1 is loudest at the apex. S_2: Occurs at end of systole; is the closure of the aortic (A_2) and pulmonic valves (P_2). P_2 is best heard at the L second ICS. S_2 is the loudest at R second ICS. The L second ICS is where to listen for splitting of A_2 and P_2. At end inspiration there is more pronounced splitting of the A_2 and P_2 sounds (they are further apart than at end expiration). With normal physiology M_1 occurs before T_1; A_2 occurs before P_2. (See Table 1–2, page 10)

Abdomen: Note shape (scaphoid, flat, distended, obese); examine for scars; auscultate for bowel sounds and bruits; percussion for tympani and masses; measure liver size (span in midclavicular line); note CVA tenderness; palpate for tenderness (if present, check for rebound tenderness), note hepatomegaly, splenomegaly; guarding, inguinal adenopathy.

Male Genitalia: Inspect for penile lesions, scrotal swelling, testicles (size, tenderness, masses, varicocele), and hernia, and observe for transillumination of testicular masses.

Pelvic: See Chapter 13, page 296.

Rectal: Inspect and palpate for hemorrhoids, fissures, skin tags, sphincter tone, masses, prostate (size [grade from small 1+ to massively enlarged 4+], note any nodules, tenderness); note presence or absence of stool; test stool for occult blood.

Musculoskeletal: Note amputations, deformities, visible joint swelling, and ROM; also palpate joints for swelling, tenderness, and warmth.

Peripheral Vascular: Note hair pattern; color change of skin; varicosities; cyanosis; clubbing; palpation of radial, ulnar, brachial, femoral, popliteal, posterior tibial, dorsalis pedis pulses; simultaneous radial pulses; calf tenderness; Homans' sign; edema; auscultate for femoral bruits.

Neurologic

Mental Status Examination. (If appropriate, see sections "Psychiatric History and Physical," and "Psychiatric Mental Status Examination," pages 8–9.)

Cranial Nerves. There are 12 cranial nerves, the functions of which are as follows:

- **I** Olfactory—Smell
- **II** Optic—Vision, visual fields, and fundi; afferent limb of pupillary response
- **III, IV, VI** Oculomotor, trochlear, abducens,—Efferent limb pupillary response, ptosis, volitional eye movements, pursuit eye movements
- **V** Trigeminal—Corneal reflex (afferent), *facial sensation*, masseter and temporalis muscle tested by biting down
- **VII** Facial—Raise eyebrows, close eyes tight, show teeth, smile, or whistle, corneal reflex (efferent)
- **VIII** Acoustic—Test hearing by watch tick, finger rub, Weber–Rinne test (see also page 19) to be done if hearing loss noted on history or by gross testing. (Air conduction lasts longer than bone conduction in a normal person.)
- **IX, X** Glossopharyngeal and vagus—Palate moves in midline; gag reflex; speech
- **XI** Spinal accessory—Shoulder shrug, push head against resistance.
- **XII** Hypoglossal—Stick out tongue. Strength can be tested by having the patient press tongue against the buccal mucosa on each side and the examiner can press a finger against the patient's cheek. Also look for fasciculations.

Motor. Strength should be tested in upper and lower extremities proximally and distally. (Grading system: 5 active motion against full resistance; 4 active motion against some resistance; 3 active motion against gravity; 2 active motion with gravity eliminated; 1 barely detectable motion; 0 no motion or muscular contraction detected)

Cerebellum. Romberg's test (see page 19)—heel to shin (should not be with assistance from gravity), finger to nose, heel-and-toe walking, rapid alternating movements upper and lower extremities

Sensory. Pain (sharp) or temperature distal and proximal upper and lower extremities, vibration using either a 128- or 256-Hz tuning fork or position sense distally upper and lower extremities, and stereognosis or graphesthesia. Identify any deficit using the dermatome and cutaneous innervation diagrams (Figure 1–2).

Reflexes. Brachioradialis and biceps C5–6, triceps C7–8, abdominal (upper T8–10, lower T10–12), quadriceps (knee) L3–5, ankle S1–2, (Grading system: 4+ hyperactive with clonus; 3+ brisker than usual; 2+ normal or average; 1+ decreased or less than normal; 0 absent). Check for pathologic

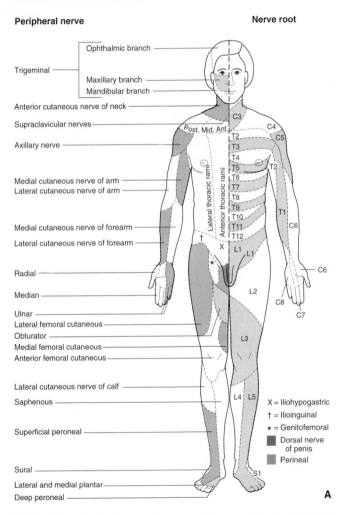

FIGURE 1–2. A: Dermatomes and cutaneous innervation patterns, anterior view. (Reproduced, with permission, from: Greenberg DA et al [eds]: *Clinical Neurology,* 5th ed, McGraw-Hill, 2002.)

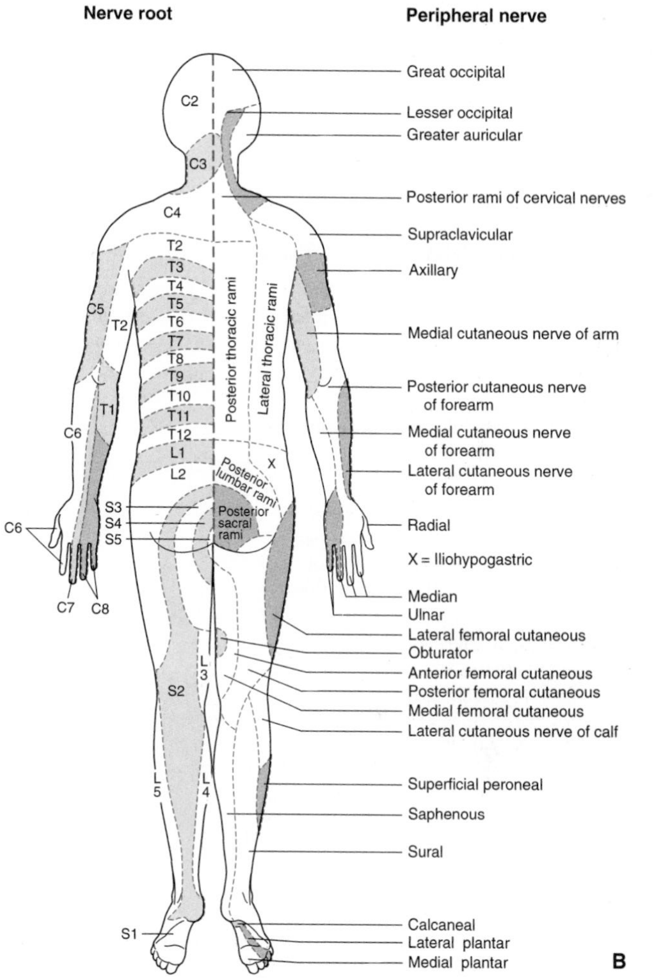
Nerve root
Peripheral nerve
Great occipital
Lesser occipital
Greater auricular
Posterior rami of cervical nerves
Supraclavicular
Axillary
Medial cutaneous nerve of arm
Posterior cutaneous nerve of forearm
Medial cutaneous nerve of forearm
Lateral cutaneous nerve of forearm
Radial
X = Iliohypogastric
Median
Ulnar
Lateral femoral cutaneous
Obturator
Anterior femoral cutaneous
Posterior femoral cutaneous
Medial femoral cutaneous
Lateral cutaneous nerve of calf
Superficial peroneal
Saphenous
Sural
Calcaneal
Lateral plantar
Medial plantar
C2
C3
C4
T2
T3
T4
T5
T6
T7
T8
T9
T10
T11
T12
L1
L2
C5
T1
C6
C7
C8
S3
S4
S5
S2
S1
L3
L4
L5
Posterior thoracic rami
Lateral thoracic rami
Posterior lumbar rami
Posterior sacral rami
X
B

FIGURE 1–2. B: Dermatomes and cutaneous innervation patterns, posterior view. (Reproduced, with permission, from: Greenberg DA et al [eds]: *Clinical Neurology,* 5th ed, McGraw-Hill, 2002.)

reflexes: Babinski's sign, Hoffmann's sign, snout, others (see pages 15 & 17 to 19). **Pediatric patients:** Moro's reflex (startle) and suck reflexes

Database

Laboratory tests, radiographs ordered as indicated by the H&P

Problem List

(See example, page 24.) Should include entry date of problem, date of problem onset, problem number. (With initial problem list, the more severe problems are numbered first. After the initial list is generated, problems are added chronologically.) List problem by status: active or inactive.

Assessment

A discussion and evaluation of the current problems with a differential diagnosis.

Plan: Additional laboratory and diagnostic tests, medical treatment, consults, etc. *Note:* The H&P should be legibly signed and your title noted. Each entry should be dated and timed.

PSYCHIATRIC HISTORY AND PHYSICAL

The elements of the psychiatric history and physical are identical to those of the basic H&P outlined earlier. The main difference involves attention to the past psychiatric history and a more detailed mental status examination as described in the following section.

Psychiatric Mental Status Examination

The following factors are evaluated as part of the psychiatric status examination.

- **Appearance:** Gestures, mannerisms, etc
- **Speech:** Coherence, flight of ideas, etc
- **Mood and Affect:** Depression, elation, anger, etc
- **Thought Process:** Blocking, evasion, etc
- **Thought Content:** Worries, hypochondriasis, lack of self-confidence, delusions, hallucinations, etc
- **Motor Activity:** Slow, rapid, purposeful, etc
- **Cognitive Functions:**

  Attention and concentration
  Memory (immediate, recent, and remote recall)
  Calculations
  Abstractions
  Judgment

Mini-Mental Status Examination

A thorough mental status exam should be done on every geriatric patient, every patient with AIDS, and any patient suspected of having dementia. The mini-mental status exam is a simple, practical test that takes only a few minutes and can be followed over time. It may show progression, improvement, or no changes in the underlying process. The mini-mental status exam developed by Folstein, Folstein, and McHugh is discussed in detail in the *Journal of Psychiatric Research,* 1975, Vol. 12, pages 189–198. The test is divided into two sections: one assessing orientation, memory, and attention, and the other testing the patient's ability to write a sentence and to copy a diagram (usually two intersecting pentagons whose intersect forms a four-sided figure. Table 1–1 page 9 is the "Mini-Mental State" Examination as outlined by Folstein and associates.

HEART MURMURS AND EXTRA HEART SOUNDS

Table 1–2 page 10 and Figure 1–1 page 4 describe the various types of heart murmurs and extra heart sounds.

TABLE 1-1
The Mini-Mental State Examination

Patient _____
Examiner _____
Date _____

"Mini-Mental State"

Maximum Score	Score	

Orientation

5   What is the (year) (season) (date) (day) (month)?

5   Where are we? (state) (county) (town) (hospital) (floor)

Registration

3   Name 3 objects: 1 second to say each. Then ask the patient all 3 after you have said them. Give 1 point for each correct answer. Then repeat until he learns all 3. Count trials and record.
Trials _____

Attention and Calculation

5   Serial 7's: One point for each correct. Stop after 5 answers. Alternatively, spell "world" backward.

Recall

3   Ask for the 3 objects repeated above. Give 1 point for each correct answer.

Language

9   Point to a pencil, and watch and ask the patient to name it. (2 points)
Repeat the following: "No if's, and's, or but's." (1 point)
Follow a 3-stage command: "Take a paper in your right hand, fold it in half, and put it on the floor." (3 points)
Read and obey the following: Close your eyes (1 point)
Write a sentence (1 point)
Copy design (two intersecting pentagrams) (1 point)

_____ Total Score

Assess level of consciousness along the following continuum

Alert   Drowsy   Stupor   Coma

Source: Based on data from: Folstein, Folstein, and McHugh: *J Psychiatr Res* 1975; **12:**189–198, 1975. Used with permission.

TABLE 1–2
Heart Murmurs and Extra Heart Sounds[a]

Type[b]	Description
A. Aortic stenosis (AS)	Heard best at second intercostal space. Systolic (medium-pitched) crescendo–decrescendo murmur with radiation to the carotid arteries. A_2 decreased, ejection click and S_4 often heard at apex. Paradoxical splitting of S_2. Narrow pulse pressure and delayed carotid upstroke and left ventricular hypertrophy (LVH) with lift at apex.
B. Aortic insufficiency (AI)	Heard best at left lower sternal border at third and fourth interspace with patient sitting up, leaning forward and fully exhaled. Diastolic (high-pitched) decrescendo murmur. Often with LVH. Widened pulse pressure, bisferious pulse, Traube's sign, Quincke's sign, and Corrigan's pulse may be seen with chronic aortic insufficiency. S_3 and pulsus alternans often present with acute aortic insufficiency.
C. Pulmonic stenosis (PS)	Heard best at left second intercostal space. Systolic crescendo–decrescendo murmur. Louder with inspiration. Click often present. P_2 delayed and soft if severe. Right ventricular hypertrophy (RVH) with parasternal lift.
D. Pulmonic insufficiency (PI)	Heard best at left second intercostal space. Diastolic decrescendo murmur. Louder with inspiration. RVH usually present.
E. Mitral stenosis (MS)	Localized at the apex. Diastolic (low-pitched rumbling sound) murmur heard best with the bell in the left lateral decubitus position. With increased or decreased S_1. Opening snap (OS) heard best at apex with diaphragm. Increased P_2, right-sided S_4, left-sided S_3 often present. RVH with parasternal lift may be present.
F. Mitral insufficiency (MI)	Heard best at apex. Holosystolic (high-pitched) murmur with radiation to axilla. Soft S_1, may be masked by murmur. S_3 and LVH often present. Midsystolic click suggests mitral valve prolapse.

(continued)

TABLE 1–2
Heart Murmurs and Extra Heart Sounds^a (continued)

Type^b	Description
G. Tricuspid insufficiency (TI)	Heard best at left lower sternal border. Holosystolic (high-pitched) murmur. Increases with inspiration. Right-sided S_3 often present. Large V wave in jugular venous pulsations.
H. Atrial septal defect (ASD)	Heard best at left upper sternal border. Systolic (medium-pitched) murmur. Fixed splitting of S_2 and RVH, often with left- and right-sided S_4.
I. Ventricular septal defect (VSD)	Heard best at left lower sternal border. Harsh holosystolic (high-pitched) murmur. S_1 and S_2 may be soft.
J. Patent ductus arteriosus (PDA)	Heard best at left first and second intercostal space. Continuous, machinery (medium-pitched) murmur. Increased P_2 and ejection click may be present.
K. Third heart sound (S_3)	Early diastolic sound caused by rapid ventricular filling. Heard best with bell. Left-sided S_3 heard at apex, right-sided S_3 heard at left lower sternal border. Left-sided S_3 seen normally in young people, also pregnancy, thyrotoxicosis, mitral regurgitation, and congestive heart failure.
L. Fourth heart sound (S_4)	Late diastolic sound caused by a noncompliant ventricle. Heard best with bell. Left-sided S_4 heard at apex, right-sided S_4 heard at left lower sternal border. Left-sided S_4 seen with hypertension, aortic stenosis, and myocardial infarction. Right-sided S_4 seen with pulmonic stenosis and pulmonary hypertension.

^aRefer to Figure 1–1 for graphic representations of murmurs (page 4).
^bCapital letters preceding type of murmur refer to graphs in Figure 1–1.

BLOOD PRESSURE GUIDELINES

There is a clear association between HTN and coronary artery and cerebrovascular disease.

Hypertension is defined as systolic BP > 140 mm Hg or a diastolic BP > 90 mm Hg in adults. Measure the BP after 5 min of rest with patient seated and arm at heart level. Use the bell of the stethoscope, the last sounds heard are the Korotkoff sounds, which are low-pitched.

Take the average of two readings separated by 2 min. Elevated readings on three separate days should be obtained prior to diagnosing HTN. Classification and measurement guidelines for adults are shown in Table 1–3.

TABLE 1–3
Guidelines for Blood Pressure Management in Adults Based on JNC7

CLASSIFICATION OF BLOOD PRESSURE (BP)

Category	SBP mmHg		DBP mmHg
Normal	<120	and	<80
Prehypertension	120–139	or	80–89
Hypertension, Stage 1	140–159	or	90–99
Hypertension, Stage 2	≥160	or	≥100

Key: SBP=systolic blood pressure; DBP=diastolic blood pressure

BLOOD PRESSURE MEASUREMENT TECHNIQUES

Method	Notes
In-office	Two readings, 5 minutes apart, sitting in chair. Confirm elevated reading in contralateral arm
Ambulatory BP monitoring	Indicated for evaluation of "white coat hypertension." Absence of 10–20 percent BP decrease during sleep may indicate increased CVD risk
Patient self-check	Provides information on response to therapy. May help improve adherence to therapy and is useful for evaluating "white coat hypertension."

The National High Blood Pressure Education Program is administered by the National Heart, Lung and Blood Institute (NHLB) at the National Institutes of Health. Copies of the JNC7 Report are available at the NHLB Website at http://www.nhlbi.nih.gov. NIH Publication 03–5233, May 2003.

In children from age 1 to 10 years, systolic BP can be calculated as follows: Lower limits (5th percentile): 70 mm Hg + (child's age in years × 2); typical (50th percentile): 90 mm Hg + (child's age in years × 2).

DENTAL EXAMINATION

The dental examination is an often overlooked part of the H&P. Many times, the patient may have some intraoral problem that is contributing to the overall medical condition (ie, the inability to eat due to a toothache, abscess, or ill-fitting denture in a poorly controlled diabetic) for which a dental consult may be necessary. Loose dentures can compromise the ability to manually maintain an open airway. In addition, in an emergency situation when intubation is necessary, complications may occur if the clinician is unfamiliar with the oral structures.

The patient may be able to give some dental history, including recent toothaches, abscesses, and loose teeth or dentures. Be sure to ask if the patient is wearing a removable partial denture (partial plate), which should be removed before intubation. As lost dentures are a chief dental complaint of hospitalized patients, care must be taken not to misplace the removed prosthesis.

A brief dental examination may be performed with gloved hand, two tongue blades, and a flashlight. Look for any obvious inflammation, erythema, edema, or ulceration of the gingiva (gums) and oral mucosa. Gently tap on any natural teeth to test for sensitivity. Place each tooth between two tongue blades and push gently to check for looseness. This is especially important for the maxillary anterior teeth, which serve as the fulcrum for the laryngoscope blade. Any abnormal dental findings should be noted and the appropriate consults obtained. Many diseases, including AIDS, STDs, pemphigus, pemphigoid, allergies, uncontrolled diabetes, leukemia, and others, may first manifest themselves in the mouth.

Hospitalized patients often have difficulty cleaning their teeth or dentures. This care should be added to the daily orders if indicated. Patients who will be receiving head and neck radiation must be examined and treated for any tooth extractions or dental infections before the initiation of the radiation therapy. Extractions after radiation to the maxilla and particularly the mandible may lead to osteoradionecrosis, a condition that may be impossible to control.

Eruption of Teeth

The eruption of teeth may be of great concern to new parents. Often, parents think something is developmentally wrong with their child if teeth have not appeared by a certain age.

The timing of tooth eruption varies tremendously. Factors contributing to this variation include family history, ethnic background, vitality during fetal development, position of teeth in the arch, size and shape of the dental arch itself, and, in the case of the eruption of permanent teeth, when the primary tooth was lost. Radiographs of the maxilla and mandible can determine whether or not the teeth are present. Figure 1–3 serves as a guide to the chronology of tooth eruption. Remember that variations may be greater than 1 year in some cases.

DERMATOLOGIC DESCRIPTIONS

Atrophy: Thinning of the surface of the skin with associated loss of normal markings. Examples: Aging, striae associated with obesity, scleroderma

Bulla: A superficial, well-circumscribed, raised, fluid-filled lesion greater than 1 cm in diameter. Examples: Bullous pemphigoid, pemphigus, dermatitis herpetiformis

Burrow: A subcutaneous linear track made by a parasite. Example: Scabies

Crust: A slightly raised lesion with irregular border and variable color resulting from dried blood, serum, or other exudate. Examples: Scab resulting from an abrasion, or impetigo

Ecchymoses: A flat, nonblanching, red-purple-blue lesion that results from extravasation of red blood cells into the skin. Differs from purpura in size; ecchymoses are large purpura. Examples: Trauma, long-term steroid use

Erosion: A depressed lesion resulting from loss of epidermis due to rupture of vesicles or bullae. Example: Rupture of herpes simplex blister

Excoriation: A linear superficial lesion, which may be covered with dried blood. Early lesions with surrounding erythema. Often self-induced. Example: Scratching associated with pruritus from any cause

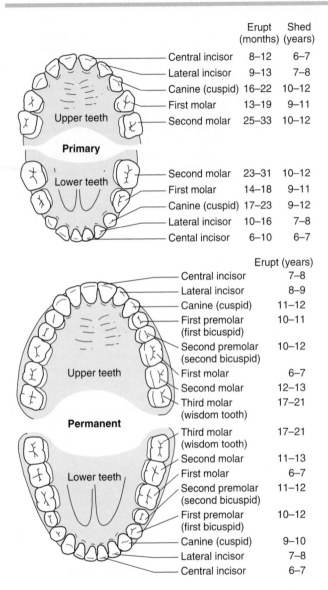

FIGURE 1–3. Dentition development sequences. There can be wide variation in the age when teeth shed and erupt. (Based on data from: McDonald RE, Avery DR [eds]: *Dentistry for the Child and Adolescent*, Mosby, St. Louis, 1994. Used with permission.)

Fissure: A deep linear lesion into the dermis. Example: Cracks seen in athlete's foot

Keloid: Irregular, raised lesion resulting from scar tissue that is hypertrophied. Examples: Often seen with burns, and African Americans are more prone to keloid formation.

Lichenification: A thickening of the skin with an increase in skin markings resulting from chronic irritation and rubbing. Example: Atopic dermatitis

Macule: A circumscribed nonpalpable discoloration of the skin less than 1 cm in diameter. Examples: Freckles, rubella, petechiae

Nodule: A solid, palpable, circumscribed lesion larger than a papule and smaller than a tumor. Examples: Erythema nodosum, gouty tophi

Papule: A solid elevated lesion less than 1 cm. Examples: Acne, warts, insect bites

Patch: A nonpalpable discoloration of the skin with an irregular border, greater than 1 cm in diameter. Example: Vitiligo

Petechiae: A flat pinhead-sized, nonblanching, red-purple lesion caused by hemorrhage into the skin. Example: Seen in DIC, ITP, SLE, meningococcemia (*Neisseria meningitidis*)

Plaque: A solid, flat, elevated lesion greater than 1 cm in diameter. Examples: Psoriasis, discoid lupus erythematosus, actinic keratosis

Purpura: A flat, nonblanching, red-purple lesion larger than petechiae caused by hemorrhage into the skin. Examples: Henoch–Schönlein purpura, TTP

Pustule: A vesicle that is filled with purulent fluid. Examples: Acne, impetigo

Scales: Partial separation of the superficial layer of skin. Examples: Psoriasis, dandruff

Scar: Replacement of normal skin with fibrous tissue, often resulting from injury. Examples: Surgical scar, burn

Telangiectasia: Dilatation of capillaries resulting in red, irregular, clustered lines that blanch. Examples: Seen in scleroderma, Osler–Weber–Rendu disease, cirrhosis

Tumor: A solid, palpable, circumscribed lesion that is greater than 2 cm in diameter. Example: Lipoma

Ulcer: A depressed lesion resulting from loss of epidermis and part of the dermis. Examples: Decubitus ulcers, primary lesion of syphilis, venous stasis ulcer

Vesicle: A superficial, well-circumscribed, raised, fluid-filled lesion that is less than 1 cm in diameter. Examples: Herpes simplex, varicella (chickenpox)

Wheal: Slightly raised, red, irregular lesions that are transient and secondary to edema of the skin. Examples: Urticaria (hives), allergic reaction to injections or insect bites

DERMATOME AND CUTANEOUS INNERVATION

The diagrams (see Figures 1–2A and B) demonstrate dermatome levels and cutaneous innervation distribution useful in the physical examination.

PHYSICAL SYMPTOMS AND EPONYMS

Allen's Test: (See Chapter 13, page 250.)

Apley's Test: Determination of meniscal tear in the knee by grinding the joint manually

Argyll Robertson Pupil: Bilaterally small, irregular, unequal pupils that react to accommodation but not to light. Seen with tertiary syphilis

Austin Flint Murmur: Late diastolic mitral murmur; associated with aortic insufficiency with a normal mitral valve

Babinski's Sign: Extension of the large toe with stimulation of the plantar surface of the foot instead of the normal flexion; indicative of upper motor neuron disease (normal in neonates)

Bainbridge's Reflex: Increased heart rate due to increased right atrial pressure

Battle's Sign: Ecchymosis behind the ear associated with basilar skull fractures

Beau's Lines: Transverse depressions in nails due to previous systemic disease

Beck's Triad: JVD, diminished or muffled heart sounds, and decreased BP associated with cardiac tamponade

Bell's Palsy: Lower motor neuron lesion of the facial nerve affecting muscles of upper and lower face. Easily distinguished from upper motor lesions, which affect predominately muscles of the lower face because upper motor neurons from each side innervate muscles on both sides of the upper face

Bergman's Triad: Altered mental status, petechiae, and dyspnea associated with fat embolus syndrome

Biot's Breathing: Abruptly alternating apnea and equally deep breaths (seen with brain injury)

Bisferious Pulse: A double-peaked pulse seen in severe chronic aortic insufficiency

Bitot's Spots: Small scleral white patches suggesting vitamin A deficiency

Blumberg' Sign: Pain felt in the abdomen when steady constant pressure is quickly released (seen with peritonitis)

Blumer's Shelf: Hardness palpable on rectal examination due to metastatic cancer of the rectouterine (pouch of Douglas) or rectovesical pouch

Bouchard's Nodes: Hard, nontender, painless nodules in the dorsolateral aspects of the proximal interphalangeal joints associated with osteoarthritis. Results from hypertrophy of the bone

Branham's Sign: Abrupt slowing of the heart rate with compression of the feeding artery (seen with large AV fistulas)

Brudzinski's Sign: Flexion of the neck causing flexion of the hips (seen in meningitis)

Chadwick's Sign: Bluish color of cervix and vagina, seen with pregnancy

Chandelier's Sign: Extreme pain elicited with movement of the cervix during bimanual pelvic examination (indicates PID)

Charcot's Triad: Right upper quadrant pain, fever (chills), and jaundice associated with cholangitis

Cheyne–Stokes Respiration: Repeating cycle of a gradual increase in depth of breathing followed by a gradual decrease to apnea (seen with CNS disorders, uremia, some normal sleep patterns)

Chvostek's Sign: Tapping over the facial nerve causes facial spasm in hypocalcemia (tetany). May be normal finding in some patients

Corrigan's Pulse: A palpable hard pulse immediately followed by sudden collapse (seen in aortic regurgitation)

Cullen's Sign: Ecchymosis around the umbilicus associated with severe intraperitoneal bleeding (seen with ruptured ectopic pregnancy and hemorrhagic pancreatitis)

Cushing's Triad: HTN, bradycardia, and irregular respiration associated with increased intracranial pressure

Darier's Sign: Stroking of the skin causes erythema and edema in mastocytosis

Doll's Eyes: Conjugated movement of eyes in one direction as head is briskly turned in the other direction in comatose patients. Tests oculocephalic reflex indicating intact brain stem

Drawer Sign: Forward (or backward) movement of the tibia with pressure, indicating laxity or a tear in the anterior (or posterior) cruciate ligament

Dupuytren's Contracture: Proliferation of fibrosis tissue of the palmar fascia resulting in contracture of the fourth and/or fifth digits, which is often bilateral. May be hereditary or seen in patients with chronic alcoholic liver disease or seizures

Duroziez's Sign: Found in aortic regurgitation a "to-and-fro" murmur when stethoscope is pressed over the femoral artery

Electrical Alternans: Beat-to-beat variation in the electrical axis (seen in large pericardial effusions), suggesting impending hemodynamic compromise

Ewart's Sign: Dullness to percussion, increased fremitus and bronchial breathing beneath the angle of the left scapula found with pericardial effusion

Fong Lesion/Syndrome: Autosomal-dominant anomalies of the nails and patella associated with renal abnormalities

Frank's Sign: Fissure of the ear lobe; may be associated with CAD, DM, and HTN

Gibbus: Angular convexity of the spine due to vertebral collapse (associated with osteoporosis or metastasis)

Gregg's Triad: Cataracts, heart defects, and deafness with congenital rubella

Grey Turner's Sign: Ecchymosis in the flank associated with retroperitoneal hemorrhage

Grocco's Sign: Triangular area of paravertebral dullness, opposite side of a pleural effusion

Heberden's Nodes: Hard, nontender, painless nodules on the dorsolateral aspects of the distal interphalangeal joints associated with osteoarthritis. Results from hypertrophy of the bone

Hegar's Sign: Softening of the distal uterus. Reliable early sign of pregnancy

Hollenhorst's Plaque: A cholesterol plaque on retina seen on funduscopic examination (associated with amaurosis fugax)

Hill's Sign: Femoral artery pressure 20 mm Hg greater than brachial pressure (seen in severe aortic regurgitation)

Hoffmann's Sign/Reflex: Flicking of the volar surface of the distal phalanx causing fingers to flex (associated with pyramidal tract disease)

Homans' Sign: Calf pain with forcible dorsiflexion of the foot (associated with DVT)

Horner's Syndrome: Unilateral miosis, ptosis, and anhidrosis (absence of sweating). From destruction of ipsilateral superior cervical ganglion often from lung carcinoma, especially squamous cell carcinoma

Janeway's Lesion: Erythematous or hemorrhagic lesion seen on the palm or sole with subacute bacterial endocarditis

Joffroy's Reflex: Inability to wrinkle the forehead when patient asked to bend head and look up (seen in hyperthyroidism)

Kayser–Fleischer Ring: Brown pigment lesion due to copper deposition (seen in Wilson's disease)

Kehr's Sign: Left shoulder and left upper quadrant pain associated with splenic rupture

Kernig's Sign: When the thigh is flexed at a right angle, complete extension of the leg is not possible because of inflammation of the meninges (seen with meningitis)

Koplik's Spots: White papules on buccal mucosa opposite molars (seen in measles)

Korotkoff's Sounds: Low-pitched sounds resulting from vibration of the artery, detected when obtaining a BP using the bell of the stethoscope. The last Korotkoff sound may be a more accurate estimate of the true diastolic BP than the diastolic BP obtained using the diaphragm.

Kussmaul's Respiration: Deep, rapid respiratory pattern (seen in coma or DKA)

Kussmaul's Sign: Paradoxical rise in the jugular venous pressure on inspiration (seen in constrictive pericarditis or COPD)

Kyphosis: Excessive rounding of the thoracic spinal convexity, associated with aging, especially in women

Lasègue's Sign/Straight-Leg-Raising Sign: The patient is extended in the supine position and raises the leg gently. Pain in the distribution of nerve root suggests lumbar disk disease.

Levine's Sign: Clenched fist over the chest while describing chest pain (associated with angina and AMI)

Lhermitte's Sign: Neck flexion results in a "shock sensation" (seen in MS)

List: Lateral tilt of the spine, frequently associated with herniated disk and muscle spasm

Lordosis: Accentuated normal concavity of the lumbar spine, normal in pregnancy

Louvel's Sign: Coughing or sneezing causes pain in the leg with DVT

Marcus–Gunn Pupil: Dilation of pupils with swinging flashlight test. Results from unilateral optic nerve disease. Normal pupillary response is elicited when light is directed from the normal eye and a subnormal response when light is quickly directed from the normal eye into the abnormal eye. When light is directed into the abnormal eye, both pupils dilate rather than maintain the previous degree of miosis.

McBurney's Point/Sign: Point located one-third of the distance from the anterior superior iliac spine to the umbilicus on the right (Tenderness at the site is associated with acute appendicitis.)

McMurray's Test: External rotation of the foot produces a palpable or audible click on the joint line, suggesting medial meniscal injury

Möbius' Sign: Weakness of convergence seen in thyrotoxicosis

Moro's Reflex (Startle Reflex): Abduction of hips and arms with extension of arms when infant's head and upper body is suddenly dropped several inches while being held. Normal reflex in early infancy

Murphy's Sign: Severe pain and inspiratory arrest with palpation of the right upper quadrant during deep inspiration (associated with cholecystitis)

Musset's or de Musset's Sign: Rhythmic nodding or movement of the head with each heart beat caused by blood flow back into the heart secondary to aortic insufficiency

Obturator Sign: Flexion and internal rotation of the thigh elicits hypogastric pain in cases of inflammation of the obturator internus (positive with pelvic abscess and appendicitis)

Ortolani's Test/Sign: Sign is hip click that suggests congenital hip dislocation. With the infant supine, point the legs toward you and flex the legs to 90 degrees at the hips and knees.

Osler's Node: Tender, red, raised lesions on the hands or feet (seen with SBE)

Pancoast's Syndrome: Carcinoma involving apex of lung, resulting in arm and or shoulder pain from involvement of brachial plexus and Horner's syndrome from involvement of the superior cervical ganglion

Pastia's Lines: Linear striations of confluent petechiae in axillary folds are antecubital fossa seen in scarlet fever

Phalen's Test: Prolonged maximum flexion of wrists while opposing dorsum of each hand against each other. A positive test results in pain and tingling in the distribution of the median nerve (seen in carpal tunnel syndrome)

Psoas Sign (Iliopsoas Test): Flexion against resistance or extension of the right hip, producing pain; seen with inflammation of the psoas muscle (positive with appendicitis)

Pulsus Alternans: Fluctuation of pulse pressure with every other beat (seen in aortic stenosis and CHF)

Queckenstedt's Test: Tests patency of the subarachnoid space; compression of the internal jugular vein during lumbar puncture; should normally immediately raise CSF pressure

Quincke's Sign: Alternating blushing and blanching of the fingernail bed following light compression (seen in chronic aortic regurgitation)

Radovici's Sign: A frontal release sign, scratching palm causes chin contractions

Raynaud's Phenomenon/Disease: Pain and tingling in fingers after exposure to cold with characteristic color changes of white to blue and then often red. May be seen with scleroderma and SLE or be idiopathic (Raynaud's disease)

Romberg's Test: Used to test position sense or cerebellar function. The patient stands with heels and toes together. Arms may be outstretched with palms facing upward or down, or arms can be at the patient's side. The patient may be lightly tapped by the examiner with the eyes open and then closed. A positive test is a loss of balance. A loss of balance with the eyes open indicates cerebellar dysfunction. Normal balance with eyes open and loss of balance with eyes closed indicates loss of position sense.

Roth's Spots: Oval retinal hemorrhages with a pale central area occurring in patients with bacterial endocarditis

Rovsing's Sign: Pain in the RLQ with deep palpation of the LLQ (seen in acute appendicitis)

Schmorl's Node: Degeneration of the intervertebral disk resulting in herniation into the adjacent vertebral body

Scoliosis: Lateral curvature of the spine

Sentinel Loop: A single dilated loop of small or large bowel, usually occurs secondary to localized inflammation such as pancreatitis

Sister Mary Joseph's Sign/Node: Metastatic cancer to umbilical lymph node

Stellwag's Sign: Infrequent ocular blinking

Tinel's Sign: Radiation of an electric shock sensation in the distal distribution of the median nerve elicited by percussion of the flexor surface of the wrist when fully extended (seen in carpal tunnel syndrome)

Traube's Sign: Booming or pistol shot sounds heard over the femoral arteries in chronic aortic insufficiency

Trendelenburg's Test: Observe patient from behind while patient shifts weight from one leg to the other; a pelvis tilt to opposite side suggests hip disease and weakness of the gluteus medius muscle. If normal, pelvis will not tilt.

Trousseau's Sign: Carpal spasm produced by inflating a BP cuff above the systolic pressure for 2–3 min, indicates hypocalcemia; also migratory thrombophlebitis associated with cancer

Turner's Sign: See Grey Turner's sign

Virchow's Node (Signal or Sentinel Node): A palpable, left supraclavicular lymph node; often first sign of a GI neoplasm, such as pancreatic or gastric carcinoma

von Graefe's Sign: Lid lag associated with thyrotoxicosis

Weber–Rinne Test: For the Weber test a 512- or 1024-Hz tuning fork is placed on the middle of the skull to determine if the sound lateralizes. For the Rinne test, the tuning fork is held against the mastoid process (BC) with the opposite ear covered. The patient indicates when the sound is gone. The tuning fork is then held next to the ear and the patient indicates whether the sound is present and when the sound (AC) disappears. Normally AC is better than BC. With sensorineural hearing loss, the Weber test lateralizes to the less affected ear and AC > BC; with conduction hearing loss, the Weber test lateralizes to the more affected ear and BC > AC.

Whipple's Triad: Hypoglycemia, CNS, and vasomotor symptoms (ie, diaphoresis, syncope); relief of symptoms with glucose (associated with insulinoma)

EXAMPLE OF A WRITTEN HISTORY AND PHYSICAL EXAMINATION

(Adult Admitted to a Medical Service)

* 12/10/03 5:30 PM

Identification: Mr. Robert Jones is a 50-year-old male referred by Dr. Harry Doyle from Whitesburg, Kentucky. The informant is the patient, who seems reliable, and a photocopy of the ER records from Whitesburg Hospital accompanies the patient.

Chief Complaint: "Squeezing chest pain for 10 h, 4 d ago"

HPI: Mr. Jones awoke at 6 AM 3 d ago with squeezing substernal chest pain that felt "like a ton of bricks" sitting on his chest. The chest pain was a 9 on a 10-point scale, with 10 being pain from a kidney stone. The pain was progressively worse after its onset and decreased in intensity after going to the Whitesburg ER. The pain radiated to his left neck and elbow and was associated with dyspnea and diaphoresis. He says he experienced no associated nausea. He notes the pain seemed to get worse with any movement, and nothing seemed to alleviate it.

He presented to the Whitesburg ER 10 h after the onset of pain and was given 3 NTG tablets SL and 2 mg morphine sulfate. ECG revealed 3 mm ST depression in leads V_1 through V_4. He was admitted to the ICU at Whitesburg Hospital and had an uneventful course. CK increased to 850 U/L at 24 h, and troponin increased to 12.5 ng/mL. He has been on aspirin 325 mg/d PO, isosorbide dinitrate 20 mg PO q6h, and metoprolol 100 mg PO q12 h. He was transferred for possible cardiac catheterization.

He notes having experienced a similar chest pain that was less intense and occurred intermittently over the last 3 mo. The pain was precipitated by exercise and relieved with rest. He sought no medical attention in the past. He reports no history of orthopnea, paroxysmal nocturnal dyspnea, dyspnea on exertion, or pedal edema.

He has smoked two packs of cigarettes per day for 35 years, notes a 2-y history of HTN for which he has been taking HCTZ 25 mg/d and reports no history of hypercholesterolemia or diabetes. He notes his BP usually runs 120–130/85 at home. The patient's father died of an MI at age 54, and his brother underwent CABG surgery last year at age 48.

PMH

Medications. As above and ranitidine 300 mg PO qhs. Occasional ibuprofen 200 mg 2–3 tabs PO for back pain and acetaminophen 500 mg PO for HA

Vitamins. One-a-day

Herbals. None

Allergies. Penicillin, rash entire body 20 years of age

Surgeries. Appendectomy age 20, Dr. Smith, Whitesburg

Hospitalization. See above.

Trauma. Roof fall in mine accident 10 years ago, injured back. Notes occasional pain, which is relieved with ibuprofen 200 mg 2–3 tabs at a time

(continued)

Transfusions. None

Illnesses. Reports no asthma, emphysema, thyroid disease, kidney disease, peptic ulcer disease, cancer, bleeding disorders, tuberculosis, or hepatitis. He notes a several-year history of water brash/heartburn and has been on ranitidine for 1 year

Routine Health Maintenance. Last diphtheria/tetanus immunization 3 y ago. Stools for guaiac were negative × 3. Refused sigmoidoscopy. He has been seen by Dr. Doyle every 3–4 mon for the last 2 y for HTN.

Family History

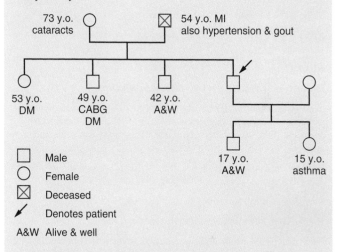

73 y.o.
cataracts

54 y.o. MI
also hypertension & gout

53 y.o.
DM

49 y.o.
CABG
DM

42 y.o.
A&W

17 y.o.
A&W

15 y.o.
asthma

☐ Male
○ Female
☒ Deceased
✔ Denotes patient
A&W Alive & well

Psychosocial History: Mr. Jones has been married for 25 years and has three children.

He and his family live in a home on 3 acres about 3 miles from Whitesburg. He worked in a coal mine until 10 years ago when he was injured in a "roof fall." He is currently employed in a local chair factory. He graduated from high school. He is Baptist and attends church regularly. Hobbies include woodworking and gardening. He eats breakfast and supper every day and has a soft drink and crackers for lunch. He currently works 8 h/d Monday through Friday. He notes going to bed every day by 10:00 PM and awakens at 5:30 AM. He drinks one to two cups of coffee per day and reports drinking no alcohol. He says he does not use drugs but smokes as noted earlier. He reports he has never been exposed to environmental toxins. He says he has no financial problems but is concerned about how his illness will affect his income. He has "good" health insurance. He denies any other stressor in his life. His sources of support are his wife, minister, and a sister who lives near the patient.

ROS: Negative unless otherwise noted.

Eyes. Has worn reading glasses since 1995; notes blurred vision for 1 year; last eye appointment 2001. Claims loss of vision, double vision, or history of cataracts.

(continued)

Respiratory. Notes cough every morning and has produced 1 teaspoon of gray sputum for years. Denies hemoptysis or pleuritic chest pain. Last CXR prior to today was 3 years ago. All other ROS negative.

PHYSICAL EXAMINATION

General: Mr. Jones is a pleasant male lying comfortably supine in bed. He appears to be the stated age.

Vital Signs: Temp 98.6°F orally. Resp 16, HR 88 and regular, BP 110/70 mm Hg left arm supine

Skin: Tattoo left arm, otherwise no lesions

Node: 1 × 1 left axillary node, nontender and mobile. No other lymphadenopathy

HEENT

Head. Normocephalic, atraumatic, nontender, no lesions

Eyes. Visual acuity 20/40 left and right corrected. External structures normal, without lesions, PERRLA. EOM intact. Visual fields intact. Funduscopic examination disks sharp bilaterally, moderate arteriolar narrowing and A-V nicking.

Ears. Hearing intact to watch tick at 3 ft bilaterally. Tympanic membranes intact with good cone of light bilaterally

Nose. Symmetrical. No lesions. Sinuses nontender

Mouth. Several dental fillings, otherwise normal dentition. No lesions

Neck. Full ROM without tenderness. No masses or lymphadenopathy. Carotids +2/4 bilaterally, no bruits. Internal jugular vein visible 2 cm above the sternal angle, patient at 30 degrees.

Chest: Symmetrical expansion. Fremitus by palpation bilaterally equal. Diaphragm moves 5.5 cm bilaterally by percussion. Lung fields clear to percussion. Breath sounds normal except end-inspiratory crackles heard at both bases that do not clear with coughing.

Breast: Normal to inspection and palpation

Heart: No cardiac impulse visible. Apical impulse palpable at the sixth intercostal space 2 cm lateral to the midclavicular line. Normal S_1, physiologically split S_2. S_4 heard at apex. No murmurs, rub, or S_3.

Abdomen: Flat, no scars. Positive bowel sounds. No bruits. Liver 10 cm midclavicular line. No CVA tenderness. No hepatomegaly or splenomegaly by palpation. No tenderness or guarding. No inguinal lymphadenopathy

Genital: Normal circumcised male, both testes descended without masses or tenderness

Rectal: Normal sphincter tone. No external lesions. Prostate smooth without tenderness or nodules. No palpable masses. Stool present, stool for occult blood negative

(continued)

Musculoskeletal: Lumbar spine decreased flexion to 75 degrees, extension to 5 degrees, decreased rotary and lateral movement. Otherwise full ROM of all joints, no erythema, tenderness, or swelling. No clubbing cyanosis or edema

Peripheral Vascular: Radial, ulnar, brachial, femoral, dorsalis pedis, and posterior tibial pulses +2/4 bilaterally. Popliteal pulses nonpalpable. No femoral bruits

Neurologic: *Cranial nerves*: I through XII intact. *Motor*: +5/5 upper and lower extremity, proximally and distally. *Sensory*: intact to pinprick upper and lower extremities proximally and distally. Vibratory sense intact in great toes and thumbs bilaterally. Stereognosis intact. *Reflexes.* Biceps, triceps, brachioradialis, quadriceps, and ankles +2/4 bilaterally. Toes down going bilaterally

Cerebellum. Romberg's sign negative. Intact finger-to-nose and heel-to-shin bilaterally; gait normal–normal heel-and-heel, toe-and-toe, and heel-to-toe gaits. Rapid alternating movements intact upper and lower extremities bilaterally

DATABASE

ECG. HR 80, NSR inverted T waves V_1 through V_5

CXR. Cardiomegaly, otherwise clear

UA. SG 1.020, protein trace otherwise negative

PT, PTT. 12.1, control 11.7, *INR* 1.1;28, control 27

Chemistry Profile. CK 250 U/L.

Troponin. 4.0 ng/mL, otherwise normal.

CBC. 6700 WBC; 49% HCT; Hbg 16 g/dL; 43 S, 5 B, 44 L, 5 M, 3 E

PROBLEM LIST

Date Entered	Date of Onset	Problem	Active	Inactive	Date Inactive
12-10-03	4-03	1	Coronary artery disease		
12-10-03	7-7-03	1a	Subendocardial MI—anterior		
12-10-03	2001	2	Hypertension		
12-10-03	1990s	3	Bronchitis		
12-10-03	2001	4	Heartburn/reflux esophagitis		
12-10-03	1993	5	Back injury		
12-10-03	7-10-03	6	Eosinophilia		
12-10-03	2002	7	Blurred vision		
12-10-03	1972	8		Appendicitis	1972

(continued)

ASSESSMENT AND PLAN

Coronary Artery Disease: Mr. Jones presented with a classic history for MI. The CK and electrocardiogram support the diagnosis. The ST depression without evolving Q waves is consistent with a nontransmural MI. Mr. Jones is at risk for further MI because it was a nontransmural MI, and he will require further evaluation before discharge.

- Continue aspirin 3275 mg/d PO and metoprolol 100 mg q12h.
- Change isosorbide to tid prior to discharge.
- Monitor by telemetry unit for next 24–48 h.
- Stress test by modified Bruce protocol prior to discharge.
- Consider cardiac catheterization especially if any further pain or if an early positive stress test.
- Continue cardiac rehabilitation.

Hypertension: In view of the patient's age, sex, and degree of HTN, and the fact that there is no evidence of a secondary cause, the HTN is most likely primary in nature. It is important that BP be well controlled after this infarct. Mr. Jones' BP has been well controlled on HCTZ alone, and he is now also on metoprolol.

- Continue metoprolol and HCTZ.
- Dietary consult to instruct patient on low-sodium as well as low-fat diet prior to discharge.
- Continue discussion of other problems as shown earlier.

Chronic Cough with Sputum Production: Most likely chronic bronchitis. Consider bronchiogenic carcinoma; however, CXR is normal except for heart size. Encourage smoking cessation.

Signature: _____

Title: _____

2

CHARTWORK

How to Write Orders	Preoperative Note
Problem-Oriented Progress Note	Operative Note
Discharge Summary/Note	Night of Surgery Note (Postop Note)
On-Service Note	Delivery Note
Off-Service Note	Outpatient Prescription Writing
Bedside Procedure Note	Shorthand for Laboratory Values

HOW TO WRITE ORDERS

The following format is useful for writing concise admission, transfer, and post-operative orders. It involves the mnemonic "A.D.C. VAAN DISSL," which stands for **A**dmit/Attending, **D**iagnosis, **C**ondition, **V**itals, **A**ctivity, **A**llergies, **N**ursing procedures, **D**iet, **I**ns and outs, **S**pecific medications, **S**ymptomatic medications and **L**abs.

A.D.C. Vaan Dissl

Admit: Admitting team, room number

Attending: The name of the attending physician (the person legally responsible for the patient's care). Also include the resident's and intern's names.

Diagnosis: List admitting diagnosis or procedure if postop orders.

Condition: Stable, critical, etc

Vitals: Determine frequency of vital signs (temperature, pulse, BP, CVP, PCWP, weight, etc).

Activity: Specify bedrest, up ad lib, ambulate qid, bathroom privileges, etc.

Allergies: Note any drug reactions or food or environmental allergies (eg, latex, adhesive tape).

Nursing Procedures

Bed Position. Elevate head of bed 30 degrees, etc

Preps. Enemas, scrubs, showers

Respiratory Care. P&PD, TC&DB, etc

Dressing Changes, Wound Care. Change dressing bid, etc

Notify House Officer If. Temperature > 101°F, BP < 90 mm Hg, etc

Diet: NPO, clear liquid, regular, etc

Ins and Outs: Refers to all "tubes" a patient may have

Record Daily I&O.

IV Fluids. Specify type and rate.

Drains.

NG Tubes, Foley Catheter, ETTs, Arterial Lines, Pulmonary-Artery Catheters. Specify care desired (eg, NG to low wall suction, Foley to gravity, suction ET q2h and PRN, etc)

Specific Medications: Specific medications (eg, diuretic, antibiotics, hormones, etc)

Symptomatic Medications: As needed medications(eg, pain medications, laxatives, "sleepers")

Labs: Indicate studies such as blood and urine, etc. Specify times if applicable. This also includes ECGs, radiographs, nuclear scans, consultation requests, etc.

PROBLEM-ORIENTED PROGRESS NOTE

(See Chapter 20 for a sample ICU progress note.)

1. List each medical, surgical, psychiatric problem separately: pneumonia, pancreatitis, CHF, etc.
2. Give each problem a call number: 1, 2, 3, \.\ (as on page 23).
3. Retain the number of each problem throughout the hospitalization.
4. When the problem is resolved, mark it as such and delete it from the daily progress note.
5. Evaluate each problem by number in the following SOAP format. Or, you may do a separate assessment and plan for each problem.

Soap

Subjective:
- How the patient feels, any complaints

Objective:
- How the patient looks
- Vital signs
- Physical examination
- Laboratory data, etc

Assessment: (for each problem)
- Evaluation of the data and any conclusions that can be drawn

Plan: (for each problem)
- Any new lab tests or medications
- Changes or additions to orders
- Discharge or transfer plans

DISCHARGE SUMMARY/NOTE

A formal discharge note is usually required for any admission that is longer than 24 h at most hospitals. This note provides a framework for the complete dictated note as well as providing a reference, if needed, before the dictated note is transcribed and filed. The following skeleton includes most of the information needed for a discharge note.

Date of Admission: Specify date.
Date of Discharge: Specify date.
Admitting Diagnosis: List main reason for initial admission.
Discharge Diagnosis: List primary diagnosis as well as any secondary diagnosis.
Attending Physician and Service Caring for Patient: Provide attending's name and service or practice group.
Referring Physician: Provide name and contact information (eg, address, phone) if available.
Procedures: Include surgery and any invasive diagnostic procedures, (eg, lumbar punctures, arteriograms).
Brief History, Pertinent Physical, and Lab Data: Briefly review the main points of the history, physical, and admission lab tests. Do not repeat what is recorded in the admission note; summarize the most important points about the patient's admission.

Hospital Course: Briefly summarize the evaluation, treatment, and progress of
the patient during the hospitalization.

Condition at Discharge: Note if improved, unchanged, etc.

Disposition: Where was the patient discharged to (eg, home, another hospital,
nursing home)? Try to give specific address if transferred to another medical institution and note who will be assuming responsibility for the patient.

Discharge Medications: List medications, dosing, refills.

Discharge Instructions and Follow-up: Clinic return date, diet instructions, activity restrictions, etc.

Problem List: List active and past medical problems.

ON-SERVICE NOTE

Also known as a "pick-up note," the on-service note is written by a new member
of the team taking over the care of a patient who has been on the service for
some time. This type of note is more common on medical services. The note
should be brief and summarize the hospital course to date as well as demonstrate
that the new team member has reviewed the patient's care to date. The following
skeleton includes most of the information needed in an on-service note.

Date of Admission:

Admitting Diagnosis:

Procedures (with Results) to Date:

Hospital Course to Date: This should be briefly summarized.

Brief Physical Examination: Pertinent to the patient's problems.

Pertinent Lab Data: Summarize key lab tests.

Problem List: Use problem numbering system.

Assessment: Describe how the patient is progressing and what problems remain.

Plan: Outline further testing or therapy planned.

OFF-SERVICE NOTE

This is written by the team member who is rotating off the service but who was
primarily responsible for the patient before the patient was ready for discharge.
The components are identical to the "on-service" note in the previous section.

BEDSIDE PROCEDURE NOTE

Procedure: LP, thoracentesis, etc

Indications: (eg, R/O meningitis, symptomatic pleural effusion)

Permit: Note risks and benefits explained and indicate if the permit is signed
and on chart.

Physicians: Note physicians present and responsible for procedure.

Description of Procedure: Indicate type of positioning, prep, anesthesia (and
amount)(eg, 2 ml 1% lidocaine). Briefly describe technique and instruments used.

Complications: List.

Estimated Blood Loss (EBL): Note as "minimal," or, if greater, estimate
amount lost.

Specimens/Findings Obtained: (eg, opening pressure for LP, CSF appearance,
and tubes sent to lab, etc)

Disposition: Describe patient's status after procedure (eg, Patient alert and oriented with no complaints; BP stable.)

PREOPERATIVE NOTE

2

The specific items in the preoperative note depend on institutional guidelines, the nature of the procedure, and the age and health of the patient. For example, an ECG and blood set-up may not be necessary for a 2-year-old child being treated for a hernia but essential for a 70-year-old scheduled for aortic valve surgery. The following list includes most of the information needed in a preoperative note.

Preop Diagnosis: Such as "acute appendicitis"
Procedure: Indicate what is the planned procedure, eg, "exploratory laparotomy."
Labs: Results of CBC, electrolytes, PT, PTT, urinalysis, etc
CXR: Note results.
ECG: Note results.
Blood: Institutional guidelines usually specify recommended quantities (eg, T&C 2 units PRBC, blood not needed, etc). See also Chapter 10)
History and Physical: Should be "on chart."
Orders: Note any special preop orders, eg, preop colon preps, vaginal douches, prophylactic antibiotics.
Permit: If completed, write "signed and on chart"; if not, indicate plans for obtaining permit. Note briefly risks and benefits explained.

OPERATIVE NOTE

The operative note is written immediately after surgery to summarize the operation for those who were not present and is meant to complement the formal operative summary dictated by the surgeon. The following list includes most of what is needed in an operative note.

Preop Diagnosis: Reason for the surgery, eg, "acute appendicitis"
Postop Diagnosis: Based on the operative findings, eg, "mesenteric lymphadenitis"
Procedure: Surgery performed, eg, "exploratory laparotomy"
Surgeons: List the attending physicians, residents, and students who scrubbed on the case, including their titles (MD, CCIV, MSII, etc). It is often helpful to identify the dictating surgeon.
Findings: Briefly note operative findings, eg, "normal appendix with marked lymphadenopathy."
Anesthesia: Specify the type of anesthesia, eg, local, spinal, general, endotracheal, etc.
Fluids: Amount and type of fluid administered during case, eg, 1500 mL NS, 1 unit PRBC, 500 mL albumin. This is usually obtained from the anesthesia records.
EBL: Usually obtained from the anesthesia or nursing records.
Drains: State location and type of drain, eg, "Jackson–Pratt drain in LUQ," "T-tube in midline," etc.
Specimens: State any samples sent to pathology and the results of examination of any intraoperative frozen sections.
Complications: Note any complications during or after the surgery.
Condition: Note where the patient is taken immediately after surgery and the patient's condition (eg, "transferred to the recovery room in stable condition").

NIGHT OF SURGERY NOTE (POSTOP NOTE)

This type of progress note is written several hours after or the night of surgery.

Procedure: Indicate the operation performed.
Level of Consciousness: Note if the patient is alert, drowsy, etc.

Vital Signs: Record BP, pulse, respiration.

I&O: Calculate amount of IV fluids, blood, urine output, and other drainage, and attempt to assess fluid balance.

Physical Examination: Examine and note the findings of the chest, heart, abdomen, extremities, and any other part of the physical examination pertinent to the surgery; examine the dressing for bleeding.

Labs: Review lab results if any were obtained since surgery.

Assessment: Evaluate the postop course thus far (stable, etc).

Plan: Note any changes in orders.

DELIVERY NOTE

__ -year-old (married or single) G __ now para __, AB __, clinic (note if patient received prenatal clinic care) patient with EDC __, and a prenatal course (uncomplicated or describe any problems). Any comments concerning labor (eg, oxytocin-induced, premature rupture) and draped in the usual sterile fashion. Under controlled conditions delivered a __ lb __ oz (__ g) viable (male , female) infant under __ (general, spinal, pudendal, none) anesthesia.

Delivery was via SVD with midline episiotomy (or forceps or cesarean section). Apgars were __ at 1 min and __ at 5 min (for Apgar scoring, see Appendix, page 625). State delivery date and time. Cord blood sent to lab and placenta expressed intact with trailing membranes. Lacerations of the __ degree repaired by standard method with good hemostasis and restoration of normal anatomy.

- EBL:
- Maternal blood type (MBT):
- HCT (predelivery and postdelivery):
- Rubella titer:
- RPR test, hepatitis B serology, HIV test, and status of other serology or cultures that could affect the mother's or the newborn's health:
- Condition of mother:

OUTPATIENT PRESCRIPTION WRITING

The format for outpatient prescription writing is outlined in the following list and illustrated in Figure 2–1. Controlled substances, such as narcotics, require a DEA number on the prescription and in some states may require that the controlled substance be written on a special type of prescription pad (see Chapter 22 for controlled drugs indicated by a [C]). For security, the DEA number should never be preprinted on a prescription pad but written by hand at the time the prescription is written.

Elements of an outpatient prescription include:

Patient's Name, Address, and Age: Print clearly where indicated.

Date: State requirements vary, but most prescriptions must be filled within 6 months.

Rx: Drug name, strength, and type (usually listed as the generic name); if you specifically want a brand name you must designate "no substitution." Rx is an abbreviation from the Latin for "recipe." List the strength of the product (usually in mg) and the form (eg, tablets, capsule, suspension, transdermal, etc).

Dispense: Amount of drug (number of capsules), or time period (1-mon supply, QS [quantity sufficient], etc).

Sig: Short for the Latin "signa," which means "mark through" on patient instructions. This part can be written out or noted in shorthand. Shorthand use is gen-

2

```
                    NICK PAVONA, MD
     BENJAMIN FRANKLIN UNIVERSITY MEDICAL CENTER
                 CHADDS FORD, PA 19317
```

LICENSE PA MD 685-488-194   **DEA** NP–3612982

NAME NICK PAVONA, Sr.   **AGE** 86

ADDRESS 34-10 75th Street   **DATE** 10/24/2003

Wilmington, DE

Rx: minioxidil (Rogaine) 2% topical solution
DISP: 60 mL
SIG: Apply BID to scalp
Brand medically necessary

REFILL X5

SUBSTITUTION PERMISSIBLE ☐   *Nick Pavona* M.D.

TO ENSURE BRAND NAME DISPENSING, PRESCRIBER MUST
SPECIFY "DISPENSE AS WRITTEN" ON THE PRESCRIPTION.*

*This can vary by state; some require that you write "Brand Medically
Necessary" to specify a brand name and not a generic.

FIGURE 2–1. Example of an outpatient prescription. As a safety feature DEA
numbers should never be preprinted on a prescription form. The "Dispense as Written" statement can vary by state requirements; this statement requests that the pharmacist fill the prescription as requested and not substitute a generic equivalent.

erally discouraged, however, because writing out the prescription decreases the
likelihood of errors. Frequently used abbreviations are noted here with a more
complete listing provided in the abbreviations list at the front of the book.

ad lib = freely at pleasure

PO = by mouth

PR = by rectum

OS = left eye

OD = right eye

qd = daily (this is a dangerous abbreviation and **should not be used;** see "Dangerous Practices," page 31)

PRN = as needed

$\dot{T}$ = one

$\ddot{T}$ = two

$\dddot{T}$ = three

qhs = every night at bedtime

bid = twice a day

tid = three times a day

q6h = every 6 h

qid = four times a day. Note that qid and q6h are NOT the same orders: qid
means that the medication is given four times a day while awake (eg, 8 AM,
12 noon, 6 PM, and 10 PM); q6h means that the medication is given four
times a day but by the clock (eg, 6 AM, 12 noon, 6 PM, 12 midnight).

Refills: Indicate how many times this prescription can be refilled.

Substitution: Can a generic drug be used instead of the one prescribed?

Tips for Safe Prescription Writing

Legibility

1. Take time to write legibly.
2. Print if this would be more legible than handwriting.
3. Use a typewriter or computer if necessary. In the near future, physicians will generate all prescriptions by computer to eliminate legibility problems.
4. Carefully print the order to avoid misreading. There are many "sound alike" drugs and medications that have similar spellings (ie, Celexa and Celebrex).

Dangerous Prescription Writing Practices

1. **Never** use a trailing zero.
   Correct: 1 mg; Dangerous: 1.0 mg. If the decimal is not seen, a 10-fold overdose can occur.
2. **Never** leave a decimal point "naked." Correct: 0.5 mL; Dangerous: .5 mL. If the decimal point is not seen, a 10-fold overdose can occur.
3. **Never** abbreviate a drug name because the abbreviation may be misunderstood or have multiple meanings.
4. **Never** abbreviate U for units as it can easily be read as a zero, thus "6 U regular insulin" can be misread as 60 units. The order should be written as "6 units regular insulin."
5. **Never** use qd (abbreviation for once a day). When poorly written, the tail of the "q" can make it read qid or four times a day.

SHORTHAND FOR LABORATORY VALUES

(See Figure 2–2 below)

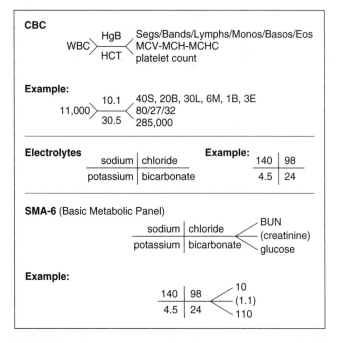

FIGURE 2–2. Shorthand notation for recording laboratory values. The basic metabolic panel is similar to the SMA-6 except that the creatinine is also listed.

DIFFERENTIAL DIAGNOSIS: SYMPTOMS, SIGNS, AND CONDITIONS

Abdominal Distention
Abdominal Pain
Adrenal Mass
Alopecia
Amenorrhea
Anorexia
Anuria
Arthritis
Ascites
Back Pain
Breast Lump
Chest Pain
Chills
Clubbing
Coma
Constipation
Cough
Cyanosis
Delirium
Dementia
Diarrhea
Diplopia
Dizziness
Dysphagia
Dyspnea
Dysuria
Earache
Edema
Epistaxis
Failure to Thrive
Fever
Fever of Unknown Origin (FUO)
Flatulence
Frequency
Galactorrhea
Gynecomastia
Headache
Heartburn (Pyrosis)
Hematemesis, Melenemesis, and Melena
Hematochezia
Hematuria
Hemoptysis
Hepatomegaly
Hiccups (Singultus)
Hirsutism
Impotence (Erectile Dysfunction)
Incontinence (Urinary)
Jaundice
Lymphadenopathy and Splenomegaly
Melena
Nausea and Vomiting
Nystagmus
Oliguria and Anuria
Pleural Effusion
Pruritus
Seizures
Splenomegaly
Syncope
Tremors
Vaginal Bleeding
Vaginal Discharge
Vertigo
Vomiting
Weight Loss
Wheezing

This chapter provides a general guide to commonly encountered symptoms and conditions and their frequent causes. Remember: "There are more uncommon presentations of common diseases than common presentations of uncommon diseases."

ABDOMINAL DISTENTION

Ascites, intestinal obstruction, cysts (ovarian or renal), tumors, hepatosplenomegaly, aortic aneurysm, uterine enlargement (pregnancy), bladder distention, inflammatory mass

ABDOMINAL PAIN

Diffuse: Intestinal angina, early appendicitis, colitis, diabetic ketoacidosis, hereditary angioedema, gastroenteritis, mesenteric thrombosis, mesenteric lymphadenitis, peritonitis, porphyria, sickle cell crisis, uremia, renal colic, renal infarct, pancreatitis

Right Upper Quadrant: Dissecting aneurysm, gallbladder disease (cholecystitis, cholangitis, choledocholithiasis), hepatitis, hepatomegaly, pancreatitis, PUD, pneumonia, PE, pyelonephritis, renal colic, renal infarct, appendicitis (retroperitoneal)

Left Upper Quadrant: Dissecting aneurysm, esophagitis, hiatal hernia, esophageal rupture, gastritis, pancreatitis, PUD, MI, pericarditis, pneumonia, PE, pyelonephritis, renal colic, renal infarct, splenic rupture or infarction

Lower Abdomen: Aortic aneurysm, colitis, diverticulitis including Meckel's, intestinal obstruction, hernias, perforated viscus, pregnancy, ectopic pregnancy, dysmenorrhea, endometriosis, mittelschmerz (ovulation), ovarian cyst or tumor (especially with torsion), PID, renal colic, UTI, rectal hematoma, bladder distention

Right Lower Quadrant: Appendicitis, ectopic pregnancy, ovarian cyst or tumor, salpingitis, mittelschmerz, cholecystitis, perforated duodenal ulcer, Crohn's disease

ADRENAL MASS

Adrenal adenoma, adrenal hyperplasia (unilateral or bilateral), adrenal metastasis (solid tumors, lymphoma, leukemia), adrenocortical carcinoma, pheochromocytoma, adrenal myelolipoma, adrenal cyst, Wolman's disease, adrenal varices, hemorrhage, congenital adrenal hyperplasia, ganglioneuroma, micronodular adrenal disease

ALOPECIA

Male pattern baldness (alopecia, androgenic type in both men and women), trauma and hair pulling, congenital, tinea capitis, bacterial folliculitis, telogen arrest, anagen arrest (chemotherapy/radiation therapy), alopecia areata, discoid lupus

AMENORRHEA

Pregnancy, menopause (physiologic or premature), severe illness, weight loss, stress, excessive athletic training, "physiologically delayed puberty," anatomic (imperforate hymen, uterine agenesis, etc), gonadal dysgenesis (Turner's syndrome, etc), hypothalamic and pituitary tumors, virilizing syndromes (polycystic ovaries, idiopathic hirsutism, etc). Amenorrhea is categorized as primary (never had menses) or secondary (cessation of menses).

ANOREXIA

Hepatitis, carcinoma (most types, especially advanced), anorexia nervosa, generalized debilitating diseases, digitalis toxicity, uremia, depression, CHF, pulmonary failure, radiation exposure, chemotherapy

ANURIA

See Oliguria, page 42

ARTHRITIS

3

Osteoarthritis, bursitis, tendonitis, connective tissue disease (RA, SLE, rheumatic fever, scleroderma, gout, pseudogout, rheumatoid variants [ankylosing spondylitis, psoriatic arthritis, Reiter's syndrome]), infection (bacterial, viral, TB, fungal Lyme disease), trauma, sarcoidosis, sickle cell anemia, hemochromatosis, amyloidosis, coagulopathy

ASCITES

(See Chapter 13, page 306, under "Peritoneal Paracentesis" for more details.) CHF, tricuspid insufficiency, constrictive pericarditis, venous occlusion (including Budd–Chiari syndrome), cirrhosis, pancreatitis, peritonitis (ruptured viscus, TB, bile leak, spontaneous bacterial), tumors (most common ovarian, gastric, uterine, unknown primary, breast, lymphoma), trauma, Meigs' syndrome (ovarian fibroma associated with hydrothorax and ascites), myxedema, anasarca (hypoalbuminemia)

BACK PAIN

Herniated disk, spinal stenosis, ankylosing spondylitis, metastatic tumor, multiple myeloma, mechanical back sprain, referred pain (visceral, vascular), vertebral body fracture, osteoporosis-induced fracture, infectious processes (diskitis, osteomyelitis, epidural abscess)

BREAST LUMP

Cancer, fibroadenoma, fibrocystic breast disease, fat necrosis, gynecomastia (males, alcoholics)

CHEST PAIN

Deep, Dull, Poorly Localized: Angina, variant angina, unstable angina, AMI, aortic aneurysm, PE, tumor, gallbladder disease, pulmonary HTN

Sharp, Well Localized: PE, pneumothorax, epidemic pleurodynia, pericarditis, atypical MI, hyperventilation, hiatal hernia, esophagitis, esophageal spasm, herpes zoster (pain may precede rash by 2–3 days), aortic aneurysm, breast lesions, variety of bony and soft tissue abnormalities (rib fractures, costochondritis, muscle damage), perforated ulcer, acute cholecystitis, pancreatitis

CHILLS

Infection (bacterial with bacteremia, viral, TB, fungal, malaria), neoplasm (Hodgkin's disease), drug and transfusion reactions, hypothermia

CLUBBING

Pulmonary causes (bronchiectasis, lung abscesses, tuberculosis, neoplasms, fibrosis), AV malformations, cardiac (congenital cyanotic heart diseases, bacterial endocarditis), GI (ulcerative and regional enteritis, cirrhosis), hereditary, thyrotoxicosis

COMA

Use the mnemonic **AEIOU TIPS: A**lcohol; **E**ncephalitis (other CNS causes—epilepsy, hemorrhage, mass), **I**nsulin (hypoglycemia, hyperglycemia), **O**piates (drugs), **U**remia (and other metabolic conditions, eg, hypernatremia, hyponatremia, hypercalcemia, hepatic failure, and thiamine deficiency), **T**rauma, **I**nfection, **P**sychiatric causes, **S**yncope (or decreased cardiac output, eg, from arrhythmias or aortic stenosis).

CONSTIPATION

Dehydration, lack of exercise, bedrest, medications (narcotics, anticholinergics, antidepressants, calcium channel blockers—verapamil, diuretics, clonidine, aluminum- or calcium-containing antacids), laxative abuse, megacolon, spastic colon, chronic suppression of the urge to defecate, fecal impaction (often with paradoxical diarrhea), neoplasm, intestinal obstruction, vascular occlusion to the bowel, inflammatory lesions (diverticulitis, proctitis), hemorrhoids, anal fissures, neurologic disorders, depression, porphyria, hypothyroidism, hypercalcemia

COUGH

Acute: Tracheobronchitis, pneumonia, sinusitis, pulmonary edema, foreign body, toxic inhalation, allergy, pharyngitis (viral or bacterial), asthma, GERD, ACE inhibitors, impacted cerumen or foreign body in ear

Chronic: Bronchitis (smoker), chronic sinusitis, emphysema, cancer (bronchogenic, head and neck, and esophageal), TB, sarcoidosis, fungal infection, bronchiectasis, mediastinal lymphadenopathy, thoracic aneurysm, GERD, ACE inhibitors

CYANOSIS

Peripheral: Arterial occlusion and insufficiency, vasospasm/Raynaud's disease, venous stasis, venous obstruction

Central: Hypoxia, congenital heart disease (right to left shunt), PE, pseudocyanosis (eg, polycythemia vera), methemoglobinemia

DELIRIUM

Metabolic: Hypoglycemia, hypoxia, sodium and calcium disorders, hypercarbia, uremia

Neurologic: Stroke, subdural and epidural hematoma, subarachnoid hemorrhage, postictal, concussion and contusion, meningitis, encephalitis, brain tumor

Drug or Toxin-Induced: Lithium intoxication, ethanol, steroids, anticholinergics, sympathomimetics, poisons (eg, mushrooms, carbon monoxide), drugs of abuse

DEMENTIA

Chronic CNS Disease: Alzheimer's, senile dementia, Pick's disease, Parkinson's, chronic demyelinating disease (MS), ALS, brain tumor, normal pressure hydrocephalus, Wilson's disease, Huntington's disease, lipid storage diseases (eg, Tay–Sachs)

Metabolic: Usually chronic (hypoxia, hypoglycemia, hypocalcemia), hyper-ammonemia, dialysis, heavy-metal intoxication, pernicious anemia (B_{12} deficiency), niacin and thiamine deficiency (usually chronic alcoholic), posthepatic coma, medications (barbiturates, phenothiazines, lithium, benzodiazepines, many others)

Infectious: AIDS encephalopathy, brain abscess, chronic meningoencephalitis (eg, fungal, neurosyphilis), encephalitis, Jakob–Creutzfeldt disease

Vascular: Vasculitis, multicerebral/cerebellar infarcts

Traumatic: Contusion, hemorrhage, subdural hematoma

Psychiatric: Sensory deprivation, depression (pseudodementia)

DIARRHEA

Acute: Infections (bacterial, viral, fungal, protozoan, parasitic), toxic (food poisoning, chemical), drugs (antibiotics, cholinergic agents, lactulose, magnesium-containing antacids, quinidine, reserpine, guanethidine, metoclopramide, bethanechol, SSRIs, metformin), appendicitis, diverticular disease, GI bleeding, ischemic colitis, food intolerance, fecal impaction (paradoxical diarrhea), pseudomembranous colitis

Chronic: Postoperative (gastrectomy, vagotomy, extensive bowel resection or resection of ileocecal valve) ZE syndrome, regional enteritis, ulcerative colitis, malabsorption, diverticular disease, carcinoma, villous adenoma, gastrinomas, lymphoma of the bowel, functional bowel disorders (irritable colon, mucous colitis), pseudomembranous colitis, endocrine disease (carcinoid, hyperthyroidism, Addison's disease), radiation enteritis, drugs, Whipple's disease, amyloidosis, AIDS

DIPLOPIA

Problems with the third, fourth, or sixth cranial nerve, eg, from vascular disturbances, meningitis, tumor, demyelination, orbital blow-out fracture, hyperthyroidism, ocular myopathy

DIZZINESS

Hyperventilation, depression, hypoglycemia, anemia, volume depletion, hypoxia, trauma, Ménière's disease, benign positional vertigo, aminoglycoside toxicity, vestibular neuronitis, MS, brainstem ischemia or stroke, posterior fossa lesions, cerebellar ischemia or stroke, arrhythmias, aortic stenosis, carotid sinus hypersensitivity

DYSPHAGIA

Loss of tongue function, pharyngeal dysfunction (myasthenia gravis), Zenker's diverticulum, tumors (bronchogenic, head and neck, and esophageal), stricture, esophageal web, Schatzki's ring, lower esophageal sphincter spasm, foreign body, aortic aneurysm, achalasia, scleroderma, diabetic neuropathy, amyloidosis, infection (especially candidiasis), dermatomyositis, polymyositis, MS, brainstem infarctions

3

DYSPNEA

Laryngeal and tracheal infections and foreign bodies, tumors (both intrinsic and extrinsic), COPD, asthma, pneumonia, lung carcinoma, atelectasis, pneumothorax, pleural effusion, hemothorax, PE, pulmonary infarction, carbon monoxide poisoning, any cause of pain from respiratory movements, cardiac and noncardiac pulmonary edema, AMI, pericardial tamponade, anemia, abdominal distention, anxiety

DYSURIA

Urethral stricture, stones, blood clot, tumor (bladder, prostate, urethral), prostatic enlargement, infection (urethritis, cystitis, vaginitis, prostatitis), trauma, bladder spasm, dehydration

EARACHE

Otitis media and externa, mastoiditis, serous otitis, otic barotrauma, foreign body, impacted cerumen, referred pain (dental or TMJ)

EDEMA

CHF, constrictive pericarditis, liver disease (cirrhosis), nephrotic syndrome, nephritic syndrome, hypoalbuminemia, malnutrition, myxedema, hemiplegia, volume overload, thrombophlebitis, lymphatic obstruction, medications (nifedipine), venous stasis

EPISTAXIS

Trauma (nose picking, blunt trauma), neoplasm, polyps, foreign body, desiccation, coagulopathy, medications (use of cocaine, nasal sprays), infections (sinusitis), uremia, hypertension (more often a result rather than a cause of epistaxis)

FAILURE TO THRIVE

Environmental: Social deprivation, decreased food intake

Organic: CNS disorder, intestinal malabsorption, CF, parasites, cleft palate, heart failure, endocrine diseases, hypercalcemia, Turner's syndrome, renal disease, chronic infection, malignancies

FEVER

Based on adult population studies, an AM temperature above 98.8°F (37.2°C) or PM above 99.9°F (37.7°C) is generally defined as a fever. Rectal temperatures are generally 1°F (0.6°C) higher and reflect core temperature, whereas axillary temperatures are about 1°F (0.6°C) lower than oral temperatures. Infections (viral, bacterial, mycobacterial, fungal, parasitic), neoplasm (lymphoma, leukemia, renal and hepatic carcinoma), connective tissue disease (SLE, vasculitis, RA, adult Still's disease, temporal arteritis), heat stroke, malignant hyperthermia, thyroid storm, adrenal insufficiency, PE, MI, atrial myxoma, inflammatory bowel disease, factitious, drugs (most commonly: amphotericin, bleomycin, barbiturates, cephalosporins, methyldopa, penicillins, phenytoin, procainamide, sulfonamides, quinidine, cocaine, LSD, phencyclidine and amphetamines)

FEVER OF UNKNOWN ORIGIN (FUO)

Defined as a temperature of 101°F (38.3°C) or greater for at least 3 wk and for which a diagnosis is not established after 1 wk of hospitalization. In children, the minimum duration is 2 wk and the temperature is at least 101.3°F (38.5°C): TB, fungal infection, endocarditis, abscess (especially hepatic), neoplasm (lymphoma, renal cell, hepatoma, preleukemia), atrial myxoma, connective tissue disease, drugs (see Fever, previous listing), PE, Crohn's disease, ulcerative colitis, hypothalamic injury, factitious; in elderly consider temporal arteritis

FLATULENCE

Aerophagia, food intolerance, disturbances in bowel motility (diabetes, uremia), lactose intolerance, gallbladder disease

FREQUENCY

Infection (bladder, prostate), excessive fluid intake, use of diuretics (also coffee, tea, or colas), diabetes mellitus, diabetes insipidus, prostatic obstruction, bladder stones, bladder tumors, pregnancy, psychogenic bladder syndrome, neurogenic bladder, interstitial cystitis

GALACTORRHEA

Hyperprolactinemia, prolonged breast feeding, major stress, pituitary tumors, breast lesions (benign, cancer, inflammatory), idiopathic with menses and after oral contraceptive use

GYNECOMASTIA

Normal (Physiologic):   Newborn, adolescence, aging

Pathologic: Medications or drug use (cimetidine, spironolactone, estrogens, gonadotropins, antiandrogens [bicalutamide, others], marijuana), decreased testosterone (Klinefelter's syndrome, testicular failure or absence), increased estrogen production (hermaphroditism, testicular or lung cancers, adrenal and liver diseases)

HEADACHE

General Classification

Cluster: Severe, sharp, stabbing, usually unilateral "clustered" over 1–4 mon

Tension: Steady, nonpulsatile "band-like distribution" around head, stress-related, increases as day progresses

Migraine: Precipitated by some factor (ie, menses, foods), and preceded by aura; photophobia, N/V, neurologic complaints, unilateral deep, throbbing severe parietal–temporal pain

Other Types: Benign exertional, benign cough headache, vascular (menstruation, hypertension), eye strain, acute glaucoma, sinusitis, dental problems, TMJ dysfunction, trauma, subarachnoid hemorrhage, intracranial mass, fever, meningitis, pseudo-tumor cerebri, trigeminal neuralgia, temporal arteritis (especially in elderly), hypoglycemia, toxin exposure (carbon monoxide poisoning), drugs (vasodilators—nifedipine [Procardia]), vasculitis

HEARTBURN (PYROSIS)

GERD, esophagitis, hiatal hernia, peptic ulcer, gallbladder disease, medications (eg, alendronate), tumors, scleroderma, food intolerance. Myocardial ischemia may be mistaken for heartburn.

HEMATEMESIS, MELENEMESIS, AND MELENA

Melena: "Black tarry stools" caused by stomach acid or intestinal bacterial conversion of hemoglobin to the black pigment hematin; suggests blood loss of > 50–100 mL.

Hematemesis: Vomiting blood.

Melenemesis: Vomiting "coffee ground" material. *Note:* These conditions suggest bleeding site in upper GI tract (ie, proximal to ligament of Treitz) but can be as distal as the right colon. Swallowed blood (eg, epistaxis), esophageal varices, esophagitis, Mallory–Weiss syndrome, hiatal hernia, gastritis, duodenal or gastric ulcer, duodenitis, carcinoma of the stomach, tumors (small and large bowel), ischemic colitis, aortoenteric fistula, bleeding diathesis, anticoagulation (may unmask GI tract pathology), medications (false appearance of dark stools, eg, bismuth-containing mediations and iron supplements)

HEMATOCHEZIA

Grossly bloody stool. Massive upper GI bleeding (rapid GI transit), hemorrhoids, anal fissure, diverticular disease, angiodysplasia, polyps, carcinoma, inflammatory bowel disease, ischemic colitis

HEMATURIA (SEE ALSO PAGE 107)

First, rule out false-positives: myoglobinuria, hemoglobinuria, porphyria. GU neoplasms (malignant and benign), polycystic kidneys, trauma, infection (urethral, bladder, prostate, etc), stones, glomerulonephritis, renal infarction, renal vein thrombosis, anticoagulation (may unmask GU tract pathology), bleeding diathesis, enterovesical fistula, sickle cell anemia, vigorous exercise ("runners' hematuria"), accelerated hypertension, factitious, and vaginal and rectal bleeding

HEMOPTYSIS

Infection (pneumonia, bronchitis, fungal, TB), bronchiectasis, cancer (usually bronchogenic), PE, arteriovenous malformations, Wegener's granulomatosus, Goodpasture's syndrome, SLE, pulmonary hemosiderosis, foreign body, trauma, bleeding diatheses, excessive anticoagulation (may unmask respiratory tract pathology), pulmonary edema, mitral stenosis

HEPATOMEGALY

CHF, hepatitis (viral, alcoholic, drug-induced, autoimmune), cirrhosis (alcoholic, etc), tumors (primary and metastatic), amyloid, biliary obstruction, hemochromatosis, chronic granulomatous disease, infections (schistosomiasis, liver abscess). Riedel's lobe is a normal variant, elongated right lobe of the liver with normal total liver volume.

HICCUPS (SINGULTUS)

Uremia, electrolyte disorders, diabetes, medications (benzodiazepines, barbiturates, others), emotionally induced (excitement, fright), gastric distention, CNS disorders, psychogenic, thoracic and diaphragmatic disorders (pneumonia, MI, diaphragmatic irritation), alcohol ingestion

HIRSUTISM

Idiopathic, familial, adrenal causes (Cushing's disease, congenital adrenal hyperplasia, virilizing adenoma or carcinoma), polycystic ovaries, medications (minoxidil, androgens)

IMPOTENCE (ERECTILE DYSFUNCTION)

Psychogenic, vascular, neurologic (cord injury, radical prostatectomy, rectal surgery, aortic bypass), pelvic radiation, medications (common drugs: antihypertensives especially thiazide diuretics, beta-blockers and methyldopa; antidepressants especially the SSRIs, anticholinergics; addictive medications: alcohol, narcotics; antipsychotics; antiandrogens: histamine H_2 blockers, finasteride, LHRH analogues, spironolactone, others); history of priapism, Peyronie's disease, testicular failure, hyperprolactinemia

INCONTINENCE (URINARY)

Cystitis, dementia and delirium, stroke, prostatic hypertrophy, fecal impaction, peripheral or autonomic neuropathy, medications (diuretics, sedatives, alpha-blockers), diabetes, spinal cord trauma or lesions, MS, childbirth, surgery (prostate, rectal), aging, acute and chronic medical conditions, estrogen deficiency

JAUNDICE

Hepatitis (alcoholic, viral, drug-induced, autoimmune), Gilbert's disease, Crigler–Najjar syndrome, Dubin–Johnson syndrome, Wilson's disease, drug-induced cholestasis (phenothiazines and estrogen), gallbladder and biliary tract disease (including inflammation, infection, obstruction, and tumors—primary hepatic and metastatic), hemolysis, neonatal jaundice, cholestatic jaundice of pregnancy, TPN

LYMPHADENOPATHY AND SPLENOMEGALY

Infection (bacterial, fungal, viral, parasitic), benign neoplasm (histiocytosis), malignant neoplasm (primary lymphoma, metastatic), sarcoid, connective tissue disease, drugs (phenytoin, etc), HIV and AIDS, splenomegaly without lymphadenopathy (cirrhosis, hereditary spherocytosis, hemoglobinopathies, hairy cell leukemia, histiocytosis X, and amyloidosis)

MELENA

(See Hematemesis, page 40.)

NAUSEA AND VOMITING

Appendicitis, acute cholecystitis, chronic gallbladder disease, PUD, gastritis (especially alcoholic), pancreatitis, gastric distention (diabetic atony, pyloric obstruction), intestinal obstruction, peritonitis, food intolerance, intestinal infection (bacterial, viral, parasitic), acute systemic infections (especially in children), hepatitis, toxins (food poisoning), CNS disorders ([increased intracranial pressure often cause vomiting without nausea], tumor, hemorrhagic stroke, hydrocephalus, meningitis, labyrinthitis, Ménière's disease, migraine headaches) AMI, CHF, endocrine disorders (DKA, adrenal crisis), hypercalcemia, hyperkalemia, hypokalemia, pyelonephritis, nephrolithiasis, uremia, hepatic failure, pregnancy, PID, drugs (opiates, digitalis, chemotherapeutic agents, L-dopa, NSAIDs), psychogenic vomiting, porphyria, radiation therapy

NYSTAGMUS

Congenital, vision loss early in life, MS, neoplasms, infarction, toxic or metabolic encephalopathy, alcohol intoxication, thiamine (B_1) deficiency, cerebellar degeneration, medications (anticonvulsants, barbiturates, phenothiazines, lithium, others), encephalitis, vascular brainstem lesions, Arnold–Chiari malformation, nonpathologic (extreme lateral gaze), opticokinetic nystagmus (attempt to fix gaze on rapidly moving object, eg, train)

OLIGURIA AND ANURIA

(See also Urinary Indices, page 115.)
    Oliguria is < 500 mL urine/24 h; **anuria** is < 100 mL urine/24 h in adults.

Prerenal: Volume depletion, shock, heart failure, fluids in the third space, renal artery compromise

Renal: Glomerular disease, acute tubular necrosis, bilateral cortical necrosis, interstitial disease (acute and chronic interstitial nephritis, urate or hypercalcemic nephropathy), transfusion reaction, myoglobulinuria, radiographic contrast media (especially in diabetics, dehydration, multiple myeloma and elderly), ESRD, drugs (aminoglycosides, amphotericin B, vancomycin, NSAIDs, cephalosporins, penicillins, and sulfonamides), emboli, thrombosis, TTP, HUS, and DIC

Postrenal: Bilateral ureteral obstruction, prostatic obstruction, neurogenic bladder

PLEURAL EFFUSION

(See Chapter 13, page 310, Thoracentesis, for more details.)

Transudate: (Pleural to serum protein ratio < 0.5, and pleural to serum LDH ratio < 0.6 and pleural LDH < ⅔ the upper limits of normal for serum LDH), CHF, cirrhosis, nephrotic syndrome, peritoneal dialysis

Exudate: (Pleural to serum protein ratio > 0.5, or pleural to serum LDH ratio > 0.6, or pleural LDH > ⅔ the upper limits of normal for serum LDH), bacterial or viral pneumonia, pulmonary infarction, TB, RA, SLE, malignancy (most common, breast, lung lymphoma, leukemia, ovarian, unknown primary, GI, mesothelioma, others), pancreatitis, pneumothorax, chest trauma, uremia

Chylothorax: Traumatic or postoperative complication

Empyema: Bacteria, fungi, TB, trauma, surgery

Hydrothorax: Usually iatrogenic (central venous catheter complication)

PRURITUS

Skin lesions (papulosquamous, vesicobullous, contact dermatitis, urticaria, infestations [scabies, etc], infections), xerosis [dry skin] (especially in winter), liver disease, uremia, diabetes, gout, iron deficiency anemia, Hodgkin's disease, leukemias, polycythemia vera, systemic mastocytosis, intestinal parasites, drug reactions with or without a rash (without a rash consider allopurinol, birth control pills, captopril, cephalosporins, cimetidine, clonidine, diuretics, HMG-CoA reductase inhibitors, narcotics, penicillin, phenothiazines and phenytoin), pregnancy, psychosomatic, neurologic, or circulatory disturbances

SEIZURES

Generalized: Grand mal and petit mal (absence), febrile

Partial Seizures: Partial motor, partial sensory, partial complex (psychomotor or temporal lobe, déjà vu, automatisms)

Causes: Primary, CNS tumors (primary, metastatic), trauma, metabolic (hypoglycemia, hyponatremia, hypernatremia, acidosis, alkalosis, porphyria, uremia, etc), fever (especially in children), infection (meningitis, encephalitis, and abscess), anoxia (arrhythmias, stroke, carbon monoxide poisoning), drugs (alcohol or barbiturate withdrawal, cocaine, amphetamines), collagen-vascular disease (SLE), chronic renal failure, trauma, hypertensive encephalopathy, toxemia of pregnancy, psychogenic

SPLENOMEGALY

(See Lymphadenopathy and Splenomegaly, page 41.)

SYNCOPE

Includes vasovagal (simple faint), orthostatic (volume depletion, sympathectomy [either functional or surgical], diabetes, Shy–Drager [idiopathic], TCAs and diuretics) and hysterical. Cardiac syncope including PAT, AF, VT, sinoatrial or atrioventricular block, pacemaker malfunction, aortic stenosis, IHSS, primary pulmonary hypertension, atrial myxoma, cough syncope, micturition, hypoglycemia, seizure disorder, subclavian steal syndrome, cerebrovascular accident, AMI, alcohol-related

TREMORS

Resting (Decrease with Movement): Parkinson's disease, Wilson's disease, brain tumors (rare), medications (SSRI antidepressants, metoclopramide, phenothiazines [tardive dyskinesia])

Action (Present with Movement): Benign essential tremor (familial and senile), cerebellar diseases, withdrawal syndromes (alcohol, benzodiazepines, opiates), normal/physiologic (induced by anxiety, fatigue)

Ataxic (Worse at End of Voluntary Movement): MS, cerebellar diseases

Others: Medication-induced (caffeine [coffee, tea], steroids, valproic acid, bronchodilators) febrile, hypoglycemic, hyperthyroidism, pheochromocytoma

VAGINAL BLEEDING

Normal menstrual period, dysfunctional uterine bleeding (premenopausal bleeding, oral contraceptives, luteal phase defect), anovulatory abnormal uterine bleeding (hypothalamic/pituitary disorders, stress, thyroid and adrenal disease, endometriosis), pregnancy-related (ectopic pregnancy, threatened/spontaneous abortion, retained products of gestation), neoplasia (uterine fibroids; cervical polyps; and endometrial, cervical, ovarian, and vulvar carcinoma)

VAGINAL DISCHARGE

Vaginitis due to *Candida albicans, Trichomonas vaginalis, Gardnerella vaginalis, Neisseria gonorrhoeae, Chlamydia trachomatis, Ureaplasma urealyticum, Mycoplasma genitalium,* herpesvirus, chronic cervicitis, tumors, irritants, foreign bodies, estrogen deficiency

VERTIGO

Ménière's disease (recurrent vertigo, deafness and tinnitus), labyrinthitis, aminoglycoside toxicity, benign positional vertigo, vestibular neuronitis, brainstem ischemia and infarction, basilar artery migraine, cerebellar infarction, acoustic neuroma, motion sickness, excess of ethanol, quinine, and salicylic acid

VOMITING

(See Nausea and Vomiting page 41)

WEIGHT LOSS

Normal or Increased Appetite: Diabetes, hyperthyroidism, anxiety, drugs (thyroid), carcinoid, malabsorption (sprue, pancreatic deficiency), parasites

Decreased Appetite: Depression, anorexia nervosa, GI obstruction, neoplasm, liver disease, severe infection, severe cardiopulmonary disease including end-stage COPD, uremia, adrenal insufficiency, hypercalcemia, hypokalemia, intoxication (alcohol, lead), old age, drugs (amphetamines, digitalis, SSRIs, such as fluoxetine [Prozac]), HIV and AIDS

WHEEZING

Large airway difficulty (laryngeal stridor, tracheal stenosis, foreign body), endobronchial tumor, asthma, bronchitis, emphysema, pulmonary edema, PE, anaphylactic reactions, myocardial ischemia

LABORATORY DIAGNOSIS: CHEMISTRY, IMMUNOLOGY, AND SEROLOGY

Acetoacetate
Acid Phosphatase
ACTH
ACTH Stimulation Test
Albumin
Albumin/Globulin Ratio
Aldosterone
Alkaline Phosphatase
Alpha-fetoprotein (AFP)
ALT
Ammonia
Amylase
ASO Titer
AST
Autoantibodies
Base Excess/Deficit
Bicarbonate
Bilirubin
Blood Urea Nitrogen (BUN)
BUN/Creatinine Ratio
C-Peptide
C-Reactive Protein
CA 15-3
CA 19-9
CA-125
Calcitonin
Calcium, Serum
Captopril Test
Carbon Dioxide
Carboxyhemoglobin
Carcinoembryonic Antigen (CEA)
Catecholamines, Fractionated Serum
Chloride, Serum
Cholesterol
Clostridium difficile Toxin Assay, Fecal
Cold Agglutinins
Complement (C3, C4, CH$_{50}$)
Cortisol, Serum
Counterimmunoelectrophoresis
Creatine Phosphokinase
Creatinine, Serum
Cryoglobulins, Serum
Cytomegalovirus Antibodies
D-Dimer
Dehydroepiandrosterone
Dehydroepiandrosterone Sulfate
Dexamethasone Suppression Test
Erythropoietin
Estradiol, Serum

Estrogen/Progesterone Receptors
Ethanol
Fecal Fat
Ferritin
First Trimester Screening
Folic Acid
Follicle-Stimulating Hormone (FSH)
FTA-ABS
Fungal Serologies
Gastrin, Serum
GGT
Glucola
Glucose
Glucose Tolerance Test, Oral
Glycohemoglobin
Haptoglobin
Helicobacter pylori Antibody Titers
Hepatitis Testing
High-Density Lipoprotein Cholesterol
HLA
Homocysteine, Serum
Human Chorionic Gonadotropin
 (HCG)
Human Immunodeficiency Antibody
 Testing (HIV)
Immunoglobulins, Quantitative
Iron
Iron-Binding Capacity, Total
Lactate Dehydrogenase (LDH)
Lactic Acid
LAP Score
LE Preparation
Lead, Blood
Legionella Antibody
Lipase
Lipid Profile
Low-Density Lipoprotein—Cholesterol
Luteinizing Hormone
Lyme Disease Serology
Magnesium
MHA-TP
β_2-Microglobulin
Monospot
Myoglobin
B-Type Natriuretic Peptide
Newborn Screening Panel
5'-Nucleotidase
Oligoclonal Banding, CSF
Osmolality, Serum

(continued)

Oxygen
P-24 Antigen (HIV Antigen)
Parathyroid Hormone
Phosphorus
Potassium, Serum
Prealbumin
Progesterone, Serum
Prolactin
Prostate-Specific Antigen (PSA)
Protein Electrophoresis, Serum and
    Urine
Protein, Serum
Renin
    Plasma
    Renal Vein
Retinol-Binding Protein
Rheumatoid Factor
Rocky Mountain Spotted Fever
    Antibodies
Semen Analysis
SGGT
SGOT

SGPT
Sodium, Serum
Stool for Occult Blood
Sweat Chloride
T_3 RU
N-Telopeptide (NTx) (Urine and Serum)
Testosterone
Thyroglobulin
Thyroid-Stimulating Hormone
Thyroxine
Thyroxine-Binding Globulin
Thyroxine Index, Free
TORCH Battery
Transferrin
Triglycerides
Triiodothyronine
Triple Screen
Troponin, Cardiac-Specific
Uric Acid
VDRL Test
Vitamin B_{12}
Zinc

This chapter outlines commonly ordered blood chemistry, immunology, and serology tests with normal values and a guide to the diagnosis of common abnormalities. Other laboratory tests can be found in the following chapters: Hematology, Chapter 5; Urine Studies, Chapter 6; Microbiology, Chapter 7; and Blood Gases, Chapter 8. If an increased or decreased value is not clinically useful, it is usually not listed. Because each laboratory has its own set of normal reference values, the normals given should only be used as a guide. The range for common normal values is given in parentheses. Unless specified, values reflect normal adult levels. This section includes the method of collection since laboratories have attempted to standardize collection methods; however, be aware that some labs may have alternative collection methods. Blood specimen tubes are listed in Chapter 13, page 316.

The Système International (SI) is a metric-based laboratory data-reporting system that is now used internationally. The mole is the unit used most extensively in the system. Most countries have adopted units per liter (U/L) as an measure of enzymatic activity. For most lab values, representative SI units have been included; however, each individual laboratory should be consulted for its "normal" values.

Most laboratories offer AMA recommended "panel" tests, whereby multiple determinations are performed on a single sample. Although your lab may vary, some common chemistry panels include:

- **AMA Electrolyte Panel:** Sodium, potassium, chloride, CO_2, (carbon dioxide)
- **AMA Basic Metabolic Panel:** Calcium, CO_2(carbon dioxide), chloride, creatinine, glucose, potassium, sodium, BUN
- **AMA Comprehensive Metabolic Panel:** (ALT) SGPT, albumin, total bilirubin, calcium, chloride, creatinine, glucose, alkaline, phosphatase, potassium, total protein, sodium, (AST) SGOT, urea nitrogen (BUN), CO_2 (carbon dioxide)

- **AMA Renal Function Panel:** Albumin, calcium, CO_2 (carbon dioxide), chloride, creatinine, glucose, phosphorus serum, potassium, sodium, urea nitrogen (BUN)
- **AMA Hepatic Function Panel:** Total protein, albumin, total bilirubin, direct bilirubin, alkaline phosphate, SGOT (AST), SGPT (ALT)
- **AMA Lipid Panel:** Cholesterol, HDL, LDL (*calculated from cholesterol and HC*), triglycerides

Other Common Panel Tests

Chem-7 Panel/SMA-7: BUN, creatinine, electrolytes (Na, K, Cl, CO_2), glucose
Health Screen-12/SMA-12: Albumin, alkaline phosphatase, AST (SGOT), bilirubin (total), calcium, cholesterol, creatinine, glucose, LDH, phosphate, protein (total), uric acid
Cardiac Enzymes: CK-MB (if total CK > 150 IU/L), troponin

ACETOACETATE (KETONE BODIES, ACETONE)

- Normal = negative • Collection: Red top tube

Positive: DKA, starvation, emesis, stress, alcoholism, infantile organic acidemias, isopropyl alcohol ingestion

ACID PHOSPHATASE (PROSTATIC ACID PHOSPHATASE, PAP)

- < 3.0 ng/mL by RIA, or < 0.8 IU/L by enzymatic • Collection: Tiger top tube
    Not a useful screening test for cancer; most useful as a marker of response to therapy or in confirming metastatic disease. PSA is more sensitive in diagnosis of cancer.

Increased: Carcinoma of the prostate (usually outside of prostate), prostatic surgery or trauma (including prostatic massage), rarely in infiltrative bone disease (Gaucher's disease, myeloid leukemia), prostatitis, or BPH

ACTH (ADRENOCORTICOTROPIC HORMONE)

- 8 AM 20–140 pg/mL (SI: 20–140 ng/L), midnight, approximately 50% of AM value • Collection: Tiger top tube

Increased: Addison's disease (primary adrenal hypofunction), ectopic ACTH production (small [oat]- cell lung carcinoma, pancreatic islet cell tumors, thymic tumors, renal cell carcinoma, bronchial carcinoid), Cushing's disease (pituitary adenoma), congenital adrenal hyperplasia (adrenogenital syndrome)

Decreased: Adrenal adenoma or carcinoma, nodular adrenal hyperplasia, pituitary insufficiency, corticosteroid use

ACTH STIMULATION TEST (CORTROSYN STIMULATION TEST)

- Collection: Tiger top tube
    Used to diagnose adrenal insufficiency. Cortrosyn (an ACTH analogue) is given at a dose of 0.25 mg IM or IV in adults or 0.125 mg in children < 2 y. Collect blood at time 0, 30, and 60 min for cortisol and aldosterone.

Normal Response: Three criteria are required: basal cortisol of at least 5 mg/dL, an incremental increase after cosyntropin (Cortrosyn) injection of at least 7 mg/dL, and a final serum cortisol of at least 16 mg/dL at 30 or 18 mg/dL at 60 min or cortisol increase of > 10 mg/dL. Aldosterone increases > 5 ng/dL over baseline.

Addison's Disease (Primary Adrenal Insufficiency):   Neither cortisol nor al-dosterone increase over baseline.

Secondary Adrenal Insufficiency: Caused by pituitary insufficiency or sup-pression by exogenous steroids, cortisol does not increase, but aldosterone does.

ALBUMIN

• Adult 3.5–5.0 g/dL (SI: 35–50 g/L), child 3.8–5.4 g/dL (SI: 38–54 g/L)
• Collection: Tiger top tube; part of SMA-12

Decreased: Malnutrition (see page 204), overhydration, nephrotic syndrome, CF, multiple myeloma, Hodgkin's disease, leukemia, metastatic cancer, protein-losing enteropathies, chronic glomerulonephritis, alcoholic cirrhosis, inflamma-tory bowel disease, collagen-vascular diseases, hyperthyroidism

ALBUMIN/GLOBULIN RATIO (A/G RATIO)

• Normal > 1
   A calculated value (Total protein minus albumin = globulins. Albumin di-vided by globulins = A/G ratio). Serum protein electrophoresis is a more inform-ative test (see page 80–82).

Decreased: Cirrhosis, liver diseases, nephrotic syndrome, chronic glomeru-lonephritis, cachexia, burns, chronic infections and inflammatory states, myeloma

ALDOSTERONE

• Serum: Supine 3–10 ng/dL (SI: 0.083–0.28 nmol/L) early AM, normal sodium intake [3 g sodium/d] • Upright 5–30 ng/dL (SI: 0.138–0.83 nmol/L); urinary 2–16 mg/24 h (SI: 5.4–44.3 nmol/d) • Collection: Green or lavender top tube
   Discontinue antihypertensives and diuretics 2 wk prior to test. Upright sam-ples should be drawn after 2 h. Primarily used to screen hypertensive patients for possible Conn's syndrome (adrenal adenoma producing excess aldosterone).

Increased: Primary hyperaldosteronism, secondary hyperaldosteronism (CHF, sodium depletion, nephrotic syndrome, cirrhosis with ascites, others), upright posture

Decreased: Adrenal insufficiency, panhypopituitarism, supine posture

ALKALINE PHOSPHATASE

• Adult 20–70 U/L, child 20–150 U/L • Collection: Tiger top tube; part of SMA-12
   A fractionated alkaline phosphatase was formerly used to differentiate the origin of the enzyme in the bone from that in the liver. Replaced by the GGT and 5′-nucleotidase determinations

Increased: (Highest levels in biliary obstruction and infiltrative liver disease) Increased calcium deposition in bone (hyperparathyroidism), Paget's disease, osteoblastic bone tumors (metastatic or osteogenic sarcoma), osteomalacia, rickets, PRG, childhood, healing fracture, liver disease, eg, biliary obstruction (masses, drug therapy), hyperthyroidism

Decreased: Malnutrition, excess vitamin D ingestion, pernicious anemia, Wilson's disease, hypothyroidism, zinc deficiency

ALPHA-FETOPROTEIN (AFP)

* (< 16 ng/mL (SI: < 16 mL) • Third trimester of PRG maximum 550 ng/mL (SI: 550 mL) • Collection: Tiger top tube

Increased: Hepatoma (hepatocellular carcinoma), testicular tumor (embryonal carcinoma, malignant teratoma), neural tube defects (in mother's serum [spina bifida, anencephaly, myelomeningocele]), fetal death, multiple gestations, ataxia–telangiectasia, some cases of benign hepatic diseases (alcoholic cirrhosis, hepatitis, necrosis)

Decreased: Trisomy 21 (Down syndrome) in maternal serum

ALT (ALANINE AMINOTRANSFERASE, ALAT) OR SGPT

* 0–35 U/L (SI: 0–0.58 mkat/L), higher in newborns • Collection: Tiger top tube

Increased: Liver disease, liver metastasis, biliary obstruction, pancreatitis, liver congestion (ALT is more elevated than AST in viral hepatitis; AST elevated more than ALT in alcoholic hepatitis.)

AMMONIA

* Adult 10–80 mg/dL (SI: 5–50 mmol/L) • To convert mg/dL to mmol/L, multiply by 0.5872 • Collection: Green top tube, on ice, analyze immediately

Increased: Liver failure, Reye's syndrome, inborn errors of metabolism, normal neonates (normalizes within 48 h of birth)

AMYLASE

* 50–150 Somogyi units/dL (SI: 100–300 U/L) • Collection: Tiger top tube

Increased: Acute pancreatitis, pancreatic duct obstruction (stones, stricture, tumor, sphincter spasm secondary to drugs), pancreatic pseudo-cyst or abscess, alcohol ingestion, mumps, parotiditis, renal disease, macroamylasemia, cholecystitis, peptic ulcers, intestinal obstruction, mesenteric thrombosis, after surgery

Decreased: Pancreatic destruction (pancreatitis, cystic fibrosis), liver damage (hepatitis, cirrhosis), normal newborns in the first year of life

ASO (ANTISTREPTOLYSIN O/ANTISTREPTOCOCCAL O) TITER (STREPTOZYME)

* < 200 IU/mL (Todd units) school-age children • < 100 IU/mL preschool and adults • Varies with lab • Collection: Tiger top tube

Increased: Streptococcal infections (pharyngitis, scarlet fever, rheumatic fever, poststreptococcal glomerulonephritis), RA, and other collagen diseases

AST (ASPARTATE AMINOTRANSFERASE, ASAT) OR SGOT

- 8–20 U/L (SI: 0–0.58 mkat/L) • Collection: Tiger top tube; part of SMA-12 Generally parallels changes in ALT in liver disease.

Increased: AMI, liver disease, Reye's syndrome, muscle trauma and injection, pancreatitis, intestinal injury or surgery, factitious increase (erythromycin, opiates), burns, cardiac catheterization, brain damage, renal infarction

Decreased: Beriberi (vitamin B_6 deficiency), severe diabetes with ketoacidosis, liver disease, chronic hemodialysis

AUTOANTIBODIES

- Normal = negative • Collection: Tiger top tube

Antinuclear Antibody (ANA, FANA)

A useful screening test in patients with symptoms suggesting collagen–vascular disease, especially if titer is > 1:160. 5% normal individuals can have positive test.

Positive: SLE, drug-induced lupus-like syndromes (procainamide, hydralazine, isoniazid, etc), scleroderma, MCTD, RA, polymyositis, juvenile RA (5–20%). Low titers are also seen in non-collagen–vascular disease.

Specific Immunofluorescent ANA Patterns
Homogenous. Nonspecific, from antibodies to DNP and native double-stranded DNA. Seen in SLE and a variety of other diseases. Antihistone is consistent with drug-induced lupus.
Speckled. Pattern seen in many connective tissue disorders. From antibodies to ENA, including anti-RNP, anti-Sm, anti-PM-1, and anti-SS. Anti-RNP is positive in MCTD and SLE. Anti-Sm is very sensitive for SLE. Anti-SS-A and anti-SS-B are seen in Sjögren's syndrome and subacute cutaneous lupus. The speckled pattern is also seen with scleroderma.
Peripheral Rim Pattern. From antibodies to native double-stranded DNA and DNP. Seen in SLE
Nucleolar Pattern. From antibodies to nucleolar RNA. Positive in Sjögren's syndrome and scleroderma

Anticentromere: Scleroderma, Raynaud's disease, CREST syndrome

Anti-DNA (Antidouble-stranded DNA):   SLE (but negative in drug-induced lupus), chronic active hepatitis, mononucleosis

Antimitochondrial: Primary biliary cirrhosis, autoimmune diseases, eg, SLE

Antineutrophil Cytoplasmic (ANCA):
c-ANCA: Wegener's granulomatosus (high titers ≥ 1:80, very predictive for Wegner's)
p-ANCA: Polyarteritis nodosa, and other vasculitides including Churg–Strauss and microscopic polyarteritis
Anti-SCL 70:   Scleroderma

Antismooth Muscle: Low titers are seen in a variety of illnesses; high titers (> 1:100) are suggestive of chronic active hepatitis.

Sjögren Syndrome Antibody (SS-A):   Sjögren syndrome, SLE, RA

Antimicrosomal: Hashimoto's thyroiditis

BASE EXCESS/DEFICIT

• –2 to +2 • See Chapter 8, page 160

BICARBONATE (OR "TOTAL CO$_2$")

• 23–29 mmol/L • See Carbon Dioxide, page 53

4

BILIRUBIN

• Total, 0.3–1.0 mg/dL (SI: 3.4–17.1 mmol/L) • Direct, < 0.2 mg/dL (SI: < 3.4 mmol/L) • Indirect, < 0.8 mg/dL (SI: < 3.4 mmol/L) • To convert mg/dL to mmol/L, multiply by 17.10 • Collection: Tiger top tube

Increased Total: Hepatic damage (hepatitis, toxins, cirrhosis), biliary obstruction (stone or tumor), hemolysis, fasting.

Increased Direct (Conjugated): *Note:* Determination of the direct bilirubin is usually unnecessary with total bilirubin levels < 1.2 mg/dL (SI: 21 mmol/L); biliary obstruction/cholestasis (gallstone, tumor, stricture), drug-induced cholestasis, Dubin–Johnson and Rotor's syndromes

Increased Indirect (Unconjugated): *Note:* This is calculated as total minus direct bilirubin. So-called hemolytic jaundice caused by any type of hemolytic anemia (transfusion reaction, sickle cell, etc), Gilbert's disease, physiologic jaundice of the newborn, Crigler–Najjar syndrome

Bilirubin, Neonatal("Baby Bilirubin")

• Normal levels dependent on prematurity and age in days • "Panic levels" usually > 15–20 mg/dL (SI: > 257–342 mmol/L in full-term infants) • Collection: Capillary tube

Increased: Erythroblastosis fetalis, physiologic jaundice (may be due to breast-feeding), resorption of hematoma or hemorrhage, obstructive jaundice, others

BLOOD UREA NITROGEN (BUN)

• Birth–1 y: 4–16 mg/dL (SI: 1.4–5.7 mmol/L) • 1–40 y 5–20 mg/dL (SI: 8–7.1 mmol/L) • Gradual slight increase with age • To convert mg/dL to mmol/L, multiply by 0.3570 • Collection: Tiger top tube
   Less useful measure of GFR than creatinine because BUN is also related to protein metabolism

Increased: Renal failure (including drug-induced from aminoglycosides, NSAIDs), prerenal azotemia (decreased renal perfusion secondary to CHF, shock, volume depletion), postrenal (obstruction), GI bleeding, stress, drugs (especially aminoglycosides)

Decreased: Starvation, liver failure (hepatitis, drugs), PRG, infancy, nephrotic syndrome, overhydration

BUN/CREATININE RATIO (BUN/CR)

• Mean 10, range 6–20;
Calculated based on serum levels

Increased: Prerenal azotemia (renal hypoperfusion can be due to decreased volume, CHF, cirrhosis/ascites, nephrosis), GI bleed (ratio often > 30), high-protein diet, sepsis/hypermetabolic state, ileal conduit, drugs (steroids, tetracycline)

Decreased: Malnutrition, PRG, low-protein diet, ketoacidosis, hemodialysis, SIADH, drugs

C-PEPTIDE, INSULIN ("CONNECTING PEPTIDE")

• Fasting, < 4.0 ng/mL (SI: < 4.0 mg/L) • Male > 60 y, 1.5–5.0 ng/mL (SI: 1.5–5.0 mg/L) • Female 1.4–5.5 ng/mL (SI: 1.4–5.5 mg/L) • Collection: Tiger top tube

Differentiates exogenous and endogenous insulin production/administration; liberated when proinsulin is split to insulin; levels suggest endogenous production of insulin

Decreased: Diabetes (decreased endogenous insulin), insulin administration (factitious or therapeutic), hypoglycemia

C-REACTIVE PROTEIN (CRP)

• Normal = none detected • Collection: Tiger top tube

A nonspecific screen for infectious and inflammatory diseases, correlates well with ESR. In the first 24 h, however, ESR may be normal and CRP elevated. Also, CRP will return to normal much quicker than the ESR in response to therapy.

Increased: Bacterial infections, inflammatory conditions (acute rheumatic fever, acute RA, MI, unstable angina, transplant rejection, embolus, inflammatory bowel disease), last half of PRG, oral contraceptives, some malignancies

CA 15-3

Used to detect breast cancer recurrence in asymptomatic patients and monitor therapy. Levels related to stage of disease

Increased: Progressive breast cancer, benign breast disease and liver disease

Decreased: Response to therapy (25% change considered significant)

CA 19-9

• < 37 U/mL (SI:< 37 kU/L) • Collection: Tiger top tube

Primarily used to determine resectability of pancreatic cancers (ie, > 1000U/mL 95% unresectable)

Increased: GI cancers, eg, pancreas, stomach, liver, colorectal, hepatobiliary, some cases of lung and prostate, pancreatitis

CA-125

• < 35 U/mL (SI: < 35 kU/L) • Collection: Tiger top tube

Not a useful screening test for ovarian cancer when used alone; best used in conjunction with ultrasound and physical examination. Rising levels after resection predictive for recurrence

Increased: Ovarian, endometrial, and colon cancer; endometriosis; inflammatory bowel disease; PID; PRG; breast lesions; and benign abdominal masses (teratomas)

CALCITONIN (THYROCALCITONIN)

- < 19 pg/mL (SI: < 19 ng/L) • Collection: Tiger top tube

Increased: Medullary carcinoma of the thyroid, C-cell hyperplasia (precursor of medullary carcinoma), small (oat) cell carcinoma of the lung, newborns, PRG, chronic renal insufficiency, Zollinger Ellison syndrome, pernicious anemia

CALCIUM, SERUM

- Infants<1 mon: 7–11.5 mg/dL (SI: 1.75–2.87 mmol/L) • 1 mon–1 y: 8.6–11.2 mg/dL (SI: 2.15–2.79 mmol/L) • < 1 y and adults: 8.2–10.2 mg/dL (SI: 2.05–2.54 mmol/L) • Ionized: 4.75–5.2 mg/dL (SI: 1.19–1.30 mmol/L) • To convert mg/dL to mmol/L, multiply by 0.2495 • Collection: Tiger top tube; ionized requires green or red tube

When interpreting a total calcium value, albumin must be known. If it is not within normal limits, a corrected calcium can be roughly calculated by the following formula. Values for ionized calcium need no special corrections.

Corrected total Ca = 0.8 (Normal albumin − Measured albumin) + Reported Ca

Increased: (*Note:* Levels > 12 mg/dL [2.99 mmol/L] may lead to coma and death.) Primary hyperparathyroidism, PTH-secreting tumors, vitamin D excess, metastatic bone tumors, osteoporosis, immobilization, milk–alkali syndrome, Paget's disease, idiopathic hypercalcemia of infants, infantile hypophosphatasia, thiazide diuretics, chronic renal failure, sarcoidosis, multiple myeloma

Decreased: (*Note:* Levels < 7 mg/dL [> 1.75 mmol/L] may lead to tetany and death.) Hypoparathyroidism (surgical, idiopathic), pseudo-hypoparathyroidism, insufficient vitamin D, calcium and phosphorus ingestion (PRG, osteomalacia, rickets), hypomagnesemia, renal tubular acidosis, hypoalbuminemia (cachexia, nephrotic syndrome, CF), chronic renal failure (phosphate retention), acute pancreatitis, factitious decrease because of low protein and albumin

CAPTOPRIL TEST

- See Aldosterone, page 48, and renin (plasma rennin activity, PRA), page 83, for normal values

Used to evaluate renovascular hypotension, captopril is an ACE inhibitor, blocks angiotensin II. Captopril is administered (25 mg IV at 8AM). Aldosterone decreases 2 h later from baseline in normals or essential HTN but does not suppress in patients with hyperaldosteronism. For renovascular HTN, the PRA increases > 12 ng/mL/h and an absolute increase of 10 ng/mL/h plus a 400% increase in PRA if pretest level < 3 ng/mL/h and > 150% over baseline if the pretest PRA was > 3 ng/mL/h. Test now also combined with nuclear renal scan to identify renal artery stenosis

CARBON DIOXIDE ("TOTAL CO$_2$" OR BICARBONATE)

- Adult 23–29 mmol/L, child 20–28 mmol/L • (See Chapter 8 for pco$_2$ values
- Collection: Tiger top tube, do not expose sample to air

Increased: Compensation for respiratory acidosis (emphysema) and metabolic alkalosis (severe vomiting, primary aldosteronism, volume contraction, Bartter's syndrome)

Decreased: Compensation for respiratory alkalosis, and metabolic acidosis (starvation, DKA, lactic acidosis, alcoholic ketoacidosis, toxins [methanol, ethylene glycol, paraldehyde], severe diarrhea, renal failure, drugs [salicylates, acetazolamide], dehydration, adrenal insufficiency)

CARBOXYHEMOGLOBIN (CARBON MONOXIDE)

• Nonsmoker < 2%; smoker < 9%; toxic > 15% • Collection: Gray or lavender top tube; confirm with lab

Increased: Smokers, smoke inhalation, automobile exhaust inhalation, normal newborns

CARCINOEMBRYONIC ANTIGEN (CEA)

• Nonsmoker < 3.0 ng/mL (SI: < 3.0 mcg/L) • Smoker < 5.0 ng/mL (SI: < 5.0 mcg/L) • Collection: Tiger top tube
   Not a screening test; useful for monitoring response to treatment and tumor recurrence of adenocarcinomas of the GI tract

Increased: Carcinoma (colon, pancreas, lung, stomach), smokers, nonneoplastic liver disease, Crohn's disease, and ulcerative colitis

CATECHOLAMINES, FRACTIONATED SERUM

• Collection: Green or lavender tube; check with lab
Values vary and depend on the lab and method of assay used. Normal levels shown here are based on a HPLC technique. Patient must be supine in a non-stimulating environment with IV access to obtain sample.

Catecholamine	Plasma (Supine) Levels
Norepinephrine	70–750 pg/mL (SI: 414–435 pmol/L)
Epinephrine	0–100 pg/mL (SI: 0–546 pmol/L)
Dopamine	< 30 pg/mL (SI: 196 pmol/L)

Increased: Pheochromocytoma, neural CREST tumors (neuroblastoma), with extraadrenal pheochromocytoma, norepinephrine may be markedly elevated compared with epinephrine.

CHLORIDE, SERUM

• 97–107 mEq/L (SI: 97–107 mmol/L) • Collection: Tiger top tube

Increased: Diarrhea, RTA, mineralocorticoid deficiency, hyperalimentation, medications (acetazolamide, ammonium chloride)

Decreased: Vomiting, DM with ketoacidosis, mineralocorticoid excess, renal disease with sodium loss

CHOLESTEROL

• Total • Normal, see Table 4–1; see also Lipid profile/Cholesterol screening, page 55, and Table 4–4, see page 75. • To convert mg/dL to mmol/L, multiply by 0.02586 • Collection: Tiger top tube

Table 4–1
National Cholesterol Education Program's New Clinical Guidelines for Cholesterol Testing and Management

STEP 1: Complete lipoprotein profile LDL, total, and HDL cholesterol (mg/dL) after 9- to 12-h fast.

LDL Cholesterol (Primary Target of Therapy)

<100	Optimal
100–129	Near optimal/above optimal
130–159	Borderline high
160–189	High
≥190	Very high

Total Cholesterol

<200	Desirable
200–239	Borderline high
≥240	High

HDL Cholesterol

<40	Low
≥60	High

STEP 2: Identify presence of clinical atherosclerotic disease that confers high risk for CHD events (CHD risk equivalent):

Clinical CHD or symptomatic CAD or peripheral arterial disease or AAA or diabetes.

STEP 3: Determine presence of major risk factors (other than LDL):

Cigarette smoking; HTN (BP ≥140/90 mm Hg or on BP medications); HDL <40 mg/dL (if ≥60 mg/dL remove one risk factor from count); Family history of premature CHD (CHD in male relative <55 y; CHD in female relative <65 y); Age (men ≥45 years; women ≥55 y)

STEP 4: If 2+ risk factors (other than LDL) are present without CHD or CHD risk equivalent, assess 10-y (short-term) CHD risk (see Framingham tables @ http://www. nhlbi.nih.gov/guidelines/cholesterol/risk_tbl.htm).

Three levels of 10-y risk: >20%
—CHD risk equivalent, 10–20% <10%

STEP 5: Establish LDL goal of therapy, determine need for TLC, determine level for drug consideration

(continued)

Table 4–1 (continued)

Risk Category	LDL Goal	LDL Level to Initiate TLC	LDL Level to Consider Drug Therapy
CHD or CHD risk equivalents (10-y risk >20%)	<100 mg/dL	≥100 mg/dL	≥130 mg/dL (100–129 mg/dL: drug optional)[a]
2+ Risk factors (10-y risk ≤20%)	<130 mg/dL	≥130 mg/dL	10-y risk 10–20%: ≥130 mg/dL
0–1 Risk factor[b]	<160 mg/dL	≥160 mg/dL	≥190 mg/dL (160–189 mg/dL: LDL-lowering drug optional)

[a]Some use LDL-lowering drugs in this category if an LDL cholesterol <100 mg/dL cannot be achieved by lifestyle changes. Others use drugs that modify triglycerides and HDL, eg, nicotinic acid or fibrate.
[b]Almost all people with 0–1 risk factor have a 10-y risk <10%, thus 10-y risk assessment in people with 0–1 risk factor is not necessary.

STEP 6: Initiate TLC if LDL is above goal.

TLC diet: Saturated fat <7% of calories, cholesterol <200 mg/d, increased viscous (soluble) fiber (10–25 g/d) and plant stanols/sterols (2 g/d), weight management and increased physical activity.

STEP 7: Consider adding drug therapy if LDL exceeds levels shown in Step 5 table: HMG-CoA reductase inhibitors (statins); bile acid sequestrants; nicotinic acid.

STEP 8: Identify metabolic syndrome and treat, if present, after 3 mon of TLC. Metabolic syndrome present if any 3 of the following present:

Risk Factor	Defining Level
Abdominal obesity	Waist circumference[a]
Men	>102 cm (>40 in.)
Women	>88 cm (>35 in.)
Triglycerides	≥150 mg/dL
HDL cholesterol	
Men	<40 mg/dL
Women	<50 mg/dL
BP	≥130/≥85 mm Hg
Fasting glucose	≥110 mg/dL

[a]Overweight and obesity are associated with insulin resistance and the metabolic syndrome.

(continued)

Table 4–1 (continued)

Treat the Metabolic Syndrome: treat underlying causes (overweight/obesity and physical inactivity); treat lipid and non-lipid risk factors if they persist despite these lifestyle therapies; treat HTN, aspirin for CHD prevention; treat elevated triglycerides and/or low HDL (as shown in Step 9)

4

STEP 9: Treat elevated triglycerides (≥150 mg/dL): Primary aim of therapy is to reach LDL goal; Intensify weight management, increase physical activity; If triglycerides ≥200 mg/dL after LDL goal is reached, set secondary goal for non HDL-cholesterol (total HDL) 30 mg/dL higher than LDL goal.

Classification of Serum Triglycerides (mg/dL)	
<150	Normal
150–199	Borderline high
200–499	High
≥500	Very high

Comparison of LDL Cholesterol and Non-HDL Cholesterol Goals for Three Risk Categories

Risk Category	LDL Goal (mg/dL)	Non-HDL Goal (mg/dL)
CHD and CHD risk equivalent (10-y risk for CHD >20%)	<100	<130
Multiple (2+) risk factors and 10-y risks 20%	<130	<160
0–1 Risk factor	<160	<190

- **If triglycerides 200–499 mg/dL after LDL goal is reached, consider adding drug if needed to reach non-HDL goal:** Intensify therapy with LDL-lowering drug, or, add nicotinic acid or fibrate to further lower VLDL.

- **If Triglycerides ≥500 mg/dL, first lower triglycerides to prevent pancreatitis:** Very low-fat diet (≤15% of calories from fat), weight management and physical activity, fibrate or nicotinic acid, when triglycerides <500 mg/dL, turn to LDL-lowering therapy.

- **Treatment of low HDL cholesterol (<40 mg/dL):** First reach LDL goal, then: weight management and increase physical activity; If triglycerides 200–499 mg/dL, achieve non-HDL goal. If triglycerides <200 mg/dL (isolated low HDL) in CHD or CHD equivalent, consider nicotinic acid or fibrate.

(continued)

Table 4–1 (continued)

LDL = low-density lipoprotein; HDL = high-density lipoprotein; CHD = coronary heart disease; CAD = carotid artery disease; AAA = abdominal aortic aneurysm; HTN = hypertension; BP = blood pressure; TLC = therapeutic lifestyle changes; HMG-CoA = hydroxymethylglutaryl coenzyme A

Based on the Third Report of the Expert Panel on Detection, Evaluation, and Treatment of High Blood Cholesterol in Adults (Adult Treatment Panel or ATP III), (http://www.nhlbi.nih.gov/guidelines/cholesterol/accessed March, 10, 2003) U.S. Department of Health and Human Services, National Institutes of Health, National Heart, Lung, and Blood Institute, Bethesda, MD.

Increased: Idiopathic hypercholesterolemia, biliary obstruction, nephrosis, hypothyroidism, pancreatic disease (diabetes), PRG, oral contraceptives, hyperlipoproteinemia (types IIb, III, V)

Decreased: Liver disease (hepatitis, etc), hyperthyroidism, malnutrition (cancer, starvation), chronic anemias, steroid therapy, lipoproteinemias, AMI

High-Density Lipoprotein Cholesterol (HDL, HDL-C)

• Fasting male 30–70 mg/dL (SI: 0.8–1.80 mmol/L) • Female 30–90 mg/dL (SI: 0.80–2.35)
   HDL-C: Best correlation with the development of CAD; decreased HDL-C in males leads to an increased risk. Levels < 40 mg/dL associated with increased risk of CAD. Levels > 60 mg/dL associated with a decreased risk of CAD.

Increased: Estrogen (menstruating females), regular exercise, small ethanol intake, medications (nicotinic acid, gemfibrozil, others)

Decreased: Males, smoking, uremia, obesity, diabetes, liver disease, Tangier disease

Low-Density Lipoprotein Cholesterol (LDL, LDL-C)

• 50–190 mg/dL (SI: 1.30–4.90 mmol/L)
   Elevated levels correlate with CAD risk

Increased: Excess dietary saturated fats, hyperlipoproteinemia, biliary cirrhosis, endocrine disease (diabetes, hypothyroidism)

Decreased: Malabsorption, severe liver disease, abetalipoproteinemia

CLOSTRIDIUM DIFFICILE TOXIN ASSAY, FECAL

• Normal= negative
Majority of patients with pseudo-membranous colitis have positive *C. difficile*. A positive is found as follows:> 90% of pseudo-membranous colitis; 30–40% antibiotic associated colitis, and 6–10% cases of antibiotic-associated diarrhea. False-positive in some normals and neonates

COLD AGGLUTININS

• < 1:32 • Collection: Lavender or blue top tube
Most frequently used to screen for atypical pneumonias.

Increased: Atypical pneumonia (mycoplasmal pneumonia), other viral infections (especially mononucleosis, measles, mumps), cirrhosis, parasitic infections, Waldenström's macroglobulinemia, lymphomas and leukemias, multiple myeloma

COMPLEMENT

- Collection: Tiger or lavender top tube

Complement describes a series of sequentially reacting serum proteins that participate in pathogenic processes and lead to inflammatory injury.

Complement C3

- 85–155 mg/dL, (SI: 800–1500 ng/L)

Decreased levels suggest activation of the classical or alternative pathway, or both.

Increased: RA (variable finding), rheumatic fever, various neoplasms (GI, prostate, others), acute viral hepatitic, MI, PRG, amyloidosis

Decreased: SLE, glomerulonephritis (poststreptococcal and membranoproliferative), sepsis, SBE, chronic active hepatitis, malnutrition, DIC, gram-negative sepsis

Complement C4

- 20–50 mg/dL (SI: 200–500 ng/L)

Increased: RA (variable finding), neoplasia (GI, lung, others)

Decreased: SLE, chronic active hepatitis, cirrhosis, glomerulonephritis, hereditary angioedema (test of choice)

Complement CH$_{50}$ (Total)

- 33–61 mg/mL (SI: 330–610 ng/L)

Tests for complement deficiency in the classical pathway.

Increased: Acute-phase reactants (tissue injury, infections, etc)

Decreased: Hereditary complement deficiencies

CORTISOL, SERUM

- 8 AM, 5.0–23.0 mg/dL (SI: 138–365 nmol/L) • 4 PM, 3.0–15.0 mg/dL (SI: 83–414 nmol/L) • Collection: Green or red top tube

Increased: Adrenal adenoma, adrenal carcinoma, Cushing's disease, nonpituitary ACTH-producing tumor, steroid therapy, oral contraceptives

Decreased: Primary adrenal insufficiency (Addison's disease), congenital adrenal hyperplasia, Waterhouse–Friderichsen syndrome, ACTH deficiency

COUNTERIMMUNOELECTROPHORESIS (CIEP, CEP)

- Normal = negative

An immunologic technique that allows for rapid identification of infecting organisms from fluids, including serum, urine, CSF, and other body fluids. Organisms identified include *Neisseria meningitidis, Streptococcus pneumoniae, Haemophilus influenzae,* and group B *Streptococcus.*

CREATINE PHOSPHOKINASE (KINASE) (CP, CPK)

- 25–145 mU/mL (SI: 25–145 U/L) • Collection: Tiger top tube
  Used in suspected MI or muscle diseases. Heart, skeletal muscle, and brain have high levels

Increased: Muscle damage (AMI, myocarditis, muscular dystrophy, muscle trauma [including injections], after surgery), brain infarction, defibrillation, cardiac catheterization and surgery, rhabdomyolysis, polymyositis, hypothyroidism

CPK Isoenzymes

MB: (Normal < 6%, heart origin) increased in AMI (begins in 2–12 h, peaks at 12–40 h, returns to normal in 24–72 h), pericarditis with myocarditis, rhabdomyolysis, crush injury, Duchenne's muscular dystrophy, polymyositis, malignant hyperthermia, and cardiac surgery

MM: (Normal 94–100%, skeletal muscle origin) increased in crush injury, malignant hyperthermia, seizures, IM injections

BB: (Normal 0%, brain origin) brain injury (CVA, trauma), metastatic neoplasms (prostate), malignant hyperthermia, colonic infarction

CREATININE, SERUM (SCr)

- Adult male < 1.2 mg/dL (SI: 106 mmol/L) • Adult female < 1.1 mg/dL (SI: 97 mmol/L) • Child 0.5–0.8 mg/dL (SI: 44–71 mmol/L) • To convert mg/dL to μmol/L, multiply by 88.40 • Collection: Tiger top tube
  A clinically useful estimate of GFR. As a rule of thumb, SCr doubles with each 50% reduction in the GFR. Creatine clearance is discussed in Chapter 6.

Increased: Renal failure (prerenal, renal, or postrenal obstruction or medication-induced [aminoglycosides, NSAIDs, others]), gigantism, acromegaly, ingestion of roasted meat, false-positive with DKA

Decreased: PRG, decreased muscle mass, severe liver disease

CRYOGLOBULINS (CRYOCRIT)

< 0.4% (or negative if qualitative) • Collection: Tiger top tube, process immediately
  These abnormal proteins precipitate out of serum at low temperatures. Cryocrit, a quantitative measure, is preferred over the qualitative method. Should be collected in tubes without anticoagulant and transported at body temperature. Positive samples can be analyzed for immunoglobulin class, and light-chain type on request.

Monoclonal: Multiple myeloma, Waldenström's macroglobulinemia, lymphoma, CLL

Mixed Polyclonal or Mixed Monoclonal: Infectious diseases (viral, bacterial, parasitic), eg, SBE or malaria; SLE; RA; essential cryoglobulinemia; lymphoproliferative diseases; sarcoidosis; chronic liver disease (cirrhosis)

CYTOMEGALOVIRUS (CMV) ANTIBODIES

• IgM < 1:8, IgG < 1:16 • Collection: Tiger top tube

Used in neonates (CMV is the most common intrauterine infection), post-transfusion CMV infection, and organ donors and recipients. Most of adults will have detectable titers.

Increased: Serial measurements 10–14 d apart with a 4 × increase in titers or a single IgM > 1:8 is suggestive for acute infection. Universally increased titers in AIDS. IgM most useful in neonatal infections

d-DIMER (SEE ALSO CHAPTER 5, PAGE 101)

• Negative • Collection: Blue top tube

D-Dimers are proteins released when the fibrinolytic system breaks down fibrin; used to evaluate suspected DVTs and PEs; levels return to normal if clot stabilized (ie, treated with heparin) and not undergoing any further fibrin deposition or plasmin activation

Increased: DVT, PE, MI, CVA, sickle cell crisis, cancer, renal failure, CHF, life-threatening infections

DEHYDROEPIANDROSTERONE (DHEA)

• Male 2.0–3.4 ng/mL (SI: 5.2–8.7 mmol/L) • Female, premenopausal 0.8–3.4 ng/mL (SI: 2.1–8.8 mmol/L) • Postmenopausal 0.1–0.6 ng/mL (SI: 0.3–1.6 mmol/L) • Collection: Tiger top tube

Increased: Anovulation, polycystic ovaries, adrenal hyperplasia, adrenal tumors

Decreased: Menopause

DEHYDROEPIANDROSTERONE SULFATE (DHEAS)

• Male 1.7–4.2 ng/mL (SI: 6–15 mmol/L) • Female 2.0–5.2 ng/mL (SI: 7–18 mmol/L) • Collection: Tiger top tube

Increased: Hyperprolactinemia, adrenal hyperplasia, adrenal tumor, polycystic ovaries, lipoid ovarian tumors

Decreased: Menopause

DEXAMETHASONE SUPPRESSION TEST

Used in the differential diagnosis of Cushing's syndrome (elevated cortisol)

Overnight Test: In the "rapid" version of this test, a patient takes 1 mg of dexamethasone PO at 11 PM and a fasting 8 AM plasma cortisol is obtained. Normally the cortisol level should be 5.0 mg/dL [138 nmol/L]. A value that is > 5 mg/dL [138 nmol/L] usually confirms the diagnosis of Cushing's syndrome; however, obesity, alcoholism, or depression may occasionally show the same result. In these patients, the best screening test is a 24-h urine for free cortisol.

Low-Dose Test: After collection of baseline serum cortisol and 24-h urine-free cortisol levels, dexamethasone 0.5 mg is administered PO q6h for eight doses. Serum and urine cortisol are repeated on the second day. Failure to suppress to a serum cortisol of < 5.0 mg/dL [138 nmol/L] and a urine-free cortisol of < 30 mcg/dL (82 nmol/L) confirms Cushing's syndrome.

High-Dose Test: After the low-dose test, dexamethasone, 2 mg PO q6h for eight doses will cause a fall in urinary-free cortisol to 50% of the baseline value in bilateral adrenal hyperplasia (Cushing's disease) but not in adrenal tumors or ectopic ACTH production.

ERYTHROPOIETIN (EPO)

- 5–36 mU/L (5–36 IU/L) • Collection: Tiger top tube
  EPO is a renal hormone that stimulates RBC production.

Increased: PRG, secondary polycythemia (high altitude, COPD, etc), tumors (renal cell carcinoma, cerebellar hemangioblastoma, hepatoma, others), PCKD, anemias with bone marrow unresponsiveness (aplastic anemia, iron deficiency, etc)

Decreased: Bilateral nephrectomy, anemia of chronic disease (ie, renal failure, nephrotic syndrome), primary polycythemia (**Note:** The determination of EPO levels before administration of recombinant EPO for renal failure is not usually necessary.)

ESTRADIOL, SERUM

- Collection: Tiger top tube
  Serial measurements useful in assessing fetal well-being, especially in high-risk PRG. Also useful in evaluation of amenorrhea and gynecomastia in males.

Female	**Normal Values**
Follicular phase	25–75 pg/mL
Midcycle peak	200–600 pg/mL
Luteal phase	100–300 pg/mL
Pregnancy	
1st trimester	1–5 ng/mL
2nd trimester	5–15 ng/mL
3rd trimester	10–40 ng/mL
Postmenopause	5–25 pg/mL
Oral contraceptives	<50 pg/mL
Male	
Prepubertal	2–8 pg/mL
Adult	10–60 pg/mL

ESTROGEN/PROGESTERONE RECEPTORS

These are typically determined on fresh surgical (breast cancer) specimens. The presence of the receptors is associated with a longer disease-free interval, survival from breast cancer, and increased likelihood of responding to endocrine therapy. Fifty to seventy-five percent of breast cancers are estrogen-receptor-positive.

ETHANOL (BLOOD ALCOHOL)

- 0 mg/dL (0 mmol/L) • Collection: Tiger top tube; do not use alcohol to clean venipuncture site, use povidone-iodine

  Physiologic changes can vary with degree of alcohol tolerance of an individual.

  - < 50 mg/dL [< 10.85 mmol/L]: Limited muscular incoordination
  - 50–100 [10.85–21.71]: Pronounced incoordination
  - 100–150 [21.71–32.57]: Mood and personality changes; legally intoxicated in most states
  - 150–400 [32.57–87]: Nausea, vomiting, marked ataxia, amnesia, dysarthria
  - ≥ 400: Coma, respiratory insufficiency and death

FECAL FAT

- 2–6 g/d on an 80–100 g/d fat diet • 72-h collection time • Sudan III stain, random < 60 droplets fat/hpf

Increased: CF, pancreatic insufficiency, Crohn's disease, chronic pancreatitis, sprue

FERRITIN

- Male 15–200 ng/mL (SI: 15–200 mg/L) • Female 12–150 ng/mL (SI: 12–150 mg/L) • Collection: Tiger top tube

Increased: Hemochromatosis, hemosiderosis, sideroblastic anemia

Decreased: Iron deficiency (earliest and most sensitive test before red cells show any morphologic change), severe liver disease

FIRST TRIMESTER SCREENING (MATERNAL SERUM BHCG, AND PAPP-A)

- Normal levels based on gestational age • Collection: Dry Paper

  Screens for fetal trisomy 21 and other common chromosome disorders. Mostly used in combination with ultrasonographic assessment of fetal nuchal translucency. Done at 11-14 wk.

FOLIC ACID (SERUM)

- > 2.0 ng/mL (SI: > 5 nmol/L) (See RBC Folic Acid)

RBC FOLIC ACID

- 125–600 ng/mL (283–1360 nmol/L) • Collection: Lavender top tube

  Serum folate can fluctuate with diet. RBC levels are more indicative of tissue stores. Vitamin B_{12} deficiency can result in the RBC unable to take up folate in spite of normal serum folate levels.

Increased: Folic acid administration

Decreased: Malnutrition/malabsorption (folic acid deficiency), massive cellular growth (cancer) or cell turnover, ongoing hemolysis, medications (trimethoprim, some anticonvulsants, oral contraceptives), vitamin B_{12} deficiency (low RBC levels), PRG

FOLLICLE-STIMULATING HORMONE (FSH)

• Males: < 22 IU/L • Females: nonmidcycle < 20 IU/L, midcycle surge < 40 IU/L Midcycle peak should be 2 × basal level • Postmenopausal 40–160 IU/L • Collection: Tiger top tube

Used in the workup of impotence, infertility in men, and amenorrhea in women

Increased: (Hypergonadotropic > 40 IU/L) postmenopausal, surgical castration, gonadal failure, gonadotropin-secreting pituitary adenoma

Decreased: (Hypogonadotropic < 5 IU/L) prepubertal, hypothalamic and pituitary dysfunction, PRG

FTA-ABS (FLUORESCENT TREPONEMAL ANTIBODY ABSORBED)

• Normal = nonreactive • Collection: Tiger top tube

FTA-ABS may be negative in early primary syphilis and remain positive in spite of adequate treatment.

Positive: Syphilis (test of choice to confirm diagnosis after a reactive VDRL test), other treponemal infections can cause false-positive (Lyme disease, leprosy, malaria)

FUNGAL SEROLOGIES

• Negative < 1:8 • Collection: Tiger top tube

This is a screening technique for complement-fixed fungal antibodies, which usually detects antibodies to *Histoplasma capsulatum, Blastomyces dermatitidis, Cryptococcus neoformans, Aspergillus* species, *Candida* species, and *Coccidioides immitis.*

GASTRIN, SERUM

• Fasting < 100 pg/mL (SI: 47.7 pmol/L) • Postprandial 95–140 pg/mL (SI: 45.3–66.7 pmol/L) • Collection: Tiger top tube, freeze immediately

Make sure patient is not on H_2 blockers or antacids.

Increased: Zollinger–Ellison syndrome, medications (antacids, H_2 blockers and PPIs) pyloric stenosis, pernicious anemia, atrophic gastritis, ulcerative colitis, renal insufficiency, and steroid and calcium administration

Decreased: Vagotomy and antrectomy

GGT (SERUM GAMMA-GLUTAMYL TRANSPEPTIDASE, SGGT)

• Male 9–50 U/L • Female 8–40 U/L • Collection: Tiger top tube

Generally parallels changes in serum alkaline phosphatase and 5′-nucleotidase in liver disease. Sensitive indicator of alcoholic liver disease

Increased: Liver disease (hepatitis, cirrhosis, obstructive jaundice), pancreatitis.

GLUCOLA (1-H GLUCOSE TOLERANCE TEST)

• Collection: Red top tube

Screening test for gestational diabetes. 50 mg of glucose given orally. A level > 135 mg/dL (or > 140) at 1 h is elevated and must be followed by a glucose tolerance test.

GLUCOSE

• Fasting, 70–105 mg/dL (SI: 3.89–5.83 nmol/L) • 2 h postprandial 140 mg/dL (SI: < 7.8 nmol/L) • To convert mg/dL to nmol/L, multiply by 0.05551 • Collection: Tiger top tube

American Diabetes Association Diagnostic Criterion for Diabetes: normal fasting < 110, impaired fasting 110–126, diabetes > 126 or any random level > 200 when associated with other symptoms. Confirm with repeat testing.

Increased: DM, Cushing's syndrome, acromegaly, increased epinephrine (injection, pheochromocytoma, stress, burns, etc), acute and chronic pancreatitis, ACTH administration, spurious increase caused by drawing blood from a site above an IV line containing dextrose, elderly patients, pancreatic glucagonoma, drugs (glucocorticoids, thiazide diuretics)

Decreased: Pancreatic disorders (islet cell tumors), extrapancreatic tumors (carcinoma of the adrenals, stomach), hepatic disease (hepatitis, cirrhosis, tumors), endocrine disorders (early diabetes, hypothyroidism, hypopituitarism), functional disorders (after gastrectomy), pediatric problems (prematurity, infant of a diabetic mother, ketotic hypoglycemia, enzyme diseases), exogenous insulin, oral hypoglycemic agents, malnutrition, sepsis

GLUCOSE TOLERANCE TEST (GTT), ORAL (OGTT)

A fasting plasma glucose level > 126 mg/dl (7.0 mmol/L) or a casual plasma glucose > 200 mg/dL (11.1 mmol/L) meets the threshold for the diagnosis of diabetes, if confirmed on a subsequent day, and precludes the need for any glucose challenge. GTT is usually unnecessary to diagnose asymptomatic DM; it may be useful in gestational diabetes. GTT is unreliable in the presence of severe infection, prolonged fasting, or after the injection of insulin. After an overnight fast, a fasting blood glucose is drawn, and the patient is given a 75-g oral glucose load (100 g for gestational diabetes screening, 1.75 mg/kg ideal body weight in children up to a dose of 75 g). Plasma glucose is then drawn at 30, 60, 120, and 180 min.

Interpretation of GTT

Adult-Onset Diabetes: Any fasting blood sugar > 126, or > 200 at both 120 min and one other time interval measured

Gestational Diabetes: Any degree or glucose intolerance with onset or first recognition during PRG. Diagnosis requires at least two abnormal plasma glucose values on a 3-h oral glucose tolerance test (100 g of glucose).Fasting: 95 mg/dL; 1 h: 180 mg/dL; 2 h: 155 mg/dL;3 h: 140 mg/dL

GLYCOHEMOGLOBIN (GHB, GLYCATED HEMOGLOBIN, GLYCOHEMOGLOBIN, HBA$_{1C}$, HBA$_1$ HEMOGLOBIN A$_{1C}$, GLYCOSYLATED HEMOGLOBIN)

• 4.6–6.4% or new standard: Nondiabetic < 6, near normal 6–7 • Excellent glucose control < 7 • Good control 7–8 • Fair control 8-9 • Poor control > 10 • Collection: Lavender top tube

The mean plasma glucose is equal to the (HbA$_{1c}$ × 35.6) – 77.3. Useful in long-term monitoring control of blood sugar in diabetics; reflects levels over preceding 3–4 mon. Glycated serum protein (GSP) under study and may reflect serum glucose over the preceding 1–2 weeks

Increased: DM (uncontrolled), lead intoxication

Decreased: Chronic renal failure, hemolytic anemia, PRG, chronic blood loss

HAPTOGLOBIN

- 40–180 mg/dL (SI: 0.4–1.8 g/L) • Collection: Tiger top tube

Increased: Obstructive liver disease, any cause of increased ESR (inflammation, collagen-vascular diseases)

Decreased: Any type of hemolysis (transfusion reaction, etc), liver disease, anemia, oral contraceptives, children and infants

HELICOBACTER PYLORI ANTIBODY TITERS

- IgG < 0.17 = negative

Most patients with gastritis and ulcer disease (gastric or duodenal) have chronic *H. pylori* infection that should be treated. Positive in 35–50% asymptomatic patients (increases with age). Use in dyspepsia controversial. Four diagnostic methods are available to test for *H. pylori*, the organism associated with gastritis and ulcers. These include noninvasive (serology and a ^{13}C breath test) and invasive (gastric mucosal biopsy and the *Campylobacter*-like organism test). The IgG subclass is found in all patient populations; occasionally only IgA antibodies can be detected. Serology most useful in newly diagnosed *H. pylori* infection or monitoring response to therapy. IgG levels decrease slowly after treatment and can remain elevated after clearing infection.

Positive: Active or recent *H. pylori* infection, some asymptomatic carriers

HEPATITIS TESTING

Recommended hepatitis panel tests based on clinical settings is shown in Table 4–2 page 67. Interpretation of testing patterns is shown in Table 4–3 page 68. Profile patterns of hepatitis A and B are shown in Figures 4–1 and 4–2 page 69, respectively.

- Hepatitis tests • Collection: Tiger top tube

Hepatitis A

Anti-HAV Ab: Total antibody to hepatitis A virus; confirms previous exposure to hepatitis A virus, elevated for life.

Anti-HAV IgM: IgM antibody to hepatitis A virus; indicative of recent infection with hepatitis A virus; declines typically 1–6 mon after symptoms

Hepatitis B

HBsAg: Hepatitis B surface antigen. Earliest marker of HBV infection. Indicates either chronic or acute infection with hepatitis B virus. Used by blood banks to screen donors; vaccination does not affect this test

Anti-HBc-Total: IgG and IgM antibody to hepatitis B core antigen; confirms either previous exposure to hepatitis B virus (HBV) or ongoing infection. Used by blood banks to screen donors

Anti-HBc IgM: IgM antibody to hepatitis B core antigen. Early and best indicator of acute infection with hepatitis B

TABLE 4-2
Hepatitis Panel Testing to Guide the Ordering
of Hepatitis Profiles for Given Clinical Settings

Clinical Setting	Test	Purpose
SCREENING TESTS		
Pregnancy	HBsAg[a]	All expectant mothers should be screened during third trimester
High-risk patients on admission (homosexuals, dialysis patients)	HBsAg	To screen for chronic or active infection
Percutaneous inoculation		
Donor	HBsAg Anti-HBc IgM Anti-Hep C	To test patient's blood (esp. dialysis and HIV patients) for infectivity with hepatitis B and C if a health care worker is exposed
Victim	HBsAg Anti-HBc Anti-Hep C	To test exposed health care worker for immunity or chronic infection
Pre-HBV vaccine	Anti-HBc Anti-HBs	To determine if a high risk individual is infected or has antibodies to HBV
Screening blood donors	HBsAg Anti-HBc Anti-Hep C	Used by blood banks to screen donors for hepatitis B and C
DIAGNOSTIC TESTS		
Differential diagnosis of acute jaundice, hepatitis, or fulminant liver failure	HBsAg Anti-HBc IgM Anti-HAV IgM Anti-Hep C	To differentiate between HBV, HAV, and hepatitis C in an acutely jaundiced patient with hepatitis or fulminant liver failure
Chronic hepatitis	HBsAg HBeAg Anti-HBe Anti-HDV (total + IgM)	To diagnose HBV infection: if positive for HBsAg to determine infectivity If HBsAg patient worsens or is very ill, to diagnose concomitant infection with hepatitis delta virus

(continued)

Table 4–2 (*continued*)

Clinical Setting	Test	Purpose
MONITORING		
Infant follow-up	HBsAg Anti-HBc Anti-HBs	To monitor the success of vaccination and passive immunization for perinatal transmission of HBV 12–15 mo after birth
Postvaccination screening	Anti-HBs	To ensure immunity has been achieved after vaccination (CDC recommends "titer" determination, but usually qualitative assay is adequate)
Sexual contact	HBsAg Anti-HBc Anti-Hep C	To monitor sexual partners of a patient with chronic HBV or hepatitis C

*See Abbreviations list on page xiii for definition of abbreviations.

TABLE 4–3
Interpretation of Viral Hepatitis Serologic Testing Patterns

Anti-HAV (IgM)	HBsAg	Anti-HBc (IgM)	Anti-HBc (Total)	Anti-C (ELISA)	Interpretation
+	–	–	–	–	Acute hepatitis A
+	+	–	+	–	Acute hepatitis A in hepatitis B carrier
–	+	–	+	–	Chronic hepatitis B[a]
–	–	+	+	–	Acute hepatitis B
–	+	+	+	–	Acute hepatitis B
–	–	–	+	–	Past hepatitis B infection
–	–	–	–	+	Hepatitis C[b]
–	–	–	–	–	Early hepatitis C or other cause (other virus, toxin)

[a]Patients with chronic hepatitis B (either active hepatitis or carrier state) should have HBeAg and anti-HBe checked to determine activity of infection and relative infectivity. Anti-HBs is used to determine response to hepatitis B vaccination.
[b]Anti-C often takes 3–6 mon before being positive. PCR may allow earlier detection.

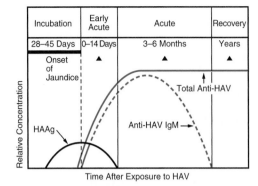

FIGURE 4–1. Hepatitis A diagnostic profile. (Based on data from Abbott Laboratories, Diagnostic Division, North Chicago, Illinois. Used with permission.)

HBeAg: Hepatitis Be antigen; when present, indicates high degree of infectivity. Order only when evaluating for chronic HBV infection

HBV-DNA: Most sensitive and specific for early evaluation of hepatitis B and may be detected when all other markers are negative

Anti-HBe: Antibody to hepatitis Be antigen; associated with resolution of active inflammation

Anti-HBs: Antibody to hepatitis B surface antigen; when present, typically indicates immunity associated with clinical recovery from HBV infection or previ-

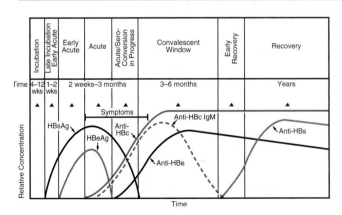

FIGURE 4–2. Hepatitis B diagnostic profile. (Based on data from Abbott Laboratories, Diagnostic Division, North Chicago, Illinois. Used with permission.)

ous immunization with hepatitis B vaccine. Order only to assess effectiveness of vaccine and request titer levels

Anti-HDV: Total antibody to delta hepatitis; confirms previous exposure. Order only in patients with known acute or chronic HBV infection.

Anti-HDV IgM: IgM antibody to delta hepatitis; indicates recent infection. Order only in cases of known acute or chronic HBV infection

Hepatitis C

Anti-HCV: Antibody against hepatitis C. Indicative of active viral replication and infectivity. Used by blood banks to screen donors. Many false-positives

HCV-RNA: Nucleic acid probe detection of current HCV infection

HIGH-DENSITY LIPOPROTEIN CHOLESTEROL

• See Cholesterol, page 54.

HLA (HUMAN LEUKOCYTE ANTIGENS; HLA TYPING)

• Collection: Green top tube

This test identifies a group of antigens on the cell surface that are the primary determinants of histocompatibility and useful in assessing transplantation compatibility. Some are associated with specific diseases but are not diagnostic of these diseases.

HLA-B27: Ankylosing spondylitis, psoriatic arthritis, Reiter's syndrome, juvenile RA

HLA-DR4/HLA DR2: Chronic Lyme disease arthritis

HLA-DRw2: MS

HLA-B8: Addison's disease, juvenile-onset diabetes, Grave's disease, gluten-sensitive enteropathy

HOMOCYSTEINE, SERUM

• Normal fasting 5 and 15 μmol/L • Fasting target < 10 μmol/L

Under investigation as a risk factor for CAD and atherosclerosis. Moderate, intermediate, and severe hyperhomocystinemia refer to concentrations between 16 and 30, between 31 and 100, and > 100 μmol/L, respectively. May be useful to screen high-risk patients and recommend strategies to obtain target of < 10 (ie, dietary, lifestyle changes, vitamin supplementation)

Increased: Vitamin B_{12}, B_6 and folate deficiency, kidney and renal failure, medications (nicotinic acid, theophylline, methotrexate, L-dopa, anticonvulsants) advanced age, hypothyroidism, impaired kidney function, SLE, and certain medications

HUMAN CHORIONIC GONADOTROPIN, SERUM (HCG, BETA SUBUNIT)

• Normal, < 3.0 mIU/mL • 10 d after conception, > 3 mIU/mL • 30 d, 100–5000 mIU/mL • 10 wk, 50,000–140,000 mIU/mL • > 16 wk,

10,000–50,000 mIU/mL • Thereafter, levels slowly decline (SI units IU/L equivalent to mIU/mL) • Collection: Tiger top tube

Increased: PRG, some testicular tumors (nonseminomatous germ cell tumors, but not seminoma), trophoblastic disease (hydatidiform mole, choriocarcinoma levels usually > 100,000 mIU/mL)

4

HUMAN IMMUNODEFICIENCY VIRUS (HIV) TESTING

See Figure 4–3 below, CDC guidelines. Any HIV-positive person over 13 y of age with a CD4+ T-cell level < 200/mL or an HIV-positive patient with a CDC-defined indicator conditions (eg, pulmonary candidiasis, disseminated histoplasmosis, HIV wasting, Kaposi's sarcoma, TB, various lymphomas, PCP, and others) is considered to have AIDS.(*Note:* Confidentiality issues in HIV testing are regulated by law. Most states require that the patient sign a release for HIV testing. Release of HIV information by phone is likewise prohibited in most states and is normally only released in writing to the ordering attending physician on a confidential basis.)

HIV Antibody

• Normal = negative • Collection: Tiger top tube

Assay kits recognize both HIV-1 and HIV-2 antibodies. Used in the diagnosis of AIDS and to screen blood for use in transfusion. Antibodies appear in blood 1–4 mon after infection in most cases.

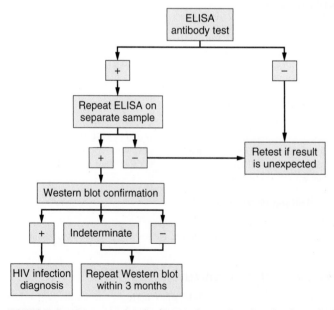

FIGURE 4–3. Diagnostic algorithm for HIV infection. (Based on data from Glaxo-Wellcome Company, Research Triangle Park, North Carolina. Used with permission.)

HIV Antibody, ELISA

- Normal = negative

    Initial screen to detect HIV antibody; a positive test is often repeated or confirmed by Western blot.

Positive: AIDS, asymptomatic HIV infection

4

False-Positive: Flu vaccine within 3 mon, hemophilia, rheumatoid factor, alcoholic hepatitis, dialysis patients

HIV Western Blot

- Normal = negative

    The technique is used as the reference procedure for confirming the presence or absence of HIV antibody, usually after a positive test result

HIV Antibody by ELISA Determination

Positive: AIDS, asymptomatic HIV infection (if indeterminate, repeat in 1 mon or perform PCR for HIV-1 DNA or RNA)

False-Positive: Autoimmune or connective tissue diseases, hyperbilirubinemia, HLA antibodies, others

HIV DNA PCR

- Normal = negative

    Performed on peripheral blood mononuclear cells. Preferred test to diagnose HIV infection in children < 18 mon of age

HIV RNA PCR

- Normal = < 400 copies/mL

    Quantifies "viral load." Establishes diagnosis before antibody production or when HIV antibody indeterminate. Obtained at baseline, an important parameter to initiate or modify HIV therapy (see viral load). Not recommended for routine testing of children < 18 mon

HIV Viral Load

- Normal < 50 copies/mL

    Best predictor of progression to AIDS and death among HIV-infected. Used as a baseline and for initiation/modification of HIV therapy, but not for diagnosis (eg, antiretroviral therapy is uniformly initiated when viral load > 20,000 copies/mL RNA or RT PCR.)

HIV Antigen (P-24 antigen)

- Normal = negative

    Detects early HIV infection before antibody conversion, used along with PCR testing

IMMUNOGLOBULINS, QUANTITATIVE

- **IgG:** 65–1500 mg/dL or 6.5–15 g/L • **IgM:** 40–345 mg/dL or 0.4–3.45 mg/L • **IgA:** 76–390 mg/dL or 0.76–3.90 g/L • **IgE:** 0–380 IU/mL or KIU/L • **IgD:** 0–8 mg/dL or 0–80 mg/L • Collection: Tiger top tube

Levels are determined in the evaluation of immunodeficiency diseases, during replacement therapy, and to evaluate humoral immunity.

Increased: Multiple myeloma (myeloma immunoglobulin increased, other immunoglobulins decreased); Waldenström's macroglobulinemia (IgM increased, others decreased); lymphoma; carcinoma; bacterial infection; liver disease; sarcoidosis; amyloidosis; myeloproliferative disorders

Decreased: Hereditary immunodeficiency, leukemia, lymphoma, nephrotic syndrome, protein-losing enteropathy, malnutrition, transient hypogammaglobulinemia of infancy

IRON

• Males 65–175 mg/dL (SI: 11.64–31.33 mmol/L) • Females 50–170 mg/dL (SI: 8.95–30.43 mmol/L) • To convert mg/dL to mmol/L, multiply by 0.1791 • Collection: Tiger top tube

Increased: Hemochromatosis, hemosiderosis caused by excessive iron intake, excess destruction or decreased production of erythrocytes, liver necrosis

Decreased: Iron deficiency anemia, nephrosis (loss of iron-binding proteins), normochromic anemia of chronic diseases and infections

IRON-BINDING CAPACITY, TOTAL (TIBC)

• 250–450 mg/dL (SI: 44.75–80.55 mmol/L) • Collection: Tiger top tube

The normal iron/TIBC ratio is 20–50%. Decreased ratio (< 10%) is almost diagnostic of iron deficiency anemia. Increased ratio is seen with hemochromatosis.

Increased: Acute and chronic blood loss, iron deficiency anemia, hepatitis, oral contraceptives

Decreased: Anemia of chronic diseases, cirrhosis, nephrosis/uremia, hemochromatosis, iron therapy overload, hemolytic anemia, aplastic anemia, thalassemia, megaloblastic anemia

LACTATE DEHYDROGENASE (LD, LDH)

• Adults < 230 U/L, (< 3.82 mkat/L) • Higher levels in childhood • Collection: Tiger top tube; carefully avoid hemolysis because this can increase LDH levels

Increased: AMI, cardiac surgery, prosthetic valve, hepatitis, pernicious anemia, malignant tumors, PE, hemolysis (anemias or factitious), renal infarction, muscle injury, megaloblastic anemia, liver disease

LDH Isoenzymes (LDH 1 to LDH 5)

Normally, the ratio LDH 1/LDH 2 is < 0.6–0.7. If the ratio becomes > 1 (also termed "flipped"), suspect a recent MI (change in ratio can also be seen in pernicious or hemolytic anemia). With an AMI, the LDH will begin to rise at 12–48 h, peak at 3–6 d, and return to normal at 8–14 d. LDH 5 is > LDH 4 in liver diseases. (Largely replaced by troponin.)

LACTIC ACID (LACTATE)

- 4.5–19.8 mg/dL (SI: 0.5–2.2 mmol/L) • Collection: Gray top tube on ice
  Suspect lactic acidosis with elevated anion gap in the absence of other causes
(renal failure, ethanol or methanol ingestion)

Increased: Lactic acidosis due to hypoxia, hemorrhage, shock, sepsis, cirrhosis, exercise, ethanol, DKA, regional ischemia (extremity, bowel) spurious (prolonged use of a tourniquet)

LAP SCORE (LEUKOCYTE ALKALINE PHOSPHATASE SCORE/STAIN)

- 50-150 • Collection: Finger stick blood sample directly on slide; air dry
  Used to differentiate among various hematologic conditions

Increased: Leukemoid reaction, acute inflammation, Hodgkin's disease, PRG, liver disease

Decreased: Chronic myelogenous leukemia, nephrotic syndrome

LE (LUPUS ERYTHEMATOSUS) PREPARATION

- Normal = no cells seen

Positive: SLE, scleroderma, RA, drug-induced lupus (procainamide, others)

LEAD, BLOOD

- Adult < 40 mg/dL (1.93 mmol/L) • Child < 25 mg/dL (1.21 mmol/L) • Collection: Lavender, navy, or green top tube; lab-specific
  Neurologic findings can be detected at 15 mg/dL in children and 30 mg/dL in adults; severe symptoms (lethargy, ataxia, coma) are present > 60 mg/dL.

Increased: Lead poisoning, occupational exposure

LEGIONELLA ANTIBODY

- < 1:32 titers
  Obtain two sera, acute (within 2 wk of onset) and convalescent (at least 3 wk after onset of fever). A fourfold rise in titers or a single titer of 1:256 is diagnostic.

Increased: *Legionella* infection; false-positives with *Bacteroides fragilis, Francisella tularensis, Mycoplasma pneumoniae.*

LIPASE

- 0–1.5 U/mL (SI: 10–150 U/L) by turbidimetric method • Collection: Tiger top tube

Increased: Acute or chronic pancreatitis, pseudo-cyst, pancreatic duct obstruction (stone, stricture, tumor, drug-induced spasm), fat embolus syndrome, renal failure, dialysis (usually normal in mumps) gastric malignancy, intestinal perforation, diabetes (usually in DKA only)

LIPID PROFILE/LIPOPROTEIN PROFILE/LIPOPROTEIN ANALYSIS

- See also Cholesterol, page 54, and TriglycerideS, page 87.

Usually includes cholesterol, HDL cholesterol, LDL cholesterol (calculated), triglycerides. Useful in the evaluation of CAD and allows classification of dyslipoproteinemias to direct treatment. Initial screening for cardiac risk includes total cholesterol, LDL, and HDL as outlined in Table 4–1. The main lipids in the blood are cholesterol and triglycerides. These lipids are carried by lipoproteins. Lipoproteins are further classified by density (least dense to most dense):

- **Chylomicrons** (least dense, rise to surface of unspun serum) and are normally found only after a fatty meal is eaten (a "lipemic specimen" on a lab report usually refers to these chylomicrons).
- **VLDL** consist mainly of triglycerides. With triglycerides < 400, the ratio of cholesterol to triglycerides is 1 to 5 in VLDL.
- **LDL** in the fasting state; the LDL carry most cholesterol.
- **HDL** are the densest and consist of mostly apoproteins and cholesterol.

Table 4–4 (see page 76) indicates the dyslipoproteinemias based on the lipid profile.

LOW-DENSITY LIPOPROTEIN-CHOLESTEROL (LDL, LDL-C)

- See Cholesterol, page 54.

LUTEINIZING HORMONE, SERUM (LH)

- Male 7–24 IU/L • Female 6–30 IU/L, midcycle peak increase two- to three-fold over baseline, postmenopausal > 35 IU/L • Collection: Tiger top tube

Increased: (Hypergonadotropic > 40 IU/L) postmenopausal, surgical or radiation castration, ovarian or testicular failure, polycystic ovaries

Decreased: (Hypogonadotropic < 40 IU/L prepubertal) hypothalamic, and pituitary dysfunction, Kallmann's syndrome, LHRH analogue therapy

LYME DISEASE SEROLOGY

- Normal varies with assay, ELISA < 1:8 • Western blot nonreactive

Most useful when comparing acute and convalescent serum levels for relative titers. Normal values differ among labs. IgM antibody becomes detectable 2–4 wk after onset of rash; IgG rises in 4–6 wk and peaks up to 6 mon after infection and may stay elevated for months to years.

Positive: Infection with *Borrelia burgdorferi,* syphilis, and other rickettsial diseases

Negative: After antibiotic therapy or during first few weeks of disease

MAGNESIUM

- 1.6–2.6 mg/dL (SI: 0.80–1.20 mmol/L) • Collection: Tiger top tube

Increased: Renal failure, hypothyroidism, magnesium-containing antacids, Addison's disease, diabetic coma, severe dehydration, lithium intoxication

Decreased: Malabsorption, steatorrhea, alcoholism and cirrhosis, hyperthyroidism, aldosteronism, diuretics, acute pancreatitis, hyperparathyroidism, hy-

TABLE 4–4
Lipoproteins

Fredrickson Classification System	Type I (Rare)	Type IIa (Common)	Type IIb (Common)	Type III (Uncommon)	Type IV (Uncommon)	Type V (Uncommon)
Cholesterol	N or slightly ↑	Very ↑	Very ↑	Very ↑	N or slightly ↑	↑
LDL	N	↑	↑	↑	N	N
HDL	N or ↓	N or ↓	N or ↓	N or ↓	N or ↓	N or ↓
Triglycerides	Very ↑	N	↑	Very ↑	Very ↑	↑
Increased lipoproteins	Chylomicrons	LDL	LDL, VLDL	LDL	VLDL	VLDL and chylomicrons
Atherogenesis risk	No increase	Very ↑	↑	↑	No increase	No increase

peralimentation, NG suctioning, chronic dialysis, renal tubular acidosis, drugs (cisplatin, amphotericin B, aminoglycosides), hungry bone syndrome, hypophosphatemia, intracellular shifts with respiratory or metabolic acidosis

MHA-TP (MICROHEMAGGLUTINATION, *TREPONEMA PALLIDUM*)

• Normal < 1:160 • Collection: Tiger top tube

Confirmatory test for syphilis, similar to FTA-ABS. Once positive, remains so, therefore cannot be used to judge effect of treatment. False-positives with other treponemal infections (pinta, yaws, etc), mononucleosis, and SLE

B$_2$-MICROGLOBULIN

• 0.1–0.26 mg/dL (1–2.6 mg/L) • Collection: Tiger top tube

A portion of the class I MHC antigen. A useful marker to follow the progression of HIV infections

Increased: HIV infection, especially during periods of exacerbation, lymphoid malignancies, renal diseases (diabetic nephropathy, pyelonephritis, ATN, nephrotoxicity from medications), transplant rejection, inflammatory conditions

Decreased: Treatment of HIV with AZT (zidovudine)

MONOSPOT

• Normal = negative • Collection: Tiger top tube

Positive: Mononucleosis, rarely in leukemia, serum sickness, Burkitt's lymphoma, viral hepatitis, RA

MYOGLOBIN

• 30–90 ng/mL • Collection: Tiger top tube

Increased: Skeletal muscle injury (crush, injection, surgical procedures), delirium tremens, rhabdomyolysis (burns, seizures, sepsis, hypokalemia, others)

B-TYPE NATRIURETIC PEPTIDE (BNP)

• < 100 pg/mL normal • Collection: Lavender top tube on ice

BNP is released by the ventricular myocardium secondary to volume and pressure overload. BNP increases sodium and water excretion (inhibits sodium reabsorption in the distal nephron). The severity of CHF correlates with the level of BNP. Levels < 100 rule out CHF, levels of 100–400 are borderline and levels > 400 are highly suggestive of CHF. BNP is very helpful in distinguishing between CHF and other causes of dyspnea (COPD).

Increased: CHF/left ventricular dysfunction

NEWBORN SCREENING PANEL

The screening required varies by state law and is obtained in the newborn period to evaluate for a variety of inherited conditions: Phenylalanine (for phenylketonuria); leucine (for branched-chain ketonuria); galactose-1-phosphate uridyl transferase (for galactosemia); methionine (for homocystinuria); thyroxine, TSH (for hypothyroidism); hemoglobin electrophoresis (for sickle cell); biotinidase (for biotinidase deficiency)

5'-NUCLEOTIDASE

- 2–15 U/L

    Used in the work-up of increased alkaline phosphatase and biliary obstruction

Increased: Obstructive or cholestatic liver disease, liver metastasis, biliary cirrhosis

OLIGOCLONAL BANDING, CSF

- Normal = negative • Collection: Serum tiger top tube and simultaneous CSF sample collected in a plain tube by LP

    This is performed simultaneously on CSF and serum samples when MS is clinically suspected. Agarose gel electrophoresis will reveal multiple bands in the IgG region not seen in the serum. Oligoclonal banding is present in up to 90% of patients with MS. Occasionally seen in other CNS inflammatory conditions and CNS syphilis

OSMOLALITY, SERUM

- 278–298 mOsm/kg (SI: 278–298 mmol/kg) • Collection: Tiger top tube

    A rough estimation of osmolality is [2(Na) + BUN/2.8 + glucose/18]. Measured value is usually less than calculated value. If measured value is 15 mOsm/kg less than calculated, consider methanol, ethanol, or ethylene glycol ingestion or some other unmeasured substance.

Increased: Hyperglycemia; ethanol, methanol, mannitol, or ethylene glycol ingestion; increased sodium because of water loss (diabetes, hypercalcemia, diuresis)

Decreased: Low serum sodium, diuretics, Addison's disease, SIADH (seen in bronchogenic carcinoma, hypothyroidism), iatrogenic causes (poor fluid balance)

OXYGEN

- See Chapter 8, Table 8–1, page 160

P-24 ANTIGEN (HIV CORE ANTIGEN)

- Normal = negative • Collection: Tiger top tube • See also Human Immunodeficiency Virus Testing, page 71

    Used to diagnose recent acute HIV infection; becomes positive earlier than HIV antibodies. Decreases "window" period. Can be positive as early as 2–4 wk but becomes undetectable during antibody seroconversion (periods of latency). With progression of disease, P-24 usually becomes evident again. Used to screen blood donors

PARATHYROID HORMONE (PTH)

- Normal based on relationship to serum calcium, usually provided on the lab report • Also, reference values vary depending on the laboratory and whether the N-terminal, C-terminal or midmolecule is measured. • PTH midmolecule: 0.29–0.85 ng/mL (SI: 29–85 pmol/L) • With calcium: 8.4–10.2 mg/dL (SI: 2.1–2.55 mmol/L) • Collection: Tiger top tube

Increased: Primary hyperparathyroidism, secondary hyperparathyroidism (hypocalcemic states, eg, chronic renal failure, others)

Decreased: Hypercalcemia not due to hyperparathyroidism, hypoparathyroidism

PHOSPHORUS

• Adult 2.5–4.5 mg/dL (SI: 0.81–1.45 mmol/L) • Child 4.0–6.0 mg/dL (SI: 1.29–1.95 mmol/L) • To convert mg/dL to mmol/L, multiply by 0.3229 • Collection: Tiger top tube

Increased: Hypoparathyroidism (surgical, pseudo-hypoparathyroidism), excess vitamin D, secondary hyperparathyroidism, renal failure, bone disease (healing fractures), Addison's disease, childhood, factitious increase (hemolysis of specimen)

Decreased: Hyperparathyroidism, alcoholism, diabetes, hyperalimentation, acidosis, alkalosis, gout, salicylate poisoning, IV steroid, glucose or insulin administration, hypokalemia, hypomagnesemia, diuretics, vitamin D deficiency, phosphate-binding antacids

POTASSIUM, SERUM

• 3.5–5 mEq/L (SI: 3.5–5 mmol/L) • Collection: Tiger top tube

Increased: Factitious increase (hemolysis of specimen, thrombocytosis), renal failure, Addison's disease, acidosis, spironolactone, triamterene, ACE inhibitors, dehydration, hemolysis, massive tissue damage, excess intake (oral or IV), potassium-containing medications, acidosis

Decreased: Diuretics, decreased intake, vomiting, NG suctioning, villous adenoma, diarrhea, ZE syndrome, chronic pyelonephritis, RTA, metabolic alkalosis (primary aldosteronism, Cushing's syndrome)

PREALBUMIN

• See Chapter 11, page 201 & 205

PROGESTERONE

• Collection: Tiger top tube
  Used to confirm ovulation and corpus luteum function

Sample Collection	Normal Values (female)
Follicular phase	<1 ng/mL
Luteal phase	5–20 ng/mL
Pregnancy	
1st trimester	10–30 ng/mL
2nd trimester	50–100 ng/mL
3rd trimester	100–400 ng/mL
Postmenopause	<1 ng/mL

PROLACTIN

• Males 1–20 ng/mL (SI: 1–20 mg/L) • Females 1–25 ng/mL (SI: 1–25 mg/L)
• Collection: Tiger top tube
  Used in the work-up of infertility, impotence, hirsutism, amenorrhea, and pituitary neoplasm

Increased: PRG, nursing after PRG, prolactinoma, hypothalamic tumors, sarcoidosis or granulomatous disease of the hypothalamus, hypothyroidism, renal failure, Addison's disease, phenothiazines, haloperidol

PROSTATE-SPECIFIC ANTIGEN (PSA)

- < 4 ng/dL by monoclonal, eg, Hybritech assay

Most useful as a measure of response to therapy of prostate cancer; approved for screening for prostate cancer. Although any elevation increases suspicion of prostate cancer, levels > 10.0 ng/dL are frequently associated with carcinoma. Age-corrected levels popular (40–50 y 2.5 ng/dL; 50–60 y 3.5 ng/dL; 60–70 y 4.5 ng/dL; > 70 y 6.5 ng/dL.)

Increased: Prostate cancer, acute prostatitis, some cases of BPH, prostatic infarction, prostate surgery (biopsy, resection), vigorous prostatic massage (routine rectal exam does not elevate levels), rarely postejaculation

Decreased: Radical prostatectomy, response to therapy of prostatic carcinoma (radiation or hormonal therapy)

PSA Velocity

A rate of rise in PSA of 0.75 ng/mL or greater per year is suggestive of prostate cancer based on at least three separate assays 6 mon apart.

PSA Free and Total

Patients with prostate cancer tend to have lower free PSA levels in proportion to total PSA. Measurement of the free/total PSA can improve the specificity of PSA in the range of total PSA from 2.0–10.0 ng/mL. Some recommend prostate biopsy only if the free PSA percentage is low. Threshold for biopsy is controversial, ranging from a ratio of < 15% to < 25%, with a higher threshold having improved sensitivity and lower threshold having improved specificity.

PROTEIN ELECTROPHORESIS, SERUM AND URINE (SERUM PROTEIN ELECTROPHORESIS, SPEP) (URINE PROTEIN ELECTROPHORESIS, UPEP)

Qualitative analysis of the serum proteins is often used in the work-up of hypoglobulinemia, macroglobulinemia, α_1-antitrypsin deficiency, collagen disease, liver disease, myeloma, and occasionally in nutritional assessment. Serum electrophoresis yields five different bands (Figure 4–4 and Table 4–5, pages 81 and 82). If a monoclonal gammopathy or a low globulin fraction is detected, quantitative immunoglobulins should be ordered. Urine protein electrophoresis can be used to evaluate proteinuria and can detect Bence Jones protein (light chain) that is associated with myeloma, Waldenström's macroglobulinemia, and Fanconi's syndrome.

PROTEIN, SERUM

- 6.0–8.0 g/dL • See also Serum Protein Electrophoresis, above. • Collection: Tiger top tube

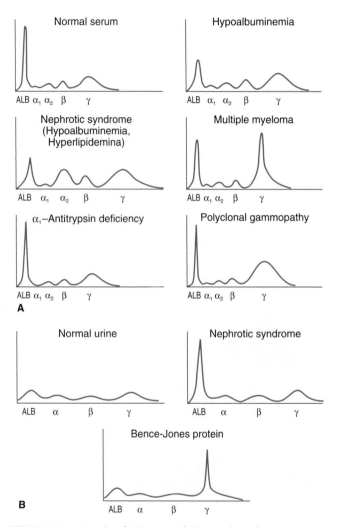

FIGURE 4–4. Examples of (**A**) serum and (**B**) urine electrophoresis patterns. See also Table 4–5, page 82. (Courtesy of Dr. Steven Haist.)

Increased: Multiple myeloma, Waldenström's macroglobulinemia, benign monoclonal gammopathy, lymphoma, chronic inflammatory disease, sarcoidosis, viral illnesses

Decreased: Malnutrition, inflammatory bowel disease, Hodgkin's disease, leukemias, any cause of decreased albumin

TABLE 4–5
Normal Serum Protein Components and Fractions as Determined by Electrophoresis, Along with Associated Conditions[a]

Protein Fraction	Percentage of Total Protein	Constituents	Increased	Decreased
Albumin	52–68	Albumin	Dehydration (only known cause)	Nephrosis, malnutrition, chronic liver disease
Alpha-1 (α_1) globulin	2.4–4.4	Thyroxine-binding globulin, antitrypsin, lipoproteins, glycoprotein, transcortin	Inflammation, neoplasia	Nephrosis, α_1-antitrypsin deficiency (emphysema related)
Alpha-2 (α_2) globulin	6.1–10.1	Haptoglobin, glycoprotein, macroglobulin, ceruloplasmin	Inflammation, infection, neoplasia, cirrhosis	Severe liver disease, acute hemolytic anemia
Beta (β) globulin	8.5–14.5	Transferrin, glycoprotein, lipoprotein	Cirrhosis, obstructive jaundice	Nephrosis
Gamma (γ) globulins (immunoglobulins)	10–21	IgA, IgG, IgM, IgD, IgE	Infections, collagen vascular diseases, leukemia, myeloma	Agammaglobulinemia, hypogammaglobulineia, nephrosis

[a](See also Figure 4–4, page 81).

RENIN

Plasma (Plasma Renin Activity [PRA])

• Adults, Normal sodium diet, upright 1–6 ng/mL/h (SI: 0.77–4.6 nmol/L/h) • Renal vein renin: L & R should be equal

Useful in the diagnosis of HTN associated with hypokalemia. Values highly dependent on salt intake and position. Stop diuretics, estrogens for 2–4 wk before testing.

4

Increased: Medications (ACE inhibitors, diuretics, oral contraceptives, estrogens), PRG, dehydration, renal artery stenosis, adrenal insufficiency, chronic hypokalemia, upright posture, salt-restricted diet, edematous conditions (CHF, nephrotic syndrome), secondary hyperaldosteronism

Decreased: Primary aldosteronism (renin will not increase with relative volume depletion, upright posture)

Renal Vein Renins

• Normal L & R should be equal

A ratio of > 1.5 (affected/nonaffected) suggestive of renovascular hypertension

RETINOL-BINDING PROTEIN (RBP)

• Adults 3–6 mg/dL • Children 1.5–3.0 mg/dL • Collection: Tiger top tube

Decreased: Malnutrition, vitamin A deficiency, intestinal malabsorption of fats, chronic liver disease

RHEUMATOID FACTOR (RA LATEX TEST)

• < 15 IU by Microscan kit or > 1:40 • Collection: Tiger top tube

Increased: Collagen-vascular diseases (RA, SLE, scleroderma, polyarteritis nodosa, others), infections (TB, syphilis, viral hepatitis), chronic inflammation, SBE, some lung diseases, MI (*Note:* 15% of patients with RA are negative for rheumatoid factor.)

ROCKY MOUNTAIN SPOTTED FEVER ANTIBODIES (RMSF)

• Normal: < 4(times) increase in paired acute and convalescent sera • IgG < 1:64 • IgM < 1:8 • Collection: Tiger top tube acute and convalescent

The diagnosis of RMSF is made by acute and convalescent titers that demonstrate a 4 × rise or a single convalescent titer > 1:64 in the clinical setting of RMSF. Occasional false-positives in late PRG

SEMEN ANALYSIS

• Volume 2–5 mL • Sperm count > 20–40 × 10^6/mL • Motility > 60% • Forward migration • Morphology > 60% normal

Specimen must be collected after 48–72 h abstinence and analyzed within 1–2 h. Test may not be valid after a recent illness or high fever. Verify abnormal analysis by serial tests.

Decreased: After vasectomy (should be 0 sperm after 3 mon), varicocele, primary testicular failure (ie, Klinefelter's syndrome), secondary testicular failure (chemotherapy, radiation, infections),varicocele, after recent illness, congenital obstruction of the vas, retrograde ejaculation, endocrine causes (hyperprolactinemia, low testosterone, others)

SGGT (SERUM GAMMA-GLUTAMYL TRANSPEPTIDASE)

• See GGT, page 64.

SGOT (SERUM GLUTAMIC-OXALOACETIC TRANSAMINASE)

• See AST, page 50.

SGPT SERUM (GLUTAMIC-PYRUVIC TRANSAMINASE)

• See ALT, page 49.

SODIUM, SERUM

• 136–145 mmol/L • Collection: Tiger top tube

In factitious hyponatremia due to hyperglycemia, for every 100 mmol/L blood glucose above normal, serum sodium decreases 2.4. For example, a blood glucose of 800 and a sodium of 125 would factitiously lower the sodium value by about (800–100) % 100 = 7 × 2.4, or 16.8. Corrected serum sodium would therefore be 125 + 17 = 142.

Increased: Associated with low total body sodium (glycosuria, mannitol, or lactulose use, urea, excess sweating), normal total body sodium (diabetes insipidus [central and nephrogenic], respiratory losses, and sweating), and increased total body sodium (administration of hypertonic sodium bicarbonate, Cushing's syndrome, hyperaldosteronism)

Decreased: Associated with excess total body sodium and water (nephrotic syndrome, CHF, cirrhosis, renal failure), excess body water (SIADH [small-cell lung cancer; pulmonary disease including TB, lung cancer, pneumonia; CNS disease including trauma, tumors, and infections; perioperative stress; drugs including SSRIs and ACE inhibitors; and after colonoscopy], hypothyroidism, adrenal insufficiency, psychogenic polydipsia, beer potomania), decreased total body water and sodium (diuretic use, renal tubular acidosis, use of mannitol or urea, mineralocorticoid deficiency, cerebral salt wasting, vomiting, diarrhea, pancreatitis), and pseudo-hyponatremia (hyperlipidemia, hyperglycemia, and multiple myeloma)

STOOL FOR OCCULT BLOOD (FECAL OCCULT BLOOD TESTING [FOBT], HEMOCCULT TEST)

Normal-Negative: Apply small amount of stool to test site on Hemoccult card and close. Open test panel on other side of card and apply 2–3 gtt developer to the test and the positive control panels; read in 30 s. Blue color is positive. Detects > 5 mg hemoglobin/g feces. Repeat 3 × for maximum yield. (A positive test more informative than a negative test)

Positive: Any GI tract ulcerated lesion (ulcer, carcinoma, polyp, diverticulosis, inflammatory bowel disease), hemorrhoids, telangiectasias, drugs that cause GI irritation (eg, NSAIDs) swallowed blood, ingestion of rare red meat, certain foods (horseradish, turnips) (vitamin C [> 500 mg/d], antacids may result in false-negative test)

SWEAT CHLORIDE

• 5–40 mEq/L (SI: 5–40 mmol/L) • Collection: 100–200 mg sweat on filter paper after electrical stimulation of sweating by pilocarpine iontophoresis on an extremity

Increased: CF (not valid on children < 3 wk); Addison's disease, meconium ileus, and renal failure can occasionally raise levels.

N-TELOPEPTIDE (NTX) (URINE AND SERUM)
Urine

• Normal adult female: Premenopausal: 17–94 nM BCE/mM creatinine; Postmenopausal: 26–124 nM BCE/mM creatinine • Normal adult male: 21–83 nM BCE/mM creatinine

Serum

• Premenopausal, adult female: 6.2–19.0 nM BCE • Male > 25 y: 5.4–24.2 nM BCE

N-Telopeptides of type I collagen (NTx), are end-products of bone resorption and allow monitoring of bone metabolism. Reported as nanomolar bone collagen equivalents per liter (nM BCE/L). In urine, values are corrected per millimolars of creatinine per liter (mM creatinine/L). Serum NTx provides a quantitative measurement of bone resorption. A baseline NTx level is obtained before antiresorptive therapy (ie, bisphosphonate, eg, alendronate) with periodic testing until decrease in NTx achieved

Increased: Osteoporosis, Paget's disease, primary hyperparathyroidism, bony metastasis

Decreased: Response to bisphosphonate therapy; (decrease of 30–40% from baseline after 3 mon of therapy is a typical for bisphonate therapy.)

T_3 RU (RESIN UPTAKE; THYROXINE-BINDING GLOBULIN RATIO)

• 30–40%

Used in conjunction with a T_4 to yield the free T_4 index [FTI], an estimate of the free T_4.

Increased: Hyperthyroidism, medications (phenytoin, steroids, heparin, aspirin, others), nephrotic syndrome

Decreased: Hypothyroidism, medications (iodine, propylthiouracil, others), any cause of increased TBG, eg, oral estrogen or PRG

TESTOSTERONE

• Male free: 9–30 ng/dL, total 300–1200 ng/dL • Female, see following table

Sample Collection	**Normal Values (female)**
Follicular phase	20–80 ng/dL
Midcycle peak	20–80 ng/dL
Luteal phase	20–80 ng/dL
Postmenopause	10–40 ng/dL

Increased: Adrenogenital syndrome, ovarian stromal hyperthecosis, polycystic ovaries, menopause, ovarian tumors

Decreased: Hypogonadism, hypopituitarism, Klinefelter's syndrome, male andropause

THYROGLOBULIN

- 1–20 ng/mL (mg/L) • Collection: Tiger top tube
  Useful for following patients with nonmedullary thyroid carcinomas

Increased: Differentiated thyroid carcinomas (papillary, follicular), Graves' disease, nontoxic goiter

Decreased: Hypothyroidism, testosterone, steroids, phenytoin

THYROID-STIMULATING HORMONE (TSH)

- 0.7–5.3 mU/mL • Collection: Tiger top tube
  Excellent screening test for hyperthyroidism as well as hypothyroidism. Differentiates between a low normal and a decreased TSH

Increased: Hypothyroidism

Decreased: Hyperthyroidism. Less than 1% of hypothyroidism is from pituitary or hypothalamic disease resulting in a decreased TSH.

THYROXINE (T$_4$ TOTAL)

- 5–12 mg/dL (SI: 65–155 nmol/L) • Males: > 60 y, 5–10 mg/dL (SI: 65–129 nmol) • Females: 5.5–10.5 mcg/dL (SI: 71–135 nmol/L) • Collection: Tiger top tube
  Good screening test for hyperthyroidism. Measures both bound and free T$_4$, therefore, can be affected by TBG levels.

Increased: Hyperthyroidism, exogenous thyroid hormone, estrogens, PRG, severe illness, euthyroid sick syndrome

Decreased: Hypothyroidism, euthyroid sick syndrome, any cause of decreased TBG

THYROXINE-BINDING GLOBULIN (TBG)

- 21–52 mg/dL (270–669 nmol/L) • Collection: Tiger top tube

Increased: Hypothyroidism, PRG, oral contraceptives, estrogens, hepatic disease, acute porphyria

Decreased: Hyperthyroidism, androgens, anabolic steroids, prednisone, nephrotic syndrome, severe illness, surgical stress, phenytoin, hepatic disease

THYROXINE INDEX, FREE (FTI)

- 6.5–1.25

Practically speaking, the FTI is equivalent to the free thyroxine. Useful in patients with clinically suspected hyper- or hypothyroidism. Determined as follows:

$$\text{Thyroxine (Total } T_4) \times T_3 \text{ RU}$$

Increased: Hyperthyroidism, high-dose beta-blockers, psychiatric illnesses

Decreased: Hypothyroidism, phenytoin (Dilantin)

TORCH BATTERY

- Normal = negative • Collection: Tiger top tube

Serial determinations best (acute and convalescent titers).

Test is based on serologic evidence of exposure to toxoplasmosis, rubella, cytomegalovirus, and herpesviruses.

TRANSFERRIN

- 220–400 mg/dL (SI: 2.20–4.0 g/L) • Collection: Tiger top tube, avoid hemolysis

Used in the work–up of anemias; transferrin levels can also be assessed by the total iron-binding capacity.

Increased: Acute and chronic blood loss, iron deficiency, hemolysis, oral contraceptives, PRG, viral hepatitis

Decreased: Anemia of chronic disease, cirrhosis, nephrosis, hemochromatosis, malignancy

TRIGLYCERIDES

- Recommended values: • Males: 40–160 mg/dL (SI: 0.45–1.81 mmol/L) • Females: 35–135 mg/dL (SI: 0.40–1.53 mmol/L) • Can vary with age. • Collection: Tiger top tube • Fasting preferred • See also Lipid Profile, page 75 and Table 4–1, page 55.

Increased: Nonfasting specimen, hyperlipoproteinemias (types I, IIb, III, IV, V), hypothyroidism, liver diseases, poorly controlled DM, alcoholism, pancreatitis, AMI, nephrotic syndrome, familial, medications (oral contraceptives, estrogens, beta-blockers, cholestyramine)

Decreased: Malnutrition, malabsorption, hyperthyroidism, Tangier disease, medications (nicotinic acid, clofibrate, gemfibrozil) congenital abetalipoproteinemia

TRIIODOTHYRONINE (T_3 RIA)

- 120–195 ng/dL (SI: 1.85–3.00 nmol/L) • Collection: Tiger top tube

Useful when hyperthyroidism is suspected, but T_4 is normal (T_3 thyrotoxicosis); not useful in the diagnosis of hypothyroidism

Increased: Hyperthyroidism, T_3 thyrotoxicosis, PRG, exogenous T_4, any cause of increased TBG, eg, oral estrogen or PRG

Decreased: Hypothyroidism and euthyroid sick state, any cause of decreased TBG

TRIPLE SCREEN (MATERNAL SERUM ALPHA-FETOPROTEIN [MM-SAFP], B-HCG, AND ESTRIOL [E3]

* Normal levels based on gestational age • Collection: Red top tube
  Screens for fetal trisomy 21, trisomy 18, and neural tube defects. Done at 14–21 wk; best sensitivity at 16–18 wk.

TROPONIN, CARDIAC-SPECIFIC

* Troponin I (TI) < 0.35 ng/mL • Troponin T (TT) < 0.2 mcg/L
  Used to diagnose AMI; increases rapidly 3–12 h, peak at 24 h and may stay elevated for several days (TI 5–7 d, TT up to 14 d). More cardiac-specific than CK-MB

Positive: Myocardial damage, including MI, myocarditis (false-positive: renal failure)

URIC ACID (URATE)

* Males: 3.4–7 mg/dL (SI: 202–416 mmol/L) • Females: 2.4–6 mg/dL (SI: 143–357 mmol/L) • To convert mg/dL to mmol/L, multiply by 59.48 • Collection: Tiger top tube
  Increased uric acid is associated with increased catabolism, nucleoprotein synthesis, or decreased renal clearing of uric acid (ie, thiazide diuretics or renal failure).

Increased: Gout, renal failure, destruction of massive amounts of nucleoproteins (leukemia, anemia, chemotherapy, toxemia of PRG), drugs (especially diuretics), lactic acidosis, hypothyroidism, PCKD, parathyroid diseases

Decreased: Uricosuric drugs (salicylates, probenecid, allopurinol), Wilson's disease, Fanconi's syndrome

VDRL TEST (VENEREAL DISEASE RESEARCH LABORATORY) OR RAPID PLASMA REAGIN (RPR)

* Normal = nonreactive • Collection: Tiger top tube
  Good screening for syphilis. Almost always positive in secondary syphilis, but frequently becomes negative in late syphilis. Also, in some patients with HIV infection, the VDRL can be negative in primary and secondary syphilis.

Positive (Reactive): Syphilis, SLE, PRG and drug addiction. If reactive, confirm with FTA-ABS (false-positives with bacterial or viral illnesses).

VITAMIN B$_{12}$ (EXTRINSIC FACTOR, CYANOCOBALAMIN)

* > 100–700 pg/mL (SI: 74–516 pmol/L) • Collection: Tiger top tube

Increased: Excessive intake, myeloproliferative disorders

Decreased: Inadequate intake (especially strict vegetarians), malabsorption, hyperthyroidism, PRG

ZINC

• 60–130 mg/dL (SI: 9–20 mmol/L) • Collection: Check with lab; special collection to limit contamination

Increased: Atherosclerosis, CAD

Decreased: Inadequate dietary intake (parenteral nutrition, alcoholism); malabsorption; increased needs, eg, PRG or wound healing; acrodermatitis enteropathica; dwarfism

4

LABORATORY DIAGNOSIS: CLINICAL HEMATOLOGY

BLOOD COLLECTION

Venipuncture is discussed in detail in Chapter 13, page 316. The best CBC sample is venous blood drawn with at least a 22-gauge or larger needle. For a routine CBC, venous blood needs to be placed in a special hematology lab tube, usually a purple top tube, that has an anticoagulant (EDTA) and that is mixed gently. Blood for a CBC should be fresh,< 3 h old. Most coagulation studies are submitted in a blue top (citrate) tube. (See page 317 for detailed description of blood collection tubes.) If a **capillary fingerstick** or **heelstick** (see page 279) is used, the hematocrit may be falsely low. If the finger needs to be "milked," sludging of the RBCs can create a falsely high hematocrit. Wright's staining can also be done and viewed as outlined in the next section.

BLOOD SMEARS: WRIGHT'S STAIN

Today, most clinical labs perform automated cell counts. The formal blood smear and Wright's stain can provide a manual differential leukocyte count for the evaluation of anemia or other conditions. The slide is usually available for review by the students or house staff. The main benefit is to allow the identification of abnormal cells or other subtleties that may not be detected by automated systems (Figure 5–1).

Viewing the Film: The Differential WBC

1. Examine the smear in an area where the red cells approximate but do not overlap.
2. If the film is too thin or if a rough-edged spreader is used, up to 50% of the WBCs may accumulate in the edges and tail (See Figure 5–1).
3. WBCs are *not* randomly dispersed even in a well-made smear. Polys and monos predominate at the margins and tail, and lymphs are prevalent in the middle of the film. To overcome this problem, use the "high dry" or oil immersion objective and count cells in a strip running the whole length of the film. Avoid the lateral edges of the film.
4. If fewer than 200 cells are counted in a strip, count another strip until at least 200 are seen. The special white cell counter found in most labs is

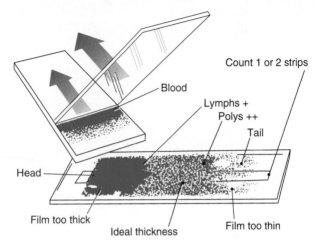

FIGURE 5–1. The technique of preparing a blood smear for staining and the distribution of white blood cells on the standard smear.

ideal for this purpose. In patients receiving chemotherapy, the total count may be so small that only a 25–50 cell differential is possible.

5. In smears of blood from patients with very high white counts, such as those with leukemia, count the cells in any well-spread area where the different cell types are easy to identify. Table 5–1 shows the correlation between the number of cells in a smear and the estimated white cell count. A platelet count can be estimated by averaging the number of platelets seen in 10 hpf (under oil immersion) and multiplying by 20,000.

NORMAL CBC VALUES

A CBC panel generally includes WBC count, RBC count, Hgb, HCT, MCH, MCHC, MCV, and the RDW and platelets (usually). The differential is usually ordered separately. Normal CBC, differential, and platelet values are outlined in Tables 5–2 and 5–3.

TABLE 5–1
Estimated WBC Based on Cells Counted in a Blood Smear

WBC/hpf (high dry or 40×)	Estimated WBC (per mm³)
2–4	4000–7000
4–6	7000–10,000
6–10	10,000–13,000
10–20	13,000–18,000

WBC = white blood cell; hpf = high-power field.

TABLE 5–2
Normal CBC for Selected Age Ranges

Age	WBC Count (cells/mm³) [SI: 10⁹/L]	RBC Count (10⁶/µL) [SI: 10¹²/L]	Hemoglobin (g/dL) [SI: g/L]	Hematocrit (%)	MCH (pg) [SI: pg]	MCHC (g/dL)[a] [SI: g/L]	MCV (µm³) [SI: fL]	RDW
Adult ♂	4500–11,000 [4.5–11.0]	4.73–5.49 [4.73–5.49]	14.40–16.60 [144–166]	42.9–49.1	27–31	33–37	76–100	11.5–14.5
Adult ♀	As above	4.15–4.87 [4.15–5.49]	12.2–14.7 [122–147]	37.9–43.9	As above	As above	As above	As above
11–15 years	4500–13,500	4.8	13.4	39	28	34	82	
6–10 years	5000–14,500	4.7	12.9	37.5	27	34	80	
4–6 years	5500–15,500	4.6	12.6	37.0	27	34	80	
2–4 years	6000–17,000	4.5	12.5	35.5	25	32	77	
4 mon–2 y	6000–17,500	4.6	11.2	35.0	25	33	77	
1 wk–4 mon	5500–18,000	4.7±0.9	14.0±3.3	42.0±7.0	30	33	90	
24 hr–1 wk	5000–21,000	5.1	18.3±4.0	52.5	36	35	103	
First day	9400–34,000	5.1±1.0	19.5±5.0	54.0±10.0	38	36	106	

[a]To convert standard reference value to SI units, multiply by 10.
WBC = white blood cell; MCH = mean cell hemoglobin; MCHC = mean cell hemoglobin concentration; MCV = mean cell volume; RDW = red cell distribution width.

TABLE 5–3
Normal CBC for Selected Age Ranges

Age	Platelet Count (10³/µL) [SI: 10⁹/L]	Lymphocytes, Total (% WBC count)	Neutrophils, Band (% WBC count)	Neutrophils, Segmented (% WBC count)	Eosinophils (% WBC count)	Basophils (% WBC count)	Monocytes (% WBC count)
Adult ♂	238±49	34	3.0	56	2.7	0.5	4.0
Adult ♀	270±58	As above	As above	As above	As above	As above	As above
11–15 y	282±63	38	3.0	51	2.4	0.5	4.3
6–10 y	351±85	39	3.0	50	2.4	0.6	4.2
4–6 y	357±70	42	3.0	39	2.8	0.6	5.0
2–4 y	357±70	59	3.0	30	2.6	0.5	5.0
4 mon–2 y	As above	61	3.1	28	2.6	0.4	4.8
1 wk–4 mon	As above	56	4.5	30	2.8	0.5	6.5
24 hr–1 wk	240–380	24–41	6.8–9.2	39–52	2.4–4.1	0.5	5.8–9.1
First day	As above	24	10.2	58	2.0	0.6	5.8

CBC = complete blood count; WBC = white blood cell.

NORMAL CBC VARIATIONS

Hbg and HCT are highest at birth (20 g/100 mL and 60%, respectively). The values fall steeply to a minimum at 3 mon (9.5 g/100 mL and 32%). Then they slowly rise to near adult levels at puberty, and thereafter both values are higher in males. A normal decrease occurs in pregnancy. The number of WBCs is highest at birth (mean of 25,000/mm^3) and slowly falls to adult levels by puberty. Lymphs predominate (up to 60% from the second week of life until age 5–7 y when polys begin to predominate.

HEMATOCRIT

An equal amount of plasma and red cells are lost in acute blood loss, the HCT will not reflect the loss until sometime later (sometimes 2–3 h). In anemia, the red cell indices and reticulocyte count should be checked.

THE "LEFT SHIFT"

The degree of nuclear lobulation of PMNs is thought to give some indication of cell age. A predominance of immature cells with only one or two nuclear lobes separated by a thick chromatin band is called a **"shift to the left."** Conversely, a predominance of cells with four nuclear lobes is called a **"shift to the right."** (For historical information, left and right designations come from the formerly used manual lab counters, in which the keys for entering the stabs were located on the left of the keyboard.) As a general rule, 55–80% of PMNs have two to four lobes. More than 20 five-lobed cells/100 WBCs suggests megaloblastic anemia, with a six- or seven-lobed poly being diagnostic.

"Bands" or "stabs," the more immature forms of PMNs (the more mature are called "segs"), are identified by the fact that the connections between ends or lobes of a nucleus are greater than one-half the width of the hypothetical round nucleus. In bands or stabs, the connection between the lobes of the nucleus is by a thick band; in segs, by a thin filament. A band is defined as a connecting strip wide enough to reveal two distinct margins with nuclear material in between. A filament is so narrow that no intervening nuclear material is present.

For practical purposes, **a left shift is present in the CBC when more than 10–12% bands are seen or when the total PMN count (segs plus bands) is greater than 80.**

Left Shift: Bacterial infection, toxemia, hemorrhage

Right Shift: Liver disease, megaloblastic anemia, iron deficiency anemia, glucocorticoid use, stress reaction

RETICULOCYTE COUNT

• Collection: Lavender top tube

The reticulocyte count is not a part of the routine CBC. The count is used in the initial work-up of anemia (especially unexplained) and in monitoring the effect of hematinic or erythropoietin therapy, monitoring the recovery from myelosuppression or monitoring engraftment following bone marrow transplant. Reticulocytes are juvenile RBCs with remnants of cytoplasmic basophilic RNA. These are suggested by **basophilia** of the RBC cytoplasm on Wright's stain; however, confirmation requires a special reticulocyte stain. The result is reported as a percentage, and you should calculate the **corrected reticulocyte count** for interpretation of the results

$$\text{Corrected reticulocyte count} = \frac{\text{Reported count} \times \text{Patient's HCT}}{\text{Normal HCT}}$$

This corrected count is an excellent indicator of erythropoietic activity. The **normal corrected reticulocyte count is < 1.5.**

Normal bone marrow responds to a decrease in erythrocytes (shown by a decreased HCT) with an increase in the production of reticulocytes. Lack of increase in a reticulocyte count with an anemia suggests a chronic disease, a deficiency disease, marrow replacement, or marrow failure.

CBC DIFFERENTIAL DIAGNOSIS

• See Tables 5–2 and 5–3 for normal age and sex-specific ranges.

Basophils

• 0–1%

Increased: Chronic myeloid leukemia, after splenectomy, polycythemia, Hodgkin's disease, and, rarely, in recovery from infection and from hypothyroidism

Decreased: Acute rheumatic fever, pregnancy, after radiation, steroid therapy, thyrotoxicosis, stress

Eosinophils

• 1–3%

Increased: Allergy, parasites, skin diseases, malignancy, drugs, asthma, Addison's disease, collagen–vascular diseases (handy mnemonic **NAACP:** **N**eoplasm, **A**llergy/asthma, **A**ddison's disease, **C**ollagen–vascular diseases, **P**arasites), pulmonary diseases including Löffler's syndrome and PIE

Decreased: Steroids, ACTH, after stress (infection, trauma, burns), Cushing's syndrome

Hematocrit (Male 40–54%; Female 37–47%)

Decreased: Megaloblastic anemia (folate or B_{12} deficiency); iron deficiency anemia; sickle cell anemia or other hemoglobinopathies; acute or chronic blood loss; sideroblastic anemia, hemolysis; anemia due to chronic disease, dilution, alcohol, or drugs

Increased: Primary polycythemia (polycythemia vera), secondary polycythemia (reduced fluid intake or excess fluid loss, congenital and acquired heart disease, lung disease, high altitudes, heavy smoking, tumors [renal cell carcinoma, hepatoma], renal cysts)

Lymphocytes

• 24–44% • See also Lymphocyte Subsets, page 98

Increased: Viral infection (AIDS, measles, rubella, mumps, whooping cough, smallpox, chickenpox, influenza, hepatitis, infectious mononucleosis), acute infectious lymphocytosis in children, acute and chronic lymphocytic leukemias

Decreased: (Normal finding in 22% of population.) Stress, burns, trauma, uremia, some viral infections, HIV and AIDS, bone marrow suppression after chemotherapy, steroids, MS

Atypical Lymphocytes

> 20%: Infectious mononucleosis, CMV infection, infectious hepatitis, toxoplasmosis

< 20%: Viral infections (mumps, rubeola, varicella), rickettsial infections, TB

MCH (Mean Cellular [Corpuscular] Hemoglobin)

• 27–31 pg (SI: pg) The weight of hemoglobin of the average red cell. Calculated by

$$MCH = \frac{Hemoglobin\ (g\,/\,L)}{RBC\ (10^6\,/\,\mu L)}$$

Increased: Macrocytosis (megaloblastic anemias, high reticulocyte counts)

Decreased: Microcytosis (iron deficiency, sideroblastic anemia, thalassemia)

MCHC (Mean Cellular [Corpuscular] Hemoglobin Concentration)

• 33–37 g/dL (SI:330–370 g/L) The average concentration of Hbg in a given volume of red cells. Calculated by the formula

$$MCHC = \frac{Hemoglobin\ (g\,/\,dL)}{Hematocrit}$$

Increased: Very severe, prolonged dehydration; spherocytosis

Decreased: Iron deficiency anemia, overhydration, thalassemia, sideroblastic anemia

MCV (Mean Cell [Corpuscular] Volume)

• 78–98 μm^3 (SI: fL) The average volume of red blood cells. Calculated by the formula

$$MCV = \frac{Hematocrit \times 1000}{RBC\ (10^6\,/\,\mu L)}$$

Increased/Macrocytosis: Megaloblastic anemia (B_{12}, folate deficiency), macrocytic (normoblastic) anemia, reticulocytosis, myelodysplasias, Down syndrome, chronic liver disease, treatment of AIDS with AZT, chronic alcoholism, cytotoxic chemotherapy, radiation therapy, Dilantin use, hypothyroidism, newborns

Decreased/Microcytosis: Iron deficiency, thalassemia, some cases of lead poisoning or polycythemia

Monocytes

• 3–7%

Increased: Bacterial infection (TB, SBE, brucellosis, typhoid, recovery from an acute infection), protozoan infections, infectious mononucleosis, leukemia, Hodgkin's disease, ulcerative colitis, regional enteritis

Decreased: Lymphocytic leukemia, aplastic anemia, steroid use

Platelets

- 150–450,000 µL

Platelet counts may be normal in number but abnormal in function, as occurs in aspirin therapy. Abnormalities of platelet function are assessed by bleeding time.

Increased: Sudden exercise, trauma, fracture, after asphyxia, after surgery (especially splenectomy), acute hemorrhage, polycythemia vera, primary thrombocytosis, leukemias, after childbirth, carcinoma, cirrhosis, myeloproliferative disorders, iron deficiency

Decreased: DIC, ITP, TTP, HUS, congenital disease, marrow suppressants (chemotherapy, alcohol, radiation), burns, snake and insect bites, leukemias, aplastic anemias, hypersplenism, infectious mononucleosis, viral infections, cirrhosis, massive transfusions, HELLP syndrome (a severe form of preeclampsia with microangiopathic **h**emolysis, **e**levated **l**iver function tests, and **l**ow **p**latelet counts), preeclampsia and eclampsia, prosthetic heart valve, more than 30 different drugs (NSAIDs, cimetidine, aspirins, thiazides, others)

PMNs (Polymorphonuclear Neutrophils) (Neutrophils)

- 40–76% • See also the "Left Shift" page 95.

Increased

Physiologic (Normal). Severe exercise, last months of pregnancy, labor, surgery, newborns, steroid therapy

Pathologic. Bacterial infections, noninfective tissue damage (MI, pulmonary infarction, pancreatitis, crush injury, burn injury), metabolic disorders (eclampsia, DKA, uremia, acute gout), leukemias

Decreased: Pancytopenia, aplastic anemia, PMN depression (a mild decrease is referred to as **neutropenia,** severe is called **agranulocytosis**), marrow damage (x-rays, poisoning with benzene or antitumor drugs), severe overwhelming infections (disseminated TB, septicemia), acute malaria, severe osteomyelitis, infectious mononucleosis, atypical pneumonias, some viral infections, marrow obliteration (osteosclerosis, myelofibrosis, malignant infiltrate), drugs (more than 70, including chloramphenicol, phenylbutazone, chlorpromazine, quinine), B_{12} and folate deficiencies, hypoadrenalism, hypopituitarism, dialysis, familial decrease, idiopathic causes

RDW (Red Cell Distribution Width)

- 11.5–14.5 RDW is a measure of the degree of **anisocytosis** (variation in RBC size) and is measured by the automated hematology counters.

Increased: Many anemias (iron deficiency, pernicious, folate deficiency, thalassemias), liver disease

LYMPHOCYTE SUBSETS

Specific monoclonal antibodies are used to identify specific T and B cells. Lymphocyte subsets (also called lymphocyte marker assays, or T- and B-cell assay) are useful in the diagnosis of AIDS and various leukemias and lymphomas. The designation **CD ("clusters of differentiation")** has largely replaced the older antibody designations (eg, Leu 3a or OKT3). Results are most reliable when reported as an absolute number of cells/µL rather than a percentage of cells. A

CD4/CD8 ratio < 1 is seen in patients with AIDS. Absolute CD4 count is used to determine when to initiate therapy with antiretrovirals or prophylaxis for certain infections, eg, PCP. The CDC includes in the category of AIDS any HIV-positive patient with a CD4 count < 200.

Normal Lymphocyte Subsets

- Total lymphocytes 0.66–4.60 thousand/μL
- T cell 644–2201 μL (60–88%)
- B cell 82–392 μL (3–20%)
- T helper/inducer cell (CD4, Leu 3a, OKT4) 493–1191 μL (34–67%)
- Suppressor/cytotoxic T cell (CD8, Leu 2, OKT8) 182–785 μL (10–42%)
- CD4/CD8 ratio > 1

RBC MORPHOLOGY DIFFERENTIAL DIAGNOSIS

The following lists some erythrocyte abnormalities and the associated conditions. General terms include **poikilocytosis** (irregular RBC shape such as sickle or burr) and
anisocytosis (irregular RBC size such as microcytes and macrocytes).
Basophilic Stippling: Lead or heavy-metal poisoning, thalassemia, severe anemia
Blister Cell: DIC, microangiopathic anemia, sickle cell, hemolysis
Burr Cells (Acanthocytes): Severe liver disease; high levels of bile, fatty acids, or toxins
Heinz Bodies: Drug-induced hemolysis
Helmet Cells (Schistocytes): Microangiopathic hemolysis, hemolytic transfusion reaction, transplant rejection, other severe anemias, TTP
Howell–Jolly Bodies: After splenectomy, some severe hemolytic anemias, pernicious anemia, leukemia, thalassemia
Nucleated RBCs: Severe bone marrow stress (hemorrhage, hemolysis, etc), marrow replacement by tumor, extramedullary hematopoiesis
Polychromasia (Basophilia): A bluish gray red cell on routine Wright's stain suggests reticulocytes
Sickling: Sickle cell disease and trait
Spherocytes: Hereditary spherocytosis, immune or microangiopathic hemolysis, severe burns, ABO transfusion reactions
Target Cells (Leptocytes): Thalassemia, hemoglobinopathies, obstructive jaundice, any hypochromic anemia, after splenectomy

WBC MORPHOLOGY DIFFERENTIAL DIAGNOSIS

The following are conditions associated with certain changes in the normal morphology of WBCs.

Auer Rods: AML
Döhle's Inclusion Bodies: Severe infection, burns, malignancy, pregnancy
Hypersegmentation: Megaloblastic anemias
Toxic Granulation: Severe illness (sepsis, burn, high temperature)

COAGULATION AND OTHER HEMATOLOGIC TESTS

Megaloblastic anemias
The coagulation cascade is shown in Figure 5–2, page 100. A variety of coagulation-related and other blood tests follow.

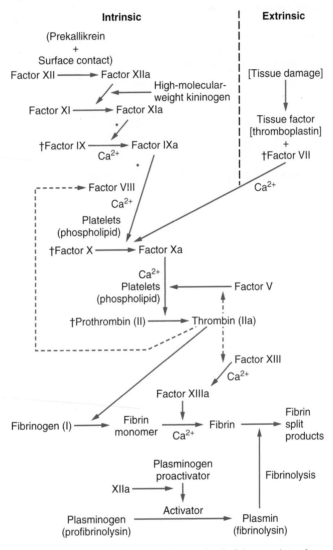

FIGURE 5–2. Blood coagulation cascade. Nearly all of the coagulation factors apparently exist as inactive proenzymes (Roman numeral) that, when activated (Roman numeral + a), serve to activate the next proenzyme in the sequence. * = Heparin acts to inhibit. ⍖ = Plasma content decreased by warfarin.

Activated Clotting Time (ACT)

- 114–186 s • Collection: Black top tube from instrument manufacturer

This is a bedside test used in the operating room, dialysis unit, or other facility to document neutralization of heparin (ie, after CSBG, heparin is reversed.)

Increased: Heparin, some platelet disorders, severe clotting factor deficiency

Antithrombin-III (AT-III)

• 17–30 mg/dL or 80–120% of control • Collection: Blue top tube, patient must be off heparin for 6 h

Used in the evaluation of thrombosis. Heparin must interact with AT-III to produce anticoagulation effect.

Decreased: Autosomal-dominant familial AT-III deficiency, PE, severe liver disease, late pregnancy, oral contraceptives, nephrotic syndrome, heparin therapy (> 3 d)

Increased: Warfarin (Coumadin), after MI

Bleeding Time

• Duke, Ivy < 6 min; Template < 10 min • Collection: Specialized bedside test performed by technicians. A small incision is made, and the wound is wicked with filter paper every 30 s until the fluid is clear

In vivo test of hemostasis, tests platelet function, local tissue factors, and clotting factors. Nonsteroidal medications should be stopped 5–7 d before the test because these agents can affect platelet function.

Increased: Thrombocytopenia (DIC, TTP, ITP), von Willebrand's disease, defective platelet function (NSAIDs such as aspirin)

Coombs' Test, Direct (Direct Antiglobulin Test)

• Normal = negative • Collection: Purple top tube

Uses patient's erythrocytes; tests for the presence of antibody on the patient's cells and used in the screening for autoimmune hemolytic anemia.

Positive: Autoimmune hemolytic anemia (leukemia, lymphoma, collagen–vascular diseases), hemolytic transfusion reaction, some drug sensitizations (methyldopa, levodopa, cephalosporins, penicillin, quinidine), hemolytic disease of the newborn (erythroblastosis fetalis)

Coombs' Test, Indirect (Indirect Antiglobulin Test/Autoantibody Test)

• Normal = negative • Collection: Purple top tube

Uses serum that contains antibody, usually from the patient. Used to check cross-match prior to blood transfusion in the blood bank.

Positive: Isoimmunization from previous transfusion, incompatible blood due to improper cross-matching or medications such as methyldopa.

Fibrin d-Dimers (See also Chapter 4, page 61)

• Negative or < 0.5 mcg/mL • Collection: Blue, green, or purple top tube

Fibrin broken into various D-dimer fragments by plasmin.

Increased: DIC, thromboembolic diseases (PE, arterial or venous thrombosis)

Fibrin Degradation Products (FDP), Fibrin Split Products (FSP)

• < 10 mcg/mL • Collection: Blue top tube

Generally replaced by the fibrin D-dimer as a screen for DIC

Increased: DIC (usually > 40 mcg/mL), any thromboembolic condition (DVT, MI, PE), hepatic dysfunction

Fibrinogen

• 123–370 mg/dL (SI:1.23–3.7 g/L) • (Panic levels < 100 or > 500) • Collection: Blue top tube

   Most useful in the diagnosis of DIC and congenital hypofibrinogenemia. Fibrinogen is cleaved by thrombin to form insoluble fragments that polymerize to form a stable clot.

Increased: Inflammatory reactions, oral contraceptives, pregnancy, cancer (kidney, stomach, breast)

Decreased: DIC (sepsis, amniotic fluid embolism, abruptio placentae), surgery (prostate, open heart), neoplastic and hematologic conditions, acute severe bleeding, burns, venomous snake bite, congenital

Lee–White Clotting Time

• 5–15 min • Collection: Draw into plain plastic syringe; clotting time measured in separate tube

Increased: Heparin therapy, plasma-clotting factor deficiency (except Factors VII and XIII). (*Note:* Not a sensitive test, not considered a good screening test.)

Mixing Study

Used to evaluate prolonged coagulation times. Add normal plasma to patient sample. If problem corrects, a factor deficiency exists (VII,VIII, IX,XI). If not, an inhibitor is present (ie, lupus anticoagulant/antiphospholipid). Prolonged **RVVT (Russell viper venom time)** confirms lupus anticoagulant.

Partial Thromboplastin Time (Activated Partial Thromboplastin Time, PTT, APTT)

• 27–38 s • Collection: Blue top tube

   Evaluates the intrinsic coagulation system (See Figure 5–2). Most commonly used to monitor heparin therapy

Increased: Heparin and any defect in the **intrinsic coagulation system** (includes factors I, II, V, VIII, IX, X, XI, and XII), prolonged use of a tourniquet before drawing a blood sample, hemophilia A and B

Prothrombin Time (PT)

• 11.5–13.5 s (INR, normal = 0.8–1.4) • Collection: Blue top tube

   Evaluates the **extrinsic coagulation system** (see Figure 5–2, page 100) that includes factors I, II, V, VII, and X. The use of **INR** instead of the patient/control ratio to guide anticoagulant (Coumadin) therapy is now the standard. **INR provides a more universal and standardized result because it measures the control against a WHO standard reference reagent.** Therapeutic INR levels are 2–3 for DVT, PE, TIAs, and atrial fibrillation. Mechanical heart valves require an INR of 2.5–3.5 (See also Chapter 22, Table 22–10 [page 622].)

Increased: Drugs (sodium warfarin [Coumadin]), vitamin K deficiency, fat malabsorption, liver disease, prolonged use of a tourniquet before drawing a blood sample, DIC

Sedimentation Rate (Erythrocyte Sedimentation Rate, ESR)

• Collection: Lavender top tube

   A nonspecific test with a high sensitivity and a low specificity. Most useful in serial measurement to follow the course of disease (eg, polymyalgia rheumatica or temporal arteritis). ZETA rate is not affected by anemia. ESR correlates well with C-reactive protein levels.

Wintrobe Scale: Males, 0–9 mm/h, females, 0–20 mm/h

ZETA Scale: 40–54% normal, 55–59% mildly elevated, 60–64% moderately elevated, > 65% markedly elevated

Westergren Scale: Males < 50 years 15 mm/h, > 50 years 20 mm/h; female < 50 years 20 mm/h, > 50 years 30 mm/h

Increased: Any type of infection, inflammation, rheumatic fever, endocarditis, neoplasm, AMI

Thrombin Time

• 10–14 s • Collection: Blue top tube

   Measures conversion of fibrinogen to fibrin and fibrin polymerization. Detects the presence of heparin and hypofibrinogenemia; an aid in the evaluation of prolonged PTT

Increased: Systemic heparin, DIC, fibrinogen deficiency, congenitally abnormal fibrinogen molecules

LABORATORY DIAGNOSIS: URINE STUDIES

URINALYSIS PROCEDURE

For a routine urinalysis, a fresh (less than 1-h old), clean-catch urine is acceptable. If it cannot be performed immediately, refrigerate the sample (urine standing at room temperature for long periods causes lysis of casts and red cells and becomes alkalinized.) See Chapter 13 under Urinary Tract Procedures, page 313, for the different ways to collect the sample.

1. Pour 5–10 mL of well-mixed urine into a centrifuge tube.
2. Check for appearance (color, turbidity, odor).
3. Spin the capped sample at 3000 rpm (450 g) for 3 min.
4. While the sample is in the centrifuge and using the dipstick (Chemstrip, etc) supplied by your lab, perform the dipstick evaluation on the remaining portion of the sample. Read the results according to the color chart and instructions on the bottle. Make sure to allow the correct amount of time before reading the test because reading before the proper amount of time has elapsed (up to 120 s) may yield false results. Record specific gravity, glucose, ketones, blood, protein, pH, nitrite, and leukocyte esterase if available. Agents that color the urine (phenazopyridine [Pyridium]) may interfere with the results of the dipstick.
5. Decant and discard the supernatant. Mix the remaining sediment by flicking it with your finger and pour or pipette one or two drops on a microscope slide. Cover with a coverslip. If a urine sample looks very grossly cloudy, it is sometimes advisable to examine an unspun sample. If an unspun sample is used, make note of this. In general, for routine urinalysis, a spun sample is more desirable.
6. Examine 10 lpf (10× objective) for epithelial cells, casts, crystals, and mucus. Casts are usually reported per low-power field. Casts tend to collect around the periphery of the coverslip.
7. Examine several high-power fields (40× objective) for epithelial cells, crystals, RBCs, WBCs, bacteria, and parasites (trichomonads). RBCs, WBCs, and bacteria are usually reported per high-power field. Two reporting systems are commonly used:

System One	System Two
Rare = < 2/field	Trace = < ¼ of field
Occasional = 3–5/field	1+ = ¼ of field
Frequent = 5–9/field	2+ = ½ of field
Many = "large number"/field	3+ = ¾ of field
TNTC = too numerous to count	4+ = field is full

URINALYSIS, NORMAL VALUES

1. *Appearance:* "Yellow, clear," or "straw-colored, clear"
2. *Specific Gravity*
   a. Neonate: 1.012
   b. Infant: 1.002–1.006
   c. Child and Adult: 1.001–1.035 (typical with normal fluid intake 1.016–1.022)
3. *pH*
   a. Newborn/Neonate: 5–7
   b. Child and Adult: 4.6–8.0
4. *Negative for:* Bilirubin, blood, acetone, glucose, protein, nitrite, leukocyte esterase, reducing substances
5. *Trace:* Urobilinogen
6. *RBC:* Male 0–3/hpf, female 0–5/hpf
7. *WBC:* 0–4/hpf
8. *Epithelial Cells:* Occasional
9. *Hyaline Casts:* Occasional
10. *Bacteria:* None
11. *Crystals:* Some limited crystals based on urine pH (see following section)

DIFFERENTIAL DIAGNOSIS FOR ROUTINE URINALYSIS

Appearance

Colorless: Diabetes insipidus, diuretics, excess fluid intake
Dark: Acute intermittent porphyria, advanced malignant melanoma
Cloudy: UTI (pyuria), amorphous phosphate salts (normal in alkaline urine), blood, mucus, bilirubin
Pink/Red:
Heme(+). Blood, Hbg, sepsis, dialysis, myoglobin
Heme(−). Food coloring, beets, sulfa drugs, nitrofurantoin, salicylates
Orange/Yellow: Dehydration, phenazopyridine (Pyridium), rifampin, bile pigments
Brown/Black: Myoglobin, bile pigments, melanin, cascara, iron, nitrofurantoin, alkaptonuria
Green/Blue: Urinary bile pigments, indigo carmine, methylene blue
Foamy: Proteinuria, bile salts

pH

Acidic: High-protein (meat) diet, ammonium chloride, mandelic acid and other medications, acidosis, (due to ketoacidosis [starvation, diabetic], COPD)

Basic: UTI, renal tubular acidosis, diet (high-vegetable, milk, immediately after meals), sodium bicarbonate therapy, vomiting, metabolic alkalosis

Specific Gravity

Usually corresponds with osmolarity except with osmotic diuresis. Value > 1.023 indicates normal renal concentrating ability. Random value 1.003–1.030

Increased: Volume depletion; CHF; adrenal insufficiency; DM; SIADH; increased proteins (nephrosis); if markedly increased (1.040–1.050), suspect artifact or excretion of radiographic contrast media

Decreased: Diabetes insipidus, pyelonephritis, glomerulonephritis, water load with normal renal function

Bilirubin

Positive: Obstructive jaundice (intrahepatic and extrahepatic), hepatitis. (*Note:* False-positives occur with stool contamination.)

Blood (Hematuria)

Note: If the dipstick is positive for blood, but no red cells are seen, free Hbg may be present; a transfusion reaction may have occurred, from lysis of RBCs (RBCs will lyse if the pH is < 5 or > 8); or myoglobin may be present because of a crush injury, burn, or tissue ischemia.

Positive: Stones, trauma, tumors (benign and malignant, anywhere in the urinary tract), BPH urethral strictures, coagulopathy, infection, menses (contamination), polycystic kidneys, interstitial nephritis, hemolytic anemia, transfusion reaction, instrumentation (Foley catheter, etc)

Glucose

Positive: DM, pancreatitis, pancreatic carcinoma, pheochromocytoma, Cushing's disease, shock, burns, pain, steroids, hyperthyroidism, renal tubular disease, iatrogenic causes. (*Note:* Glucose oxidase technique in many kits is specific for glucose and will not react with lactose, fructose, or galactose.)

Ketones

Detects primarily acetone and acetoacetic acid and not β-hydroxybutyric acid.

Positive: Starvation, high-fat diet, DKA, vomiting, diarrhea, hyperthyroidism, PRG, febrile states (especially in children)

Nitrite

Many bacteria will convert nitrates to nitrite. (See also the section on leukocyte esterase, page 108)

Positive: Infection (negative test does not rule out infection because some organisms, such as *S. faecalis* and other gram-positive cocci, do not produce nitrite, and the urine must also be retained in the bladder for several hours to allow the nitrite reaction to take place.)

Protein

Indication by dipstick of persistent proteinuria should be quantified by 24-h urine studies.

Positive: Pyelonephritis, glomerulonephritis, glomerular sclerosis (diabetes), nephrotic syndrome, myeloma, postural causes, preeclampsia, inflammation and malignancies of the lower tract, functional causes (fever, stress, heavy exercise), malignant hypertension, CHF

Leukocyte Esterase

Test detects 5 WBC/hpf or lysed WBCs. When combined with the nitrite test, it has a positive predictive value of 74% for UTI if both tests are positive and a negative predictive value of > 97% if both tests are negative.

Positive: UTI (false-positive: vaginal/fecal contamination)

Reducing Substances

Positive: Glucose, fructose, galactose, false-positives (vitamin C, salicylates, antibiotics, etc)

Urobilinogen

Positive: Cirrhosis, CHF with hepatic congestion, hepatitis, hyperthyroidism, suppression of gut flora with antibiotics

URINE SEDIMENT

Many labs no longer do microscopic examinations unless specifically requested or if evidence exists for an abnormal finding on dipstick test (eg, positive leukocyte esterase).
Figure 6–1 is a pictorial representation of materials found in urine sediments.

Red Blood Cells (RBCs):   Trauma, pyelonephritis, genitourinary TB, cystitis, prostatitis, stones, tumors (malignant and benign), coagulopathy, and any cause of blood on dipstick test (See previous section on routine urinalysis blood, page 107.)

White Blood Cells (WBCs):   Infection anywhere in the urinary tract, TB, renal tumors, acute glomerulonephritis, radiation, interstitial nephritis (analgesic abuse)

Epithelial Cells: ATN, necrotizing papillitis. (Most epithelial cells are from an otherwise unremarkable urethra.)

Parasites: *Trichomonas vaginalis, Schistosoma haematobium* infection

Yeast: *Candida albicans* infection (especially in diabetics, immunosuppressed patients, or if a vaginal yeast infection is present)

Spermatozoa: Normal in males immediately after intercourse or nocturnal emission

Crystals
Abnormal. Cystine, sulfonamide, leucine, tyrosine, cholesterol
Normal. Acid urine: Oxalate (small square crystals with a central cross), uric
    acid. *Alkaline urine:* Calcium carbonate, triple phosphate (resemble coffin
    lids)

Contaminants: Cotton threads, hair, wood fibers, amorphous substances (all usually unimportant)

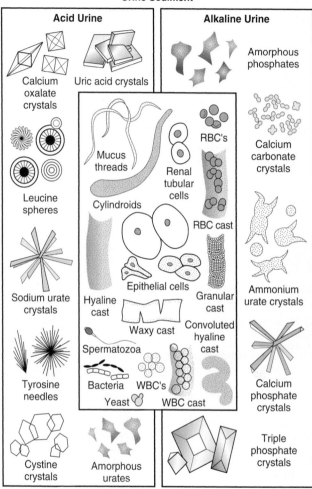

FIGURE 6–1. Urine sediment as seen under the microscope. (Revised with permission, from: Greene MG [ed]: *The Harriet Lane Handbook: A Manual for Pediatric House Officers,* 12th ed., Yearbook Medical Publishers, Chicago, IL, 1991.)

Mucus: Large amounts suggest urethral disease (normal from ileal conduit or other forms of urinary diversion)

Glitter Cells: WBCs lysed in hypotonic solution

Casts: Localizes some or all of the disease process to the kidney itself.

Hyaline Casts. (Acceptable unless they are "numerous"), benign hypertension, nephrotic syndrome, after exercise

RBC Casts. Acute glomerulonephritis, lupus nephritis, SBE, Goodpasture's disease, after a streptococcal infection (poststreptococcal glomerulonephritis), vasculitis, malignant hypertension

WBC Casts. Pyelonephritis, acute interstitial nephritis, glomerulonephritis

Epithelial (Tubular) Casts. Tubular damage, nephrotoxin, virus

Granular Casts. Breakdown of cellular casts, leads to waxy casts; "dirty brown granular casts" typical for ATN

Waxy Casts. (End stage of granular cast). Severe chronic renal disease, amyloidosis

Fatty Casts. Nephrotic syndrome, DM, damaged renal tubular epithelial cells

Broad Casts. Chronic renal disease

6 SPOT OR RANDOM URINE STUDIES

The so-called spot urine, which is often ordered to aid in diagnosing various conditions, relies on only a small sample (10–20 mL) of urine.

Spot Urine for β_2-Microglobulin

• < 0.3 mg/L A marker for renal tubular injury

Increased: Diseases of the proximal tubule (ATN, interstitial nephritis, pyelonephritis), drug-induced nephropathy (aminoglycosides), diabetes, trauma, sepsis, HIV, lymphoproliferative and lymphodestructive diseases

Spot Urine for Electrolytes

The usefulness of this assay is limited because of large variations in daily fluid and salt intake, and the results are usually indeterminate if a diuretic has been given.

1. **Sodium < 10 mEq/L (mmol/L):** Volume depletion, hyponatremic states, prerenal azotemia (CHF, shock, etc), hepatorenal syndrome, glucocorticoid excess
2. **Sodium > 20 mEq/L (mmol/L):** SIADH, ATN (usually > 40 mEq/L), postobstructive diuresis, high salt intake, Addison's disease, hypothyroidism, interstitial nephritis
3. **Chloride < 10 mEq/L (mmol/L):** Chloride-sensitive metabolic alkalosis (vomiting, excessive diuretic use), volume depletion
4. **Potassium < 10 mEq/L (mmol/L):** Hypokalemia, potassium depletion, extrarenal loss

Spot Urine for Erythrocyte Morphology

The morphology of red blood cells in a sample of urine that tests positive for blood may give some indication of the nature of the hematuria. **Eumorphic red cells** are typically seen in cases of postrenal, nonglomerular bleeding. **Dysmorphic red cells** are more likely associated with glomerular causes of bleeding. Labs vary, but > 90% dysmorphic erythrocytes with asymptomatic hematuria indicates a renal glomerular source of bleeding, especially if associated with proteinuria and or casts (ie, IgA nephropathy, poststreptococcal glomerular, sickle cell disease or trait, etc). If there are 90% eumorphic erythrocytes or even "mixed" results (10–90% eumorphic erythrocytes), a postrenal cause of hematuria requires urologic evaluation (ie, hypercalciuria, urolithiasis, cystitis, trauma, tumors, hemangioma, exercise induced, BPH, etc).

Spot Urine for Microalbumin

- Normal < 30 µg albumin/mg creatinine (timed collection < 20 µg/min)

   To determine which patients with diabetes are at risk for nephropathy. Clinical albuminuria occurs at > 300 µg albumin/mg creatinine. Repeat two or three separate determinations over 6 mon. Diabetics with levels between 30–300 µg have microalbuminuria and are usually initiated on ACE inhibitor or angiotensin receptor blocker.

Spot Urine for Myoglobin

- Qualitative negative

Positive: Skeletal muscle conditions (crush injury, electrical burns, carbon monoxide poisoning, delirium tremens, surgical procedures, malignant hyperthermia), polymyositis.

Spot Urine for Osmolality

- 75–300 mOsm/kg (mmol/kg), varies with water intake

   Patients with normal renal function should concentrate > 800 mOsm/kg (mmol/kg) after a 14-h fluid restriction; < 400 mOsm/kg (mmol/kg) is a sign of renal impairment.

Increased: Dehydration, SIADH, adrenal insufficiency, glycosuria, high-protein diet

Decreased: Excessive fluid intake, diabetes insipidus, acute renal failure, medications (acetohexamide, glyburide, lithium)

Spot Urine for Protein

- Normal < 10 mg/dL (0.1 g/L) or < 20 mg/dL (0.2 g/L) for a sample taken in the early AM

   See page 107 for the differential diagnosis of protein in the urine.

CREATININE AND CREATININE CLEARANCE

Normal
Adult Male. Total creatinine 1–2 g/24 h (8.8–17.7 mmol/d); clearance 85–125 mL/min/1.73 m^2
Adult Female. Total creatinine 0.8–1.8 g/24 h (7.1–15.9 mmol/d); clearance 75–115 mL/min 1.73 m^2 (1.25–1.92 mL/s/1.73 m^2)
Child. Total creatinine (> 3 y) 12–30 mg/kg/24 h; clearance 70–140 mL/min/1.73 m^2 (1.17–2.33 mL/s/1.73 m^2)

Decreased: A decreased creatinine clearance results in an increase in serum creatinine usually secondary to renal insufficiency. See Chapter 4, page 60, for differential diagnosis of increased serum creatinine.

Increased: Early DM, pregnancy

Creatinine Clearance (CrCl) Determination

CrCl is one of the most sensitive indicators of early renal insufficiency. Clearances are ordered for patients with suspected renal disease and monitoring patients on nephrotoxic medications, (eg, gentamicin). CrCl decreases with age. A

CrCl of 10–20 mL/min indicates severe renal failure, and usually the need for dialysis. To determine CrCl, order a concurrent SCr and a 24-h urine creatinine. A shorter time interval can be used, for example, 12 h, but the formula must be corrected for this change and a 24-h sample is less prone to collection error.

Example: The following are calculations of (a) CrCl from a 24-h urine sample with a volume of 1000 mL, (b) a urine creatinine of 108 mg/100 mL, and (c) a SCr of 1 mg/100 mL (1 mg/dL).

$$\text{Clearance} = \frac{\text{Urine creatinine} \times \text{Total urine volume}}{\text{Plasma creatinine} \times \text{Time}}$$

where time = 1440 min if 24-h collection.

$$\text{Clearance} = \frac{(108 \text{ mg} / 100 \text{ mL}) \ (1000 \text{ mL})}{(1 \text{ mg} / 100 \text{ mL}) \ (1440 \text{ min})} = 75 \text{ mL} / \text{min}$$

To determine if the urine sample is valid (ie, a full 24-h collection), it should contain 18–25 mg/kg/24 h of creatinine for adult males or 12–20 mg/kg/24 h for adult females. If the patient is an adult (150 lb = body surface area of 1.73 m^2), adjustment of the clearance for body size is not routinely done. Adjustment for pediatric patients is a necessity.

If the values in the previous example were for a 10-year-old boy who weighed 70 lb (1.1 m^2), the clearance would be:

$$75 \text{ mL} / \text{min} \times \frac{1.73 \text{ m}^2}{1.1 \text{ m}^2} = 118 \text{ mL} / \text{min}$$

A rapid determination can be made by a formula:

$$\text{CRCl (male)} = \frac{(140 - \text{Age}) \times (\text{wgt in KG})}{\text{Scr} \times 72}$$
$$\text{CRCl (female)} = 0.85 \times (\text{CRCl male})$$

24-HOUR URINE STUDIES

A wide variety of diseases, most of them endocrine, can be diagnosed by assays of 24-h urine samples.

Calcium, Urine

Normal: On a calcium-free diet < 150 mg/24 h (3.7 mmol/d), average calcium diet (600–800 mg/24 h) 100–250 mg/24 h (2.5–6.2 mmol/d)

Increased: Hyperparathyroidism, hyperthyroidism, hypervitaminosis D, distal renal tubular acidosis (type I), sarcoidosis, immobilization, osteolytic lesions (bony metastasis, multiple myeloma), Paget's disease, glucocorticoid excess, immobilization, furosemide

Decreased: Medications (thiazide diuretics, estrogens, oral contraceptives), hypothyroidism, renal failure, steatorrhea, rickets, osteomalacia

Catecholamines, Fractionated

Used to evaluate neuroendocrine tumors, including pheochromocytoma and neuroblastoma. Avoid caffeine and methyldopa (Aldomet) prior to test

Normal: Values are variable and depend on the assay method used. Norepinephrine 15–80 mg/24 h [SI: 89–473 nmol/24 h], epinephrine 0–20 mg/24 h [0–118 nmol/24 h], dopamine 65–400 mg/24 h [SI: 384–2364 nmol/24 h].

Increased: Pheochromocytoma, neuroblastoma, epinephrine administration, presence of drugs (methyldopa, tetracyclines cause false increases)

Cortisol, Free

Used to evaluate adrenal cortical hyperfunction, screening test of choice for Cushing's syndrome

Normal: 10–110 mg/24 h [SI: 30–300 nmol]

Increased: Cushing's syndrome (adrenal hyperfunction), stress during collection, oral contraceptives, pregnancy

Creatinine

• See pages 60 and 111

Cysteine

Used to detect cystinuria, homocystinuria, monitor response to therapy

Normal: 40–60 mg/g creatinine

Increased: Heterozygotes < 300 mg/g creatinine; homozygotes > 250 mg/g creatinine

5-HIAA (5-Hydroxyindoleacetic Acid)

5-HIAA is a serotonin metabolite useful in diagnosing carcinoid syndrome.

Normal: (2–8 mg [SI: 10.4–41.6] mmol/24-h urine collection)

Increased: Carcinoid tumors (except rectal), certain foods (banana, pineapple, tomato, walnuts, avocado), phenothiazine derivatives

Metanephrines

Detects metabolic products of epinephrine and norepinephrine, a primary screening test for pheochromocytoma

Normal: < 1.3 mg/24 h (7.1 mmol/L) for adults, but variable in children

Increased: Pheochromocytoma, neuroblastoma (neural crest tumors), false-positive with drugs (phenobarbital, guanethidine, hydrocortisone, MAO inhibitors)

Protein

• See also Urine Protein Electrophoresis, pages 80 and 81.

Normal: < 150 mg/24 h (< 0.15 g/d)

Increased: Nephrotic syndrome usually associated with > 3.5 g/1.73 m^2 per 24 h

17-Ketogenic Steroids (17-KGS, Corticosteroids)

Overall adrenal function test, largely replaced by serum or urine cortisol levels

Normal: Males 5–24 mg/24 h (17–83 mmol/24 h); females 4–15 mg/24 h (14–52 mmol/24 h)

Increased: Adrenal hyperplasia (Cushing's syndrome), adrenogenital syndrome

Decreased: Panhypopituitarism, Addison's disease, acute steroid withdrawal

17-Ketosteroids, Total (17-KS)

Measures DHEA, androstenedione (adrenal androgens); largely replaced by assay of individual elements

Normal: Adult males 8–20 mg/24 h (28–69 mmol/L); adult female 6–15 mg/dL (21–52 mmol/L). *Note:* Low values in prepubertal children

Increased: Adrenal cortex abnormalities (hyperplasia [Cushing's disease], adenoma, carcinoma, adrenogenital syndrome), severe stress, ACTH or pituitary tumor, testicular interstitial tumor and arrhenoblastoma (both produce testosterone)

Decreased: Panhypopituitarism, Addison's disease, castration in men

Vanillylmandelic Acid (VMA)

VMA is the urinary product of both epinephrine and norepinephrine; good screening test for pheochromocytoma, also used to diagnose and follow up neuroblastoma and ganglioneuroma

Normal: < 7–9 mg/24 h (35–45 mmol/L)

Increased: Pheochromocytoma, other neural crest tumors (ganglioneuroma, neuroblastoma), factitious (chocolate, coffee, tea, methyldopa)

OTHER URINE STUDIES
Drug Abuse Screen

• Normal = negative.

Tests for common drugs of abuse, often used for employment screening for critical jobs. Assay will vary by facility and may include tests for amphetamines, barbiturates, benzodiazepines, marijuana (cannabinoid metabolites), cocaine metabolites, opiates, phencyclidine.

Xylose Tolerance Test (D-Xylose Absorption Test)

• 5 g xylose in 5-h urine specimen after 25 g oral dose of xylose or 1.2 g after 5-g oral dose • Collection: Patient is NPO after midnight except for water • After 8 AM void, 25 g of D-xylose (or 5 g if GI irritation is a concern) is dissolved in 250 mL water • An additional 750 mL water is drunk and the urine collected for the next 5 h.

Used to assess proximal bowel function; differentiates between malabsorption due to pancreatic insufficiency or intestinal problems.

TABLE 6–1
Urinary Indices Useful in the Differential Diagnosis of Oliguria

Index	Prerenal	Renal (ATN)[a]
Urine osmolality	>500	<350
Urinary sodium	<20	>40
Urine/serum creatinine	>40	<20
Urine/serum osmolarity	>1.2	<1.2
Fractional excreted sodium[b]	<1	>1
Renal failure index (RFI)[c]	<1	>1

[a]Acute tubular necrosis (intrinsic renal failure).

$$^b\text{Fractional excreted sodium} = \frac{\text{Urine / Serum sodium}}{\text{Urine / Serum creatinine}} \times 100$$

$$^c\text{Renal failure index} = \frac{\text{Urine sodium} \times \text{Serum creatinine}}{\text{Urine creatinine}}$$

6

Decreased: Celiac disease (nontropical sprue, gluten-sensitive enteropathy), false decrease with renal disease

URINARY INDICES IN RENAL FAILURE

Use Table 6–1 to help differentiate the causes (renal or prerenal) of oliguria. (See also Oliguria and Anuria, page 42.)

URINE OUTPUT

Although clinical situations vary greatly, the usual, minimal acceptable urine output for an adult is 0.5–1.0 mL/kg/h (daily volume normally 1000–1600 mL/d).

URINE PROTEIN ELECTROPHORESIS

See Protein Electrophoresis, Serum and Urine, page 80, and Figure 4–5, page 81.

CLINICAL MICROBIOLOGY

STAINING TECHNIQUES

Acid-Fast Stain (AFB Smear, Kinyoun Stain)

Clinical microbiology labs can also perform a "modified" acid-fast stain for organisms that are weakly acid-fast-staining (eg, *Nocardia* spp.).

Procedure
1. Spread the smear on a slide, allow it to air dry, and then gently heat fix it.
2. Stain the smear for 3–5 min with terpinol in carbol-fuchsin red solution.
3. Rinse the slide with tap water.
4. Decolorize with acid–alcohol solution for no longer than 30 s.
5. Rinse with tap water.
6. Counterstain with methylene blue for 1 min.
7. Rinse the slide with tap water and allow it to air dry.
8. Examine the smear with high dry and oil immersion lenses; search for the acid-fast bacilli that stain red to bright pink against the light blue background (*Mycobacterium tuberculosis* [TB], *M. scrofulaceum, M. avium-intracellulare,* others). These organisms have a beaded rod appearance under oil immersion.
9. These organisms must be cultured on specialized media. Rapid-growing AFB include *M. abscessus, M. chelonae, and M. fortuitum* and can usually be cultured in fewer than 7 d. Most other AFB (*M. tuberculosis, M. avium* complex, *M. kansasii, M. marinum*) require at least 7–10 d to grow. *M. gordonae* is thought to be nonpathogenic.

Darkfield Examination

Darkfield examination is used to identify *Treponema pallidum,* the organism responsible for syphilis. Rectal and oral lesions cannot be examined by this technique due to the presence of nonpathogenic spirochetes.

Procedure

1. The chancre is cleansed with a saline-moistened swab, and a slide is touched on the lesion and examined under darkfield illumination within 15 min of applying the specimen to the slide.

2. The organisms resemble tight corkscrews and are $1-1\frac{1}{2} \times$ the diameter of an RBC in length.

Giemsa Stain

Used to identify intracellular organisms such as chlamydiae, *Plasmodium* (malaria), and other parasites.

Gonorrhea Smear (See page 124 Gonorrhea [GC] Cultures)
Gram Stain

The Gram stain is used to determine whether an organism can be decolorized with alcohol after being stained with crystal violet. This determination is based on the organism's cell wall characteristics. Gram staining is performed on bacteria from a variety of body fluids, including exudates, abscesses, sputum, and others as clinically indicated.

Procedure

1. Smear the specimen (sputum, peritoneal fluid, etc) on a glass slide in a fairly thin coat. If time permits, allow the specimen to air dry. The smear may also be fixed under very low heat (excessive heat can cause artifacts). If a Bunsen burner is not available, other possible methods for heating the sample include using a hot light bulb or setting an alcohol swab on fire. Heat the slide until it is warm, but not hot, when touched to the back of the hand.

2. Timing for the stain is not critical, but allow at least 10 s for each set of reagents.

3. Apply the **crystal violet (Gram stain)**, rinse the slide with tap water, apply iodine solution, and rinse with water.

4. Decolorize the slide carefully with the acetone–alcohol solution until the blue color is barely visible in the runoff. (Be careful; this is the step where most Gram stains are ruined.)

5. Counterstain with a few drops of safranin, rinse the slide with water, and blot it dry with lint-free bibulous or filter paper.

6. Use the high dry and oil immersion lenses on the microscope to examine the slide. If the Gram stain is satisfactory, any polys on the slide should be pink with light blue nuclei. On a Gram stain of **sputum,** an excessive number of epithelial cells (> 25/hpf) means the sample contained more saliva than sputum. **Gram-positive organisms stain dark blue to purple; gram-negative ones stain red.**

Gram Stain Characteristics of Common Pathogens

Initial lab reports identify the Gram stain characteristics of the organisms. Complete identification usually requires culturing the organism. The lab algorithms for gram-positive and gram-negative organisms are shown in Figures 7–1 and 7–2, respectively. Gram stain characteristics of clinically important bacteria are shown in Table 7–1, page 121.

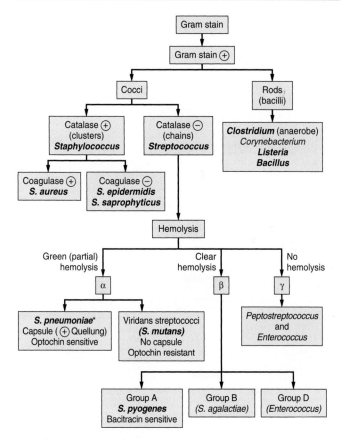

*Important pathogens are in **bold type**.
 Note: Enterococcus is Group D but it is not β-hemolytic; it is α- or γ-hemolytic.

FIGURE 7–1 Lab algorithm for the identification of gram-positive organisms. (Reprinted, with permission, from: Bhushan, V [ed]: *First Aid for the USMLE, Step 1,* McGraw-Hill, 2003.)

India Ink Preparation

India ink is used primarily on CSF to identify fungal organisms (especially cryptococci).

KOH Preparation

KOH (potassium hydroxide) preps are used to diagnose fungal infections. Vaginal KOH preps are discussed in detail in Chapter 13, page 298.

Procedure

1. Apply the specimen (vaginal secretion, sputum, hair, skin scrapings) to a slide. Skin scrapings of a lesion are usually obtained by gentle scraping with a No. 15 scalpel blade (see page 247 for description).

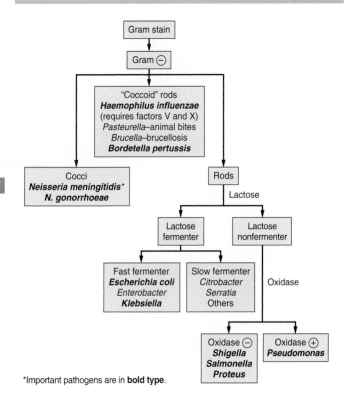

FIGURE 7–2 Lab algorithm for the identification of gram-negative organisms. (Reprinted, with permission, from: Bhushan, V [ed]: *First Aid for the USMLE, Step 1*, McGraw-Hill, 2003.)

2. Add 1–2 gtt of 10% KOH solution and mix. Gentle heating (optional) may accelerate dissolution of the keratin. A fishy odor from a vaginal prep suggests the presence of *Gardnerella vaginalis* (see page 298)

3. Put a coverslip over the specimen, and examine the slide for the branching hyphae and blastospores that indicate the presence of a fungus. KOH should destroy most elements other than fungus. If dense keratin and debris are present, allow the slide to sit for several hours and then repeat the microscopic examination. Lowering the substage condenser provides better contrast between organisms and the background.

Stool Leukocyte Stain (Fecal Leukocytes, Löffler Methylene Blue Stain)

Differentiates treatable diarrhea (ie, bacterial) from other causes. This method detects causes from Crohn's disease, ulcerative colitis, TB, and amebic infection as well, but many causes of severe diarrhea are viral. The positive predictive value of a bacterial pathogen as a cause for the diarrhea is 70%.

TABLE 7–1
Gram Stain Characteristics and Key Features of Common Organisms[a]

Gram Staining Pattern and Organisms	Identifying Key Features
Gram-Positive Cocci	
Enterococcus spp. (*E. faecalis*) (*Note:* These are equivalent group D *Streptococcus*)	Pairs, chains; catalase-negative
Peptostreptococcus spp.	Anaerobic
Staphylococcus spp.	Clusters; catalase-positive
Staphylococcus aureus	Clusters; catalase-positive; coagulase-positive; beta-hemolytic; yellow pigment
Staphylococcus epidermidis	Clusters; catalase-positive; coagulase-negative; skin flora
Staphylococcus saprophyticus	Clusters; catalase-positive; coagulase-negative
Streptococcus spp.	Pairs, chains; catalase-negative
Streptococcus agalactiae (group B)	Pairs, chains; catalase-negative; vaginal flora
Streptococcus bovis (group D *Enterococcus*)	Pairs, chains; catalase-negative
Streptococcus faecalis (group D *Enterococcus*)	Pairs, chains; catalase-negative
Streptococcus pneumoniae (*Pneumococcus*, group B)	Pairs, lancet-shaped; alpha-hemolytic; optochin-sensitive
Streptococcus pyogenes (group A)	Beta-hemolytic
Streptococcus viridans	Pairs, chains; catalase-negative; alpha-hemolytic, optochin-resistant
Gram-Negative Cocci	
Acinetobacter spp.	Filamentous, branching pattern
Moraxella (*Branhamella*) *catarrhalis*	Diplococci in pairs
Neisseria gonorrhoeae (gonococcus)	Diplococci in pairs, often intracellular; ferments glucose but not maltose
Neisseria meningitidis (meningococcus)	Diplococci in pairs; ferments glucose and maltose
Veillonella spp.	Anaerobic

(continued)

TABLE 7–1
(Continued)

Gram Staining Pattern and Organisms	Identifying Key Features
Gram-Positive Bacilli	
Actinomyces	Branching, beaded, rods; anaerobic
Bacilli anthracis (anthrax)	Spore-forming rod
Clostridium spp. (*C. difficile, C. botulinum, C. tetani*)	Large, with spores; anaerobic
Corynebacterium spp. (*C. diphtheriae*)	Small, pleomorphic diphtheroid; skin flora
Eubacterium spp.	Anaerobic
Lactobacillus spp.	Common vaginal bacterium; anaerobic
Listeria monocytogenes	Beta-hemolytic
Mycobacterium spp. (limited staining)	Only rapidly growing species gram stain (*M. abscessus, M. chelonae, M. fortuitum*)
Nocardia	Beaded, branched rods; partially acid-fast-staining
Propionibacterium acne	Small, pleomorphic diphtheroid; anaerobic
Gram-Negative Bacilli	
Acinetobacter spp.	Lactose-negative, oxidase-negative
Aeromonas hydrophilia	Lactose-negative (usually), oxidase-positive
Bacteroides fragilis	Anaerobic
Bordetella pertussis	Coccoid rod
Brucella (brucellosis)	Coccoid rod
Citrobacter spp.	Lactose-positive (usually)
Enterobacter spp.	Lactose-positive (usually)
Escherichia coli	Lactose-positive
Fusobacterium spp.	Long, pointed shape; anaerobic
Haemophilus ducreyi (chancroid)	Gram-negative bacilli
Haemophilus influenzae	Coccoid rod, requires chocolate agar to support growth
Klebsiella spp.	Lactose-positive
Legionella pneumophila	Stains poorly, use silver stain and special medium
Morganella morganii	Lactose-negative, oxidase-negative

(continued)

TABLE 7–1
(Continued)

Gram Staining Pattern and Organisms	Identifying Key Features
Gram-Negative Bacilli	
Proteus mirabilis	Lactose-negative, oxidase-negative, indole-negative
Proteus vulgaris	Lactose-negative, oxidase-negative, indole-positive
Providencia spp.	Lactose-negative, oxidase-negative
Pseudomonas aeruginosa	Lactose-negative, oxidase-positive blue-green pigment
Salmonella spp.	Lactose-negative, oxidase-negative
Serratia spp.	Lactose-negative, oxidase-negative
Serratia marcescens	Lactose-negative, oxidative-negative, red pigment
Shigella spp.	Lactose-negative, oxidase-negative
Stenotrophomonas (Xanthomonas) maltophilia	Lactose-negative, oxidase-negative
Vibrio cholerae (cholera)	Gram-negative bacilli
Yersinia enterocolitica	Gram-negative bacilli
Yersinia pestis (bubonic plague)	Gram-negative bacilli

ᵃOrganisms are aerobic unless otherwise specified.

Procedure
1. Mix a small amount of stool or mucus on a slide with 2 gtt of Löffler (methylene blue) stain. Mucus is preferred; if no mucus is present, use a small amount of stool from the outside of a formed stool.
2. Place a coverslip and then examine the smear after 2–3 min to allow the white cells to take up the stain. The presence of many leukocytes suggests a bacterial cause. Increased white cells (usually polys) are seen in *Shigella, Salmonella, Campylobacter, Clostridium difficile,* and enteropathogenic *Escherichia coli* infections, as well as ulcerative colitis and pseudomembranous colitis. White cells are absent in cholera and in *Giardia* and viral (rotavirus, Norwalk virus, etc) infections.

Tzanck Smear

This technique (named after Arnault Tzanck) is used in the diagnosis of herpesvirus infections (ie, herpes zoster or simplex).

Procedure
1. Clean a vesicle (not a pustule or crusted lesion) with alcohol, allow it to air dry, and gently unroof it with a No. 15 scalpel blade. Scrape the base with the blade, and place the material on a glass slide.
2. Allow the sample to air dry, and stain with Wright's stain as used for peripheral blood. Giemsa stain can also be used; however, the sample must be fixed for 10 min with methyl alcohol before the Giemsa is applied.
3. Scan the slide under low power, and identify cellular areas. Then use high-power oil immersion to identify multinucleated giant cells (epithelial cells infected with herpes viruses). This strongly suggests viral infection; culture is necessary to identify the specific virus.

Vaginal Wet Preparation

- See Chapter 13, page 298

Wayson Stain

Wayson stain is a good quick scout stain that colors most bacteria.

Procedure
1. Spread the smear on a slide, and air or heat dry it.
2. Pour freshly filtered Wayson stain onto the slide, and allow it to stand for 10–20 s (timing is not critical).
3. Rinse the slide gently with tap water, and dry it with filter paper.
4. Use the high dry and oil immersion lenses to examine the slide.

GONORRHEA (GC) CULTURES AND SMEAR

Neisseria gonorrhea can be cultured from many different sites, including female genital tract (endocervix is the preferred site), male urethra, urine, anorectum, throat, and synovial fluid, and the specimen is plated on selective (**Thayer–Martin** or **Transgrow**) media. Due to the high incidence of coinfection with *Chlamydia* and *T. pallidum* (syphilis), *Chlamydia* cultures and syphilis serology should also be performed, especially in females with genital infections with GC. Anorectal stains may contain nonpathogenic *Neisseria* spp.; avoid fecal contact; apply swab to anal crypts. In males with a urethral discharge, insert a **calcium alginate swab (Calgiswab)** into the urethra to collect the specimen and then plate.

The GC smear (see Chapter 13, page 298) has a low sensitivity (< 50% in female endocervical smear), but is fairly reliable (> 95%) in males with urethral discharge. A rapid enzyme immunoassay (**gonococcal antigen assay [Gonozyme]**) is available to diagnose cervical or urethral GC (not throat or anus) infections in less than 1 h. DNA probe testing is becoming widespread for rapid diagnosis.

NASOPHARYNGEAL CULTURES

Specimen for culture should be obtained from deep in the nasopharynx and not the anterior nares, and the swab should not touch the skin. Cultures of nasopharyngeal specimens are useful in identifying *Staphylococcus aureus* and *N. meningitidis* infections. Normal nasal flora include *Staphylococcus epidermidis* and *S. aureus*, *Streptococcus pneumoniae*, *Haemophilus influenzae*, and several others.

BLOOD CULTURES

Blood cultures are not usually indicated for the routine work-up of fever. The best use is for

1. Fever of unknown origin, especially in adults with WBC > 15,000/mm^3 and no localizing signs or symptoms to suggest the source. Remember, a normal white count or leukopenia with a bandemia can be present with sepsis.
2. Clinical situations in which the diagnosis is established by a positive blood culture (eg, acute and SBE).
3. Febrile elderly, neutropenic, or immunocompromised patients.

Chills and fever usually ensue from $\frac{1}{2}$–2 h after sudden entry of bacteria into the circulation (bacteremia). If bacteremia is suspected, several sets of cultures are usually needed to improve the chances of culturing the offending organism. Ideally, more than one set of cultures should be done at least 1 h apart; drawing more than three sets of specimens a day does not usually increase the yield. Obtain the blood through venipuncture, and avoid sampling through venous lines. Each "set" of specimens for blood culture consists of both an aerobic and anaerobic culture bottle. If possible, culture the specimens before antibiotics are initiated; if the patient is already on antibiotics, use **ARD** culture bottles, which absorb the antibiotic that may otherwise destroy any bacteria. *Legionella, Mycobacterium, Bordetella,* and *Histoplasma* may require special blood collection devices.

Procedure

1. Review the section on the technique of venipuncture (Chapter 13 page 316). Apply a tourniquet above the chosen vein.
2. Paint the venipuncture site with a povidone-iodine solution. Repeat this procedure 3 × with a different pad. Then wipe the area around the vein with alcohol and allow the alcohol to dry.
3. Use an 18–22-gauge needle (or smaller if needed) and a 10–20-mL syringe. Enter the skin over the prepped vein, and aspirate a sufficient volume of blood (10–20 mL in adults, 1–5 mL in children); adequate volume will increase the detection rate. **Be careful not to touch the needle or the prepped skin site.** Draw about 10 mL of blood. Remove the tourniquet, compress the venipuncture site, and apply an adhesive bandage.
4. Discard the needle used in the puncture and replace it with a **new, sterile** 20–22-gauge needle. Place the blood in each of the bottles by allowing the vacuum to draw in the appropriate volume, usually specified on the collection device. Submit the samples to the lab promptly with the appropriate lab slips completed, including current antibiotics being given.

Interpretation

Preliminary results are usually available in 12–48 h; cultures should not be formally reported as negative before 4 d. A single blood culture that is positive for one of the following organisms usually suggests contamination; however, on rare occasions these agents are the causative pathogen: *Staphylococcus epidermidis, Staphylococcus hominis, Bacillus* spp., *Corynebacterium diphtheriae* (and other diphtheroids). Negative results do not rule out bacteremia, and false-positives can result from contamination. Gram-negative organisms, fungi, and anaerobes are considered to be pathogenic until proven otherwise.

SPUTUM CULTURES

Cultures of sputum remain controversial. Many clinicians do not even order sputum cultures and treat only based on the Gram stain and clinical findings. One problem is that "sputum" samples often contain only saliva. If you do a Gram stain on the specimen and see only a few squamous cells, with many polys and histiocytes, the sample is good, and the culture will probably be reliable. Excessive numbers of squamous cells (see previous section on Gram stain, page 118) suggests that the sample is more saliva than sputum. An early morning sample is most likely to be from deep within the bronchial tree.

Steps to Improve the Quality of the Sputum Collection

1. Careful instructions to the patient.
2. If the patient cannot mobilize the secretions, P&PD along with nebulizer treatments may help.
3. Careful nasotracheal suctioning using a specimen trap.

Most labs will not accept anaerobic sputum cultures (critical in the diagnosis of aspiration pneumonia and lung abscesses) unless obtained by **transtracheal aspirate** or **endobronchial endoscopic collection** and submitted in special anaerobic transport media.

Viral, *Legionella, Mycoplasma,* and TB cultures require special culture materials available at most labs. **PCP** can be diagnosed by expectorated sputum about 10% of the time; therefore open-lung biopsy, endobronchial lavage, or other invasive techniques must be used to demonstrate the organisms. Specialized staining techniques for identifying ***Pneumocystis carinii*** include the methenamine silver, Giemsa, and toluidine blue stains.

STOOL CULTURES

A fresh stool sample is cultured to diagnose the cause of diarrhea or to identify disease carriers. Most common pathogens (*Salmonella, Shigella,* enteropathogenic *E. coli,* etc) can be grown on standard media. *Yersinia* and *Campylobacter* require a special culture medium.

A quick bedside test for bacterial causes of diarrhea is to check the stool for white cells (fecal leukocyte smear; see page 120).

Clostridium difficile Assay

Clostridium difficile is usually best diagnosed by determining the presence of *C. difficile* enterotoxin in the stool (See Chapter 4) and not by culture.

Stool for Ova and Parasites

With toxic diarrhea, the possibility of parasitic disease must be considered, and stool for **"ova and parasites"** should be ordered. Protozoa (ameba [*Entamoeba histolytica,* others] and *Blastocystis, Giardia*) cannot be cultured and are identified by seeing mature, mobile organisms or cysts on microscopic examination of freshly passed feces. Immunosuppressed (eg, HIV-positive) individuals may demonstrate *Cryptosporidium, Microsporidia,* and *Isospora belli. Strongyloides* often causes GI symptoms in immunocompetent individuals.

The ova are most frequently identified in the stool of parasites such as nematodes (*Ascaris, Strongyloides*), cestodes (*Taenia, Hymenolepis*), and trematodes (*Schistosoma*).

THROAT CULTURES

Used to differentiate viral from bacterial (usually group A beta-hemolytic streptococci, eg, *Streptococcus pyogenes*) pharyngitis.

Procedure

1. The best culture is obtained with the help of a tongue blade and a good
    light source.
2. **If epiglottitis (croup) is suspected (stridor, drooling), a culture should
    not be attempted.**
3. Use the culture swab and try not to touch the oral mucosa or tongue, but
    only the involved area. In the uncooperative patient, an arch-like swath
    touching both the tonsillar areas and posterior pharynx should be at-
    tempted.

Many labs perform a specific **"strep screen"** to rapidly identify group A
beta-hemolytic streptococci. Normal flora on routine culture can include alpha-
hemolytic strep, nonhemolytic Staph, saprophytic *Neisseria* spp., *Haemophilus,
Klebsiella, Candida,* and diphtheroids.

Other pathogens can cause pharyngitis. If **Neisseria gonorrhoeae** is suspected, use Thayer–Martin medium. Diphtheria (**C. diphtheriae**) with its characteristic pseudo-membrane, should be cultured on special media and the lab
notified.

URINE CULTURES

As is true for sputum cultures, culturing for urinary tract pathogens is often controversial. Some clinicians base their decision to treat only when the culture is
positive, whereas others rely on the presence of WBC or bacteria in the urinalysis, using cultures only for sensitivities in refractory infections. The introduction
of urine dipsticks to detect leukocytes (by the detection of leukocyte esterase)
aids in the decision-making when cultures are not obtained or are confusing.
Routine cultures fail to diagnose other urinary tract pathogens such as *N. gonorrhea* or *Chlamydia.*

A clean-catch urine (see Chapter 13, page 313) is about 85% accurate in females and uncircumcised males. In general, a positive culture is a colony count
of > 100,000 bacteria/mL of urine or a count from 10,000–100,000 bacteria/mL
of urine in the presence of pyuria. If the culture is critical for diagnosis, obtain
an in-and-out catheterized urine (page 314) or suprapubic aspiration in children
(page 316). Any growth of bacteria on an in-and-out catheterized or suprapubic
specimen is considered to represent a true infection.

If a urine specimen cannot be taken to the lab within 60 min, refrigerate it.
The lab assumes that more than three organisms growing on a culture represents
a contaminant and the specimen collection should be repeated. The exception
occurs in patients with a chronic indwelling Foley catheter that may be colo-
nized with multiple bacterial or fungal organisms; the lab should be told to "culture all organisms" in such cases.

VIRAL CULTURES AND SEROLOGY

The laboratory provides the proper collection container for the specific virus.
Common pathogenic viruses cultured include **herpes simplex** (from genital
vesicles, throat), **CMV** (from urine or throat), **varicella-zoster** (from skin vesi-

cles in children with chickenpox and adults with shingles), and enterovirus (rectal swab, throat).

For serologic testing, obtain an **acute specimen (titer)** as early as possible in the course of the illness, and take a **convalescent specimen (titer)** 2–4 wk later. A fourfold or greater rise in the convalescent titer compared with the acute titer indicates an active infection (see Chapter 4 for selected viral antibody titers). With the development of PCR techniques, biopsies performed on older lesions may yield useful information when cultures might be negative.

SCOTCH TAPE TEST

Also known as a "pinworm preparation," this method is used to identify infestation with *Enterobius vermicularis*. A 3-in. piece of *clear* Scotch tape is attached around a glass slide (sticky side out). The slide is applied to the perianal skin in four quadrants and examined under the microscope for pinworm eggs. The best sample is collected either in the early morning prior to bathing or several hours after retiring.

MOLECULAR MICROBIOLOGY

Molecular techniques can now identify many bacterial and viral organisms without culturing. Many tests rely on DNA probes to identify the pathogens. The following includes some microbes commonly identified from clinical specimens (ie, swab, serum, tissue). Availability varies with each clinical facility.

Common Microorganisms Identifiable by PCR/DNA Probe

- *Chlamydia trachomatis*
- *Borrelia burgdorferi* (Lyme disease)
- HIV
- *Mycoplasma pneumoniae*
- *Mycobacterium tuberculosis*
- *Neisseria gonorrhoeae*
- Hepatitis B
- HPV
- Many others under development

SUSCEPTIBILITY TESTING

To more effectively treat a specific infection by choosing the right antibiotic, many labs routinely provide the MIC or MBC. For more complex infections (endocarditis), Schlichter testing is sometimes used.

MIC (Minimum Inhibitory Concentration)

This is the lowest concentration of antibiotic that prevents an in vitro growth of bacteria.

The organism is tested against a battery of antimicrobials in concentrations normally achieved in vivo and reported as

Susceptible (S):   The organism is inhibited by the agent in the usual dose and route, and the drug should be effective.

Intermediate (I):   Sometimes also reported as "indeterminate," this implies that high doses of the drug, such as those achieved with parenteral therapy (IM, IV), most likely inhibit the organism.

Resistant (R):   The organism is resistant to the usual levels achieved by the drug.

MBC (Minimum Bactericidal Concentration)

Similar to the MIC, but indicates the lowest antibiotic concentration that will kill 99.9% of the organisms. The MBC results in killing the organisms, and the MIC prevents growth but may not kill the organism.

Schlichter Test (Serum Bacteriocidal Level)

Used to determine the antibacterial level of the serum or CSF of patients who are receiving antibiotic therapy. The test uses eight serial dilutions of the patient's serum (1:1 through 1:128) to determine what dilution is bactericidal to the infecting organism. The test is usually coordinated through the microbiology laboratory. One set of blood or CSF cultures must be negative for the infecting organism before the test is performed. Opinion varies greatly as to interpretation of the results. Optimal killing of the organism occurs at dilutions of blood (and CSF) ranging anywhere from a trough of 1:4 to a peak of 1:8. That is, a result such as "*S. aureus* bactericidal level = 1:8" means the infecting organism was killed at a serum dilution of 1:8. Some data suggest higher titers (1:32) are needed to treat bacterial endocarditis. For the test to be performed, the organisms responsible for the infection must be isolated from a patient specimen before the test can be run.

DIFFERENTIAL DIAGNOSIS OF COMMON INFECTIONS AND EMPIRIC THERAPY

The pathogens causing common infectious diseases are outlined in Table 7–2 along with some empiric therapeutic recommendations. The antimicrobial drug of choice for the treatment of infection is usually the most active drug against the pathogenic organism or the least toxic alternative among several effective agents. The choice of drugs is modified by the site of infection, clinical status (allergy, renal disease, pregnancy, etc), and susceptibility testing.

Tables 7–3 through 7–7 provide empiric treatment guidelines for some common infectious diseases, including bacterial, fungal, viral, HIV, parasitic, and tick-borne diseases.

SBE PROPHYLAXIS

The following recommendations are based on guidelines published by the American Heart Association (*JAMA* 1997;**277**:1794). The guidelines specify which patients are at high, moderate, or low risk of bacteremia and indicate which procedures are more likely to be associated with bacterial endocarditis. **SBE prophylaxis is recommended only for patients who are at high or moderate risk.** See Tables 7–8 page 155 and 7–9 page 156 for regimens.

High-Risk: Prosthetic cardiac valves, history of bacterial endocarditis, complex cyanotic congenital heart disease, surgically constructed systemic pulmonary shunts

Moderate-Risk: Most other congenital cardiac malformations (other than those in the previous or following lists), acquired valvular disease (eg, rheumatic heart disease), hypertrophic cardiomyopathy, mitral valve prolapse with regurgitation or thickened leaflets

Low-Risk: Isolated ASD secundum; repair of atrial/ventricular septal defect, or PDA; prior CABG; mitral valve prolapse without regurgitation; innocent heart murmurs; previous Kawasaki disease or rheumatic fever without valve dysfunction; pacemakers or implanted defibrillator

TABLE 7-2
Organisms Responsible for Common Infectious Diseases with Recommended Empiric Therapy[a]

Site/Condition	Common Uncommon but Important	Common Empiric Therapy (Modify based on clinical factors such as Gram stain)
BONES AND JOINTS		
Osteomyelitis	*Staphylococcus aureus* Enterobacteriaceae If nail puncture: *Pseudomonas* spp.	Oxacillin, nafcillin
Joint, septic arthritis	*S. aureus* Group A strep Enterobacteriaceae Gonococci	Oxacillin; ceftriaxone if gonococci
Joint, prosthetic	*S. aureus, S. epididymis, Streptococcus* spp.	Vancomycin plus ciprofloxacin
BREAST		
Mastitis, postpartum	*S. aureus*	Cefazolin, nafcillin, oxacillin
BRONCHITIS	In adolescent/young patient: *Mycoplasma pneumoniae* Respiratory viruses In chronic adult infection: *Streptococcus pneumoniae Haemophilus influenzae Moraxella catarrhalis Chlamydia pneumoniae*	Treatment controversial because most infections are viral; treat if febrile, or associated with sinusitis, positive sputum culture in patients with COPD or if duration >7 days; doxycycline, eryhromycin, azithromycin, clarithromycin

(continued)

TABLE 7-2
(Continued)

Site/Condition	Common Uncommon but Important	Common Empiric Therapy (Modify based on clinical factors such as Gram stain)
CERVICITIS (nongonococcal) *CHANCHROID* *CHLAMYDIA*	*Chlamydia, Mycoplasma hominis,* *Ureaplasma,* others *Haemophilus ducreyi*	Azithromycin single dose, doxycycline (evaluate and treat partner) Ceftriaxone or azithromycin as single dose
Urethritis, cervicitis, conjunctivitis, proctitis	*Chlamydia trachomatis*	Azithromycin, doxycycline (amoxicillin if pregnant)
Neonatal ophthalmia, pneumonia		Erythromycin
lymphogranuloma venereum	*C. trachomatis* (specific serotypes, L1, L2, L3)	Doxycycline
DIVERTICULITIS (no perforation or peritonitis)	Enterobacteriaceae, enterococci, bacteroids	TMP–SMX, ciprofloxacin plus metronidazole
EAR		
Acute mastoiditis	*S. pneumoniae* Group A strep *S. aureus*	Amoxicillin, ampicillin/clavulanic acid, cefuroxime
Chronic mastoiditis	Polymicrobial: Anaerobes Enterobacteriaceae Rarely: *Mycobacterium tuberculosis*	Ticarcillin/clavulanic acid, imipenem

(continued)

131

TABLE 7-2
(Continued)

Site/Condition	Common Uncommon but Important	Common Empiric Therapy (Modify based on clinical factors such as Gram stain)
EAR		
Otitis externa	Pseudomonas spp. Enterobacteriaceae In diabetic or malignant otitis: Pseudomonas spp.	Topical agents such as Cortisporin otic, TobraDex Malignant otitis externa: acutely aminoglycoside, plus ceftazidime, imipenem or piperacillin
Otitis media	S. pneumoniae, H. influenzae, M. catarrhalis, viral causes S. aureus, group A strep In nasal intubation: Enterobacteriaceae, Pseudomonas spp.	Amoxicillin, ampicillin/clavulanic acid, cefuroxime
EMPYEMA ENDOCARDITIS		
Native valve	S. pneumoniae, S. aureus S. viridans S. pneumoniae Enterococci S. bovis	Cefotaxime, ceftriaxone Parenteral: penicillin or ampicillin or oxacillin or nafcillin plus gentamicin; vancomycin plus gentamicin
IV drug user	S. aureus Pseudomonas spp.	Nafcillin plus gentamicin

(continued)

TABLE 7-2
(Continued)

Site/Condition	Common Uncommon but Important	Common Empiric Therapy (Modify based on clinical factors such as Gram stain)
EMPYEMA ENDOCARDITIS		

Prosthetic valve	If early (<6 mon after implant)
	  S. epidermidis
	  S. aureus
	  Enterobacteriaceae
	If late (>6 mon after implant)
	  S. viridans
	  Enterococci
	  S. epidermidis
	  S. aureus
		Vancomycin plus rifampin plus gentamicin

EPIGLOTTITIS	H. influenzae S. pneumoniae S. aureus Group A strep	Ceftriaxone, cefotaxime, cefuroxime ampicillin/sulbactam, trimethoprime/sulfamethoxazole or TMP/SMX
GALL BLADDER		
Cholecystitis	Acute: E. Coli, Klebsiella, Enterococcus Chronic obstruction: anaerobes, coliforms, Clostridium	Ampicillin plus gentamicin w/wo metronidazole, imipenem
Cholangitis	E. coli, Klebsiella, Enterococcus	

(continued)

7

133

TABLE 7-2
(Continued)

Site/Condition	Common Uncommon but Important	Common Empiric Therapy (Modify based on clinical factor such as Gram stain)
GASTROENTERITIS		
Afebrile, no gross blood or no WBC in stool	Virus, mild bacterial infection	Supportive care only
Febrile, gross blood, and WBC in stool	Enteropathogenic *E. coli* *Shigella* *Salmonella* *Campylobacter* *Vibrio* *C. difficile* *Listeria monocytogenes*	Empiric treatment pending cultures: ciprofloxacin, levofloxacin
GRANULOMA INGUINALE	*Calymmatobacterium granulomatis*	Doxycycline, trimethoprim/sulfamethoxazole
GONORRHEA (urethra, cervix, rectal, pharyngeal)	*Neisseria gonorrhea*	Cefixime, ciprofloxacin, ofloxacin, ceftriaxone all as single dose; (treat also for *Chlamydia*)
MENINGITIS (Empiric therapy before cultures)		
Neonate	Group B strep, *E. coli*, *L. monocytogenes*	Ampicillin plus cefotaxime

(continued)

TABLE 7-2
(Continued)

Site/Condition	Common / Uncommon but Important	Common Empiric Therapy (Modify based on clinical factors such as Gram stain)
Meningitis (continued)		
Infant 1–3 mon	S. pneumoniae N. meningitidis	Vancomycin plus ceftriaxone
Child/adult, community acquired	S. pneumoniae N. meningitidis, H. influenzae	Vancomycin plus ceftriaxone
Postoperative or traumatic	S. epidermitis, S. aureus, S. pneumoniae, Pseudomonas	Vancomycin plus ceftazidime
Immunosuppressed (ie, steroids)	Gram-negative bacilli, L. monocytogenes S. pneumoniae	Ampicillin plus ceftazidime
History of alcohol abuse	N. meningitidis, gram-negative bacilli Pseudomonas spp. H. influenzae	Ampicillin plus ceftriaxone or cefotaxime plus vancomycin
HIV infection	Cryptococcus	Amphotericin B (acutely), fluconazole
NOCARDIOSIS	Nocardia asteroides	Sulfisoxazole, TMP–SMX

(continued)

TABLE 7-2
(Continued)

Site/Condition	Common Uncommon but Important	Common Empiric Therapy (Modify based on clinical factors such as Gram stain)
PELVIC INFLAMMATORY DISEASE	Gonococci Enterobacteriaceae *Bacteroides* spp. *Chlamydia* Enterococci *M. hominis*	Ofloxacin and metronidazole or ceftriaxone (single dose) plus doxycycline; parenteral cefotetan or cefoxitin plus doxycycline
PERITONITIS Primary (spontaneous)	*S. pneumoniae* Enterobacteriaceae	Cefotaxime or ceftriaxone
Secondary to (bowel perforation, etc)	Enterobacteriaceae, *Bacteroides* spp. Enterococci *Pseudomonas* spp.	Suspect small bowel: piperacillin, mezlocillin, meropenem, cefoxitin Suspect large bowel: clindamycin plus aminoglycoside
Peritoneal dialysis-related	*S. epidermidis* *S. aureus* Enterobacteriaceae *Candida*	Based on culture

(continued)

TABLE 7-2
(Continued)

Site/Condition	Common Uncommon but Important	Common Empiric Therapy (Modify based on clinical factors such as Gram stain)
PHARYNGITIS	Respiratory virus Group A strep Gonococci C. diphtheria Epstein–Barr virus (infectious mono); spirochetes, anaerobes	Exudative (group A strep): benzathine penicillin G, erythromycin, loracarbef, azithromycin
PNEUMONIA Neonate	Viral (CMV, herpes), bacterial (group B strep, L. monocytogenes, coliforms, S. aureus, Chlamydia)	Ampicillin or nafcillin plus gentamicin
Infant (1–24 mon)	Most viral such as RSV; S. pneumonia, Chlamydia, Mycoplasma	Cefuroxime; if critically ill, cefotaxime, ceftriaxone plus cloxacillin
Child (3 mon– 5 y)	As above	Erythromycin, clarithromycin; if critically ill, cefuroxime plus erythromycin
Child (5–18 y)	Mycoplasma, respiratory viruses, S. pneumoniae, C. pneumoniae	Clarithromycin, azithromycin; erythromycin

(continued)

TABLE 7-2
(Continued)

Site/Condition	Common / Uncommon but Important	Common Empiric Therapy (Modify based on clinical factors such as Gram stain)
Adult community-acquired	M. pneumoniae, C. pneumoniae, S. pneumoniae Smokers: As above plus M. catarrhalis, H. influenzae	Clarithromycin, azithromycin If hospitalized, third-generation cephalosporin plus erythromycin or azithromycin
Adult community-acquired aspiration	S. pneumoniae oral flora, including anaerobes (eg, Fusobacterium, Bacteroides sp.) Enterobacteriaceae	Clindamycin
Adult hospital-acquired or ventilator-associated	S. pneumonia, coliforms, Pseudomonas, Legionella	Imipenem, meropenem
HIV-associated	Pneumocystis Others as above TB, fungi	Pneumocystis: TMP–SMX; may require steroids
SINUSITIS	S. pneumoniae H. influenzae M. catarrhalis Anaerobes	Acute: TMP-SMX ampicillin, amoxicillin/clavulanic acid, clarithromycin

(continued)

138

TABLE 7-2
(Continued)

Site/Condition	Common Uncommon but Important	Common Empiric Therapy (Modify based on clinical factors such as Gram stain)
SINUSITIS (continued)	In nosocomial, nasal intubations, etc:	
	S. aureus	
	Pseudomonas spp.	
	Enterobacteriaceae	
SKIN/SOFT TISSUE		
Acne	Propionibacterium acne	Tetracycline, minocycline, topical clindamycin
Acne rosacea	Possible skin mite	Topical: metronidazole, doxycycline
Burns	S. aureus, Enterobacteriaceae, Pseudomonas, Proteus	Topical: silver sulfadiazine
	Herpes simplex virus, Providencia, Serratia, Candida	Sepsis: Aztreonam or tobramycin plus cefoperazone, ceftazidime or piperacillin
Bite (human and animal)	Anaerobes	Ampicillin/sulbactam IV or amoxicillin/clavulanic acid PO
	P. multiloculada	
Cellulitis	Streptococcus spp. (group A, B, C, G)	Diabetic: nafcillin, oxacillin with or without penicillin; if anaerobic, high-dose penicillin G, cefoxitin, cefotetan
	S. aureus	
	Anaerobic	

(continued)

7

139

TABLE 7-2
(Continued)

Site/Condition	Common Uncommon but Important	Common Empiric Therapy (Modify based on clinical factors such as Gram stain)
Decubitus	Group A strep (S. pyogenes) Anaerobes, S. aureus, Enterobacteria Polymicrobial anaerobic	If acutely ill: imipenem, meropenem, ticarcillin/ clavulanic acid
Erysipelas	Group A strep (S. pyogenes)	Nafcillin, oxacillin, dicloxacillin, cefazolin
Impetigo	Group A strep S. arueus	Penicillin, erythromycin; oxacillin or nafcillin if S. aureus
Tinea capitis (scalp) "ringworm"	Fungus: Trichophyton spp., Microsporum spp.	Terbinafine, itraconazole, fluconazole,
Tinea corporis (body)	Fungus: Trichophyton spp., Epidermophyton	Topical: ciclopirox, clotrimazole, econazole, ketocona- zole, miconazole, terconazole, others
Tinea unguium	Various fungi	Itraconazole, fluconazole, terbinafine
SYPHILIS (less than 1 y duration)	Treponema pallidum	Benzathine penicillin G one dose; doxycycline, tetracycline, ceftriaxone
TUBERCULOSIS Pulmonary, HIV (–)	Mycobacterium tuberculosis	INH, rifampin ethambutol plus pyrazinamide at least 6 mo (+/– pyridoxine)

(continued)

TABLE 7-2
(Continued)

Site/Condition	Common Uncommon but Important	Common Empiric Therapy (Modify based on clinical factors such as Gram stain)
TB exposure, PPD (–)		Children <5 INH X3 mo (+/– pyridoxine), others observe
Prophylaxis in high-risk patients (diabetics, IV drug users, immunosuppressed, etc)		INH 6–12 mo (+/– pyridoxine)
PPD + conversion		INH 6–12 mo (+/– pyridoxine)
URINARY TRACT INFECTIONS		
Cystitis	Enterobacteriaceae (*E. coli* most common)	Quinolone, TMP–SMX
	Staphylococcus saprophyticus (young female)	
	Candida	Candida: fluconazole or amphotericin B bladder irrigation
Urethritis	Gonococci, *C. trachomatis*, *Trichomonas*	Ceftriaxone, cefixime, ciprofloxacin, ofloxacin (all one dose) plus azithromycin (single dose) or doxycycline (treat partner)
	Herpesvirus	
	Ureaplasma urealyticum	

(continued)

141

TABLE 7-2
(Continued)

Site/Condition	Common Uncommon but Important	Common Empiric Therapy (Modify based on clinical factors such as Gram stain)
Prostatitis, acute <35 y	C. trachomatis Gonococci Coliforms Cryptococcus (AIDS)	Ofloxacin
Prostatitis, acute >35 y	Coliforms	Quinolone, TMP–SMX; if acutely ill gentamicin/ampicillin IV
Prostatitis, chronic bacterial	Coliforms, enterococci, Pseudomonas	Long-term ciprofloxacin or ofloxacin
Pyelonephritis	Enterobacteriaceae (E. coli) Enterococci Pseudomonas spp.	If acutely ill, gentamicin/ampicillin IV; quinolone, TMP–SMX
ULCER DISEASE (duodenal or gastric, not NSAID related)	Helicobacter pylori	Omeprazole plus amoxicillin plus clarithromycin
VAGINA Candidiasis	C. albicans C. glabrata, C. tropicalis	Fluconazole, itraconazole

(continued)

142

TABLE 7-2
(Continued)

Site/Condition	Common Uncommon but Important	Common Empiric Therapy (Modify based on clinical factors such as Gram stain)
Trichomonas	*Trichomonas vaginalis*	Metronidazole (treat partner)
Vaginosis, bacterial	Polymicrobial (*Gardnerella vaginalis, Bacteroides, M. hominis*	Metronidazole (PO or vaginal gel); clindamycin, PO or intravaginally

[a]All antimichrobial therapy should be based on complete clinical data, including results of Gram's stains and cultures. See also Tables 7–3 (Viral), page 144, 7–4 (HIV) page 148, 7–5 (Fungal) page 148, and 7–6 (Parasitic) page 149, and 7–7 (Tick-Borne) page 153.
Note: These guidelines are based on agents commonly involved in adult infections. Actual anti-microbial treatment should be guided by microbiologic studies interpreted in the clinical setting.

AIDS = acquired immunodeficiency syndrome; COPD = chronic obstructive pulmonary disease; HIV = human immunodeficiency virus; INH = isoniazid; IV = intravenous; NSAID = nonsteroidal antiinflammatory drug; PO = by mouth; PPD = purified protein derivative; TB = tuberculosis; TMP-SMX = trimethoprim–sulfamethoxazole.

7

TABLE 7–3
Pathogens and Drugs of Choice for Treating Common Viral Infections[a]

Viral Infection	Drug of Choice	Adult Dosage
CMV		
Retinitis, colitis, esophagitis	Ganciclovir (*Cytovene*)[b]	5 mg/kg IV q12h × 14–21d, 5 mg/kg/d IV or 6 mg/kg IV 5×/wk or 1 g PO tid
	(*Vitrasert*[b]) implants or Foscarnet (*Foscavir*)	4.5 mg intraocularly q 5–8 mon 60 mg/kg IV q8h or 90 mg/kg IV q1–2 h × 14–21 d followed by 90–120 mg/kg/d IV
	or Cidofovir (*Vistide*)	5 mg/kg/wk IV × 2 wk, then 5 mg/kg IV q2 wk
	or Fomivirsen (*Vitravene*)	330 μg intravitreally q2 wk × 2 then 1/mon
EBV		
Infectious mononucleosis	None	
HAV	None, but gamma globulin within 2 wk of exposure may limit infection	0.2 mL/kg IM × 1
HBV		
Chronic hepatitis	Lamivudine (*Epivir HBV*) Interferon alfa-2b (*Intron A*)	100 mg PO 1×/d × 1–3 y 5 million units/d or 10 million units 3×/wk SC or IM × 4 mon

(*continued*)

7

144

TABLE 7-3
(Continued)

Viral Infection	Drug of Choice	Adult Dosage
HCV		
Chronic hepatitis	Interferon alfa-2b plus Ribavirin (*Rebetron*)	3 million units 3×/wk SC plus ribavirin 1000–1200 mg/d PO × 12 mon
	Interferon alfa-2b (*Intron A*)	3 million units SC or IM 3×/wk × 12–24 mo
	Interferon alfa-2a (*Roferon-A*)	3 million units SC or IM 3×/wk × 12–24 mo
	Interferon alfacon-1 (*Infergen*)	9 µg 3×/wk × 6 mo
HSV		
Orolabial herpes in the immunocompetent with multiple recurrences	Penciclovir (*Denavir*)	1% cream applied q2h while awake × 4 d
Genital herpes		
first episode	Acyclovir (*Zovirax*)	400 mg PO tid or 200 mg PO 5×/d × 7–10 d
	or Famciclovir (*Famvir*)	250 mg PO tid × 5–10 d
	or Valacyclovir (*Valtrex*)	1 g PO bid × 7–10 d
recurrence	Acyclovir (*Zovirax*)	400 mg PO tid × 5 d
	or Famciclovir (*Famvir*)	125 mg PO bid × 5 d 17
	or Valacyclovir (*Valtrex*)	500 mg PO bid × 5 d

(continued)

TABLE 7–3
(Continued)

Viral Infection	Drug of Choice	Adult Dosage
Genital herpes (continued) chronic suppression	Acyclovir (Zovirax)	400 mg PO bid
	or Valacyclovir (Valtrex)	500–1000 mg PO 1×/d
	or Famciclovir (Famvir)	250 mg PO bid
Mucocutaneous in the immunocompromised	Acyclovir (Zovirax)	5 mg/kg IV q8h × 7–14 d
	or Acyclovir (Zovirax)	400 mg PO 5×/d × 7–14 d
Encephalitis	Acyclovir (Zovirax)	10–15 mg/kg IV q8h × 14–21 d
Neonatal	Acyclovir (Zovirax)	20 mg/kg IV q8h × 14–21 d
Acyclovir-resistant	Foscarnet (Foscavir)	40 mg/kg IV q8h × 14–21 d
Keratoconjunctivitis	Trifluridine (Viroptic)	1 drop 1% solution topically, q2h, up to 9 gtt/d × 10 d
HIV (See Table 7–4 page 148)		
INFLUENZA A AND B VIRUS		
	Zanamivir (Relenza)	10 mg bid × 5d by inhaler
	Oseltamivir (Tamiflu)	75 mg PO bid × 5 d
INFLUENZA A VIRUS		
	Rimantadine (Flumadine)	200 mg PO 1×/d or 100 mg PO bid × 5 d
	Amantadine (Symmetrel)	100 mg PO bid × 5 d
MEASLES		
Children	None (immunize, See Table 22–9)	
Adults	None or ribavirin	20–35 mg/kg/d × 7 d

(continued)

TABLE 7-3
(Continued)

Viral Infection	Drug of Choice	Adult Dosage
PAPILLOMA VIRUS (HPV) Anogenital warts	Podofilox or podophyllin Interferon alfa-2b (*Intron A*) Imiquimod, 5% cream (*Aldara*)	Topical application (see Chapter 22) 1 million units intralesional 3×/wk × 3 wk Apply 3/wk hs, remove 6–10 h later up to 16 wk
RSV Bronchiolitis	Ribavirin (*Virazole*)	Aerosol treatment 12–18 h/d × 3–7 d
VZV Exposure prophylaxis in the immunocompromised (HIV, steroids, etc)	VZIG, varicella-zoster immune globulin	See package insert
Varicella (>12 y old)	Acyclovir (*Zovirax*)	20 mg/kg (800 mg max) PO qid × 5 d
Herpes zoster	Valacyclovir (*Valtrex*) or Famciclovir (*Famvir*) or Acyclovir (*Zovirax*)	1 g PO tid × 7 d 500 mg PO tid × 7 d 800 mg PO 5×/d × 7–10 d
Varicella or zoster in the immunocompromised	Acyclovir (*Zovirax*)	10 mg/kg IV q8h × 7 d
Acyclovir-resistant	Foscarnet (*Foscavir*)	40 mg/kg IV q8h × 10 d

^aBased on Guidelines from the CDC published in *MMWR* and the *Medical Letter* Vol. 41 December 3, 1999.
^bThe generic drug name appears in regular type; the trade name appears in parentheses afterward in *italics*.
CMV = cytomegalovirus; EBV = Epstein–Barr virus; HAV = hepatitis A virus; HBV = hepatitis B virus; HCV = hepatitis C virus; HIV = human immunodeficiency virus;
HPV = human papilloma virus; HSV = herpes simplex virus; RSV = respiratory syncytial virus; VZV = varicella-zoster virus.

7

TABLE 7–4
Drugs of Choice for HIV Infection in Adults

Drugs of Choice
2 NRTIs[a] + 1 protease inhibitor[b]
2 NRTIs[a] + 1 NNRTI[c]
2 NRTIs[a] + ritonavir[d] + another protease inhibitor[d]
Abacavir + 2 other NRTIs[a]

ALTERNATIVES
1 protease inhibitor[b] + 1 NRTI + NNRTI[c]
2 protease inhibitors[d] + 1 NRTI + NNRTI[c]

[a]One of the following is recommended: zidovudine + lamivudine; zidovudine + didanosine; stavudine + lamivudine; stavudine + didanosine; lamivudine + didanosine. The combination of zidovudine and zalcitabine is an alternative.
[b]Nelfinavir, indinavir, saquinavir soft gel capsules, amprenavir or lopinavir/ritonavir. Full doses of ritonavir are used less frequently because of troublesome adverse effects.
[c]Efavirenz is often preferred. In most patients, nevirapine causes more adverse effects. Nevirapine and delavirdine require more doses. Combinations of efavirenz or nevirapine with protease inhibitors require increasing the dosage of the protease inhibitor.
[d]Ritonavir is usually given in dosage of 100–400 mg bid when used with another protease inhibitor. Protease inhibitors that have been combined with ritonavir 100–400 mg bid include, in addition to lopinavir, indinavir 400–800 mg bid, amprenavir 600–800 mg bid, saquinavir 400–600 mg bid and nelfinavir 500–750 mg bid.
NRTI = Nucleoside reverse transcriptase inhibitors
Reproduced, with permission, from The Medical Letter, Vol. 43 (Issue 1119) November 26, 2001, New Rochelle, NY.

7

TABLE 7–5
Systemic Drugs for Treating Fungal Infections

Infection	Drug of Choice	Alternatives
ASPERGILLOSIS	Amphotericin B or itraconazole	Amphotericin B lipid complex, amphotericin cholesteryl complex liposomal amphotericin B
BLASTOMYCOSIS	Itraconazole or amphotericin B	Fluconazole
CANDIDIASIS		
Oral (thrush)	Fluconazole or itraconazole	Nystatin lozenge or swish and swallow
Stomatitis, eosphagitis, vaginitis in AIDS	Fluconazole or itraconazole	Parenteral or oral amphotericin B
Systemic	Amphotericin B or fluconazole	
Cystitis/vaginitis	See Table 7–2, page 141	
COCCIDIOIDOMYCOSIS		
Pulmonary (normal individual)	No drug usually recommended	
Pulmonary (high risk)	Itraconazole or fluconazole	Amphotericin B
CRYPTOCOCCOSIS		
In non-AIDS patient	Amphotericin B or fluconazole	Amphotericin B fluconazole
Meningitis (HIV/AIDS)	Amphotericin B plus 5-flucytosine; then long-term suppression with fluconazole	Amphotericin B lipid complex

(continued)

7

TABLE 7-5
(Continued)

Infection	Drug of Choice	Alternatives
HISTOPLASMOSIS		
Pulmonary, disseminated		
Normal individual	Moderate disease: itraconazole	Severe: amphotericin B
HIV/AIDS	Amphotericin B, followed by itraconazole suppression	Itraconazole
MUCORMYCOSIS	Amphotericin B	No dependable alternative
PARACOCCIDIOIDOMYCOSIS	Itraconazole	Amphotericin B
SPOROTRICHOSIS		
Cutaneous	Itraconazole	Potassium iodide 1–5 mL tid
Systemic	Itraconazole	Amphotericin B

Abbreviations: AIDS = acquired immunodeficiency syndrome; HIV = human immunodeficiency virus.

TABLE 7–6
Drugs for Treating Selected Parasitic Infections

Infection	Drug
Amebiasis (*Entamoeba histolytica*)	
Asymptomatic	Iodoquinol or paramomycin
Mild to moderate intestinal disease	Metronidazole or tinidazole
Severe intestinal disease, hepatic abscess	Metronidazole or tinidazole
Ascariasis (*Ascaris lumbricoides,* roundworm)	Albendazole, mebendazole or pyrantel pamoate
Cryptosporidiosis (*Cryptosporidium*)	Paromomycin
Cutaneous larva migrans (creeping eruption, dog and cat hookworm)	Albendazole, thiabendazole or ivermectin
***Cyclospora* infection**	Trimethoprim–sulfamethoxazole
Enterobius vermicularis (pinworm)	Pyrantel pamoate, mebendazole or albendazole
Filariasis (*Wuchereria bancrofti, Brugia malayi, Loa loa*)	Diethylcarbamazine
Giardiasis (*Giardia lamblia*)	Metronidazole
Hookworm infection (*Ancylostoma duodenale, Necator americanus*)	Albendazole, mebendazole, or pyrantel pamoate
Isosporiasis (*Isospora belli*)	Trimethoprim–sulfamethoxazole
Lice (*Pediculus humanus, P. capitis, Phthirus pubis*)	1% permethrin (topical) or 0.5% malathion
Malaria (*Plasmodium falciparum, P. ovale, P. vivax,* and *P. malariae*)	
Chloroquine-resistant *P. falciparum*	Quinine sulfate plus doxycycline, tetracycline, clindamycin or pyrimethamine–sulfadoxine (oral)
Chloroquine-resistant *P. vivax*	Quinine sulfate plus doxycycline, or pyrimethamine–sulfadoxine (oral)
All *Plasmodium* except chloroquine-resistant *P. falciparum*	Chloroquine phosphate (oral)
All *Plasmodium* (parenteral)	Quinine gluconate or quinine dihydrochloride
Prevention of relapses: *P. vivax,* and *P. ovale* only	Primaquine phosphate
Malaria, prevention	
Chloroquine-sensitive areas	Chloroquine phosphate
Chloroquine-resistant areas	Mefloquine or doxycycline

(*continued*)

TABLE 7–6
(Continued)

Infection	Drug
Mites, see Scabies	
Pinworm, see *Enterobius*	
Pneumocystis carinii **pneumonia**	Trimethoprim–sulfamethoxazole
	Alternative: pentamidine
Primary and secondary prophylaxis	Trimethoprim–sulfamethoxazole
Roundworm, see Ascariasis	
Scabies (*Sarcoptes scabiei*)	5% Permethrin topically
	Alternatives: ivermectin, 10% crotamiton
Strongyloidiasis (*Strongyloides stercoralis*)	Ivermectin
Tapeworm infection	
Adult (intestinal stage)	
Diphyllobothrium latum (fish), *Taenia saginata* (beef), *Taenia solium* (pork), *Dipylidium caninum* (dog), *Hymenolepis nana* (dwarf tapeworm)	Praziquantel
Larval (tissue stage)	
Echinococcus granulosus (hydatid cyst)	Albendazole
Cysticercus cellulosae (cysticercosis)	Albendazole or praziquantel
Toxoplasmosis (*Toxoplasma gondii*)	Pyrimethamine plus sulfadiazine
Trichinosis (*Trichinella spiralis*)	Steroids for severe symptoms plus mebendazole
Trichomoniasis (*Trichomonas vaginalis*)	Metronidazole or tinidazole
Hairworm infection (*Trichostrongylus colubriformis*)	Pyrantel pamoate
Trypanosomiasis (*Trypanosoma cruzi,* Chagas' disease)	Benznidazole
Trichuriasis (*Trichuris trichiuria,* whipworm)	Mebendazole or albendazole
Visceral larva migrans, toxocariasis (*Toxocara canis*)	Albendazole or mebendazole

Source: Based on data from *The Medical Letter* March 2000 www. medletter.com.

TABLE 7-7
Guide to Common Tick-borne Diseases

Disease	Causative Agent	Season	Vector Habits
Rocky Mountain spotted fever	*Rickettsia rickettsii* (bacterium)	Mostly spring, summer	*American Dog Tick* Found in high grass and low shrubs, fields
			Lone Star Tick Found in woodlands, forest edge, and old fields
Human granulocytic ehrlichiosis	*Ehrlichia* spp. (bacterium)	Peaks in summer, may be seen year-round	*Deer* (black-legged) *Tick* found in woodlands, old fields, landscaping with significant ground cover vegetation
Lyme disease	*Borrelia burgdorferi* (bacterium)	Mostly spring, but year-round	Same as for the deer tick
Babesiosis	*Babesia microti* (protozoan)	Mostly spring/summer	Same as for the deer tick

(continued)

TABLE 7-7
(Continued)

Classic Clinical Presentation	Incubation Period	Diagnosis	Treatment
Sudden moderate to high fever, severe headache, maculopapular rash (with planer/palmer presentation)	2–14 d	Clinical serology	Adults—doxycycline Children/pregnant women—chloramphenicol
Fever, headache, constitutional symptoms	1–30 d	Clinical serology	Adults—tetracyclines Children/pregnant women—consult specialist
EM rash, constitutional symptoms, arthritis, cardiovascular- and nervous system involvement	3–30 d	Clinical serology, culture	Doxycycline, amoxicillin, cefuroxime for 14–21 d
Fever, hemolytic anemia, constitutional symptoms	1–52 wk	Thick and thin blood smears	Clindamycin/quinine

EM = erythema multiforme.

154

7

TABLE 7–8
SBE Prophylaxis for Oral, Respiratory or Esophageal Procedures[a]

Prophylaxis	Agent	Regimen[b]
Standard prophylaxis	Amoxicillin	Adults: 2.0 g; children: 50 mg/kg PO 1 h before procedure
Unable to take oral medications	Ampicillin	Adults: 2.0 g IM or IV; children: 50 mg/kg or IV 30 min before procedure
Allergic to penicillin	Clindamycin or	Adults: 600 mg; children: 20 mg/kg PO 1 h before procedure
	Cephalexin or cefadroxil	Adults: 2.0 g; children; 50 mg/kg PO 1 h before procedure
	Azithromycin or clarithromycin	Adults: 500 mg; children: 15 mg/kg PO 1 h before procedure Adults: 600 mg; children: 20 mg/kg IV 30 min before procedure
Penicillin allergic and unable to take oral medications	Clindamycin or cefazolin	Adults: 1.0 g; children: 25 mg/kg IM or IV 30 min before procedure

[a]See text page 129 for recommended risk groups.
[b]Total children's dose should not exceed adult dose.

ISOLATION PROTOCOLS

To prevent the spread of infectious diseases from patient to patient, visitors, and hospital personnel, isolation procedures are recommended for various pathogens and clinical settings by various agencies such as the Centers for Disease Control, Atlanta, Georgia. Local hospital procedures may vary slightly from these recommendations.

Strict Isolation   (Single room, controlled airflow, handwashing, gown, gloves, mask) Varicella, herpes (localized, disseminated, neonatal), wound or burns infected with *S. aureus* or group A *Streptococcus, S. pneumoniae,* congenital rubella, rabies, smallpox, others

Contact Isolation: (Single room, controlled airflow, handwashing, gown, gloves, mask) All acute respiratory infections in infants and children (cough, cold, pneumonia, croup, pharyngitis, etc), extensive impetigo, gonococcal conjunctivitis in the newborn, others

Respiratory Isolation: (Single room, controlled airflow, handwashing, mask) TB (known or suspected), measles, mumps, rubella, pertussis, meningitis (sus-

TABLE 7–9
SBE Prophylaxis for GU/GI (Excluding Esophageal) Procedures[a]

Patient	Agents	Regimen
High-risk	Ampicillin + gentamicin	Adults: ampicillin 2.0 g IM/IV + gentamicin 1.5 mg/kg (max 120 mg) within 30 min of procedure; 6 h later, ampicillin 1 g IM/IV or amoxicillin 1 g PO Children: ampicillin 50 mg/kg IM or IV (2.0 g max) + gentamicin 1.5 mg/kg within 30 min of procedure; 6 h later, ampicillin 25 mg/kg IM/IV or amoxicillin 25 mg/kg PO
High-risk allergic to ampicillin/ amoxicillin	Vancomycin + gentamicin	Adults: vancomycin 1.0 g IV over 1–2 h + gentamicin 1.5 mg/kg IV/IM (120 mg max); dose within 30 min of starting procedure Children: vancomycin 20 mg/kg IV over 1–2 h + gentamicin 1.5 mg/kg IV/IM; complete dose within 30 min of starting procedure
Moderate-risk	Amoxicillin or ampicillin	Adults: amoxicillin 2.0 g PO 1 h before procedure, or ampicillin 2.0 g IM/IV within 30 min of starting procedure Children: amoxicillin 50 mg/kg PO 1 h before procedure, or ampicillin 50 mg/kg IM/IV within 30 min of starting procedure
Moderate-risk allergic to ampicillin/ amoxicillin	Vancomycin	Adults: vancomycin 1.0 g IV over 1–2 h complete infusion within 30 min of starting procedure Children: vancomycin 20 mg/kg IV over 1–2 h; complete infusion within 30 min of starting procedure

[a]See text page 129 for recommended risk groups.
Total children's dose should not exceed adult dose.

pected *N. meningitidis* or *H. influenzae* infection), pneumonia due to *H. influenzae*, epiglottitis, others

Wound and Skin Precautions: (Single room; handwashing; for direct contact with patient secretions: gown, gloves, mask) Major wound and skin infections, group A streptococcal endometritis, gas gangrene. Scabies and lice require only 24 h after effective therapy.

Enteric Precautions: (Single room; handwashing; for direct contact with patient secretions: gown, gloves) Known or suspected infectious gastroenteritis from rotavirus, enterovirus, *Salmonella, Shigella, E. coli, Giardia, and C. difficile* enterocolitis, acute hepatitis (all types)

Blood and Body Fluid Precautions: (Handwashing; for direct contact with patient secretions: gown, gloves) Known or suspected HIV infection, hepatitis (in acute and chronic carriers), syphilis, malaria, Lyme disease, all rickettsial infections, others

Secretion/Discharge Precautions: (Handwashing and gloves with direct patient contact) Conjunctivitis, minor skin wounds, decubiti, colonization (but not infection that requires wound and skin precautions) with MRSA, herpes, mucocutaneous candidiasis, ulcerative STDs, coccidioidomycosis, others

Pregnancy Precautions: (Handwashing) CMV, rubella, parvovirus

BLOOD GASES AND ACID–BASE DISORDERS

NORMAL BLOOD GAS VALUES

The results of testing ABG are usually given as pH, po_2, pCO_2, [HCO_3^-], base excess/deficit (difference), and oxygen saturation. This test gives information on acid–base homeostasis (pH, pCO_2, [HCO_3^-], and base difference) and on blood oxygenation (po_2, O_2 saturation). Less frequently, venous blood gases and mixed venous blood gases are measured. Normal values for blood gas analysis are given in Table 8–1, page 160, and capillary blood gases are discussed in a following section. Note that the HCO_3^- from the blood gas is a calculated value and should not be used in the interpretation of the blood gas levels, instead the HCO_3^- from a chemistry panel should be used. The ABG and the chemistry panel [HCO_3^-] should be obtained at the same time.

VENOUS BLOOD GASES

There is little difference between arterial and venous pH and bicarbonate (except in CHF and shock). Venous blood gas level may occasionally be used to assess acid–base status, but venous oxygen levels are significantly less than arterial (see Table 8–1).

CAPILLARY BLOOD GASES

A CBG is obtained from a highly vascularized capillary bed. The CBG is often used for pediatric patients (the heel) because it is easier to obtain than the ABG and is less traumatic (no risk of arterial thrombosis, hemorrhage). See Chapter 13, page 279, under Heelstick.

When interpreting a CBG, apply the following rules:

- **pH:** Same as arterial or slightly lower (Normal = 7.35–7.40)
- **pCO_2:** Same as arterial or slightly higher (Normal = 40–45)
- **po_2:** Lower than arterial (Normal = 45–60)
- **O_2 Saturation:** > 70% is acceptable. Saturation is probably more useful than the po_2 itself when interpreting a CBG.

TABLE 8–1
Normal Blood Gas Values

Measurement	Arterial Blood	Mixed Venous[a]	Venous
pH	7.40	7.36	7.36
(range)	(7.37–7.44)	(7.31–7.41)	(7.31–7.41)
pO$_2$ (mm Hg) (decreases with age)	80–100	35–40	30–50
pCO$_2$ (mm Hg)	36–44	41–51	40–52
O$_2$ saturation (decreases with age)	>95	60–80	60–85
HCO$_3^-$(mEq/L) [SI: mmol/L]	22–26	22–26	22–28
Base difference (deficit/excess)	–2 to +2	–2 to +2	–2 to +2

[a] Obtained from the right atrium, usually through a pulmonary artery catheter.

8

GENERAL PRINCIPLES OF BLOOD GAS DETERMINATIONS

(Oxygen values are discussed on page 160 & 168.)

1. The blood gas analyzers in most labs actually measure the pH and the pCO$_2$ (as well as the pO$_2$). The [HCO$_3^-$] and the base difference are calculated values using the **Henderson–Hasselbalch equation:**

$$\text{pH} = pK_a + \frac{\log[\text{HCO}_3^-] \text{ in mEq / L}}{0.03 \times \text{pco}_2 \text{ in mmHg}}$$

or the **Henderson equation:**

$$[\text{H}^+] \text{ in mEq / L} = \frac{24 \times \text{pco}_2 \text{ in mm Hg}}{[\text{HCO}_3^-] \text{ in mEq / L}}$$

2. For a rough estimate of [H⁺], [H⁺] = (7.80 – pH) × 100 (accurate from a pH 7.25 – 7.48); 40 mEq/L = [H⁺] at the normal pH of 7.40. pH is a log scale; for every change of 0.3 in pH from 7.40 the [H⁺] doubles or halves. For pH 7.10 the [H⁺] = 2 × 40, or 80 nmol/L, and for pH 7.70 the [H⁺] = ½ × 40, or 20 nmol/L.

3. The calculated [HCO$_3^-$] should be within 2 mEq/L of the bicarbonate concentration from a venous chemistry determination (eg, BMP) drawn at the same time. If not, an error has been made in the collection or the determination of the values, and the blood gas and serum bicarbonate should be recollected.

4. Two additional relationships that are derived from the Henderson–Hasselbalch equation should be committed to memory. These two rules are helpful in interpreting blood gas results, particularly in defining a simple versus a mixed blood gas disorder:

Rule I: A change in pCO_2 up or down 10 mm Hg is associated with an increase or decrease in pH of 0.08 units. As the pCO_2 decreases, the pH increases; as the pCO_2 increases, the pH decreases.

Rule II: A pH change of 0.15 is equivalent to a base change of 10 mEq/L. A decrease in base (ie, $[HCO_3^-]$) is termed a **base deficit,** and an increase in base is termed a **base excess.**

ACID–BASE DISORDERS: DEFINITION

1. Acid–base disorders are very common clinical problems. **Acidemia** is a pH < 7.37, and alkalemia is a pH > 7.44. **Acidosis and alkalosis** are used to describe how the pH changes. The primary causes of acid–base disturbances are abnormalities in the respiratory system and in the metabolic or renal system. As from the Henderson–Hasselbalch equation, a respiratory disturbance leading to an abnormal pCO_2 alters the pH, and similarly a metabolic disturbance altering the $[HCO_3^-]$ changes the pH.
2. Any primary disturbance in acid–base homeostasis invokes a **normal compensatory response.** A primary metabolic disorder leads to respiratory compensation, and a primary respiratory disorder leads to an acute metabolic response due to the buffering capacity of body fluids, *and* a more chronic compensation (1–2 days) due to alterations in renal function.
3. The degree of compensation is well known and can be expressed in terms of the degree of the primary acid–base disturbance. Table 8–2, page 162, lists the major categories of primary acid–base disorders, the primary abnormality, the secondary compensatory response, and the expected degree of compensation in terms of the magnitude of the primary abnormality. These changes are defined graphically in Figure 8–1, page 163. The types of simple acid–base disorders are discussed in the following sections.

MIXED ACID–BASE DISORDERS

1. Most acid–base disorders result from a single primary disturbance with the normal physiologic compensatory response and are called **simple acid–base disorders.** In certain cases, however, particularly in seriously ill patients, two or more different primary disorders may occur simultaneously, resulting in a **mixed acid–base disorder.** The net effect of mixed disorders may be additive (eg, metabolic acidosis and respiratory acidosis) and result in extreme alteration of pH; or they may be opposite (eg, metabolic acidosis and respiratory alkalosis) and nullify each other's effects on the pH.
2. To determine a mixed acid–base disorder from a blood gas value, follow the six steps in the Interpretation of Blood Gases (in the following section). Alterations in either $[HCO_3^-]$ or pCO_2 that differ from expected compensation levels indicate a second process. Two of the examples given in the following section illustrate the strategies employed in identifying a mixed acid–base disorder.

INTERPRETATION OF BLOOD GASES

Use a uniform, stepwise approach to the interpretation of blood gases. (See also Figure 8–1, page 163.)

Step 1: Determine if the numbers fit.

TABLE 8-2
Simple Acid–Base Disturbances

Acid–Base Disorder	Primary Abnormality	Expected Compensation	Expected Degree of Compensation
Metabolic acidosis	$\downarrow\downarrow\downarrow[HCO_3^-]$	$\downarrow\downarrow pCO_2$	$pCO_2 = (1.5 \times [HCO_3]) + 8$
Metabolic alkalosis	$\uparrow\uparrow\uparrow[HCO_3^-]$	$\uparrow\uparrow pCO_2$	$\uparrow$ in $pCO_2 = \Delta\,[HCO_3^-] \times 0.6$
Acute respiratory acidosis	$\uparrow\uparrow\uparrow pCO_2$	$\uparrow[HCO_3^-]$	$\uparrow$ in $[HCO_3^-] = \Delta pCO_2/10$
Chronic respiratory acidosis	$\uparrow\uparrow\uparrow pCO_2$	$\uparrow\uparrow[HCO_3^-]$	$\uparrow$ in $[HCO_3^-] = 4 \times \Delta pCO_2/10$
Acute respiratory alkalosis	$\downarrow\downarrow\downarrow pCO_2$	$\downarrow[HCO_3^-]$	$\downarrow$ in $[HCO_3^-] = 2 \times \Delta pCO_2/10$
Chronic respiratory alkalosis	$\downarrow\downarrow\downarrow pCO_2$	$\downarrow\downarrow[HCO_3^-]$	$\downarrow$ in $[HCO_3^-] = 5 \times \Delta pCO_2/10$

8

162

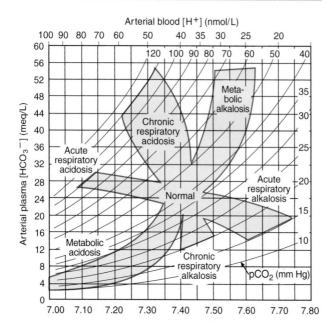

FIGURE 8-1. Nomogram for acid-base disorders. (Reprinted, with permission, from: Cogan MG: *Fluid and Electrolytes,* Originally published by Appleton & Lange, Copyright © 1991 by the McGraw-Hill Companies, Inc.)

$$[H^+] = \frac{24 \times pCO_2}{[HCO_3^-]}$$

The right side of the equation should be within about 10% of the left side. If the numbers do not fit, you need to obtain another ABG and chemistry panel for $[HCO_3^-]$.

Example. pH 7.25, pCO_2 48, $[HCO_3^-]$ 29 mmol/L.

$$56 = 24 \times \frac{48}{29}$$

$$56 \neq 40$$

The blood gas is uninterpretable, and the ABG and $[HCO_3^-]$ need to be recollected. The most common reason for the numbers not fitting is that the ABG and the chemistry panel $[HCO_3^-]$ were obtained at different times.

Step 2: Next, determine if an acidemia (pH < 7.37) or an alkalemia (pH > 7.44) is present.

Step 3: Identify the primary disturbance as metabolic or respiratory. For example, if acidemia is present, is the pCO_2 > 44 mm Hg (respiratory acidosis), or is the $[HCO_3^-]$ < 22 mmol/L (metabolic acidosis)? In other words, identify which component, respiratory or metabolic, is altered in the same direction as the pH abnormality. If both components act in the same direction (eg, both respiratory

[$pCO_2 > 44$ mm Hg] and metabolic [HCO_3^-] < 22 mmol/L] acidosis are present), then this is a **mixed acid–base problem,** discussed later in this section. The primary disturbance will be the one that varies from normal the greatest, that is, with a [HCO_3^-] = 6 mmol/L and pCO_2 = 50 mm Hg, the primary disturbance would be a metabolic acidosis, the [HCO_3^-] is about one-quarter normal, whereas the increase in pCO_2 is only 25%.

Step 4: After identifying the primary disturbance, use the equations in Table 8–2, page 162, to calculate the expected compensatory response. If the difference between the actual value and the calculated value is significant, then a mixed acid–base disturbance is present.

Step 5: Calculate the anion gap. Anion gap = Na^+ − (Cl^- + [HCO_3^-]). Normal anion gap is 8–12 mmol. If the anion gap is increased, proceed to step 6.

Step 6: If the anion gap is elevated, compare the changes from normal between the anion gap and [HCO_3^-]. If the change in the anion gap is greater than the change in the [HCO_3^-] from normal, then a metabolic alkalosis is present in addition to a gap metabolic acidosis. If the change in the anion gap is less than the change in the [HCO_3^-] from normal, then a nongap metabolic acidosis is present in addition to a gap metabolic acidosis. See Examples 5, 6, and 7, pages 171–172.

Finally, be sure the interpretation of the blood gas is consistent with the clinical setting.

METABOLIC ACIDOSIS: DIAGNOSIS AND TREATMENT

Metabolic acidosis represents an increase in acid in body fluids reflected by a decrease in [HCO_3^-] and a compensatory decrease in pCO_2.

Differential Diagnosis

The diagnosis of metabolic acidosis (Figure 8–2, page 163) can be classified as an anion gap or a nonanion gap acidosis. The **anion gap** (Normal range, 8–12 mmol/L) is calculated as:

$$Anion\ gap = [Na^+] - ([Cl^-] + [HCO_3^-])$$

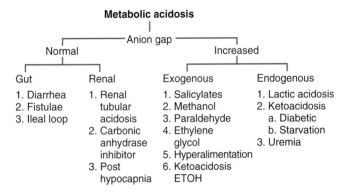

Metabolic acidosis

Anion gap

Normal		Increased	
Gut	Renal	Exogenous	Endogenous
1. Diarrhea	1. Renal	1. Salicylates	1. Lactic acidosis
2. Fistulae	tubular	2. Methanol	2. Ketoacidosis
3. Ileal loop	acidosis	3. Paraldehyde	a. Diabetic
	2. Carbonic	4. Ethylene	b. Starvation
	anhydrase	glycol	3. Uremia
	inhibitor	5. Hyperalimentation	
	3. Post	6. Ketoacidosis	
	hypocapnia	ETOH	

FIGURE 8–2. Differential diagnosis of metabolic acidosis.

Anion Gap Acidosis: Anion gap > 12 mmol/L; caused by a decrease in [HCO$_3^-$] balanced by an increase in an unmeasured acid ion from either endogenous production or exogenous ingestion (**normochloremic acidosis**).

Nonanion Gap Acidosis: Anion gap = 8–12 mmol/L; caused by a decrease in [HCO$_3^-$] balanced by an increase in chloride (**hyperchloremic acidosis**). Renal tubular acidosis is a type of nongap acidosis that can be associated with a variety of pathologic conditions (Table 8–3, page 166). The anion gap is helpful in identifying metabolic gap acidosis, nongap acidosis, mixed metabolic gap and nongap acidosis. If an elevated anion gap is present, a closer look at the anion gap and the bicarbonate helps differentiate among (a) a pure metabolic gap acidosis, (b) a metabolic nongap acidosis, (c) mixed metabolic gap and nongap acidosis, and (d) a metabolic gap acidosis and metabolic alkalosis.

Treatment of Metabolic Acidosis

1. Correct any underlying disorder (control diarrhea, etc).
2. Treatment with bicarbonate should be reserved for severe metabolic gap acidosis. If the pH < 7.20, correct with sodium bicarbonate. The total replacement dose of [HCO$_3^-$] can be calculated as follows:

$$[\text{HCO}_3^-] \text{ needed in mEq} = \frac{\text{Base deficit (mEq)} \times \text{Patient's weight (kg)}}{4}$$

3. Replace with **one-half the total amount of bicarbonate over 8–12 h** and reevaluate. Be aware of sodium and volume overload during replacement. Normal or isotonic bicarbonate drip is made with 3 amp NaHCO$_3$ (50 mmol NaHCO$_3$/amp) in 1 L D$_5$W.

METABOLIC ALKALOSIS: DIAGNOSIS AND TREATMENT

Metabolic alkalosis represents an increase in [HCO$_3^-$] with a compensatory rise in pCO$_2$.

Differential Diagnosis

In two basic categories of diseases the kidneys retain [HCO$_3^-$] (Figure 8–3). They can be differentiated in terms of response to treatment with sodium chloride and also by the level of urinary [Cl$^-$] as determined by ordering a "spot," or "random" urine for chloride (U$_{Cl}$).

Chloride-Sensitive (Responsive) Metabolic Alkalosis: The initial problem is a sustained loss of chloride out of proportion to the loss of sodium (either by renal or GI losses). This chloride depletion results in renal sodium conservation leading to a corresponding reabsorption of [HCO$_3^-$] by the kidney. In this category of metabolic alkalosis, the urinary [Cl$^-$] is < 10 mEq/L, and the disorders respond to treatment with intravenous NaCl.

Chloride-Insensitive (Resistant) Metabolic Alkalosis: The pathogenesis in this category is direct stimulation of the kidneys to retain bicarbonate irrespective of electrolyte intake and losses. The urinary [Cl$^-$] > 10 mEq/L, and these disorders do not respond to NaCl administration.

TABLE 8–3
Renal Tubular Acidosis: Diagnosis and Management

Clinical Condition	Renal Defect	GFR	Serum [HCO₃⁻] (mEq/L)	Serum [K⁺] (mEq/L)	Minimal Urine pH	Associated Disease States	Treatment
Normal	None	N	24–28	3.5–5	4.8–5.2	None	N/A
Proximal RTA (type II RTA)	Proximal H⁺ secretion	N	15–18	↓	<5.5	Drugs, Fanconi's syndrome, various genetic disorders, dysproteinemic states, secondary hyperparathyroidism, toxins (heavy metals), tubulointerstitial diseases, nephrotic syndrome, paroxysmal nocturnal hemoglobinuria	NaHCO₃ or KHCO₃ (10–15 mEq/kg/d), thiazide diuretics
Classic distal RTA (type I RTA)	Distal H⁺ secretion	N	20–30	↓	>5.5	Various genetic disorders, autoimmune diseases, nephrocalcinosis, drugs, toxins, tubulointerstitial diseases, hepatic cirrhosis, empty sella syndrome	NaHCO₃ (1–3 mEq/kg/d)
Buffer deficiency (type III RTA)	Distal NH₃ delivery	↓	15–18	N	<5.5	Chronic renal insufficiency, renal osteodystrophy, severe hypophosphatemia	NaHCO₃ (1–3 mEq/kg/d)
Generalized distal RTA (type IV RTA)	Distal Na⁺ reabsorption, K⁺ secretion, and H⁺ secretion	↓	24–28	↑	<5.5	Primary mineralocorticoid deficiency (eg, Addison's disease), hyporeninemic hypoaldosteronism, diabetes mellitus, tubulointerstitial diseases, nephrosclerosis, drugs), salt-wasting mineralocorticoid-resistant hyperkalemia	Fludrocortisone (0.1–0.5 mg/d) dietary K⁺ restriction, NaHCO₃ (1–3 mEq/kg/d) furosemide (40–160 mg/d)

8

166

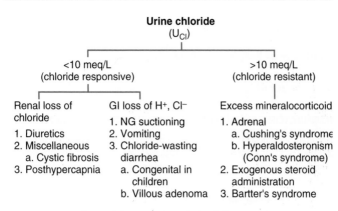

FIGURE 8–3. Differential diagnosis of metabolic alkalosis.

Treatment of Metabolic Alkalosis

Correct the underlying disorder.

1. **Chloride-responsive**
   a. Replace volume with NaCl if depleted.
   b. Correct hypokalemia if present.
   c. NH_4Cl and HCl should be reserved for extreme cases.
2. **Chloride-resistant**
   a. Treat underlying problem, such as stopping exogenous steroids.

RESPIRATORY ACIDOSIS: DIAGNOSIS AND TREATMENT

Respiratory acidosis is a primary rise in pCO_2 with a compensatory rise in plasma $[HCO_3^-]$. Increased pCO_2 occurs in clinical situations in which decreased alveolar ventilation occurs.

Differential Diagnosis

1. **Neuromuscular Abnormalities with Ventilatory Failure**
   a. Muscular dystrophy, myasthenia gravis, Guillain–Barré syndrome, hypophosphatemia
2. **Central Nervous System**
   a. Drugs: Sedatives, analgesics, tranquilizers, ethanol
   b. CVA
   c. Central sleep apnea
   d. Spinal cord injury (cervical)
3. **Airway Obstruction**
   a. Chronic (COPD)
   b. Acute (asthma)
   c. Upper airway obstruction
   d. Obstructive sleep apnea
4. **Thoracic–Pulmonary Disorders**
   a. Bony thoracic cage: Flail chest, kyphoscoliosis
   b. Parenchymal lesions: Pneumothorax, severe pulmonary edema, severe pneumonia

  c. Large pleural effusions
  d. Scleroderma
  e. Marked obesity (Pickwickian syndrome)

Treatment of Respiratory Acidosis

Improve Ventilation: Intubate patient and place on ventilator, increase ventilator rate, reverse narcotic sedation with naloxone (Narcan), etc

RESPIRATORY ALKALOSIS: DIAGNOSIS AND TREATMENT

Respiratory alkalosis is a primary fall in pCO_2 with a compensatory decrease in plasma $[HCO_3^-]$. Respiratory alkalosis occurs with increased alveolar ventilation.

Differential Diagnosis

1. **Central Stimulation**
  a. Anxiety, hyperventilation syndrome, pain
  b. Head trauma or CVA with central neurogenic hyperventilation
  c. Tumors
  d. Salicylate overdose
  e. Fever, early sepsis
2. **Peripheral Stimulation**
  a. PE
  b. CHF (mild)
  c. Interstitial lung disease
  d. Pneumonia
  e. Altitude
  f. Hypoxemia: Any cause (See the section on Hypoxia, below.)
3. **Miscellaneous**
  a. Hepatic insufficiency
  b. Pregnancy
  c. Progesterone
  d. Hyperthyroidism
  e. Iatrogenic mechanical overventilation

Treatment of Respiratory Alkalosis

Correct the underlying disorder.

Hyperventilation Syndrome: Best treated by having the patient rebreathe into a paper bag to increase pCO_2, decrease ventilator rate, increase amount of dead space with ventilator, or treat underlying cause.

HYPOXIA

1. The second type of information gained from a blood gas level, in addition to acid–base results, pertains to the level of oxygenation. Usually, results are given as po_2 and oxygen saturation (See Table 8–1 for normal values on page 160). These two parameters are related to each other.
2. Oxygen saturation at any given po_2 is influenced by temperature, pH, and the level of 2,3-DPG as shown in Figure 8–4, page 169.

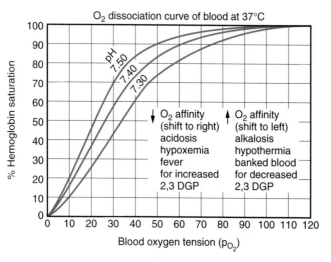

FIGURE 8–4. Oxyhemoglobin dissociation curve.

Differential Diagnosis

1. **V̇/Q̇ Abnormalities**
   a. COPD: Emphysema, chronic bronchitis
   b. Asthma
   c. Atelectasis
   d. Pneumonia
   e. PE
   f. ARDS
   g. Pneumothorax
   h. Pneumoconiosis
   i. CF
   j. Obstructed airway
2. **Alveolar Hypoventilation**
   a. Skeletal abnormalities
   b. Neuromuscular disorders
   c. Pickwickian syndrome
   d. Sleep apnea
3. **Decreased Pulmonary Diffusing Capacity**
   a. Pneumoconiosis
   b. Pulmonary edema
   c. Drug-induced pulmonary fibrosis (Bleomycin)
   d. Collagen-vascular diseases
4. **Right-to-Left Shunt**
   a. Congenital heart disease: Tetralogy of Fallot, transposition, etc

SAMPLE ACID–BASE PROBLEMS

In each of the following examples, use the technique for blood gas interpretation on page 160 in this chapter to identify the acid–base disorder.

Example 1

A patient with COPD has a blood gas of pH 7.34, pCO_2 55, and $[HCO_3^-]$ of 29.

Step 1:

$$46 = 24 \times \frac{55}{29}$$

$$46 \approx 45$$

The numbers fit because the difference between the calculated and observed is < 10%.

Step 2:   pH < 7.37, an acidemia.

Step 3: pCO_2 > 44 and $[HCO_3^-]$ is **not** < 22, a respiratory acidosis.

Step 4:   Normal compensation for chronic (COPD) respiratory acidosis (from Table 8–2, page 162).

$$\Delta[HCO_3^-] = 4 \times \Delta\,(pCO_2\,/10) = 4 \times \frac{15}{10} = 6$$

Expected $[HCO_3^-]$ is 24 mEq/L + 6 = 30, which is close to the measured $[HCO_3^-]$ of 29, a simple respiratory acidosis. This patient has a chronic respiratory acidosis due to hypoventilation (simple acid–base disorder).

Example 2

Immediately after a cardiac arrest a patient has a pH 7.25, pCO_2 28, and $[HCO_3^-]$ 12.

Step 1:

$$56 = 24 \times \frac{28}{12}$$

$$56 = 56$$

The numbers fit.

Step 2:   pH < 7.37, an acidemia.

Step 3: $[HCO_3^-]$ is < 22 mEq/L and pCO_2 is **not** > 44, a metabolic acidosis.

Step 4:   (See Table 8–2, page 162)

$$pCO_2 = (1.5 \times [HCO_3^-] + 8) = (1.5 \times 12) + 8 = 26$$

The expected pCO_2 of 26 mm Hg is very similar to the actual measured value of 28 mm HG, so this is a simple metabolic acidosis. This patient has a lactic acidosis following a cardiopulmonary arrest (simple acid–base disorder).

Example 3

A young man with a fever of 103.2°F and a fruity odor on his breath has a blood gas with pH = 7.36, pCO_2 = 9, and $[HCO_3^-]$ = 5.

Step 1:

$$45 = \frac{24}{5} \times 9$$

$$43 \approx 45$$

The numbers fit.

Step 2: The pH < 7.37 indicates an acidemia.

Step 3: [HCO_3^-] < 22 and pCO_2 is **not** > 44, thus a metabolic acidosis is present.

Step 4: The expected compensation in pCO_2 can be calculated as follows (see Table 8–2, page 162):

$$pCO_2 = (1.5 \times [HCO_3^-]) + 8 \pm 2$$
$$= (1.5 \times 5) + 8 \pm 2$$
$$= 17.5 \pm 2$$

The expected pCO_2 is 17.5, but the actual result is 9 mm Hg, indicating a second process, a respiratory alkalosis. This patient has a metabolic acidosis due to DKA and a concomitant respiratory alkalosis due to early sepsis and fever (mixed acid–base disorder).

Example 4

A 30-year-old female who is 30-wk pregnant presents with nausea and vomiting. Blood gas reveals a pH 7.55, $pCO_2 = 25$ and [HCO_3^-] = 22.

Step 1:

$$28 = 24 \times \frac{25}{22}$$
$$28 \approx 27$$

The numbers fit.

Step 2: pH < 7.44 indicates alkalemia.

Step 3: pCO_2 < 36 and the [HCO_3^-] is **not** > 26, thus a respiratory alkalosis is present.

Step 4: The expected compensation for a chronic respiratory alkalosis (ie, pregnancy) is calculated from Table 8–2, page 162:

$$\Delta[HCO_3^-] = 5 \times \Delta pCO_2 / 10$$
$$= 5 \times \frac{15}{10} = 7.5$$

The calculated [HCO_3^-] is 24 – 7.5, or 16–17 mmol, but the actual bicarbonate is 22, indicating a relative secondary metabolic alkalosis ([HCO_3^-] is higher than expected).This patient has a respiratory alkalosis due to pregnancy and a relative secondary metabolic alkalosis due to vomiting.

Example 5

A 19-year-old patient with diabetes has an anion gap of 29 and a [HCO_3^-] of 6.

Step 1:

29 mmol/L actual gap
−<u>10</u> mmol/L normal gap
19 mmol/L expected change in [HCO_3^-]

Step 2:

24 mmol/L normal [HCO_3^-]

$$-\underline{19} \text{ mmol/L expected change in } [HCO_3^-]$$
$$5 \text{ mmol/L expected change in } [HCO_3^-]$$

Actual bicarbonate is 6 mmol/L, close to the expected of 5 mmol/L. Thus, a pure metabolic gap acidosis is present, most likely from DKA.

Example 6

A 21-year-old patient with diabetes presents with nausea, vomiting, and abdominal pain. The anion gap is 23, and the $[HCO_3^-]$ is 18.

Step 1:

$$23 \text{ mmol/L actual gap}$$
$$-\underline{10} \text{ mmol/L normal gap}$$
$$13 \text{ mmol/L expected change in } [HCO_3^-] \text{ from normal}$$

Step 2:

$$24 \text{ mmol/L normal } [HCO_3^-]$$
$$-\underline{13} \text{ mmol/L expected change in } [HCO_3^-]$$
$$11 \text{ mmol/L expected change in } [HCO_3^-]$$

Actual bicarbonate is 18 mmol and not the 11 mmol/L expected from a pure metabolic gap acidosis. Because the actual bicarbonate was higher than expected, this is a mixed metabolic gap acidosis and metabolic alkalosis. The patient has a metabolic gap acidosis from DKA and a metabolic alkalosis from the vomiting.

Example 7

A 55-year-old patient who drinks a fifth of whiskey per day has a 2-wk history of diarrhea. The anion gap is 17, and $[HCO_3^-]$ was 10.

Step 1:

$$17 \text{ mmol/L actual gap}$$
$$-\underline{10} \text{ mmol/L normal gap}$$
$$7 \text{ mmol/L expected change in } [HCO_3^-] \text{ from normal}$$

Step 2:

$$24 \text{ mmol/L normal } [HCO_3^-]$$
$$-\underline{7} \text{ mmol/L expected change in } [HCO_3^-]$$
$$17 \text{ mmol/L expected change in } [HCO_3^-]$$

Actual bicarbonate is 10 mmol/L and not the expected 17 mmol/L in pure metabolic gap acidosis. Because the actual bicarbonate is lower than expected, there must be a mixed metabolic gap acidosis and metabolic nongap acidosis. The patient has a metabolic nongap acidosis from diarrhea and a metabolic gap acidosis from the alcoholic ketoacidosis.

FLUIDS AND ELECTROLYTES

Principles of Fluids and Electrolytes	Determining an IV Rate
Composition of Parenteral Fluids	Electrolyte Abnormalities: Diagnosis
Composition of Body Fluids	and Treatment
Ordering IV Fluids	

PRINCIPLES OF FLUIDS AND ELECTROLYTES

Fluid Compartments

- Example: 70-kg male

Total Body Water: 42,000 mL (60% of BW)
- Intracellular: 28,000 mL (40% of BW)
- Extracellular: 14,000 mL (20% of BW)
- Plasma: 3500 mL (5% of BW)
- Interstitial: 10,500 mL (15% of BW in a 70 kg male)

Total Blood Volume

Total blood volume = 5600 mL (8% of BW in a 70 kg male)

Red Blood Cell Mass

- Male, 20–36 mL/kg (1.15–1.21 L/m^2) • Female, 19–31 mL/kg (0.95–1.0 L/m^2)

Water Balance

- 70-kg male

The minimum obligate water requirement to maintain homeostasis (assuming normal temperature and renal concentrating ability and minimal solute [urea, salt] excretion) is about 800 mL/d, which would yield 500 mL of urine.

"Normal" Intake: 2500 mL/d (about 35 mL/kg/d baseline)
- Oral liquids: 1500 mL
- Oral solids: 700 mL
- Metabolic (endogenous): 300 mL

"Normal" Output: 1400–2300 mL/d
- Urine: 800–1500 mL
- Stool: 250 mL
- Insensible loss: 600–900 mL (lungs and skin). (With fever, each degree above 98.6°F adds 2.5 mL/kg/d to insensible loss; insensible losses are decreased if a patient is on a ventilator; free water gain may occur from humidified ventilation.)

Baseline Fluid Requirement

Afebrile 70-kg Adult: 35 mL/kg/24 h

If not a 70-kg Adult: Calculate the water requirement according to the following **"kg Method"**:

- For the first 10 kg of body weight: 100 mL/kg/d plus
- For the second 10 kg of body weight: 50 mL/kg/d plus
- For the weight above 20 kg: 20 mL/kg/d

Electrolyte Requirements

- 70-kg adult, unless otherwise specified

Sodium (as NaCl):   80–120 mEq (mmol)/d (Pediatrics, 3–4 mEq/kg/ 24 h [mmol/ kg/24 h])

Chloride: 80–120 mEq (mmol)/d, as NaCl

Potassium: 50–100 mEq/d (mmol/d) (Pediatrics, 2–3 mEq/kg/24 h [mmol/ kg/24 h]). In the absence of hypokalemia and with normal renal function, most of this is excreted in the urine. Of the total amount of K, 98% is intracellular, and 2% is extracellular.

   Thus, assuming the serum K level is normal, about 4.5 mEq/L (mmol/L), the total extracellular pool of $K^+ = 4.5 \times 14$ L = 63 mEq (mmol). K is easily interchanged between intracellular and extracellular stores under conditions such as acidemia or alkalemia. K demands increase with diuresis and building of new body tissues (anabolic states).

Calcium: 1–3 g/d, most of which is secreted by the GI tract. Routine administration is not needed in the absence of specific indications.

Magnesium: 20 mEq/d (mmol/d). Routine administration is not needed in the absence of specific indications, such as parenteral hyperalimentation, massive diuresis, ethanol abuse (frequently needed) or preeclampsia.

Glucose Requirements

- 100–200 g/d (65–75 g/d/m^2). During starvation, caloric needs are supplied by body fat and protein; the majority of protein comes from the skeletal muscles. Every gram of nitrogen in the urine represents 6.25 g of protein broken down. The **protein-sparing effect** is one of the goals of basic IV therapy. The administration of at least 100 g of glucose/d reduces protein loss by more than one-half. Virtually all IV fluid solutions supply glucose as dextrose (pure dextrorotatory glucose). Pediatric patients require about 100–200 mg/kg/h.

COMPOSITION OF PARENTERAL FLUIDS

Parenteral fluids are generally classified based on molecular weight and oncotic pressure. Colloids have a molecular weight of > 8000 and have high oncotic pressure; crystalloids have a molecular weight of < 8000 and have low oncotic pressure.

Colloids

- Albumin (see Table 10–2, page 296)
- Blood products (RBCs, single-donor plasma, etc) (Chapter 10, page 189)

- Plasma protein fraction (Plasmanate) (See Chapter 22)
- Synthetic colloids (hetastarch [Hespan], dextran) (Chapter 22)

Crystalloids

Table 9–1, page 176 describes common crystalloid parenteral fluids.

COMPOSITION OF BODY FLUIDS

Table 9–2, page 177 gives the average daily production and the amount of some major electrolytes present in various body fluids.

ORDERING IV FLUIDS

One of the most difficult tasks to master is choosing appropriate IV therapy for a patient. The patient's underlying illness, vital signs, serum electrolytes, and a host of other variables all must be considered. The following are general guidelines for IV therapy. Specific requirements for each patient can vary tremendously from these guidelines.

Maintenance Fluids

These amounts provide the minimum requirements for routine daily needs:
1. **70-kg Male:** Five percent dextrose in one-quarter concentration normal saline ($D_5\frac{1}{4}NS$) with 20 mEq KCl/L (20 mmol/L) at 125 mL/h. (This will deliver about 3 L of free water/d.)
2. **Other Adult Patients:** Also use $D_5\frac{1}{4}NS$ with 20 mEq KCl/L. Determine their 24-h water requirement by the "kg method" (page 174) and divide by 24 h to determine the hourly rate.
3. **Pediatric Patients:** Use the same solution, but determine the daily fluid requirements by either of the following methods:
   a. *kg Method:* (page 174)
   b. *Meter Squared Method:* Maintenance fluids are 1500 mL/m^2/d. Divide by 24 to get the flow rate per hour. To calculate the surface area, use Table 9–3, page 177 "rule of sixes nomogram." Formal body surface area charts are in the Appendix.

Specific Replacement Fluids

These fluids are used to replace excessive, nonphysiologic losses.

Gastric Loss (Nasogastric Tube, Emesis): $D_5\frac{1}{2}NS$ with 20 mEq/L (mmol/L) potassium chloride (KCl)

Diarrhea: D_5LR with 15 mEq/L (mmol/L) KCl. Use body weight as a replacement guide (about 1 L for each 1 kg, or 2.2 lb, lost)

Bile Loss: D_5LR with 25 mEq/L (½ amp) of sodium bicarbonate mL for mL

Pancreatic Loss: D_5LR with 50 mEq/L (1 amp) HCO_3^- mL for mL.

Burn Patients: Use the Parkland or "Rule of Nines" formulas:
   Parkland Formula.

$$\text{Total fluid required during the first 24 h} = (\% \text{ body burn}) \times (\text{body weight in kg}) \times 4 \text{ mL}$$

TABLE 9–1
Composition of Commonly Used Crystalloids

		Electrolytes (mEq/L)							
Fluid	Glucose (g/L)	Na^+	Cl^-	K^+	Ca^{2+}	HCO_3^{-1}	Mg^{2+}	HPO_4^{2-}	kcal/L
D_5W (5% dextrose in water)	50	—	—	—	—	—	—	—	170
$D_{10}W$ (10% dextrose in water)	100	—	—	—	—	—	—	—	340
$D_{20}W$ (20% dextrose in water)	200	—	—	—	—	—	—	—	680
$D_{50}W$ (50% dextrose in water)	500	—	—	—	—	—	—	—	1700
½ NS (0.45% NaCl)	—	77	77	—	—	—	—	—	—
3% NS	—	513	513	—	—	—	—	—	—
NS (0.9% NaCl)	—	154	154	—	—	—	—	—	—
D_5¼NS (0.22% NaCl)	50	38	38	—	—	—	—	—	170
D_5½NS (0.45% NaCl)	50	77	77	—	—	—	—	—	170
D_5NS (0.9% NaCl)	50	154	154	—	—	—	—	—	170
D_5LR (5% dextrose in lactated Ringer's)	50	130	110	4	3	27	—	—	180
Lactated Ringer's	—	130	110	4	3	27	—	—	<10
Ionosol MB	50	25	22	20	—	23	3	3	170
Normosol M	50	40	40	13	—	16	3	—	170

[a]HCO_3 is administered in these solutions as lactate that is converted to bicarbonate.

TABLE 9-2
Composition and Daily Production of Body Fluids

Fluid	Na⁺	Cl⁻	K⁺	HCO₃⁻	Average Daily Productionᵃ (mL)
	Electrolytes (mEq/L)				

Fluid	Na^+	Cl^-	K^+	HCO_3^-	Average Daily Productionᵃ (mL)
Sweat	50	40	5	0	Varies
Saliva	60	15	26	50	1500
Gastric juice	60–100	100	10	0	1500–2500
Duodenum	130	90	5	0–10	300–2000
Bile	145	100	5	15	100–800
Pancreatic juice	140	75	5	115	100–800
Ileum	140	100	2–8	30	100–9000
Diarrhea	120	90	25	45	—

ᵃIn adults.

Replace with lactated Ringer's solution over 24 h. Use

- One-half the total over first 8 h (from time of burn)
- One-quarter of the total over second 8 h. One-quarter of the total over third 8 h
- *Rule of Nines.* Used for estimating percentage of body burned in adults. See Figure 9–1 page 178 for the exact calculation for the body burn in adults and children. This is also useful for determining ongoing fluid losses from a burn until it is healed or grafted.
- Fluid losses can be estimated as

$$\text{Loss in mL} = (25 \times \% \text{ body burn}) \times m^2 \text{ body surface area}$$

TABLE 9-3
"Rule of Sixes" Nomogram for Calculating Fluids in Childrenᵃ

Weight (lb)	Body Surface Area (m²)
3	0.1
6	0.2
12	0.3
18	0.4
24	0.5
30	0.6
36	0.7
42	0.8
48	0.9
60ᵇ	1.0

ᵃOver 100 lb, treat as an adult.
ᵇAfter 60 lb, add 0.1 for each additional 10 lb.

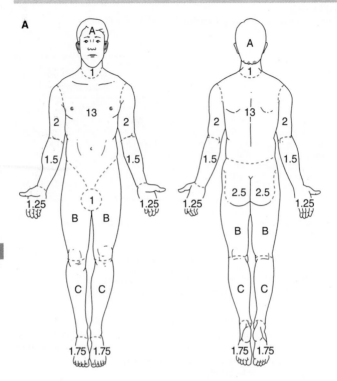

Relative Percentages of Areas Affected by Growth

Area	Age		
	10	15	Adult
A = half of head	5.5	4.5	3.5
B = half of one thigh	4.25	4.5	4.75
C = half of one leg	3	3.25	3.5

FIGURE 9–1.   Tables and graphics for estimating the extent of burns in adults **(A)** and children **(B)**. In adults, a reasonable system for calculating the percentage of the body surface burned is the "rule of nines": Each arm equals 9%, the head equals 9%, the anterior and posterior each equal 18%, and the perineum equals 1%. (Reprinted, with permission, from: Way LW, Doherty GM [eds]: *Current Surgical Diagnosis and Treatment,* 11th ed., McGraw-Hill, 2003.)

B

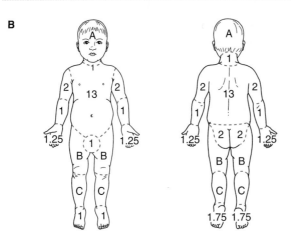

Relative Percentages of Areas Affected by Growth

Area	Age		
	0	1	5
A = half of head	9.5	8.5	6.5
B = half of one thigh	2.75	3.25	4
C = half of one leg	2.5	2.5	2.75

FIGURE 9–1. Continued.

DETERMINING AN IV RATE

Most IV infusions are regulated by infusion pumps. If a mechanical infusion device is not available, use the following formulas to determine the infusion rate.

For a MAXI Drip Chamber: Use 10 gtt/mL; thus
- 10 gtt/min = 60 mL/h or
- 16 gtt/min = 100 mL/h

For a MINI Drip Chamber: Use 60 gtt/mL; thus
- 60 gtt/min = 60 mL/h or
- 100 gtt/min = 100 mL/h

ELECTROLYTE ABNORMALITIES: DIAGNOSIS AND TREATMENT

In all of the following situations, the primary goal should be to correct the underlying condition. Unless specified, all dosages are for adults. The complete differential diagnosis of laboratory findings can be found in Chapter 4.

Hypernatremia (Na⁺ > 144 mEq/L [mmol/L])

Mechanisms: Most frequently, a deficit of total body water.

- **Combined Sodium and Water Losses ("hypovolemic hypernatremia").** Water loss in excess of Na loss results in low total body Na. Due to renal (diuretics, osmotic diuresis due to glycosuria, mannitol, postobstructive diuresis, etc) or extrarenal (sweating, GI [vomiting, NG suction], respiratory) losses

- **Excess Water Loss ("isovolemic hypernatremia").** Total body Na remains normal, but total body water is decreased. Caused by diabetes insipidus (central and nephrogenic), excess skin losses, respiratory loss, others.
- **Excess Sodium ("hypervolemic hypernatremia").** Total body Na increased, caused by iatrogenic Na administration (ie, hypertonic dialysis, hypertonic saline enemas, Na-containing medications) or other exogenous sources (sea water ingestion, salt tablets) or adrenal hyperfunction (Cushing's syndrome, hyperaldosteronism).

Symptoms: Depends on the absolute level and also how rapidly the Na$^+$ level has changed

- Confusion, irritability, lethargy, stupor, coma, muscle twitching, seizures

Signs: Hyperreflexia, mental status changes

Treatment: Check the serum Na$^+$ levels frequently while attempting to correct hypernatremia.

- **Hypovolemic Hypernatremia.** Determine if the patient volume is depleted by determining if orthostatic hypotension is present (see page 292); if volume is depleted, rehydrate with NS until patient is hemodynamically stable, then administer hypotonic saline (½NS).
- **Euvolemic/Isovolemic.** (No orthostatic hypotension) calculate the volume of free water needed to correct the Na$^+$ to normal as follows:

$$\text{Body water deficit} = \text{Normal TBW} - \text{Current TBW}$$

where

$$\text{Normal TBW} = 0.6 \times \text{Body weight in kg}$$

and

$$\text{Current TBW} = \frac{\text{Normal serum Na}^+ \times \text{TBW}}{\text{Measured serum Na}^+}$$

Give free water as D$_5$W, one-half the volume in the first 24 h and the full volume in 48 h. (**Caution:** The rapid correction of the Na$^+$ level using free water (D$_5$W) can cause cerebral edema and seizures.)
- **Hypervolemic Hypernatremia.** Avoid medications that contain excessive Na$^+$ (carbenicillin, etc).Use furosemide along with D$_5$W.

Hyponatremia (Na$^+$ < 136 mEq/L [mmol/L])

Mechanisms: Most often due to excess body water as opposed to decreased body Na$^+$. To define the cause, determine serum osmolality.

- **Isotonic Hyponatremia.** Normal osmolality
- **Pseudo-Hyponatremia.** An artifact caused by hyperlipidemia or hyperproteinemia.

- **Hypertonic Hyponatremia (dilutional).** High osmolality. Water shifts from intracellular to extracellular in response to high concentrations of such solutes as glucose or mannitol. The shift in water lowers the serum Na; however, the total body Na remains the same.
- **Hypotonic Hyponatremia.** Low osmolality. Further classified based on clinical assessment of extracellular volume status.

  Isovolemic Hyponatremia. No evidence of edema, normal BP. Caused by water intoxication (urinary osmolality < 80 mOsm), SIADH, hypothyroidism, hypoadrenalism, thiazide diuretics, beer potomania

  Hypovolemic Hyponatremia. Evidence of decreased skin turgor and an increase in heart rate and decrease in BP after going from lying to standing. Due to renal loss (urinary Na > 20 mEq/L) from diuretics, postobstructive diuresis, mineralocorticoid deficiency (Addison's disease, hypoaldosteronism) or extrarenal losses (urinary Na < 10 mEq/L) from sweating, vomiting, diarrhea, third spacing fluids (burns, pancreatitis, peritonitis, bowel obstruction, muscle trauma)

  Hypervolemic Hyponatremia. Evidence of edema (urinary Na < 10 mEq/L). Seen with CHF, nephrosis, renal failure, and liver disease

- **Excess Water Intake.** Primary (psychogenic water drinker) or secondary (large volume of sterile water used in procedures, eg, transurethral resection of the prostate or multiple tap water enemas)

Symptoms: Usually with Na^+ < 125 mEq/L (mmol/L); severity of symptoms correlates with the rate of decrease in Na^+.

- Lethargy, confusion, coma
- Muscle twitches and irritability, seizures
- Nausea, vomiting

Signs: Hyporeflexia, mental status changes

Treatment: Based on determination of volume status. Evaluate volume status by physical examination: HR and BP lying and standing after 1 min, skin turgor, edema and by determination of the plasma osmolality. Do not need to treat hyponatremia from pseudo-hyponatremia (increased protein or lipids) or hypertonic hyponatremia (hyperglycemia), treat underlying disorder (see above).

- **Life-Threatening.** (Seizures, coma) 3–5% NS can be given in the ICU setting. Attempt to raise the Na to about 125 mEq/L with 3–5% NS.
- **Isovolemic Hyponatremia.** (SIADH) Restrict fluids (1000–1500 mL/d). Demeclocycline can be used in chronic SIADH.
- **Hypervolemic Hyponatremia.** Restrict Na and fluids (1000–1500 mL/d). Treat underlying disorder. CHF may respond to a combination of ACE inhibitor and furosemide.
- **Hypovolemic Hyponatremia.** Give D_5NS or NS.

Hyperkalemia

- K^+ > 5.2 mEq/L (mmol/L)

Mechanisms: Most often due to iatrogenic or inadequate renal excretion of K.

- **Pseudo-Hyperkalemia.** Due to leukocytosis, thrombocytosis, hemolysis, poor venipuncture technique (prolonged tourniquet time)
- **Inadequate Excretion.** Renal failure, volume depletion, medications that block K^+ excretion (spironolactone, triamterene, others), hypoaldosteronism (including adrenal disorders and hyporeninemic states [such as type IV renal tubular acidosis], NSAIDs, ACE inhibitors), long-standing use of heparin, digitalis toxicity, sickle cell disease, renal transplant
- **Redistribution.** Tissue damage, acidosis (a 0.1 decrease in pH increases serum K^+ approximately 0.5–1.0 mEq/L due to extracellular shift of K^+), beta-blockers, decreased insulin, succinylcholine
- **Excess Administration.** K-containing salt substitutes, oral replacement, K^+ in IV fluids

Symptoms: Weakness, flaccid paralysis, confusion.

Signs:
- Hyperactive deep tendon reflexes, decreased motor strength
- ECG changes, such as, peaked T waves, wide QRS, loss of P wave, sine wave, asystole
- $K^+ = 7–8$ mEq/L (mmol/L) yields ventricular fibrillation in 5% of cases
- $K^+ = 10$ mEq/L (mmol/L) yields ventricular fibrillation in 90% of cases

Treatment
- Monitor patient on ECG if symptomatic or if $K^+ > 6.5$ mEq/L; discontinue all K^+ intake, including IV fluids; order a repeat stat K^+ to confirm.
- Pseudo-hyperkalemia should be ruled out. If doubt exists, obtain a plasma K^+ in a heparinized tube; the plasma K will be normal if pseudo-hyperkalemia is present.

- **Rapid Correction.** These steps only protect the heart from K^+ shifts, and total body K^+ must be reduced by one of the treatments shown under Slow Correction.

Calcium chloride, 500 mg, slow IV push (only protects heart from effect of hyperkalemia)

Alkalinize with 50 mEq (1 amp) Na bicarbonate (causes intracellular K^+ shift)

50 mL $D_{50}W$, IV push, with 10–15 units regular insulin, IV push (causes intracellular K shift)

- **Slow Correction**
  Sodium polystyrene sulfonate (Kayexalate) 20–60 g given orally with 100–200 mL of sorbitol or 40 g Kayexalate with 40 g sorbitol in 100 mL water given as an enema. Repeat doses qid as needed.
  Dialysis (hemodialysis or peritoneal)

- **Correct Underlying Cause.** Such as stopping K-sparing diuretics, ACE inhibitors, mineralocorticoid replacement for hypokalemia

Hypokalemia

- $K^+ < 3.6$ mEq/L (mmol/L)

Mechanisms: Due to inadequate intake, loss, or intracellular shifts

- **Inadequate Intake.** Oral or IV
- **GI Tract Loss.** (Urinary chloride usually < 10 mEq/d; "chloride-responsive alkalosis") vomiting, diarrhea, excess sweating, villous adenoma, fistula

- **Renal Loss.** Diuretics and other medications (amphotericin, high-dose penicillins, aminoglycosides, cisplatin), diuresis other than diuretics (osmotic, eg, hyperglycemia or ethanol-induced), vomiting (from metabolic alkalosis from volume depletion), renal tubular disease (renal tubular acidosis type II [distal], and [proximal]), Bartter's syndrome (due to increased renin and aldosterone levels), hypomagnesemia, natural licorice ingestion, mineralocorticoid excess (primary and secondary hyperaldosteronism, Cushing's syndrome, steroid use), and ureterosigmoidostomy
- **Redistribution (Intracellular Shifts).** Metabolic alkalosis (each 0.1 increase in pH lowers serum K^+ approximately 0.5–1.0 mEq/L, due to intracellular shift of K^+), insulin administration, beta-adrenergic agents, familial periodic paralysis and treatment of megaloblastic anemia

Symptoms
- Muscle weakness, cramps, tetany
- Polyuria, polydipsia

Signs
- Decreased motor strength, orthostatic hypotension, ileus
- ECG changes, such as flattening of T waves, "U" wave becomes obvious (U wave is the upward deflection after the T wave.)

Treatment: The therapy depends on the cause.
- A history of HTN, GI symptoms, or use of certain medications may suggest the diagnosis.
- A 24-h urine for K^+ may be helpful if the diagnosis is unclear. Levels < 20 mEq/d suggest extrarenal/redistribution, > 20 mEq/d suggest renal losses.
- A serum K^+ level of 2 mEq/L (mmol/L) probably represents a deficit of at least 200 mEq (mmol) in a 70-kg adult; to change K^+ from 3 mEq/L (mmol/L) to 4 mEq/L (mmol/L) takes about 100 mEq (mmol) of K^+ in a 70-kg adult.
- Treat underlying cause.
- Hypokalemia potentiates the cardiac toxicity of digitalis. In the setting of digoxin use, hypokalemia should be aggressively treated.
- Treat hypomagnesemia if present. It will be difficult to correct hypokalemia in the presence of hypomagnesemia.
- **Rapid Correction.** Give KCl IV. Monitor heart with replacement > 20 mEq/h. IV K^+ can be painful and damaging to veins.

  Patient < 40 kg: 0.25 mEq/kg/h × 2 h
  Patient > 40 kg: 10–20 mEq/h × 2 h
  Severe [< 2 mEq/L (mmol/L)]: Maximum 40 mEq/h IV in adults. In all cases check a stat K^+ following each 2–4 h of replacement.

- **Slow Correction.** Give KCl orally (see also Table 22–8, page 620) for K^+ supplements).

  Adult: 20–40 mEq two to three times a day (bid or tid)
  Pediatric patients: 1–2 mEq/kg/d in divided doses

Hypercalcemia

- $Ca^{2+} > 10.2$ mg/dL (2.55 mmol/L)

Mechanisms
- **Parathyroid-Related.** Hyperparathyroidism with secondary bone resorption
- **Malignancy-Related.** Solid tumors with metastases (breast, ovary, lung, kidney), or paraneoplastic syndromes, (squamous cell, renal cell, transitional cell carcinomas, lymphomas, and myeloma)
- **Vitamin-D-Related.** Vitamin D intoxication, sarcoidosis, other granulomatous disease
- **High Bone Turnover.** Hyperthyroidism, Paget's disease, immobilization, vitamin A intoxication
- **Renal Failure.** Secondary hyperparathyroidism, aluminum intoxication
- **Other.** Thiazide diuretics, milk–alkali syndrome, familial hypocalciuric hypercalcemia, exogenous intake

Symptoms
- Stones (renal colic), bones (osteitis fibrosa), moans (constipation), and groans (neuropsychiatric symptoms—confusion), as well as polyuria, polydipsia, fatigue, anorexia, nausea, vomiting

Signs
- HTN, hyporeflexia, mental status changes
- Shortening of the QT interval on the ECG.

Treatment: Usually emergency treatment if patient is symptomatic and $Ca^{2+} >$ 13 mEq/L (3.24 mmol/L)

Use saline diuresis: D_5NS at 250–500 mL/h.

Give furosemide (Lasix) 20–80 mg or more IV (saline and Lasix will treat most cases).

Euvolemia or hypervolemia must be maintained. Hypovolemia results in calcium reabsorption.

- **Other Second-Line Therapies**

Calcitonin 2–8 IU/kg IV or SQ q6–12h if diuresis has not worked after 2–3 h
Pamidronate 60 mg IV over 24 h (one dose only)
Gallium nitrate 200 mg/m^2 IV infusion over 24 h for 5 d
Plicamycin 25 µg/kg IV over 2–3 h (use as last resort—very potent)
Corticosteroids. Hydrocortisone 50–75 mg IV every 6 h
Hemodialysis.

- **Chronic Therapy**

Treat underlying condition, discontinue contributing medications (ie, thiazides).

Oral medications (prednisone 30 mg PO bid or P/K/Na supplement [Neutra-Phos] 250–500 mg PO qid) can be effective in chronic therapy for such diseases as breast cancer or sarcoidosis.

Hypocalcemia

- $Ca^{2+} < 8.4$ mg/dL (2.1 mmol/L)

Mechanisms: Decreased albumin can result in decreased total calcium (see discussion on page 53).

- **PTH.** Responsible for the immediate regulation of calcium levels
- **Critical Illness.** Sepsis and other ICU-related conditions can cause decreased calcium because of the fall in albumin often seen in critically ill patients, ionized calcium may be normal.
- **PTH Deficiency.** Acquired (surgical excision or injury, infiltrative diseases such as amyloidosis or hemochromatosis and irradiation) hereditary hypoparathyroidism (pseudo-hypoparathyroidism), hypomagnesemia
- **Vitamin D Deficiency.** Chronic renal failure, liver disease, use of phenytoin or phenobarbital, malnutrition, malabsorption (chronic pancreatitis, postgastrectomy)
- **Other.** Hyperphosphatemia, acute pancreatitis, osteoblastic metastases, medullary carcinoma of the thyroid, massive transfusion

Symptoms

- Hypertension, peripheral and perioral paresthesia, abdominal pain and cramps, lethargy, irritability (in infants)
- Signs
- Hyperactive DTRs, carpopedal spasm (Trousseau's sign, see page 19).
- Positive Chvostek's sign (see page 16) (facial nerve twitch, can be present in up to 25% of normal adults).
- Generalized seizures, tetany, laryngospasm
- Prolonged QT interval on ECG

Treatment

- **Acute Symptomatic**

  100–200 mg of elemental calcium IV over 10 min in 50–100 mL of D_5W followed by an infusion containing 1–2 mg/kg/h over 6–12 h 10% calcium gluconate contains 93 mg of elemental calcium. 10% calcium chloride contains 272 mg of elemental calcium. Check magnesium levels and replace if low.

- **Chronic**

  For renal insufficiency, use vitamin D along with oral calcium supplements (see the following lists) and phosphate-binding antacids (Phospho gel, AlternaGEL).
  Calcium supplements:

  Calcium carbonate (Os-Cal) 650 mg PO qid (28% calcium)
  Calcium citrate (Critical) 950-mg tablets (21% calcium)
  Calcium gluconate 500- or 1000-mg tablets (9% calcium)
  Calcium glubionate (Neo-Calglucon) syrup 115 mg/5 mL (6.4% calcium)
  Calcium lactate 325- or 650-mg tablets (13% calcium)

Hypermagnesemia

- $Mg^{2+} > 2.1$ mEq/L (mmol/L)

Mechanisms

- **Excess Administration.** Treatment of preeclampsia with magnesium sulfate
- **Renal Insufficiency.** Exacerbated by ingestion of magnesium-containing antacids
- **Others.** Rhabdomyolysis, adrenal insufficiency

Symptoms and Signs
- 3–5 mEq/L(mmol/L): Nausea, vomiting, hypotension
- 7–10 mEq/L (mmol/L): Hyperreflexia, weakness, drowsiness
- > 12 mEq/L (mmol/L): Coma, bradycardia, respiratory failure

Treatment: Clinical hypermagnesemia requiring therapy is infrequently encountered in the patient with normal renal function.

- Calcium gluconate: 10 mL of 10% solution (93 mg elemental calcium) over 10–20 min in 50–100 mL of D_5W given IV to reverse symptoms (useful in patients being treated for eclampsia).
- Stop magnesium-containing medications (hypermagnesemia is most often encountered in patients in renal failure on magnesium-containing antacids).
- Insulin and glucose as for hyperkalemia. Furosemide and saline diuresis
- Dialysis

Hypomagnesemia

- $Mg^{2+} < 1.5$ mEq/L (mmol/L)

Mechanisms
- **Decreased Intake or Absorption.** Malabsorption, chronic GI losses, deficient intake (alcoholics), TPN without adequate supplementation
- **Increased Loss.** Diuretics, other medications (gentamicin, cisplatin, amphotericin B, others), RTA, DM (especially DKA), alcoholism, hyperaldosteronism, excessive lactation
- **Other.** Acute pancreatitis, hypoalbuminemia, vitamin D therapy.

Symptoms
- Weakness, muscle twitches, asterixis, vertigo

Symptoms of hypocalcemia and hypokalemia (hypomagnesemia may cause hypocalcemia and hypokalemia)

Signs
- Tachycardia, tremor, hyperactive reflexes, tetany, seizures
- ECG may show prolongation of the PR, QT, and QRS intervals as well as ventricular ectopy, sinus tachycardia

Treatment
- **Severe: Tetany or Seizures:** Monitor patient with ECG in ICU setting. 2 g magnesium sulfate in D_5W infused over 10–20 min. Follow with magnesium sulfate: 1 g/h for 3–4 h follow DTR and levels. Repeat replacement if necessary. These patients are often hypokalemic and hypophosphatemic as well and should be supplemented. Hypocalcemia may also result from hypomagnesemia.
- **Moderate:** $Mg^{2+} < 1.0$ mg/dL but asymptomatic: Magnesium sulfate: 1 g/h for 3–4 h, follow levels and repeat replacement if necessary.
- **Mild:** Magnesium oxide: 1 g/d PO (available over the counter in 140-mg capsules, and in 400- and 420-mg tablets). May cause diarrhea.

Hyperphosphatemia

- $PO_4^{3-} > 4.5$ mg/dL (1.45 mmol/L)

Mechanisms
- **Increased Intake/Absorption.** Iatrogenic, abuse of laxatives or enemas containing phosphorus, vitamin D, granulomatous disease
- **Decreased Excretion** (Most Common Cause). Renal failure, hypoparathyroidism, adrenal insufficiency, hyperthyroidism, acromegaly, sickle cell anemia
- **Redistribution/Cellular Release.** Rhabdomyolysis, acidosis, chemotherapy-induced tumor lysis, hemolysis, plasma cell dyscrasias

Symptoms and Signs: Mostly related to tetany as a result of hypocalcemia (see page 184) caused by the hyperphosphatemia or metastatic calcification (deposition of calcium phosphate in various soft tissues)

Treatment
- Low-phosphate diet
- Phosphate binders like aluminum hydroxide gel (Amphojel) or aluminum carbonate gel (Basaljel) orally
- Acute, severe cases: Acetazolamide 15 mg/kg q4h or insulin and glucose infusion, dialysis as last resort

Hypophosphatemia

- $PO_4^{3-} < 2.5$ mg/dL (0.8 mmol/L)

Mechanisms
- **Decreased Dietary Intake.** Starvation, alcoholism, iatrogenic (hyperalimentation without adequate supplementation), malabsorption, vitamin D deficiency, phosphate-binding antacids (ie, AlternaGEL)
- **Redistribution.** Conditions associated with respiratory or metabolic alkalosis (alcohol withdrawal, salicylate poisoning, etc), endocrine (insulin, catecholamine, etc), anabolic steroids, hyper- or hypothermia, leukemias and lymphomas, hypercalcemia, hypomagnesemia
- **Renal Losses.** RTA, diuretic phase of ATN, hyperparathyroidism, hyperthyroidism, hypokalemia, diuretics, hypomagnesemia, alcohol abuse, poorly controlled DM
- **Other.** Refeeding in the setting of severe protein-calorie malnutrition, severe burns, treatment of DKA

Symptoms and Signs: < 1 mg/dL (0.32 mmol/L): Weakness, muscle pain and tenderness, paresthesia, cardiac and respiratory failure, CNS dysfunction (confusion and seizures), rhabdomyolysis, hemolysis, impaired leukocyte and platelet function

Treatment: IV therapy is reserved for severe potentially life-threatening hypophosphatemia (< 1.0–1.5 mg/dL) because too rapid correction can lead to severe hypocalcemia. With mild to moderate hypophosphatemia (1.5–2.5 mg/dL), oral replacement is preferred.

- **Severe.** (< 1.0–1.5 mg/dL) Potassium or sodium phosphate. 2 mg/kg (0.08 mmol/kg) given IV over 6 h. (**Caution:** Too rapid replacement can lead to hypocalcemic tetany.)
- **Mild to Moderate.** (Levels > 1.5 mg/dL) Sodium–potassium phosphate (Neutra-Phos) or potassium phosphate (K-Phos): 1–2 tablets (250–500 mg PO_4 or 8 mmol/tablet) PO bid or tid: Sodium phosphate (Fleet's Phospho-soda) 5 mL PO_4^{-3}, bid or tid (128 mg PO_4^{-3} or 4 mmol/mL)

BLOOD COMPONENT THERAPY

BLOOD BANKING PROCEDURES

T&S or T&H: The blood bank types the patient's blood (ABO and Rh) and screens for antibodies. If a rare antibody is found, the physician will usually be notified, and if it is likely that blood will be needed, the T&S order may be changed to a T&C. This usually takes less than 1 h.

T&C: The blood bank types and screens the patient's blood as described in the previous section and matches specific donor units for the patient. The cross-match involves testing the recipient's serum against the donor blood cells.

STAT Requests: The bank sets up blood immediately and usually holds it for 12 h. For routine requests, the blood is set up at a date and time that you specify and usually held for 36 h.

ROUTINE BLOOD DONATION

Voluntary blood donation is the mainstay of the blood system in the United States. Donors must usually be > 18 y old, in good health, afebrile. and weigh > 110 lb. Donors are usually limited to 1 unit every 8 wk and 6 donations/y. Patients with a history of hepatitis, HBsAg positivity, insulin-dependent DM, IV drug abuse, heart disease, anemia, and homosexual activity are excluded from routine donation. Patients who may have transmissible diseases are counseled about high-risk behaviors that may put the recipient of the blood at risk. Donor blood is tested for ABO, Rh, antibody screen, HBsAg, antihepatitis B core antigen, hepatitis C antibody, anti-HIV-1 and 2, and anti-HTLV-1 and 2.

AUTOLOGOUS BLOOD DONATION

Preadmission autologous blood banking (predeposit phlebotomy) is popular for some patients anticipating elective surgery in which blood may be needed. General guidelines for autologous banking include good overall health status, an HCT greater than 34%, and arm veins that can accommodate a 16-gauge needle. Patients can usually donate up to 1 unit every 3–7 d, until 3–7 d prior to surgery (individual blood banks have their own specifications), depending on the needs of the planned surgery. Iron supplements (eg, ferrous gluconate 325 mg PO tid) are usually given prior to and several months after the donation. The use of erythropoietin is being investigated in this preoperative setting. Units of whole blood can be held for up to 35 d.

DONOR-DIRECTED BLOOD PRODUCTS

This method of donation involves a relative or friend donating blood for a specific patient. This technique cannot be used in the emergency setting because it takes up to 48 h to process the blood for use.

This system has some drawbacks: Relatives may be unduly pressured to give blood, risk factors that would normally exclude the use of the blood (hepatitis or HIV positivity) become problematic, and ultimately the routine donation of blood for emergency transfusion may be adversely affected. These units are usually stored as PRBC and released into the general transfusion pool 8 h after surgery unless otherwise requested.

IRRADIATED BLOOD COMPONENTS

Transfusion-associated GVHD, a frequently fatal condition, can be minimized through the use of highly selected irradiated blood components. Patients who are at risk for GVHD include recipients of donor-directed units or HLA-matched platelets, fetal intrauterine transfusions, and selected immunocompromised and bone marrow recipients.

APHERESIS

Apheresis procedures are used to collect single-donor platelets (**plateletpheresis**) or white blood cells (**leukapheresis**); the remaining components are returned to the donor. **Therapeutic apheresis** is the separation and removal of a particular component to achieve a therapeutic effect (eg, **erythrocytapheresis** to treat polycythemia).

PREOPERATIVE BLOOD SET-UP

Most institutions have established parameters for setting up blood before surgical procedures. A number of units of PRBC or only a T&S may be needed based on the procedure. Check with the surgeon.

EMERGENCY TRANSFUSIONS

Non-cross-matched blood is rarely transfused because most blood banks can do a complete cross-match within 1 h. In cases of massive, exsanguinating hemorrhage, type-specific blood (ABO- and Rh-matched only), usually available in 10 min, can be used. If even this delay is too long, type O, Rh-negative, PRBC can be used as a last resort. When possible, it is generally preferable to support BP with colloid or crystalloid until properly cross-matched blood is available.

BLOOD GROUPS

Table 10–1 page 191 gives information on the major blood groups and their relative occurrences. O– is the **"universal donor"** and AB+ is the **"universal recipient."**

BASIC PRINCIPLES OF BLOOD COMPONENT THERAPY

Table 10–2 page 192 provides some common indications and uses for transfusion products. The following are the basic transfusion principles for adults.

TABLE 10–1
Blood Groups and Guidelines for Transfusion

Type (ABO/Rh)	Occurrences	Can Usually Receive[a] Blood From
O+	1 in 3	O (+/–)
O–	1 in 15	O (–)
A+	1 in 3	A (+/–) or O (+/–)
A–	1 in 16	A (–) or O (–)
B+	1 in 12	B (+/–) or O (+/–)
B–	1 in 67	B (–) or O (–)
AB+	1 in 29	AB, A, B, or O (all + or –)
AB–	1 in 167	AB, A, B, or O (all –)

[a]First choice is always the identical blood type, other acceptable combinations are shown. An attempt is also made to match Rh status of donor and recipient; Rh negative can usually be given to an RH+ recipient safely.

Red Cell Transfusions

Acute Blood Loss: Normal, healthy individuals can usually tolerate up to 30% blood loss without need for transfusion; patients may manifest tachycardia, mild hypotension without evidence of hypovolemic shock. Replace loss with volume (IV fluids, etc) replacement.

- Hgb > 10 g/dL, rarely needs transfusion.
- Hgb 6–10 g/dL, transfuse based on clinical symptoms, unless patient has severe medical problems (ie, CAD, severe COPD).
- Hgb < 6 g/dL usually requires transfusion.

"Allowable Blood Loss": Often used to guide acute transfusion in the operating room setting. Losses less than allowable are usually managed with IV fluid replacement.

$$\text{Weight in kg} \times 0.08 = \text{Total blood volume}$$

$$\text{Total volume} \times 0.3 = \text{Allowable blood loss (assumes normal Hbg)}$$

Example: A 70-kg adult

$$\text{Estimated allowable blood loss} = 70 \times 0.08 =$$
$$5.6\text{L or } (5600 \text{ mL}) \times 0.3 = 1680 \text{ mL}$$

Chronic Anemia: Common in certain chronic conditions such as renal failure, rarely managed with blood transfusion; typically managed with pharmacologic therapy (eg, erythropoietin). However, transfusion is generally indicated if Hgb < 6 g/dL or in the face of symptoms due to low hemoglobin.

RBC Transfusion Formula: As a guide, one unit of PRBC raises the HCT by 3% (Hgb 1 g/dL) in the average adult. To roughly determine the volume of whole blood or PRBC needed to raise a HCT to a known amount, use the following formula:

TABLE 10–2
Blood Bank Products

Product	Description	Common Indications
Whole blood (see also page 191)	No elements removed 1 unit = 450 mL ± 45 mL (HCT ≈ 40%) Contains RBC, WBC, plasma and platelets (WBC & platelets may be nonfunctional) Deficient in factors V & VII	Not for routine use Acute, massive bleeding Open heart surgery Neonatal total exchange
Packed Red Cells (PRBC) (see also page 191)	Most plasma, WBC, platelets removed; unit = 250–300 mL. (HCT ≈ 75%) 1 unit should raise HCT 3%	Replacement in chronic and acute blood loss, GI bleeding, trauma
Universal Pedi-Packs	250–300 mL divided into 3 bags Contains red cells, some white cells, some plasma and platelets	Transfusion of infants
Leukocyte-Poor (Leukocyte-reduced) Red Cells	Most WBC removed by filtration to make it less antigenic <5×10^6 WBC, few platelets, minimal plasma 1 unit = 200–250 mL	Potential renal transplant patients Previous febrile transfusion reactions Patients requiring multiple transfusions (leukemia, etc.)

(continued)

10

TABLE 10–2
(Continued)

Product	Description	Common Indications
Washed RBCs	Like leukocyte-poor red cells, but WBC almost completely removed <5 × 10⁸ WBC, no plasma 1 unit = 300 mL	As for leukocyte-poor red cells, but very expensive and much more purified
Granulocytes (pheresis)	1 unit = ≈220 mL Some RBC, >1 × 10¹⁰ PMN/unit, lymphocytes, platelets	See page 190
Platelets (see also page 197)	1 "pack" should raise count by 5000–8000 "6-pack" means a pool of platelets from 6 units of blood 1 pack = about 50 mL >5 × 10¹⁰ platelets unit, contains RBC, WBC	Decreased production or destruction (ie, aplastic anemia, acute leukemia, postchemo, etc) Counts <5000–10,000 (risk of spontaneous hemorrhage) must transfuse Counts 10,000–30,000 if risk of bleeding (headache, GI losses, contiguous petechiae) or active bleeding Counts <50,000 if life-threatening bleed Prophylactic transfusion >20,000 for minor surgery or >50,000 for major surgery Usually not indicated in ITP or TTP unless life-threatening bleeding or preoperatively

(continued)

10

**TABLE 10–2
(Continued)**

Product	Description	Common Indications
Platelets, pheresis	>3 × 10¹⁰ platelets/unit 1 unit = 300 mL	See Platelets, may be HLA matched
Platelets, leukocyte-reduced	As above, but <5 × 10⁶ WBC/unit	See Platelets, may decrease febrile reactions and CMV transmission, alloimmunization to HLA antigens
Cryoprecipitated Antihemophilic Factor ("Cryo")	Contains factor VIII, factor XIII, von Willebrand's factor, and fibrinogen 1 unit = 10 mL	Hemophilia A (factor VIII deficiency), when safer factor VIII concentrate not available; von Willebrand's disease, fibrinogen deficiency, fibrin surgical glue
Fresh-Frozen Plasma (FFP)	Contains factors II, VII, IX, X, XI, XII, XIII and heat-labile V and VII About 1 h to thaw 150–250 mL (400–600 mL if single-donor pheresis)	Emergency reversal of Warfarin Massive transfusion (>5 L in adults) Hypoglobulinemia (IV immune globulin preferred) Suspected or documented coagulopathy (congenital or acquired) with active bleeding or before surgery Clotting factor replacement when concentrate unavailable Not recommended for volume replacement If PT <22 s or PTT <70 s, 1 unit is usually sufficient

(continued)

TABLE 10–2
(Continued)

Product	Description	Common Indications
Single Donor Plasma	Like FFP, but lacks factors V and VIII About 1 h to thaw; 150–200 ml	No longer routinely used for plasma replacement Stable clotting factor replacement Warfarin reversal, hemophilia B (Christmas disease)
Rho Gam (Rho D immune globulin)	Antibody against Rh factor (volume = 1 mL)	Rh-mother with Rh+ baby, within 72 h of delivery, to prevent hemolytic disease of newborn; autoimmune thrombocytopenia

ALL OF THE AFOREMENTIONED ITEMS USUALLY REQUIRE A "CLOT TUBE" TO BE SENT FOR TYPING. THE FOLLOWING PRODUCTS ARE USUALLY DISPENSED BY MOST HOSPITAL PHARMACIES AND ARE USUALLY ORDERED AS A MEDICATION.

Product	Description	Common Indications
Factor VII (purified antihemophilic factor)	From pooled plasma, pure Factor VIII Increased hepatitis risk	Routine for hemophilia A (factor VIII deficiency)
Factor IX concentrate (prothrombin complex)	Increased hepatitis risk Factors II, VII, IX, and X Equivalent to 2 units of plasma	Active bleeding in Christmas disease (Hemophilia B or factor IX deficiency)
Immune serum globulin	Precipitate from plasma "gamma globulin"	Immune globulin deficiency Disease prophylaxis (hepatitis A, measles, etc.)

(continued)

10

TABLE 10–2
(Continued)

Product	Description	Common Indications
5% Albumin or 5% plasma protein fraction	Precipitate from plasma (see Drugs, Chapter 22)	Plasma volume expanders in acute blood loss
25% Albumin	Precipitate from plasma	Hypoalbuminemia, volume expander, burns
		Draws extravascular fluid into circulation

RBC = red blood cells; WBC = white blood cells; HCT = hematocrit; GI = gastrointestinal; ITP = idiopathic thrombocytopenic purpura; TTP = thrombotic thrombocytopenic purpura; HLA = histocompatibility locus antigen; PT = prothrombin time; PTT = partial thromboplastin time.

10

$$\text{Volume of cells} = \frac{\text{Total blood volume of patient} \times (\text{Desired HCT} - \text{Actual HCT})}{\text{HCT of transfusion product}}$$

where total blood volume is 70 mL/kg in adults, 80 mL/kg in children; the HCT of PRBC is approximately 70, and that of whole blood is approximately 40.

White Cell Transfusions

- The use of white cell transfusions is rarely indicated today due to the use of genetically engineered myeloid growth factors such as GM-CSF (see Chapter 22)
- Indicated for patients being treated for overwhelming sepsis and severe neutropenia (< 500 PMN/μL)

Platelet Transfusions

For indications, see Table 10–2, page 192

Platelet Transfusion Formula: Platelets are often transfused at a dose of 1 unit/10 kg of body weight. After administration of 1 unit of multiple-donor platelets, the count should rise 5000–8000/mm³ within 1 h of transfusion and 4500 mm³ within 24 h. Normally, stored platelets that are transfused survive in vivo 6–8 d after infusion. Clinical factors (DIC, alloimmunization) can significantly shorten these intervals. To standardize the corrected platelet count to an individual patient, use the CCI. Measure the platelet count immediately before and 1 h after the platelet infusion. If the correction is less than expected, do a work-up to determine the possible cause (antibodies, splenomegaly, etc). Many institutions are now using platelet pheresis units. One platelet pheresis unit has enough platelets to raise the count by 6000–8000/mm³. Using a single unit has the advantage of exposing the patient to only one donor versus possibly six to eight donors. This limits exposure to different HLA antigens, thus reducing the risk of antiplatelet antibody production and also reduces the risks of infection transmission.

$$\text{CCI} = \frac{\text{Posttransfusion platelet count} - \text{Pretransfusion count} \times \text{Body surface area (m}^2)}{\text{Platelets given} \times 10^{11}}$$

BLOOD BANK PRODUCTS

Table 10–2 (page 192) describes products used in blood component therapy and gives recommendations for use of these products.

TRANSFUSION PROCEDURES

1. Draw a clot tube (red top), and sign the lab slips to verify that the sample came from the correct patient. The patient should be identified by referring to the ID bracelet and asking the patient, if able, to state his or her name. Place the patient's name, hospital number, date, and your signature on the tube label. **Prestamped labels are not accepted by most blood banks.**

2. Obtain the patient's informed consent by discussing the reasons for the transfusion and the potential risks and benefits from it. Follow hospital procedure regarding the need for the patient to sign a specific consent form. At most hospitals, chart documentation is usually all that is necessary.

3. When the blood products become available, ensure good venous access for the transfusion (18-gauge needle or larger is preferred in an adult).

4. Verify the information on the request slip and blood bag with another person, such as a nurse, and with the patient's ID bracelet. Many hospitals have defined protocols for this procedure; check your institutional guidelines.

5. Mix blood products to be transfused with isotonic (0.9%) NS only. Using hypotonic products such as D_5W may result in hemolysis of the blood in the tubing. Lactated Ringer's should *not* be used because the calcium could chelate the anticoagulant citrate.

6. Red cells are infused through a special filter. Specific leukocyte reduction filters are available and may be used in very specific circumstances (history of febrile transfusion reactions, to reduce potential CMV transmission, to reduce risk of alloimmunization to WBC antigens).

7. When transfusing large volumes of PRBC (> 10 units), monitor coagulation, Mg^{2+}, Ca^{2+}, and lactate levels. It is usually necessary to also transfuse platelets and FFP. Also, a calcium replacement is sometimes needed because the preservative used in the blood is a calcium binder, and hypocalcemia can result after large amounts of blood are transfused. Also, for massive transfusions (usually > 50 mL/min in adults and 15 mL/min in children), the blood should be warmed to prevent hypothermia and cardiac arrhythmias.

10

TRANSFUSION REACTIONS

Several types of transfusion reactions are possible:

1. **Acute intravascular hemolysis.** Over 85% of adverse hemolytic reactions involving the transfusion of RBCs result from clerical error. Usually caused by ABO-incompatible transfusion. Can result in renal failure (< 1/250,000 units transfused).

2. **Nonhemolytic febrile reaction.** Usually mild, fever, chills, rigors, mild dyspnea. Due to a reaction to donor white cells (HLA) and more common in patients who have had multiple transfusions or delivered several children ($\cong$2–3:100 units transfused).

3. **Mild allergic reaction.** Urticaria or pruritus can be caused by sensitization to plasma proteins in transfusion product ($\cong$1/100 units transfused).

4. **Anaphylactic reaction.** Acute hypotension, hives, abdominal pain and respiratory distress; seen mostly in IgA-deficient recipients (< 1/1000 units transfused).

5. **Sepsis.** Usually caused by transfusion of a bacterially infected transfusion product, with platelet transfusions having the greatest risk. *E. coli, Pseudomonas, Serratia, Salmonella,* and *Yersinia* are the more commonly implicated bacteria (< 1/500,000 RBC units transfused, 1/12,000 platelet units transfused).

6. **Acute lung injury.** Fever, chills, and life-threatening respiratory failure; probably induced by antibodies from donor against recipient white cells (< 1/5000 units transfused).

7. **Volume overload.** Usually due to excess volume infusion; can exacerbate CHF.

Detection of a Transfusion Reaction

1. Spin an HCT to look for a pink plasma layer (indicates hemolysis).
2. Order serum for free Hgb and serum haptoglobin (haptoglobin decreases with a reaction) and urine for hemosiderin levels. Obtain a stat CBC to determine the presence of schistocytes, which can be present with a transfusion reaction.
3. If you suspect acute hemolysis, request a DIC screen (PT, PTT, fibrinogen, and fibrin degradation products).

Treatment of Transfusion Reactions

1. Stop the blood product immediately, and notify the blood bank.
2. Keep the IV line open with NS, and monitor the patient's vital signs and urine output carefully.
3. Save the blood bag, and have the lab verify the T&C. Verify that the proper patient received the proper transfusion. Redraw blood samples for the blood bank.
4. Make specific recommendations, using the following guidelines; modifications should be based on clinical judgment.

   - **Nonhemolytic febrile reaction:** Antipyretics can be used and the transfusion continued with monitoring. Use leukocyte-washed transfusion products in future.
   - **Mild allergic reaction:** Administer diphenhydramine (25–50 mg IM/PO/IV). Resume the transfusion carefully only if the patient improves promptly.
   - **Anaphylactic reaction.** Terminate transfusion, monitor closely, give antihistamines (diphenhydramine 25–50 mg IM/PO/IV), corticosteroids (methylprednisolone 125 mg IV, 2 mg/kg Peds IV), epinephrine (1:1000 0.3–0.5 mL SQ adults, 0.1 mL/kg Peds), and pressors as needed. Premedicate (antihistamines, steroids) for future transfusions; use only leukocyte-washed red cells.
   - **Acute lung injury.** Give ventilatory support as needed; use only leukocyte-washed red cells for future transfusions.
   - **Sepsis:** Culture the transfusion product and specimens from the patient; treat sepsis empirically by monitoring and administering pressors and antibiotics (third-/fourth-generation cephalosporin or piperacillin/tazobactam along with an aminoglycoside) until cultures return.
   - **Volume overload.** Employ a slow rate of infusion with selective use of diuretics.
   - **Acute intravascular hemolysis.** Prevent acute renal failure. Place a Foley catheter, monitor the urine output closely, and maintain a brisk diuresis with plain D_5W, mannitol (1–2 g/kg IV), furosemide (20–40 mg IV), and/or dopamine (2–10 mcg/kg/min IV) as needed. Consider alkalinization of the urine with bicarbonate (see Chapter 22). DIC may be present. A renal and hematology consult are usually indicated with a severe hemolytic reaction. Support pressure as needed (fluids, vasopressors such as dopamine).

10

TRANSFUSION-ASSOCIATED INFECTIOUS DISEASE RISKS

Hepatitis

Incidence of posttransfusion hepatitis for Hep B is 1:63,000 units transfused and for Hep C is 1:103,000 units transfused. Anicteric hepatitis is more common than hepatitis with jaundice. Screening of donors for HBsAg and hepatitis C has greatly reduced the transmission of these forms of hepatitis. Historically, the greatest risk is with pooled factor products (concentrates of factor VIII). Use of albumin and globulins involves no risk of hepatitis.

HIV

Incidence is < 1:600,000 units transfused. Antibody testing is routinely performed on the donor's blood. A positive antibody test means that the donor may be infected with the HIV virus; a confirmatory Western blot is necessary. Do a follow-up test on any donor found to be HIV-positive because false-positives can occur. With screening, AIDS transmission has decreased. Because there is a delay of approximately 22 d between HIV exposure and the development of the HIV antibody, a potential risk of HIV transmission exists even with blood from a donor who is HIV-negative. Newer molecular detection methods should decrease the window from becoming infected to being able to detect infection from 22 d to approximately 11 d.

CMV

Incidence in donors is very high (approaches 100% in many series), but clinically represents a major risk mostly for immunocompromised recipients and neonates. Leukocyte filters can reduce the risk of transmission.

HTLV-I, II

Very rare (<<1/641,000 units transfused). Use of leukocyte filters can decrease risk of transmission of HTLV.

West Nile Virus

Very, very rare. 15 cases from 10 states related to transfusion have been reported by the CDC as of the fall of 2002. As the incidence of West Nile virus increases we will likely see more cases of transfusion-related West Nile infection.

Bacteria and Parasites

Sepsis due to bacteria is discussed on page 199. Parasites are very rarely transmitted, but careful donor screening is necessary, especially in endemic regions (eg, Chagas' disease in Central America).

11

NUTRITION SUPPORT, ENTERAL NUTRITION, AND INFANT FEEDING

Nutritional Assessment
Postoperative Nutritional Support
Determining the Route of Nutritional
   Support

Nutritional Requirements
Hospital Diets
Principles of Enteral Tube Feeding
Infant Formulas and Feeding

The use of nutrition support in hospitalized patients is not to be undertaken without the same consideration given to other treatment modalities. Each patient should be individually assessed, nutritional requirements determined, and then an appropriate route of support chosen. The risks and benefits of each intervention must be carefully weighed in each individual case.

NUTRITIONAL ASSESSMENT

Nutritional screening should be incorporated into the H&P evaluation of all patients. Identifying patients at nutritional risk is crucial because malnutrition is prevalent among hospitalized patients and has been associated with adverse clinical outcomes. Situations that predispose a patient to malnutrition include recent and continuing nausea, vomiting, diarrhea, inability to feed oneself, inadequate food intake (cancer-related, others), decreased nutrient absorption or utilization, and increased nutrient losses and nutritional requirements.

Although many patients are admitted to the hospital in a nutritionally depleted state, some patients become malnourished during their hospital stay. According to guidelines from the American Society for Parenteral and Enteral Nutrition, "patients should be considered malnourished or at risk of developing malnutrition if they have inadequate nutrient intake for 7 d or more or if they have a weight loss of 10% or more of their preillness body weight." Formal evaluation is often necessary to identify patients at nutritional risk and to provide a baseline to assess whether therapeutic goals are being achieved with specialized nutritional support. The patient's history is useful in evaluating weight loss; dietary intolerance, including that for glucose or lactose; and disease states that may influence nutritional tolerance.

Anthropometric evaluations include comparisons of actual body weight to ideal and usual body weight. Other anthropometric measurements, such as MAMC and TCF, have much interobserver variability and are generally not useful unless performed by an experienced evaluator.

Absolute lymphocyte count is sometimes used as a marker of visceral proteins and immunocompetence. Visceral protein markers, such as prealbumin and transferrin, may be helpful in evaluating nutritional insult as well as catabolic stress. Although the most commonly quoted laboratory parameter of nutritional status is albumin, the albumin concentration often reflects hydration status and metabolic response to injury (ie, the acute phase response) more than the nutritional state of the patient, especially in patients with intravascular volume deficits. Due to its long half-life, albumin may be normal in the malnourished patient. Prealbumin is superior as an indicator of malnutrition only because of its shorter half-life. Use of these serum proteins as indicators of malnutrition is subject to the same limitation, however, because they are all affected by catabolic stress. Table 11–1, page 203, lists the parameters for identifying potentially malnourished patients; however, no single criterion should be used to assess a patient's nutritional status. Patients can generally be classified as mildly, moderately, or severely nutritionally depleted based on these parameters. Keep in mind the deleterious effects of malnutrition, which include, but are not limited to, increased mortality, disruption of mucosal barriers, decreased wound healing, compromised immune system, susceptibility to infection, suboptimal organ function, weakened muscles (including muscles of respiration), increased intubation time and ventilatory dependence, and prolonged hospital stay.

POSTOPERATIVE NUTRITIONAL SUPPORT

The postoperative patient is a "special case" in nutritional assessment. Most patients can be started on oral feedings postoperatively, the question though, is when to begin. One must be aware that motility is delayed in patients undergoing laparotomy, whereas motility is not hampered in patients who undergo surgery on other parts of the body, once they recover consciousness sufficiently to protect their airway. The GI tract gut recovers motility as follows: The small intestine never loses motility (peristalsis is observed in the OR), the stomach regains motility about 24 h postoperatively, and the colon is the last to recover at 72–96 h postoperatively. Thus, by the time a patient reports flatus, one can assume that the entire gut has regained motility.

Although the traditional method of postoperative feeding support initiates feeds once the entire bowel recovers motility (as indicated by the passage of flatus), there is emerging evidence that early feeding in select surgical patients is desirable. The current literature supports feeding select patients within 24–48 h postoperatively after elective colonic resection. There is no need to step through a progression from clear liquids to full liquids to a regular diet. Many surgeons offer the patient one meal of clear liquids and then advance directly to a regular diet.

DETERMINING THE ROUTE OF NUTRITIONAL SUPPORT

After a thorough assessment of a patient's nutritional state is undertaken and it is determined that the patient will likely benefit from nutritional support, the patient's nutritional requirements (as shown in the following section) must be determined as well as the most effective and appropriate route for administration. Routes of support include:

- Enteral supplementation by mouth
- Enteral support by tube feeding
- Total parenteral nutrition (TPN) (Chapter 12)

In determining the route of nutritional support, it is most important to remember the adage **"If the gut works, use it."** If the GI tract is functioning and can be used safely, tube feedings should be ordered instead of parenteral nutrition when nutrition support is necessary because it

- Is more easily absorbed physiologically
- Is associated with fewer complications than TPN

TABLE 11-1
Parameters Used to Identify the Malnourished Patient

Parameters	Measurement/Interpretation	Usefulness/Limitations
Anthropometric Measurement		
Actual body weight (ABW) compared with ideal body weight (IBW)	"Rule-of-thumb" method to determine IBW	
	Step 1	
	For men: IBW (lb) = 106 lb for 5 ft of height, plus 6 lb for each inch of height over 5 ft	
	For women: IBW (lb) = 100 lb for first 5 ft of height plus an additional 5 lb for each inch over 5 ft	
	Step 2	
	$\%\ IBW = \dfrac{ABW}{IBW} \times 100$	
	% of IBW	
	90–110 Normal nutritional status	
	80–90 Mild malnutrition	
	70–80 Moderate malnutrition	
	<70 Severe malnutrition	

(continued)

11

203

TABLE 11-1
(Continued)

Parameters	Measurement/Interpretation		Usefulness/Limitations
Actual body weight compared with usual body weight (UBW)	$\% \text{ UBW} = \dfrac{\text{ABW}}{\text{UBW}} \times 100$		Routinely available
	% of UBW		
	85–95%	Mild malnutrition	
	75–84%	Moderate malnutrition	
	<75%	Severe malnutrition	
Biochemical Parameters			
Serum albumin	3.5–5.2 g/dL	Normal	Valuable prognostic indicator: depressed levels predict increased mortality and morbidity
	2.8–3.4 g/dL	Mild depletion	Inexpensive
	2.1–2.7 g/dL	Moderate depletion	Large body stores and relatively long half-life (approximately 20 d) limit usefulness in evaluating short-term changes in nutritional status
	<2 g/dL	Severe depletion	

(continued)

11

TABLE 11–1
(Continued)

Parameters	Measurement/Interpretation		Usefulness/Limitations
Transferrin (TFN)	200–300 mg/dL	Normal	Frequently available
	150–200 mg/dL	Mild visceral depletion	Depressed levels predict increased mortality and morbidity
	100–150 mg/dL	Moderate depletion	Smaller body pool and shorter half-life (8–10 days) than serum albumin
	<100 mg/dL	Severe depletion	If TFN is calculated from TIBC, levels will be increased with the presence of iron deficiency or chronic blood loss
	TFN can be calculated from the total iron-binding capacity (TIBC) as follows:		Levels are increased during pregnancy
	$$TFN = (0.8 \times TIBC) - 43$$		Levels are decreased if iron stores are increased as a result of hemosiderosis, hemochromatosis, thalassemia

(continued)

TABLE 11-1
(Continued)

Parameters	Measurement/Interpretation		Usefulness/Limitations
Prealbumin	16–30 mg/dL	Normal	Half-life is 2 d. Thus is more sensitive indicator of acute change in nutritional status than is albumin or TFN
	10–15 mg/dL	Mild depletion	
	5–10 mg/dL	Moderate depletion	
	<5 mg/dL	Severe depletion	Not routinely available
			Levels are quickly depleted after trauma or acute infection. Also decreased in response to cirrhosis, hepatitis, and dialysis, and therefore, should be interpreted with caution
Absolute lymphocyte count (calculated as WBC × % lymphocytes)	1400–2000	Mild depletion	May not be valid in cancer patients. Not used by some nutritionists
	900–1400	Moderate depletion	
	<900	Severe depletion	

- Maintains the gut barrier to infection
- Maintains the integrity of the GI tract
- Is more cost-effective than TPN

NUTRITIONAL REQUIREMENTS

Determining the patient's nutritional requirements is one of the first steps in prescribing a modified diet order or supplementation for a patient. Monitoring the patient's progress and adjusting nutritional goals on the basis of clinical judgment is important for ensuring that the patient's specific needs are being met. It is critically important to determine both caloric and protein needs before selecting a method of nutrition support.

Determination of a patient's nutritional requirements is important not only for providing the patient with sufficient calories, but just as importantly, for avoiding overfeeding the patient. Numerous studies have demonstrated the deleterious effects of overfeeding, including; electrolyte imbalances, fatty liver (hepatic steatosis), azotemia, hyperlipidemia, hypercarbia (due to increased carbohydrate load), and prolongation or failure to wean from the ventilator.

Caloric Needs

A patient's caloric needs can be calculated by the following two methods: the Harris–Benedict equation and the rule-of-thumb method.

11

Method I. Harris–Benedict Equation (Basal Energy Expenditure or BEE)
    Men:

$$BEE = 66.47 + 13.75\,(w) + 5.00\,(h) - 6.76\,(a)$$

    Women:

$$BEE = 655.10 + 9.56\,(w) + 1.85\,(h) - 4.689\,(a)$$

w = weight in kilograms; h = height in centimeters; and a = age in years.

After the BEE has been determined from the Harris–Benedict equation, the patient's total daily maintenance energy requirements are estimated by multiplying the BEE by an activity factor and a stress factor.

    Total energy requirements = BEE × Activity factor × Stress factor

Use the following correction factors:

Activity Level	Correction Factor
Bedridden	1.2
Ambulatory	1.3

Level of Physiologic Stress	Correction Factor
Minor operation	1.2
Skeletal trauma	1.35
Major sepsis	1.60
Severe burn	2.10

II. "Rule-of-Thumb" Method

- Maintenance of the patient's nutritional status without significant metabolic stress requires 25–30 kcal/kg body weight/d.
- Maintenance needs for the hypermetabolic, severely stressed patient or for supporting weight gain in the underweight patient without significant metabolic stress requires 35–40 kcal/kg body weight/d.
- Greater than 40 kcal/kg body weight/d may be needed to meet the needs of severely burned patients.

Protein Needs

The maintenance protein requirement for nonstressed patients is 0.8 g of protein per kilogram of body weight per day. Repletion requirements for the nutritionally depleted patient are 1.2–2.5 g of protein per kilogram of body weight per day.

HOSPITAL DIETS

If a patient can take in adequate calories by mouth, then this route is preferred. The most commonly ordered standard hospital diets and their indications are listed in Table 11–2, page 209. The vast majority of patients admitted to the hospital can be given one of these hospital diets without any specific supplementation or modification. Most hospitals have diet manuals available for reference, and registered dietitians are usually on staff for nutritional consultation. A physician's order for diet instruction by a clinical dietitian is recommended for all patients being discharged with a therapeutic or modified diet.

Enteral Supplementation and Tube Feeding

Enteral nutrition encompasses both oral supplements and feedings by tube directly into the GI tract (eg, NG tube, gastrostomy tube or jejunostomy tube). If the patient's oral intake is inadequate, every effort should be made to increase intake by providing nutrient-dense foods, frequent feedings, or oral supplements. If such attempts are unsuccessful, tube feeding may be necessary. In addition, patients who have a functioning GI tract but for whom oral nutrition intake is contraindicated (eg, a patient with an esophageal fistula) should be considered for tube feedings.

PRINCIPLES OF ENTERAL TUBE FEEDING

The factors involved in choosing the route for enteral nutrition include the projected duration of feeding by this method, GI tract pathophysiology, and the risk for aspiration. Nasally placed tubes are the most frequently used. Patient comfort is maximized by using a small-bore flexible tube. When enteral feedings are started, it is often important to assess gastric residual volumes. The small-bore tubes do not allow for aspiration of residual volumes, however, which may be significant if gastric emptying is questionable. Thus, larger bore tubes are often used to start, and, once feeding tolerance is ensured, the tube is changed to a small-bore tube, which can be left in place comfortably for prolonged periods. Feeding directly into the stomach (as opposed to the bowel) is often preferable because the stomach is the best line of defense against hyperosmolarity. Patients at risk for aspiration require longer tubes into the jejunum or duodenum. Types of feeding tubes and placement procedures are discussed in detail in Chapter 13, page 276.

TABLE 11–2
Hospital Diets

Diet	Guidelines	Indications
House/regular	Adequate in all essential nutrients All foods are permitted Can be modified according to patient's food preferences	No diet restrictions or modifications
Mechanical soft	Includes soft-textured or ground foods that are easily masticated and swallowed	Decreased ability to chew or swallow Presence of oral mucositis or esophagitis May be appropriate for some patients with dysphagia
Pureed	Includes liquids as well as strained and pureed foods	Inability to chew or swallow solid foods Presence of oral mucositis or esophagitis May be appropriate for some patients with dysphagia
Full liquid	Includes foods that are liquid at body temperature Includes milk/milk products Can provide approximately: 2500–3000 ml fluid 1500–2000 Cal 60–80 g high-quality protein <10 g dietary fiber 60–80 g fat per day	May be appropriate for patients with severely impaired chewing ability Not appropriate for a lactase-deficient patient unless commercially available lactase enzyme tablets are provided

(continued)

209

11

TABLE 11–2
(Continued)

11

Diet	Guidelines	Indications
Clear liquid	Includes foods that are liquid at body temperature Foods are very low in fiber Lactose-free Virtually fat-free Can provide approximately: 2000 mL fluid 400–600 Cal <7 g low-quality protein <1 g dietary fiber <1 g fat/day This diet is inadequate in all nutrients and should not be used >3 d without supplementation	Ordered as initial diet in the transition from NPO to solids Used for bowel preparation before certain medical or surgical procedures For management of acute medical conditions warranting minimized biliary contraction or pancreatic exocrine secretion
Low-fiber	Foods that are low in indigestible carbohydrates Decreases stool volume, transit time, and frequency	Management of acute radiation enteritis and inflammatory bowel disease when narrowing or stenosis of the gut lumen is present

(continued)

TABLE 11-2
(Continued)

Diet	Guidelines	Indications
Carbohydrate controlled diet (ADA)	Calorie level should be adequate to maintain or achieve desirable body weight Total carbohydrates are limited to 50–60% of total calories Ideally fat should be limited to ≈30% of total calories	Diabetes mellitus
Acute renal failure	Protein (g/kg DBW) 0.6 Calories 35–50 Sodium (g/day) 1–3 Potassium (g/day) Variable Fluid (mL/day) Urine output + 500	For patients in renal failure who are not undergoing dialysis
Renal failure/ Hemodialysis	Protein (g/kg DBW) 1.0–1.2 Calories (per kilogram DBW) 30–35 Sodium (g/d) 1–2 Potassium (g/d) 1.5–3 Fluid (mL/d) Urine output + 500	For patients in renal failure on hemodialysis

(continued)

11

TABLE 11–2
(Continued)

Diet	Guidelines		Indications
Peritoneal dialysis	Protein (g/kg DBW)	1.2–1.6	For patients in renal failure on peritoneal dialysis
	Calories (per kilogram DBW)	25–35	
	Sodium (g/d)	3–4	
	Potassium (g/d)	3–4	
	Fluid (mL/d)	Urine output + 500	
Liver failure	In the absence of encephalopathy do not restrict protein		Management of chronic liver disorders
	In the presence of encephalopathy initially restricted protein to 40–60 g/d then liberalize in increments of 10 g/d as tolerated		
	Sodium and fluid restriction should be specified based on severity of ascites and edema		
Low lactose/ Lactose-free	Limits or restricts mild products Commercially available lactase enzyme tablets are available on the market		Lactase deficiency
Low-fat	<50 g total fat per day		Pancreatitis Fat malabsorption

(continued)

TABLE 11-2
(Continued)

Diet	Guidelines	Indications
Fat/cholesterol restricted	Total fat >30% total calories Saturated fat limited to 10% of calories <300 mg cholesterol <50% calories from complex carbohydrates	Hypercholesterolemia
Low-sodium	Sodium allowance should be as liberal as possible to maximize nutritional intake yet control symptoms "No-added salt" is 4 g/d; no added salt or highly salted food; 2 g/d avoids processed foods (ie, meats) <1 g/d is unpalatable and thus compromises adequate intake	Indicated for patients with hypertension, ascites, and edema associated with the underlying disease

11

When long-term feeding is anticipated, a tube enterostomy may be required. **PEG tubes** can usually be placed without general anesthesia. Patients with tumors, GI obstruction, adhesions, or abnormal anatomy, however, may require open surgical placement. A jejunal feeding tube may be threaded through a PEG for small-bowel feeding. The placement of a needle catheter or Witzel's jejunostomy during surgery generally allows for earlier postoperative feeding with an elemental formulation than waiting for the return of gastric emptying and colonic function.

Enteral Products

A variety of enteral products, tube feedings and supplements are available (see Table 11–3, page 215, for some examples). Check the enteral formulary for the specific products available in your facility. The protein component can be supplied as intact proteins, partially digested hydrolyzed proteins, or crystalline amino acids. Each gram of protein provides 4 kcal. The carbohydrate source may be intact complex starches, glucose polymers, or simpler disaccharides such as sucrose. Fat in enteral products is usually supplied as long-chain fatty acids. Some enteral products, however, contain MCTs, which are transported directly in the portal circulation rather than via chyle production. Because MCT oil does not contain essential fatty acids, it cannot be used as the sole fat source. Long-chain fatty acids provide 9 kcal/g, and MCT oil provides 8 kcal/g.

The osmolality of an enteral product is determined primarily by the concentration of carbohydrates, electrolytes, amino acids, or small peptides. The clinical importance of osmolality is often debated. Hyperosmolal formulations, with osmolalities exceeding 450 mOsm/L, may contribute to diarrhea by acting in a manner similar to osmotic cathartics.

Hyperosmolar feedings are well tolerated when delivered into the stomach (as opposed to the small bowel) because gastric secretions dilute the feeding before it leaves the pylorus to traverse the small bowel. Thus, feedings administered directly to the small bowel (eg, via feeding jejunostomy) should not exceed 450 mOsm/L.

Oral supplements differ from other enteral feedings in that they are designed to be more palatable so as to improve compliance. Although most enteral products do not contain lactose (Ensure, others), several oral supplements, commonly referred to as "meal replacements" (such as Compleat) contain lactose and are therefore not appropriate for patients with lactase deficiency and are not normally used for tube feedings.

Based on osmolality and macronutrient content, enteral products can be classified into several categories. Low-osmolality formulas are isotonic and contain intact macronutrients. They usually provide 1 kcal/mL and require approximately 2 L to provide the RDA for vitamins. These products are appropriate for the general patient population and include products such as Ensure.

High-density formulas may provide up to 2 kcal/mL. These concentrated solutions are hyperosmolar and also contain intact nutrients. The RDA for vitamins can be met with volumes of 1500 mL or less. These products are used for volume-restricted patients(eg, Ensure Plus HN).

Chemically defined or elemental formulas provide the macronutrients in the predigested state. These formulations are usually hyperosmolar and have poor palatability. Patients with compromised nutrient absorption abilities or GI function may benefit from elemental type feedings. Vivonex and Peptamen are two such products.

TABLE 11–3
Some Commonly Used Enteral Formulations.[a]

Product	Description	Calories
Advera	High-calorie, high-protein, low-fat, fiber-fortified liquid; designed for HIV or AIDS; oral liquid supplement, meal replacement, or for total enteral support.	1.28/mL
Alitraq	Elemental powder formula for metabolically stress patients with impaired GI function (severe trauma, IBD, burns, chemo or radiation injury)	1.0/mL
Casec	Concentrated protein powder; negligible fat and carbohydrates; supplement diets of children and adults	380/100 g
Compleat	Blenderized tube feeding formula for patients with intolerance to semisynthetic formulas; contains lactose	1.07/mL
Deliver 2.0	Supplement useful in fluid restrictions (ie, CHF, neurosurgery), high-calorie requirements (ie, cancer cachexia, COPD) liver disease with malnutrition including encephalopathy	2.0/mL
Enlive!	High-calorie, fat-free alternative to sweeter supplements; vitamin supplemented may be used in clear-liquid, pre- and postop, bowel-prep, fat malabsorptive, fat-restricted, low-sodium, or low-cholesterol diets.	1250/mL
Ensure	Complete, balanced nutrition for supplemental use with or between meals; can be used as a sole source of nutrition.	1.06/mL
Ensure Fiber with FOS	See Ensure; enhanced fiber content	1.06/mL
Ensure Plus	Concentrated calories, high protein; to gain or maintain healthy weight; a complete and balanced oral nutritional supplement; use with or between meals; useful in fluid restrictions/volume-limited feedings; lactose-free, low-fat	1.5/mL

(continued)

11

215

TABLE 11-3
(Continued)

Product	Description	Calories
Ensure Plus HN	Concentrated calories, high protein; used with or between meals or, in appropriate amounts, as a meal replacement, lactose-free, low-fat; oral (flavored or tube feed)	1.5/mL
Glucerna	Reduced-carbohydrate, modified-fat, fiber-containing; supplemental or total enteral feeding for patients with abnormal glucose tolerance (eg, type 1 and type 2 DM, abnormal glucose tolerance resulting from metabolic stress)	1.0/mL
Impact	Enteral formula containing arginine, dietary nucleotides and fish oil; immune system enhancer; may enhance recovery of critically ill patients	1.0/mL
Introlite	Fortified, half-calorie liquid formula to initiate tube feeding.	0.53/mL
Isocal	General tube-feeding needs; inadequate voluntary oral intake (cancer, anorexia, stroke); postoperative feeding, etc	1.06/mL
Jevity	Isotonic, fiber-fortified, high-nitrogen liquid formula; complete, balanced nutrition for patients requiring tube feeding; fiber helps maintain normal bowel function; reduces the potential for hyperosmotic diarrhea.	1.06/mL
Jevity Plus	High-nitrogen, fiber-fortified liquid formula; complete, balanced nutrition for patients who may benefit from a moderate increase in protein and caloric density; contains a soluble and insoluble fiber and fructooligosaccharides (FOS) to moderate bowel function.	1.2/mL
Nepro	Moderate protein, nutritionally complete formula with a vitamin–mineral profile designed for renal failure requiring dialysis; tube or oral feeding	2.0/mL
Nutrifocus	Oral nutritional supplement for use by people with, or at risk for, pressure ulcers.	1.5/mL

(continued)

TABLE 11–3
(Continued)

Product	Description	Calories
Optimental	Ready-to-feed elemental formula; for patients with malabsorptive conditions, such as Crohn's disease, metabolic stress, acute trauma.	1.0/mL
Osmolite	Isotonic, low-residue liquid; complete, balanced nutrition; useful for tube-fed patients who are sensitive to hyperosmolar feedings or oral feeding for patients with altered taste perception	1.06/mL
Osmolite HN	See Osmolite; high-nitrogen; useful in patients who require less than 2000 cal/d or for patients with elevated nitrogen requirements who require tube feeding	1.06/mL
Osmolite HN Plus	See Osmolite; higher calorie	1.2/mL
Oxepa	Low-carbohydrate, calorically dense enteral nutrition product designed for the dietary management of critically ill patients on mechanical ventilation or with lung injury; tube feeding	1.5/mL
Perative	Ready-to-feed enteral product; for metabolically stressed patients (eg, multiple fractures, wounds, burns, etc)	1.3/mL
Polycose	Easily digestible source of carbohydrate calories; use when additional calories are required; mixes easily with regular foods and beverages to provide extra calories for persons with increased caloric needs; not intended to be used as a sole-source nutritional product (contains no protein or fat) (powder and liquid)	1.0/mL (liquid)
Promod	Concentrated, protein supplement powder for increased protein needs or if unable to meet protein needs with a normal diet; not for use as a sole source of nutrition	28/5 g

(continued)

217

TABLE 11-3
(Continued)

Product	Description	Calories
Prosure	Beverage to help normalize metabolism and promote weight gain and lean body mass (LBM) in people experiencing tumor-induced weight loss	1.27/mL
Pulmocare	High-calorie, low-carbohydrate liquid; helps reduce carbon dioxide production to minimizing CO_2 retention (eg, COPD, cystic fibrosis, ventilator dependency)	1.5/mL
RE/NEPH	Snack beverage for potassium-, phosphorus-, and fluid-restricted diets (eg, dialysis patients) to maintain normal weight.	250/4 oz
Suplena	Low-protein, nutritionally complete; vitamin–mineral profile for chronic/acute renal failure patients who are not receiving dialysis	2.0/mL
Twocal HN	Nutritionally complete, high-nitrogen liquid; tube feeding for increased protein and calorie needs in severe fluid restrictions or in limited volume tolerance	2.0/mL
Tolerex	Nutritionally complete powder, elemental diet; 100% free amino acids; useful in impaired digestion and absorption and food allergies	1.0/mL
Vital High Nitrogen	Peptide-based elemental powder formula for patients with chronically impaired GI maldigestion/malabsorption (IBD, radiation enteritis, etc)	1.0/mL
Vivonex Pediatric	Nutritionally complete elemental (100% free amino acids for children ages 1–10; use as a tube feeding; powder consumed orally with Vivonex Flavor Packets	0.8/mL
Vivonex Plus	See Vivonex RTF; this product is a powder with additional free glutamine (10 g/L), enhanced arginine, and branched-chain amino acid contents	1.0/mL

(continued)

TABLE 11-3
(Continued)

Product	Description	Calories
Vivonex RTF	Is a ready-to-use, high-nitrogen, low-fat, elemental (100% free amino acids) diet for total enteral nutrition; useful in stressed, catabolic patients; may be used post-operatively as an enteral alternative to TPN and may also benefit patients with gastrointestinal impairment (see Vivonex TEN).	1.0/mL
Vivonex TEN (powder)	Very low-fat, elemental diet; 100% free amino acids and enriched with glutamine; for patients with GI impairment (eg, bowel resection, irradiated bowel, malabsorption syndrome, Crohn's disease, etc)	1.0/mL

^aSee specific hospital dietary manuals for products available at specific institutions.
HIV = human immunodeficiency virus; AIDS = acquired immune deficiency syndrome; GI = gastrointestinal; IBD = irritable bowel disease; CHF = congestive heart failure; COPD = chronic obstructive pulmonary disease; DM = diabetes mellitus

11

Disease-specific (special metabolic) enteral formulas have been developed for various disease states. Products for pulmonary patients, such as Pulmocare, contain a higher percentage of calories from fat to decrease the carbon dioxide load from the metabolism of excess glucose. A low-carbohydrate, high-fat product for persons with DM (Glucerna) is available that also contains fiber to help regulate glucose control. Other fiber-containing enteral feedings are available to help regulate bowel function (Enrich, Jevity). The clinical utility of many of the specialty products remains controversial.

Initiating Tube Feedings

Guidelines for ordering enteral feedings are outlined in Table 11–4, below. Contraindications for tube feedings are shown in Table 11–5, page 221. In summary, when using enteral feedings:

1. Determine nutritional needs.
2. Assess GI tract function and appropriateness of enteral feedings.
3. Determine fluid requirements and volume tolerance based on overall status and concurrent disease states.
4. Select an appropriate enteral feeding product and method of administration.
5. Verify that the regimen selected satisfies micronutrient requirements.
6. Monitor and assess nutritional status to evaluate the need for changes in the selected regimen.

The tube feeding can be given into the stomach (bolus, intermittent gravity drip, or continuous) or into the small intestine by continuous infusion (Table 11–6, page 222). Enteral nutrition is best tolerated when instilled into the stomach because this method produces fewer problems with osmolarity or feeding volumes. The stomach serves as a barrier to hyperosmolarity, thus the use of isotonic feedings is mandated only when instilling nutrients directly into the small intestine. The use of gastric feedings is thus preferable and should be used whenever appropriate. Patients at risk for aspiration or with impaired gastric emptying may need to be fed past the pylorus into the jejunum or the duodenum. Feedings via a jejunostomy placed at the time of surgery can often be initiated on the first postoperative day, obviating the need for parenteral nutrition.

Although enteral nutrition is generally safer than parenteral nutrition, aspiration can be a significantly morbid event in the care of these patients. Appropriate monitoring for residual volumes in addition to keeping the head of the

TABLE 11–4
Routine Orders for Enteral Nutrition Administered by Tube Feeding

1. Confirm tube placement. (Usually by radiograph)
2. Elevate head of bed to 30–45 degrees
3. Check gastric residuals in patients receiving gastric feedings. Hold feedings if >1.5–2x infusion rate. Significant residuals should be re-instilled and rechecked in 1 h. If continues to be elevated, hold tube feeding and begin NG suction.
4. Check patient weight 3x/wk.
5. Record strict I&O
6. Request routine laboratory studies

TABLE 11–5
Contraindications to Tube Feeding

Complete bowel obstruction
GI bleeding
High-output (>500 mL/d) enterocutaneous fistula or fistula not located
   in the proximal or distal GI tract
Hypovolemic or septic shock
Ileus
Inability to obtain safe enteral tube feeding access
Poor prognosis not warranting invasive nutritional support
Severe acute pancreatitis
Severe intractable diarrhea
Severe intractable nausea and vomiting
Severe malabsorption
Anticipated duration of tube feeding therapy <5 d

bed elevated can help prevent this complication. A "significant residual" may be defined as four times the instillation rate. If a patient has a large residual, it can be treated in a number of ways. Any transient postoperative ileus is best treated by waiting for the ileus to resolve. Metoclopramide or erythromycin may be useful pharmacologic therapy for postoperative ileus in some patients (Chapter 22).

Patients who have been tolerating feedings and develop intolerance should be carefully assessed for the cause. Feeding intolerance is characterized by vomiting, abdominal distention, diarrhea, or high gastric residual volumes. In these cases a global approach to assessment of the GI tract is warranted. If feeding into the stomach, gastric emptying should be evaluated. Generally, if an adult patient drains 600 mL/24-h shift on NG suction, the pylorus is functioning appropriately. Clamping of the NG tube to evaluate gastric emptying may be dangerous because it unnecessarily exposes the patient to the risk of aspiration. Tolerance to enteral feeding can be assessed with the instillation of an isotonic diet given for 24 h at 30 mL/h as a trial. Feeding intolerance is characterized by vomiting, abdominal distention, diarrhea, or high gastric residual volumes.

Complications of Enteral Nutrition

Diarrhea: Diarrhea occurs in about 10–60% of patients receiving enteral feedings. The physician must be certain to evaluate the patient for other causes of diarrhea. Formula-related causes include contamination, excessively cold temperature, lactose intolerance, osmolality, and an incorrect method or route of delivery. Eliminate potential causes before using antidiarrheal medications.

- Check medication profile for possible drug-induced cause.
- Rule out *Clostridium difficile* colitis in patients receiving antibiotics (see Chapters 4 and 7).
- Attempt to decrease the feeding rate or try an alternative regimen such as bolus feeding.

TABLE 11-6
Tube Feeding Delivery Methods

Delivery Site/Indication	Delivery Method	Notes	Suggested Feeding Progression
INTRAGASTRIC Appropriate for alert patients with intact gag and cough reflexes and for those with normal gastric emptying	Bolus	Rapid infusion of formula into the stomach by syringe or other feeding reservoir; generally 240–480 mL of formula is given every 3–6 h Feedings are usually given over a period of 5–15 min Associated symptoms of GI distress, such as bloating, nausea, and distention	Typical starter regimen: 60–120 mL of full-strength formula is generally provided Typical feeding progression: Volume of formula provided at each feeding may be increased in 60–120 mL increments every 12 h or as tolerated
INTRAGASTRIC	Intermittent gravity drip	Generally 240–480 mL of formula is allowed to drip from a feeding container through tubing over a 30–60 min period four to eight times per day Rate of formula administration is controlled with a clamp in the tubing	Typical starter regimen: 60–120 mL of full-strength formula is generally provided Typical feeding progression: Volume of formula provided at each feeding may be increased to 60–120 mL increments every 12 h or as tolerated

(continued)

11

TABLE 11-6
(Continued)

Delivery Site/ Indication	Delivery Method	Notes	Suggested Feeding Progression
INTRAGASTRIC (cont.)		May reduce the incidence of GI complications associated with bolus delivery Highly viscous formulas, such as those that contain 2 Cal/mL, may not flow through the tubing More expensive than bolus method because feeding containers are necessary Not recommended for critically ill patients	
INTRAGASTRIC	Continuous	Preferred method to administer formula if gastric feeding is necessary for a critically ill patient because it reduces risk of aspiration Use of a feeding pump to deliver precise volumes of formula at a constant rate	Typical starter regimen: Full-strength formula is generally initiated at a rate of 40 or 50 mL/h Typical feeding progression: Feeding rate is generally increased in increments of 10–15 mL/h every 12 h or as tolerated until the goal feeding rate is achieved

(continued)

11

223

TABLE 11-6
(Continued)

Delivery Site/Indication	Delivery Method	Notes	Suggested Feeding Progression
INTRAGASTRIC (cont.)		Goal feeding rates are typically between 80 and 125 mL/h, depending on the individual's nutritional requirements Volume- and rate-controlled delivery minimizes gastric emptying and reduces the incidence of osmotic diarrhea secondary to dumping syndrome In the hospital setting, the formula is usually provided over a 24-h period; home patients may cycle feedings over an 8–14-h period May be necessary to deliver formulas with high viscosity	

(continued)

11

TABLE 11-6
(Continued)

Delivery Site/ Indication	Delivery Method	Notes	Suggested Feeding Progression
		Necessity of feeding pump in addition to feeding bag and tubing increases cost	Typical starter regimen: Full-strength formula is generally initiated at a rate of 40–50 mL/h; markedly hypertonic formulas (>600 mOsm/L) occasionally may be diluted to half-strength if dumping syndrome is present or if a prolonged period without enteral nutrition has elapsed
INTRAINTESTINAL Appropriate for patients who are at high risk for aspiration, including those who cannot keep the proper position during feeding (head of bed 30 degrees upright) and those without an intact gag reflex	Continuous	Restricts ambulation in patients who are not critically ill Feeding pump required because excessively rapid formula delivery, as would occur with bolus or gravity drip administration, would probably result in dumping syndrome, allows tube feeding formula to be delivered in a more physiologic manner Goal rates are usually 80–125 mL/h, depending on the patient's nutritional needs Usually 24-h infusions are given	Typical feeding progression: Feeding rate is generally increased in increments of 10–12 mL/h every 12 h or as tolerated until the goal feeding rate is achieved; if hypertonic formula was initially diluted, the patient can be switched to

11

(continued)

TABLE 11-6
(Continued)

Delivery Site/ Indication	Delivery Method	Notes	Suggested Feeding Progression
INTRAINTESTINAL (cont.) Required feeding route when proximal (ie, oral, esophageal, or gastric) GI obstruction or impairment is present Preferred delivery site for critically ill patients		in the hospital, but cyclic infusions are an option for the ambulatory or home patient Associated with high cost because of necessity of feeding containers and infusion pump Continuous infusions may restrict patient ambulation	full-strength formula after the goal feeding rate is achieved

- Change the formulation, for example, limit lactose or reduce the osmolality.
- Use pharmacologic therapy only after eliminating treatable causes (eg, give *Lactobacillus* powder [one packet tid to replenish gut flora]; most effective in patients on antibiotics) or antidiarrheal medications (loperamide [Lomotil], calcium carbonate).

Constipation: Although less common than diarrhea, constipation can occur in the enterally fed patient. Check to ensure that adequate fluid volume is being given. Patients with additional requirements may benefit from water boluses or dilution of the enteral formulation. Fiber can be added to help regulate bowel function.

Aspiration: Aspiration is a serious complication of enteral feedings and is more likely to occur in the patient with diminished mental status. The best approach is prevention. Elevate the head of the bed and carefully monitor residual fluid volume. Further evaluate any patient who may have aspirated or who is assessed as being at increased risk for aspiration prior to instituting enteral feedings. Such patients may not be candidates for gastric feedings, and small-bowel feedings may be necessary.

Drug Interactions: The vitamin K content of various enteral products varies from 22 to 156 mg/1000 kcal. This can significantly affect the anticoagulation profile of a patient receiving warfarin therapy. Tetracycline products should not be administered 1 h before or 2 h after enteral feedings to avoid the inhibition of absorption. Similarly, enteral feedings should be stopped 2 h before and after the administration of phenytoin.

INFANT FORMULAS AND FEEDING

Bottle feeding is often chosen by the mother and, in general, commercially available formulas are recommended over homemade formulas because of their ease of preparation and their standardization of nutrients. Occasionally, special formulas are medically indicated and can only be supplied by commercially available formulas. Commonly used formulas are outlined in Table 11–7, page 278.

Principles of Infant Feeding

Criteria for Initiating Infant Feeding: Most normal full-term infants are fed within the first 4 h after birth. The following criteria should usually be met before initiating infant feedings.

- The infant should have no history of excessive oral secretions, vomiting, or bile-stained gastric aspirate.
- An examination should have been performed with particular attention to the abdomen. The examination should be normal with normal bowel sounds and a nondistended, soft abdomen.
- The infant should be clinically stable.
- At least 6 h should pass before recently extubated infants are fed. The infant should be tolerating extubation well and have little respiratory distress.
- The respiratory rate should be <60 breaths/min for oral feeding and ≤ 80 breaths/min for gavage (tube) feeding. Tachypnea increases the risk of aspiration.

TABLE 11–7
Commonly Used Infant Formulas

Formula	Indications[a]
Human milk	
Donor	Preterm infant <1200 g
Maternal	All infants
Breast milk fortifiers	
Standard formulas	
Isoosmolar	
Enfamil 20	Full-term infants: as supplement to breast milk
Similac 20	Preterm infants >1800–2000 g
SMA 20	
Higher Osmolality	
Enfamil 24	Term infants: for infants on fluid restriction or
Similac 24 & 27	who cannot handle required volumes of
SMA[b] 24 & 27	20-Cal formula to grow
Low Osmolality	
Similac 13	Preterm and term infants: for conservative initial feeding in infants who have not been fed orally for several days or weeks. Not for long-term use
Soy formulas	
ProSobee (lactose- and sucrose-free)	Term infants: milk sensitivity, galactosemia, carbohydrate intolerance. Do not use in
Isomil (lactose-free)	preterm infants. Phytates can bind calcium
Nursoy (lactose-free)	and cause rickets
Protein hydrosylate formulas	
Nutramigen	Term infants: Gut sensitivity to proteins, multiple food allergies, persistent diarrhea, galactosemia.
Pregestimil	Preterm and term infants: disaccharidase deficiency, diarrhea, GI defects, cystic fibrosis, food allergy, celiac disease, transition from TPN to oral feeding
Alimentum	Term infants: protein sensitivity, pancreatic insufficiency, diarrhea, allergies, colic, carbohydrate and fat malabsorption
Special formulas	
Portagen	Preterm and term infants: pancreatic or bile acid insufficiency, intestinal resection
Similac PM 60/40	Preterm and term infants: problem feeders on standard formula; infants with renal, cardiovascular, digestive diseases that require decreased protein and mineral levels, breastfeeding supplement, initial feeding

(continued)

TABLE 11–7
(Continued)

Formula	Indications[a]
Premature formulas	
Low osmolality	
Similac Special Care 20	Premature infants (<1800–2000 g) who are growing rapidly. These formulas promote growth at intrauterine rates. Vitamin and mineral concentrations are higher to meet the needs of growth. Usually started on 20 Cal/oz and advanced to 24 Cal/oz as tolerated.
Enfamil Premature 20	
Preemie SMA 20	
Isoosmolar	
Similac Special Care 24	Same as for low-osmolality premature formulas
Enfamil Special Care 24	
Preemie SMA 24	

[a]Multivitamin supplementation such as Polyvisol (Mead Johnson) ½ mL/d may be needed for commercial formulas if baby is taking <2 oz/d.
[b]SMA has decreased sodium content and can be used in patients with congestive heart failure, bronchopulmonary dysplasia, and cardiac disease.
Modified and produced with permission from Gomella, TL (ed) *Neonatology*, 5th ed. Mc-Graw-Hill, 2004.

11

Prematurity: Considerable controversy remains concerning the timing of initial enteral feeding for the preterm infant. For the stable larger (> 1500 g) premature infant, the first feeding may be given within the first 24 h of life. Early feeding may allow the release of enteric hormones that exert a trophic effect on the intestinal tract. On the other hand, apprehension about necrotizing enterocolitis (mostly in very low birth weight infants) in the following circumstances often precludes the initiation of enteral feeding: perinatal asphyxia, mechanical ventilation, presence of umbilical vessel catheters, patent ductus arteriosus, indomethacin treatment, sepsis, and frequent episodes of apnea and bradycardia.

No established policies are available, and delay and duration of delay in establishing feeding with those conditions varies for every institution. In general, enteral feeding is started in the first 3 d of life, with the objective of reaching full enteral feeding by 2–3 wk of life. Parenteral nutrition including amino acids and lipids should be started at the same time to provide for adequate caloric intake.

Choice of Formula: (See Table 11–7, page 228.) Human breast milk is recommended for feeding infants whenever possible. Breast-feeding has many advantages: It is ideal for virtually all infants, produces fewer infantile allergies, is immunoprotective to the infant due to the presence of immunoglobulins, is convenient and economical, and offers several theoretical psychologic benefits to both the mother and child. Occasionally, an infant cannot be breast-fed due to extreme prematurity or other problems such as a cleft palate.

If commercial infant formula is chosen, no special considerations are needed for normal full-term newborns. Selection of the best formula for preterm infants may require more care.

The majority of infant formulas are isoosmolar (Similac 20, Enfamil 20, and SMA 20 with and without iron). These formulas are used most often for healthy infants. Formulas for premature infants, containing 24 kcal/oz (Similac 24, Enfamil 24, "preemie" SMA 24), are also isoosmolar and are indicated for rapidly growing premature infants. Many other "specialty" formulas are available for such conditions as milk and protein sensitivity, among others.

Many pediatricians recommend vitamin supplements with some formulas if the infant is taking < 32 oz/d. An iron-containing formula is generally recommended.

Infant Feeding Guidelines

1. **Initial feeding.** For the initial feeding for all infants, use sterile water or 5% dextrose in water (D_5W) if the infant is not being breast-fed. Ten percent dextrose in water ($D_{10}W$) should not be used because it is a hypertonic solution.

2. **Subsequent feedings.** There is controversy over whether infant formulas should be diluted for the next several feedings if the infant tolerates the initial one. Some clinicians advocate diluting formulas with sterile water and advance as tolerated (eg, ¼ strength, increase to ½ and then ¾ strength). Others feel this is unnecessary and that full-strength formula can be used if infants tolerate the initial feeding without difficulty. Breast milk is never diluted.

Oral Rehydration Solutions: Infants with mild or moderate dehydration, often due to diarrhea or vomiting, may benefit from oral rehydration formulas. These solutions typically include glucose, sodium, potassium, and bicarbonate or citrate. Common formulations include **Pedialyte, Lytren, Infalyte, Resol, and Hydrolyte.**

12

TOTAL PARENTERAL NUTRITION (TPN)

Total parenteral nutrition, also called "hyperalimentation," is the provision of all essential nutrients—protein, carbohydrates, lipids, vitamins, electrolytes, and trace elements—by the intravenous (parenteral) route. Nutrients may be supplied by either a peripheral or central vein. To provide a patient's entire nutritional requirement by vein, however, a central venous line must be used because of the tonicity of the fluid required. Peripheral veins simply cannot tolerate these hypertonic fluids, and thus peripheral parenteral alimentation can be used only as a supplement.

The administration of TPN is considered after careful consideration of two issues:

- The patient requires nutrition support (see Chapter 11, "Nutrition Assessment") and is predicted to benefit from it.
- The patient will not tolerate enteral feedings (see Chapter 11, "Determining the Route of Nutritional Support").

Patients who do not meet these two criteria are generally not candidates for the administration of TPN. After establishing that parenteral nutritional support is indicated, the clinician determines the individual patient's nutritional requirements (see Chapter 11, "Nutritional Requirements").

The following indications, among others, are appropriate for TPN administration:

- Preoperatively, in the malnourished patient. There is no benefit for patients who are not malnourished.
- Postoperatively, for patients with a slow return of GI function in patients who also have complications that limit or prohibit the use of the GI tract. The interval between surgery and initiation of nutritional support to prevent complications is not definitively known. However, many practitioners wait 7–10 d after surgery, anticipating the return of bowel function. If this does not occur, nutritional support is begun.
- Patients with Crohn's disease, ulcerative colitis, pancreatitis, fistulas, and short bowel syndrome who cannot tolerate enteral feedings.
- Patients who are malnourished secondary to a disease or injury that results in inadequate oral intake. This may include patients with organ failure, severe metabolic stress, malignancies, burns, or trauma.

PARENTERAL NUTRITIONAL COMPONENT CONSIDERATIONS

The fundamental principle of TPN is the administration of sufficient protein to avoid catabolism of endogenous protein (muscle). Carbohydrates must be given to supply necessary calories (at a ratio of 150 kcal/g of nitrogen) to support these anabolic processes. Fat is given as a source of essential fatty acids. These few principles provide the basis for TPN as a combination of protein, carbohydrate, and fat administration. In addition, TPN includes all necessary fluids, electrolytes, vitamins, and trace elements required to support life. Studies have shown that doses between 4–7 mg/kg/min of carbohydrate (generally, do not exceed 5 mg/kg/min) provide optimal protein sparing with minimal liver toxicity. Assessment of the carbohydrate intake is important in order to limit complications from TPN.

Lipid calories should not exceed 3 g/kg/d due to increased complications. Additionally, no more than 50% of total daily calories should be administered as fat.

The best method for establishing a protein need for a given patient is the 24-h urine sample testing for urine urea nitrogen (UUN) levels. This value reflects the amount of protein catabolism occurring daily. Urinary losses of 8–12 g/d are consistent with a mild stress condition, 14–18 g/d moderate stress, and greater than 20 g/d with severe stress.

Protein dosing should be modified based on the 24-h UUN and daily nitrogen balance. Initially, however, if the patient is considered mildly stressed, 0.8–1.2 g/kg/d is appropriate. In cases of moderate and severe stress (burned and head-injured patients) 1.3–1.75 g/kg/d and 2–2.5 g/kg/d may be required, respectively. (*Note:* Generally, do not exceed 2.0 g/kg/d.) Several studies suggest that doses of protein in this range exceed the patient's utilization capacity and may increase BUN. Adequate renal function must be present to provide such high protein loads. Patients with renal failure who are not receiving dialysis may be dosed at the minimum daily allowance, 0.6 g/kg/d, until a decision for dialysis is made. Once the patient is receiving dialysis, normal dosing may be instituted.

NITROGEN BALANCE

The best method for determining the adequacy of nutritional support is the calculation of nitrogen balance. A **positive nitrogen balance** implies that the amount of protein being administered is sufficient to cover the losses of endogenous protein that occur secondary to catabolism. This is the best therapeutic goal for TPN because it is impossible to determine whether the prescribed protein is preventing muscle breakdown or not. Once positive nitrogen balance has been achieved, however, protein replacement has been optimized. In critical care patients, nitrogen losses may be very high, and an attempt should be made to at least achieve nitrogen equilibrium. This may be impossible in the acute phase of injury, in severe trauma, or in burn cases. Thus, minimizing protein loss (–2 to –4 g/d) may be the goal during this period.

A **negative nitrogen balance** is indicative of insufficient protein replacement for the degree of skeletal muscle loss. Under most circumstances, an attempt to achieve positive nitrogen balance should be made. Patients with renal dysfunction or those who are severely stressed may not be able to achieve a positive balance due to safety concerns. The efficacy of protein doses exceeding 2.5 g/kg/d has not been established. Investigational agents (growth hormone, IGF-1) and specialized formulas (branched-chain amino acids, essential amino acids, glutamine) are being studied in these populations to assess their potential in improving nitrogen retention under these circumstances. The following are key concepts in determining nitrogen balance:

- Nitrogen balance = Nitrogen input − Nitrogen output
- 1 g of nitrogen = 6.25 g of protein
- Nitrogen input = (Protein in grams/6.25 g nitrogen)
- Nitrogen output = 24-h UUN + 4 g/d (nonurine loss)
- The conditions and disease states that increase the amount of nonurine losses for nitrogen include high-output fistulas and massive diarrhea. Fecal nitrogen measurements can be obtained but are difficult for nursing staff to perform.

Sample Determination of Nitrogen Balance

A patient is receiving 2 L TPN/24 h with 27.5 g crystalline amino acid (protein) solution per liter.

1. 27.5 g protein/L × 2 L = 55 g protein/24 h.
2. Recall that 1 g of nitrogen = 6.25 g of protein.
3. Nitrogen input = 55 g protein/6.25 g protein/g N = 8.8 g.
4. Patient voided 22.5 dL urine/24 h with UUN 66 mg/dL.
5. Nitrogen lost in urine = 22.5 dL × 66 mg/dL = 1485 mg, or about 1.5 g.
6. Add 4.0 g for nonurine nitrogen loss.
7. Nitrogen output = 1.5 g + 4.0 = 5.5 g.
8. Nitrogen balance = Input − output = 8.8 − 5.5 = +3.3 g nitrogen.

12

TPN SOLUTIONS

Different strength amino acid (CAA) solutions are available (Table 12–1 below) to which the pharmacy can add varying concentrations of dextrose, electrolytes, vitamins, and trace elements. Most hospitals supply a "house," or standard, formula for patients with normal renal and hepatic function. Changes in the standard formulas can be made when necessary while a TPN solution is being infused based

TABLE 12–1
Typical TPN Solutions for Adults

Component	Solution 1	Solution 2
CAA	4.25% (42.5 g/L)	4.25% (42.5 g/L)
Dextrose	25% (250 g/L, 850 Cal/L)	12.5% (125 g/L, 425 Cal/L)
Na	50 mEq/L	50 mEq/L
K	50 mEq/L	50 mEq/L
Ca	6 mEq/L	6 mEq/L
Mg	6 mEq/L	6 mEq/L
PO_4	15 mMol/L	15 mMol/L
Cl	45 mEq/L	45 mEq/L

CAA = crystalline amino acids.

on measured laboratory parameters. Administration of TPN is never an emergency and in most cases can be provided within 24 h of prescribing. If a formula change is necessary based on a change in patient status, discontinue the TPN and replace it with $D_{10}W$ at the same rate until a new bag of TPN can be provided.

Amino acid formulas are supplied as CAA or SAA in concentrations ranging from 3.5–15%. These are diluted by the pharmacy to varying concentrations to provide for the necessary protein dose (2.75%, 4.25%, etc). The final concentrations of dextrose vary but are usually either 12.5% or 25%. Examples of typical TPN solutions for adults are provided in Table 12–1.

The maximum rate of infusion of solution 1 from Table 12–1 should be 100–125 mL/h to avoid excessive glucose administration (remember to consider the patient's weight and the dosing guidelines of 4–7 mg/kg/min). Fat emulsions should be given with solution 1 to provide essential fatty acids (10%, 500 mL 3×/wk) or as an additional calorie source. Solution 2 is designed to be given at a maximum rate of 125 mL/h, but this only provides 1275 kcal from dextrose and must be supplemented with a fat emulsion (10% 500 mL = 550 kcal, 20% 500 mL = 1000 kcal).

Many hospitals have adopted a "three-in-one" solution for the standard house formula. This involves the administration of protein, carbohydrate, and fat from the same TPN bag over a 24-h period; in other words, the fat is not administered peripherally through a separate site. Caution should be used when altering the standard formula in this situation because the fat emulsion may be less stable to additives and makes incompatibilities less visible. For example, the solution will be milky in color, and a calcium–phosphate problem, normally easily seen, would not be apparent. Additions to these formulations should be done in conjunction with a pharmacist to ensure that precautions are taken for appropriate additive concentrations.

Remember, the solutions described in Table 12–1 contain full concentrations of electrolytes and are for patients with normal renal function. For patients with renal impairment, the concentrations of potassium, magnesium, phosphorus, and protein should be reduced (see page 239).

TPN ADDITIVES

Vitamins are a necessary component of TPN solutions. A product conforming to recommendations of the American Medical Association Nutrition Advisory Group is usually used, such as multivitamin infusion-12 (MVI-12). The contents of two vials is added to 1 L of TPN solution daily (Table 12–2). In addition to

TABLE 12–2
Typical Vitamins Provided in 1 L of TPN by Adding 2 Vials of Standard MVI-12

Ascorbic acid	100 mg	Pyridoxine (B_6)	4 mg
Vitamin A	3300 IU	Dexpanthenol	15 mg
Vitamin D	200 IU	Vitamin E (α-tocopherol)	10 IU
Biotin	60 mcg	Thiamine (B_1)	3 mg
Folic acid	400 mcg	Riboflavin (B_2)	3.6 mg
Vitamin B_{12}	5 mcg	Niacin	40 mg

MVI–12 = multivitamin infusion–12.

MVI-12, 5–10 mg of vitamin K (phytonadione) must be given IM weekly. Vitamin K may also be added to the TPN and given as a 1-mg IV dose daily.

Several manufacturers sell a trace element supplement that conforms to the AMA group's guidelines. Each milliliter contains 1.0 mg zinc, 0.4 mg copper, 4.0 mg chromium, and 0.1 mg manganese. Suggested doses for trace elements are listed in Table 12–3, below.

Trace element deficiencies are rare in hospitalized patients receiving short-term TPN supplements. Supplementation should be routine, however, to ensure trace element availability for cell restoration. In patients receiving long-term support or home TPN, additional trace element supplementation may be necessary.

Iron can be given as an injectable iron–dextran complex (Dexferrum, InFeD). Note, however, that owing to the inconvenience of its administration, many clinicians avoid injectable iron–dextran. A complete medical and hematologic work-up is often indicated before instituting parenteral iron replacement. Prior to receiving the first dose, a test IV dose of 0.5 mL is recommended. Anaphylaxis is rare, but a period of 1 h should elapse before the therapeutic dose of iron is administered. Use the following equation to determine the dose of iron:

$$\text{Total replacement dose (mL)} = 0.0476 \times \text{Weight (kg)} \times$$
$$[\text{Desired hemoglobin (g/dL)} - \text{Measured hemoglobin (g/dL)}]$$
$$+ 1\text{ mL}/5\text{ kg weight (max 14 mL)}$$

Maximum Daily Dose: Adults > 50 kg: 100 mg iron; Peds < 5 kg: 25 mg iron, 5–10 kg: 50 mg iron, 0–50 kg: 100 mg iron

The iron–dextran is supplied in an injectable form of 50 mg (Fe)/mL. The calculated dose should be added to TPN at 2 mL/L until the entire dose has been given.

Insulin, when required, can be given subcutaneously as regular insulin using a sliding scale, as shown in Table 12–4, page 234. But the preferred method is to add the insulin directly to the TPN solution, once the appropriate dose is determined. This allows a constant infusion of insulin along with the infusion of dextrose, which avoids the peaks and valleys in blood glucose that occur when the sliding scale is used. The usual starting dose per liter of TPN is 10 units of regular insulin. Doses from 10 to 90 units/L may often be required. Insulin drips are not advised because TPN can be temporarily or permanently discontinued, which would then stop the insulin. Other additives include H_2 antagonists and heparin.

TABLE 12–3
Suggested Trace Element Dosing

Trace Element	Parenteral Dose per Day
Zinc	2.5–4.0 mg[a]
Copper	0.5–1.5 mg
Selenium	20–40mg
Chromium	10–15mg
Manganese	0.15–0.8 mg

[a]May be higher, up to 15 mg/d, in severe stress or in patients with high-output fistulas.

TABLE 12–4
Sliding Scale for Insulin Orders

Urine Glucose[a]	Regular Insulin Dose (Units, given SQ)
0–1+	0
2+	5
3+	10
4+	15
Any acetone: call house officer	

[a]Should be checked every 6 h as part of standing TPN orders.

FAT EMULSIONS

Lipid emulsions were initially used only to provide essential fatty acids (linoleic acid, and linolenic acid in children). This could be done with minimal supplementation; as little as 4% of total calories per day would prevent the syndrome of essential fatty acid deficiency (EFAD). Most clinicians prescribe 500 mL of 10% lipid emulsion three times weekly to prevent this syndrome. The signs and symptoms of this deficiency include scaling skin rash, alopecia, and wound healing failure.

Linoleic acid is a precursor to arachidonic acid, which is essential for prostaglandin and leukotriene synthesis. Once data became available establishing the problems associated with overfeeding of carbohydrate calories, the use of lipid for caloric supplementation became more recognized.

Commercially available intravenous fat emulsions are derived from soybean oil, with one product **(Liposyn II)** combining both soybean and safflower oil. The 10% products provide 1.1 kcal/mL, and the 20% products provide 2.0 kcal/mL. Pediatricians often prefer the Liposyn II product because of its higher percentage of linolenic acid. Because the particle size of these emulsions closely approximates naturally occurring chylomicrons, parenteral infusion is possible. In addition, the emulsions are cleared from the bloodstream in a manner and rate similar to that for chylomicrons.

Before beginning the IV fat emulsion, the serum triglyceride level should be checked to ensure that hypertriglyceridemia is not present. Provided that the serum triglyceride level is below 400 mg/dL, the fat emulsion can be given over a 6–12-h period. The longer infusion rate is preferred. The first bottle should be given slowly (1 mL/min for 15 min to check for hypersensitivity reaction). Adverse reactions can include dyspnea, fever, chills, chest tightness, wheezing, headaches, and nausea.

Currently, the only absolute contraindication to the use of IV fat emulsion is type IV hypertriglyceridemia, although isolated cases of nontype IV intolerance to the solution have been reported. To monitor for the clearing of the fat from the bloodstream, a trough serum triglyceride level should be tested 8–12 h following the daily infusion of the fat emulsion.

Because fat emulsions are primarily composed of triglycerides (essentially cholesterol-free), if the blood is mistakenly drawn while the fat is being infused or shortly thereafter, the serum triglyceride level will be markedly elevated. Other possible contraindications include lipoid nephrosis, severe hepatic failure, and allergy to eggs (egg phosphatides are used as the emulsifying agent).

Fat emulsions can be administered through peripheral veins, although the vein may be damaged and cease to be functional in 2–3 d. For this reason, it is usually recommended that the fat emulsion be infused into the central line under strict aseptic technique via a sterile Y-connector. As mentioned earlier, some institutions combine the lipid with the TPN formula in one bag for 24-h administration. This limits the clinician's ability to validate fat clearance from the blood and makes baseline triglyceride data extremely important.

STARTING TPN

In general, TPN should not be started until a patient has a stable fluid and electrolyte profile. It is usually unwise to begin TPN in a patient who requires large amounts of fluid, may need resuscitation following trauma, or is septic. Once a patient's fluid and electrolyte requirements are reasonably stable, TPN can be started safely. The initiation of TPN is never an emergency.

Placement of a deep line must be done aseptically, as outlined in Chapter 13, page 258. Infection (bacteremia, fungemia) arising from the catheter or the catheter–skin interface is the most common complication of TPN. Many hospitals now have standardized order forms for starting patients on TPN.

1. **Baseline laboratory tests:**
   a. CBC with differential and platelets
   b. PT and PTT
   c. SMA-7 and SMA-12; in particular check phosphate, glucose, and routine electrolytes (Na^+, K^+, Cl^-)
   d. Urinalysis
   e. Baseline weight
2. **Order the type of TPN** desired along with the additives and supplements. Medications are generally not added to TPN solutions except insulin and H_2 receptor blockers. A 0.22-μm filter should be used with aqueous TPN (no fat). A 1.2-μm filter should be used with three-in-one TPN.
3. **Nursing orders:**
   a. Check urine for sugar and acetone every 6–8 h, house officer should be called if sugar is > 2+ or acetone is present.
   b. Take vital signs every shift.
   c. Change tubing and deep-line dress every other day (or per hospital procedure).
   d. Weigh patient every other day.
   e. Monitor daily fluid balance.
4. **Laboratory monitoring:**
   a. SMA-7 daily until patient is stable, then every other day.
   b. CBC with differential, platelets, PT/PTT, twice weekly.
   c. SMA-12 twice weekly (especially liver function tests).
   d. Triglyceride trough level (obtained at least 6 h after infusion has stopped, preferably prior to hanging next bottle of fat) once or twice weekly.
   e. 24-h urine for nitrogen balance determinations and creatinine clearance once or twice weekly.
5. **Begin the solution at 25–50 mL/h** when using a 25% or 50–75 mL/h when using a 12.5% dextrose solution. Increase by 25 mL/h every 24 h, providing the urine sugar levels are negative. Advance to the maximum rate based on the calculated daily caloric need (page 207).

12

6. **Begin the IV fat emulsion the next day,** provided that the serum triglyceride levels are less than 400 mg/dL. Remember that glucose intolerance is the major adverse effect seen during the initial infusion period. Urine sugar and acetone levels should be less than 2+, and serum glucose values less than 180–200 mg/dL. If the sugar level rises above these levels, insulin must be given to achieve the desired level of caloric intake. If glucose intolerance develops when using a 25% dextrose solution, consider decreasing the amount of calories from dextrose and increasing the calories from fat. (Be sure to check that overfeeding is not occurring, ie, > 4–7 mg/kg/min, in this case reduce the dose of carbohydrate prior to the addition of insulin). Glucose intolerance arising once the patient has been stabilized may signify sepsis.

ASSESSING THE EFFICACY OF TPN THERAPY

Nitrogen balance is a good measure of the success of the TPN regimen because the goal is protein-sparing. Serum albumin will not change appreciably during TPN therapy lasting less than 3 wk. This is due to albumin's long half-life of 22–24 d. In stressed patients, albumin often falls due to reduced production because the body shifts to increased production of acute-phase reactant proteins.

STOPPING TPN

TPN can usually be stopped when necessary. Although widely practiced, there is rarely a need for a formal weaning schedule. If there are concerns about hypoglycemia, then a 10% dextrose solution can be administered after cessation of the TPN.

12

DISEASE-SPECIFIC TPN FORMULATIONS

Cardiac Failure: In patients with CHF, reduce water from 1 to 0.5 mL/kcal or 500 mL insensible loss plus measured water losses. This limits overloading with water from TPN. Other considerations include providing energy needs at the BEE + 30% for initiation of TPN calories, limiting protein initially to 0.8–1 g/kg and reducing sodium to 0.5–1.5 g/d.

Diabetes: Consider increasing the percentage of calories provided from fat. Ideally, blood sugar should be well controlled or at least not > 200 when initiating TPN. Remember that no more than 50% of total intake should be from fat and not > 3 g/kg/d. Fat provides 9 kcal/g. Commercial lipid emulsions provide 1.1 or 2 kcal/mL. Insulin should be added to the solution initially at 5–10 units/bag in patients requiring > 20 units of insulin daily.

Geriatrics: Patients older than 75 years have a documented need for fewer calories. Use caution in monitoring total fluids to prevent overload.

Inflammatory Bowel Disease: TPN can be initiated in these patients at approximately 1.5 × RME at 30 kcal/kg of ideal body weight. Protein needs vary from 1 to 2 g/kg of ideal body weight daily. Dose the protein based on a 24-h UUN. *Note:* Patients with fistulas lose nitrogen via this route and need additional protein. Zinc losses may be greater in this group of IBD patients also.

Liver Disease: Specialized formulas of amino acids that contain primarily branched-chain amino acids (leucine, isoleucine, and valine) are available for use in cases of liver disease. Theoretically, these products may improve arousal from hepatic encephalopathy by competing with the aromatic amino acids that are precursors for some centrally active amines. There is no definitive evidence that branched-chain formulas improve patient outcome. The specialized formulas should only be used in cases of severe hepatic disease accompanied by encephalopathy. In other clinical conditions of liver disease, standard formulas should be used. Lipid emulsions are not recommended in cases of severe hepatic failure when hypertriglyceridemia is present.

Pancreatic Disease: Total energy needs may be high in this disease (35 kcal/kg). Protein should be initiated at 1.5 g/kg/d. Intravenous fat may be administered in these cases because it is metabolized by peripheral tissue lipases. A reasonable nonprotein system would be 70% carbohydrate and 30% fat.

Pulmonary Disease: Carbohydrate metabolism produces higher amounts of CO_2 than does fat metabolism. Consequently, the patient with CO_2 retention problems often is stressed if overfed with carbohydrates. Increasing the percentage of daily nonprotein calories provided by fat (not > 60%) may decrease the CO_2 load and assist with ventilator weaning. Higher fat percentages influence oxygen diffusion capacity and are not beneficial, especially in cases of mild pulmonary compromise. Phosphate depletion is a second clinically relevant concern in this population due to the depression of the hypoxic ventilatory drive. Once patients are started on TPN, PO_4^{2-} often decreases due to the incorporation into ATP. Adequate supplementation and monitoring is very important in this group of patients.

Renal Failure: Several considerations become important in this disease. If a patient is not receiving dialysis or is not a dialysis candidate, protein must be restricted to 0.6–0.8 g/kg/d, and total energy needs must be limited to approximately 30 kcal/kg/d. Weight should be ideal or admission weight, so as to control for the influence of water retention. Specialized amino acid formulas have been developed for this group of patients. These products provide higher concentrations of essential amino acids than the standard amino acid products. Theoretically, the nitrogen waste products are recycled to make the nonessential amino acids, thereby reducing the BUN content. Risks exist, however, for elevations in ammonia when arginine is not also supplemented. Consequently, manufacturers have modified the original formulas to include several nonessential amino acids. Due to these changes, the renal products provide a very similar amino acid profile to those of the SAA solutions at very low concentrations (2.5%). The cost differential can be significant. It is therefore recommended that patients with renal dysfunction receive SAA formulas at a reduced concentration to provide the minimum daily allowance of protein. TPN should not be supplemented with potassium or magnesium, and sodium should be reduced to 40–180 mEq/d once the GFR is < 10 mL/min.

Patients receiving hemodialysis or peritoneal dialysis may be fed protein similarly to patients without renal disease. Doses of 1–1.2 g/kg/d may be used. Nitrogen balance calculations are not useful in this population due to the problem of renal clearance of urea waste inherent to kidney disease.

Sepsis or Trauma: Sepsis and trauma causes hypermetabolism and requires greater numbers of calories from nonprotein (30–35 kcal/kg) and protein (2–2.5 g/kg/d) sources. Estimates of RME should be increased by 50% initially, and some cases may support up to 100%. Note that feeding > 3000 kcal/d is not recommended. Specialized amino acid formulas are also available for this group of patients. Again, these formulas include higher concentrations of the branched-chain amino acids. The reason for their inclusion in this population is to provide substrate directly to the skeletal muscle undergoing catabolism to provide gluco-neogenic precursors. Although these formulas have been shown to normalize the amino acid profile and in some cases improve nitrogen balance, no studies have demonstrated an improved patient outcome. The additional cost of these formu-las is a deterrent to their routine use in these populations until further data are available. Additional zinc supplementation is often recommended in this group of patients. Studies have shown losses to be increased in stress; therefore, daily supplementation of up to 15 mg of zinc may be appropriate.

COMMON TPN COMPLICATIONS

Hyperosmolar Nonketotic Coma: Usually found in improperly monitored pa-tients with impaired insulin responses. Caused by excessive glucose levels, usu-ally corrected by administration of insulin and rehydration. Sustained hyper-glycemia (> 220 mg/dL) depresses monocyte activity and could compromise the immune defenses.

Infection (Sepsis):   The care of the deep-line site and tubing must be meticu-lous. Suspect sepsis if a previously stable patient becomes glucose-intolerant. If the patient becomes septic, the deep line should be considered a possible source. If no other source of infection can be identified, the deep line must be removed or changed and the tip sent for routine culture and sensitivity. *Candida albicans* is the most frequently encountered pathogen on the catheter, followed by *Staphylococcus aureus, S. epidermidis* and gram-negative rods.

Hypophosphatemia: Severe hypophosphatemia can occur in patients started on TPN after severe weight loss and those with conditions such as anorexia ner-vosa (refeeding syndrome). This may also result from increased metabolic processes requiring phosphate and can significantly hamper weaning from the ventilator.

Elevated Liver Function Tests: The usual cause is excessive glucose infusion. When the primary metabolic pathway for glucose becomes saturated, excess glucose is converted to intracellular triglycerides in the liver. This is especially seen when rates exceed 4–7 mg/kg/min. A reduction in carbohydrate calories, supplementing with fat, is recommended.

Cholestasis: This often occurs secondary to overfeeding of fat calories (> 3 g/kg/d or > 60% of total nonprotein calories).

Hyperkalemia: This is the most common electrolyte disturbance seen with TPN. Most TPN formulations contain potassium 40–50 mEq/L and are intended for patients with normal renal function. Excess potassium over and above that required for maintenance and urine losses (usually 3–5 mEq/g nitrogen) is in-cluded. Potassium must be closely followed in the elderly and those with im-paired renal function. Additionally, many drugs contribute to potassium balance problems. These include some antibiotics that are potassium salts (eg, peni-cillins); oral phosphate supplements (Neutra-Phos); ACE inhibitors, which re-duce potassium excretion (Captopril, Enalapril); and potassium-sparing diuretics (triamterene, spironolactone).

Metabolic Alkalosis: Modern SAAs are present as the acetate salt (80–100 mEq/L), which is converted to bicarbonate in vivo. In postoperative patients with NG tubes, the loss of chloride, together with the high infusion of the acetate, can lead to a metabolic alkalosis. The increased use of histamine blockers and antacids in intensive care patients has also contributed to a higher incidence of this problem. Treating this condition requires increasing the chloride level in the solution and reducing the acetate.

Hyponatremia: Serum sodium levels of 127–135 mEq/L are commonly seen in patients on TPN. The cause is controversial but is probably due to mild SIADH; therefore the problem is probably an excess of water and not deficiency of sodium. It is usually asymptomatic and does not require a change in formula unless the sodium drops below 125 mEq/L.

Hypermagnesemia: This is usually seen in patients with renal failure. Antacid therapy may also contribute to this condition. If potassium is reduced in the TPN, magnesium should also be reduced.

12

BEDSIDE PROCEDURES

Procedure Basics
Amniotic Fluid Fern Test
Arterial Line Placement
Arterial Puncture
Arthrocentesis (Diagnostic and
    Therapeutic)
Bone Marrow Aspiration and Biopsy
Central Venous Catheterization
Chest Tube Placement (Closed
    Thoracostomy, Tube Thoracostomy)
Cricothyrotomy (Needle and Surgical)
Culdocentesis
Doppler Pressures
Electrocardiogram
Endotracheal Intubation
Fever Work-up
Gastrointestinal Intubation
Heelstick and Fingersticks (Capillary
    Blood Sampling)
Internal Fetal Scalp Monitoring

Injection Techniques
Intrauterine Pressure Monitoring
IV Techniques
Lumbar Puncture
Orthostatic Blood Pressure
    Measurement
Pelvic Examination
Pericardiocentesis
Peripherally Inserted Central Catheter
    (PICC Line)
Peritoneal Lavage
Peritoneal (Abdominal) Paracentesis
Pulmonary Artery Catheterization
Pulsus Paradoxus Measurement
Skin Biopsy
Skin Testing
Thoracentesis
Urinary Tract Procedures
Venipuncture

PROCEDURE BASICS

Universal Precautions

Universal precautions should be used whenever an invasive procedure exposes the operator to potentially infectious body fluids. Not all patients infected with transmissible pathogens can be reliably identified. Because pathogens transmitted by blood and body fluids pose a hazard to personnel caring for such patients, particularly during invasive procedures, certain precautions are now *required* for *routine* care of **all** patients whether or not they have been placed on isolation precautions of any type. The CDC calls these universal precautions.

1. Wash hands before and after **all** patient contact.
2. Wash hands before and after **all** invasive procedures.
3. Wear gloves in **every** instance in which contact with blood or body fluid is certain or likely. For example, wear gloves for all venipunctures, for all IV starts, for IV manipulation, and for wound care.
4. Wear gloves once and discard. Do not wear the same pair to perform tasks on two different patients or two different tasks at different sites on the same patient.
5. Wear gloves in **every** instance in which contact with any body fluid is likely, including urine, feces, wound secretions, respiratory tract care, thoracentesis, paracentesis, etc.
6. Wear gown when splatter of blood or body fluids on clothing seems likely.
7. Additional barrier precautions may be necessary for certain invasive procedures when significant splatter or aerosol generation is likely. This does

not occur during most routine patient care activities but may occur in the OR, ER, ICU, during invasive bedside procedures, and during CPR. Always wear masks when goggles are worn and vice versa.

Accidental Needle Sticks

The FDA has recommended safer needle devices, including that a device provide a barrier between the hands and the needle after use. Needlestick injury is a cause of occupational injury among health care workers in the United States. OSHA estimates 600,000–800,000 needlestick injuries occur on the job each year. Health care workers are at risk of transmission of more than 20 different blood-borne pathogens (eg, HIV, hepatitis B and C virus). Although it is not possible to completely eliminate the risk of needlestick injury, research estimates 62–88% of sharps injuries could be reduced through the use of devices and procedures designed to protect health care workers from exposed needles. A variety of self-shielding needle devices are now on the market (See sections on Heelsticks, IV, and Venipuncture for examples).

Informed Consent

Patients should be counseled before any procedure concerning the reasons for the procedure, possible alternatives, and the potential risks and benefits. Explaining the various steps will make the patient more cooperative and the procedure easier on both parties. In general, procedures such as bladder catheterization, NG intubation, or venipuncture do not require a written informed consent beyond normal hospital sign-in protocols. More invasive procedures, such as thoracentesis or lumbar puncture, for example, require written consent and must be obtained by a licensed physician.

Latex Allergy

13

Individuals with certain medical conditions or occupations that are heavily exposed to products containing natural rubber latex (NRL) may became sensitized and develop allergic reactions to NRL. It is estimated that 7% of health care workers have allergic reactions; patients with spina bifida have a 18–40% incidence. Any group of patients frequently and intensely exposed to latex, such as those undergoing repeated surgical procedures and treatments like intermittent catheterization, are at increased risk. Local and systemic allergic reactions can often be dramatic and occasionally life-threatening. The treatment is the same as for any allergic reaction (remove exposure, epinephrine, and steroids, See Chapter 21).

If a patient has latex allergy, it should be noted on prominently displayed signs and on the patient's chart, and the patient should wear an alert bracelet. Latex is found in significant quantity in common items beyond just gloves (ie, anesthesia masks, catheters, condoms, diaphragms, douche bulbs, endotracheal tubes, hemodialysis components, NG tubes, drains, syringes, others) as well as consumer products (eg, balloons, rubber bands, SCUBA-diving equipment, underwear). Most hospitals now have an inventory of latex-free products and operating rooms have latex allergy procedures in place. Nitrile gloves are becoming commonplace in hospital settings due to this growing problem (see also page 360).

Basic Equipment

Table 13–1 lists useful collections of instruments and supplies, often packaged together, that aid in the completion of the procedures outlined in this chapter. Local anesthesia is discussed in Chapter 17.

TABLE 13–1
Instruments and Supplies Used in the Completion of Common Bedside Procedures

MINOR PROCEDURE TRAY

Sterile gloves
Sterlile towels/drapes
4×4 gauze sponges
Povidone-iodine (Betadine) prep solution
Syringes: 5-, 10-, 20-mL
Needles: 18-, 20-, 22-, 25-gauge
1% Lidocaine (with or without epinephrine)
Adhesive tape

INSTRUMENT TRAY

Scissors
Needle holder
Hemostat
Scalpel and blade (No. 10 for adult, No. 15 for children or delicate work)
Suture of choice (2-0 or 3-0 silk or nylon on cutting needle; cutting needle best for suturing to skin)

The size of various catheters, tubes, and needles is often designated by **French unit (1 Fr = ⅓ mm in diameter)** or by **needle gauge.** Reference listings for these designations can be found in Figure 13–1A page 246. Designations of surgical scalpels used in the performance of many basic bedside procedures and in the operating room are shown in Figure 13–1B page 247.

13

AMNIOTIC FLUID FERN TEST

Indication

- Assess for rupture of membranes

Materials

- Sterile speculum and swab
- Glass slide and microscope
- Nitrazine paper (optional)

Procedure

1. Using a sterile speculum, a sample of fluid "pooled" in the vaginal vault is swabbed on a glass slide and air dried.
2. Amniotic fluid yields an arborization, or "fern," pattern, seen under 10× magnification. False-positive: cervical mucus collection; however, the ferning pattern of mucus is coarser. Test is unaffected by meconium, vaginal pH, and blood-to-amniotic-fluid ratios > 1:10. Samples heavily contaminated with blood may not fern.
3. Another test for ruptured membranes uses nitrazine paper, which has a pH turning point of 6.0. Normal vaginal pH in pregnancy is 4.5–6.0; amniotic

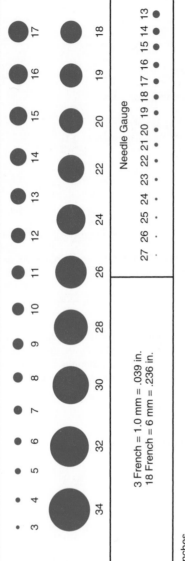

FIGURE 13–1. A: French catheter guide and needle gauge reference. (Courtesy Cook Urological.)

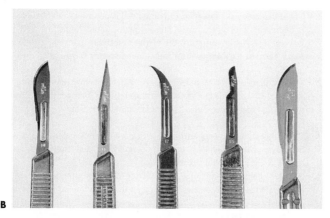

B

FIGURE 13–1B. Commonly used scalpel blades. From left to right: Number 10, 11, 12, 15, and 20. The No. 10 is the standard surgical blade; No. 11 is useful for incisions into abscesses or to open the skin for the placement of large intravenous devices; No. 12 is designed to open tubular structures; No. 15 is widely used for bedside procedures and for more delicate work; the No. 20 blade is used to make large incisions.

fluid pH is 7.0–7.5. A positive nitrazine test: color change in the paper from yellow to blue. False-positive: more common with the nitrazine test; blood, meconium, semen, alkalotic urine, cervical mucus, and vaginal infections can raise the pH.

Complication

- Bacteria may be introduced if sterile technique is not used.

ARTERIAL LINE PLACEMENT

Indications

- Continuous BP readings (eg, critically ill patient)
- Facilitate frequent ABG measurements.

Contraindications

- Arterial insufficiency with poor collateral circulation (See Allen test, page 250)
- Thrombolytic therapy or coagulopathy (relative)

Materials

- Minor procedure and instrument tray (page 245)
- Heparin flush solution (1:1000 dilution)
- Arterial line set-up per local ICU routine (transducer, tubing and pressure bag with preheparinized saline, monitor)
- Arterial line catheter kit **or** 20-gauge catheter over needle, 1½–2 in. (Insyte Autoguard shielded IV catheter, Angiocath Autoguard Shielded IV catheter) with 0.025-in. guidewire (optional)

Procedure (Figure 13–2 below)

1. The radial artery is most frequently used and is described here. Other sites, in decreasing preference: ulnar, dorsalis pedis, femoral, brachial, and axillary arteries. **Never puncture the radial and ulnar arteries in the same hand because this may compromise blood supply to the hand and fingers.**

2. Verify collateral circulation between the radial and ulnar arteries using the Allen test (page 250) or Doppler ultrasound probe. Prepare the flush bag, tubing, and transducer, paying particular attention to removing the air bubbles.

3. Place the extremity on an armboard with a roll of gauze behind the wrist to hyperextend the joint. Prep with povidone-iodine, and drape with sterile towels. Wear gloves and a mask.

4. Palpate the artery, and choose the puncture site where it appears most superficial. Raise a very small skin wheal at the puncture site with 1% lidocaine using a 25-gauge needle.

5. **a. Standard technique:** (See Figure 13–2). While palpating the path of the artery with the nondominant hand, advance the 20-gauge (preferably 1½ in. long) catheter-over-needle assembly into the artery at a low (< 30-degree) angle. Once "flash" of blood is seen in the hub, advance the entire unit 1–2 mm, so that the needle and catheter are in the artery. If blood flow in the hub stops, carefully pull the entire unit back

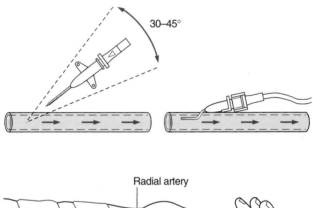

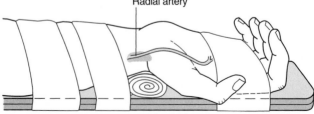

FIGURE 13–2. Technique for arterial line placement. (Reprinted, with permission, from: Gomella TL [ed] *Neonatology: Basic Management, On-Call Problems, Diseases, Drugs,* 5th ed. McGraw-Hill, 2004.)

until flow is reestablished. Once the catheter is in the artery, hold the needle steady, and advance the catheter over the needle into the artery. The catheter should slide smoothly into the artery. Activate the safety button on the catheter to automatically shield the needle. Withdraw the shielded needle completely and check for arterial blood flow from the catheter. A catheter that does not spurt blood is not in position. Briefly occlude the artery with manual pressure while the pressure tubing is being connected. *Note:* The pressure tubing system must be preflushed to clear all air bubbles prior to connection.

    b. **Prepackaged kit technique:** Kits, sometimes referred to as "quick catheters" are available with a needle and guidewire that allow the Seldinger technique (described in step 8) to be used. Place the entry needle at a 30-degree angle to the skin site, and insert until a flash of blood rises in the catheter. The catheter does not need to be advanced, but advance both the guidewire portion (orange handle in some kits) and the catheter into the vessel. Remove the wire and connect it to the pressure tubing.

6. If placement is not successful, apply pressure to the site for 5 min and reattempt one or two more times. If still not successful, move to another site.

7. Suture in place with 3-0 silk, and apply a sterile dressing. Splint the dorsum of the wrist to limit mobility and provide catheter stability.

8. If larger vessels such as the femoral artery are used, the clinician can employ the **Seldinger technique** for femoral artery cannulation: locate the vessel lumen with a small-gauge, thin-walled needle; pass a 0.035 floppy-tipped J ("J" describes the configuration of the end of the floppy wire) guidewire into the lumen; and use the guidewire to pass a larger catheter into the vessel. Use a 16-gauge catheter assembly at least 6 in. long for the femoral artery.

9. Replace arterial lines at a different site every 3–4 d (or per local protocol) to decrease risk of infection.

10. Any amount of heparin can make coagulation studies (PTT) inaccurate. If an arterial line sample is obtained and unexpectedly high results are seen, repeat the test and consider standard venipuncture (see page 316). Even with a 5–10-mL discard sample from the line, some of the heparin solution can contaminate the line.

11. Always compare the arterial line pressure with a standard cuff pressure. An occasional difference is normal (10–20 mm Hg) and should be incorporated when following the BP.

13

Complications

Thrombosis, hematoma, arterial embolism, arterial spasm, arterial insufficiency with tissue loss, infection, hemorrhage, and pseudo-aneurysm formation.

ARTERIAL PUNCTURE

Indications

- Blood gas determinations and when arterial blood is needed for chemistry determinations (eg, ammonia levels)

Materials

- Cup of ice
- Blood gas-sampling kit

or

- 3–5-mL syringe
- 23–25-gauge needle(radial artery); 20–22 (femoral artery
- Heparin (1000 U/mL), 1 mL
- Alcohol or povidone-iodine swabs

Procedure

1. Use "heparinized" syringe for blood gas and a "nonheparinized" syringe for chemistry determinations. If a blood gas kit is not available, a 3–5-mL syringe can be heparinized by drawing up 1 mL of 1:1000 solution of heparin through a small-gauge needle (23–25 gauge) into the syringe, pulling the plunger all the way back. The heparin is then expelled, leaving only a small coating.

2. In order of preference, use radial, femoral, and brachial arteries. For the radial artery, perform an **Allen test** to verify patency of the ulnar artery. You do not want to damage the radial artery if there is no flow in the ulnar artery. To perform the Allen test, the patient makes a tight fist. Occlude both the radial and ulnar arteries at the wrist and have the patient open the hand. While maintaining pressure on the radial artery, release the ulnar artery. If the ulnar artery is patent, the hand flushes red within 6 s. A radial puncture can be safely performed. If the flushing is delayed or part of the hand or remains pale, do **not** perform the radial puncture because collateral flow is inadequate. Choose an alternative site. Doppler ultrasound can also be used to determine patentcy of the ulnar artery.

3. For the femoral artery, use the mnemonic **NAVEL** to locate groin structures. Palpate the femoral artery just below the inguinal ligament. From lateral to medial the structures are Nerve, Artery, Vein, Empty space, Lymphatic (NAVEL).

4. With gloves, palpate the chosen artery carefully; lidocaine SQ can be used (small needle such as a 25–27 gauge), but this often turns a "one-stick procedure" into a "two-stick procedure." Palpate the artery proximally and distally with two fingers, or trap the artery between two fingers placed on either side of the vessel. Hyperextension of the joint brings the radial and brachial arteries closer to the surface.

5. Prep the area with either a povidone-iodine solution or alcohol swab.

6. Hold the syringe like a pencil with the needle bevel up, and enter the skin at a 60–90-degree angle. Often you can feel the arterial pulsations as you approach the artery.

7. Maintaining a slight negative pressure on the syringe, obtain blood on the downstroke or on slow withdrawal (after both sides of the artery have been punctured). Aspirate very slowly. A good arterial sample requires only minimal back pressure. If a glass syringe or special blood-gas syringe is used, the barrel usually fills spontaneously and it is not necessary to pull on the plunger.

8. If the vessel is not encountered, withdraw the needle without coming out of the skin, and redirect.

9. After obtaining the sample, withdraw the needle quickly and apply **firm** pressure at the site for **at least 5 min** (longer if the patient is receiving anti-

coagulants. Apply pressure even if a sample was not obtained in order to prevent a compartment syndrome from extravasated blood. Activate needle reshielding mechanism.

10. If the sample is for a blood-gas determination, expel any air from the syringe, mix the contents thoroughly by twirling the syringe between your fingers, remove and dispose of the needle assembly, and make the syringe airtight with a cap. Place the syringe in an ice bath if more than a few minutes will elapse before the sample is processed. Note the inspired oxygen concentration and time of day on the lab slip.

ARTHROCENTESIS (DIAGNOSTIC AND THERAPEUTIC)
Indications

- **Diagnostic.** Evaluate new-onset arthritis; to rule out infection in an acute or chronic, unremitting joint effusion.
- **Therapeutic.** Instill steroids, maintain drainage of septic arthritis; relief of tense hemarthrosis or effusion

Contraindications

Cellulitis at injection site. Relative contraindication: bleeding disorder; caution if coagulopathy or thrombocytopenia is present or if the patient is receiving anticoagulants.

Materials

- Minor procedure tray (page 245). 18- or 20-gauge needle (smaller for finger or toe)
- Ethyl chloride spray can be substituted for lidocaine.
- Two heparinized tubes for cell count and crystal examination
- Note microbiology lab preference for transporting fluid for bacterial, fungal, AFB culture, and Gram's stain; Thayer–Martin plate used for *Neisseria gonorrhoeae* (GC)
- A syringe containing a long-acting corticosteroid such as methylprednisolone (Depo-Medrol) or triamcinolone (see Chapter 22) optional for therapeutic arthrocentesis.

13

Procedures, General

1. Obtain consent after describing the procedure and complications.
2. Determine the optimal site for aspiration (see next section), identify landmarks, and mark site with indentation or sterile marking pen. Avoid injecting into tendons.
3. If aspiration is followed by corticosteroid injection, maintaining a sterile field with sterile implements minimizes infection.
4. Clean the area with povidone-iodine, dry and wipe over the aspiration site with alcohol. Povidone-iodine can render cultures negative. Let the alcohol dry before beginning procedure.
5. Anesthetize the puncture site with lidocaine using a 25-gauge needle; do **not** inject into the joint space; lidocaine is bactericidal. Avoid lidocaine preparations w/epinephrine, especially in a digit. Alternatively, spray the area with ethyl chloride ("freeze spray") just prior to needle aspiration.

6. Insert the aspirating needle, applying a small amount of vacuum to the syringe. When the capsule is entered, fluid usually flows easily. Remove as much fluid as possible, repositioning the syringe if necessary.

7. If corticosteroid is to be injected, remove the aspirating syringe from the needle, which is still in the joint space. (*Note:* Ensure that the syringe can easily be removed from the needle before step 6). Attach the syringe containing corticosteroid, pull back on the plunger to ensure you are not in a vein, and inject contents. Never inject steroids when there is any possibility of an infected joint. Remove the needle, and apply pressure to the area (leakage of SQ steroids can lead to localized atrophy of the skin). Generally, the equivalent of 40 mg of methylprednisolone is injected into large joints such as the knee and 20 mg into medium-size joints such as the ankle or wrist. Warn the patient that a postinjection "flare" (pain several hours later) is treated with ice and NSAIDs.

8. Note volume aspirated from joint. The knee typically contains 3.5 mL of synovial fluid; in inflammatory, septic, or hemorrhagic arthritis, volumes can be higher. A bedside test for viscosity is to allow a drop of fluid to fall from the tip of the needle. Normal synovial fluid is highly viscous and forms a several-inch-long string; decreased viscosity is seen in infection. A **mucin clot test** (normally forms in < 1 min; delayed result suggests inflammation) once a standard test for RA, is not now routinely performed.

9. Joint fluid is usually sent for:

   - Cell count and diff (purple or green top tube)
   - Microscopic crystal exam using polarized light microscopy (purple or green top tube); **normally** no debris, crystals, or bacteria; urate crystals present with gout; calcium pyrophosphate in pseudo-gout.
   - Glucose (red top tube) (Table 13–2 page 253)
   - Gram's stain, and cultures for bacteria, fungi, and AFB as indicated (check with your lab or deliver immediately in a sterile tube with no additives.)
   - Cytology if a malignant effusion is suspected clinically

Arthrocentesis of the Knee

1. Fully extend the knee with the patient supine. Wait until the patient has a relaxed quadriceps muscle because its contraction approximates the patella against the femur, making aspiration painful.

2. Insert the needle posterior to the *lateral* portion of the patella into the patellar–femoral groove. Direct the advancing needle slightly posteriorly and inferiorly (Figure 13–3 page 254)

Arthrocentesis of the Wrist

1. The easiest site for aspiration is between the navicular bone and radius on the dorsal wrist. Locate the distal radius between the tendons of the extensor pollicis longus and the extensor carpi radialis longus to the second finger. This site is just ulnar to the anatomic snuff box. Direct the needle perpendicular to the mark (Figure 13–4 page 255).

Arthrocentesis of the Ankle

1. The most accessible site is between the tibia and the talus. Position the angle of the foot to leg at 90 degrees. Make a mark lateral and anterior to

TABLE 13–2
Synovial Fluid Analysis and Categories for Differential Diagnosis[a]

Parameter	Normal	Noninflammatory	Inflammatory	Septic	Hemorrhagic
Viscosity	High	High	Decreased	Decreased	Variable
Clarity	Transparent	Transparent	Translucent-opaque	Opaque	Cloudy
Color	Clear	Yellow	Yellow to opalescent	Yellow to green	Pink to red
WBC (per μL)	<200	<3000	3000–50,000	>50,000[b]	Usually <2000
Polymorphonuclear leukocytes (%)	<25%	<25%	50% or more	75% or more	30%
Culture	Negative	Negative	Negative	Usually positive	Negative
Glucose (mg/dl)	Approx. serum	Approx. serum	>25, but <serum	<25, «serum	>25

[a]See page 252 for additional information.
[b]May be lower if antibiotics initiated.
WBC = white blood cells.

13

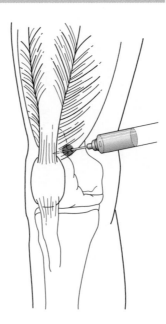

FIGURE 13–3.   Arthrocentesis of the knee. (Reprinted, with permission, from: *Internal Medicine on Call*, 3rd ed. Haist SA, Robbins JB [eds]. McGraw-Hill, New York, 2001.)

the medial malleolus and medial and posterior to the tibialis anterior tendon. Direct the advancing needle posteriorly toward the heel (Figure 13–5, page 256).

2. The **subtalar ankle joint** does not communicate with the ankle joint and is difficult to aspirate even by an expert. Be aware that "ankle pain" may originate in the subtalar joint rather than in the ankle.

Synovial Fluid Interpretation

Normal synovial fluid values and values in disease states are found in Table 13–2, page 253.

Noninflammatory Arthritis: Osteoarthritis, traumatic, aseptic necrosis, osteochondritis desiccans

Inflammatory Arthritis: Gout (usually associated with elevated serum uric acid), pseudo-gout, RA, rheumatic fever, collagen-vascular disease

Septic Arthritis: Pyogenic bacterial (*S. aureus,* GC and *S. epidermidis* most common), TB

Hemorrhagic: Hemophilia or other bleeding diathesis, trauma, with or without fracture

Complications

Infection, bleeding, pain. Postinjection flare of joint pain and swelling can occur after steroid injection and may persist for up to 24 h. This complication is felt to

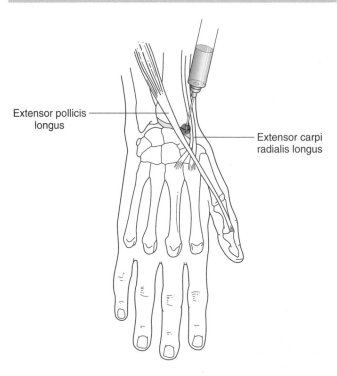

Extensor pollicis longus

Extensor carpi radialis longus

FIGURE 13–4. Arthrocentesis of the wrist. (Reprinted, with permission, from: *Internal Medicine on Call*, 3rd ed. Haist SA, Robbins JB [eds]. McGraw-Hill, New York, 2001.)

be a crystal-induced synovitis due to the crystalline suspension used in long-acting steroids.

BONE MARROW ASPIRATION AND BIOPSY
Indications

- Evaluation of unexplained anemia, thrombocytopenia, leukopenia
- Evaluation of unexplained leukocytosis, thrombocytosis, search for malignancy primary to the marrow (leukemia, myeloma) or metastatic to the marrow (small-cell lung cancer, breast cancer)
- Evaluation of iron stores; evaluation of possible disseminated infection (tuberculosis, fungal disease)
- Bone marrow donor harvesting (aspiration)

Contraindications

- Infection, osteomyelitis near the puncture site
- Relative contraindications include severe coagulopathy or thrombocytopenia (may be corrected by platelet transfusion); prior radiation to the region

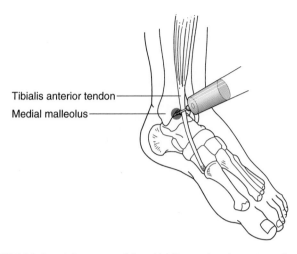

Tibialis anterior tendon
Medial malleolus

FIGURE 13–5.   Arthrocentesis of the ankle. (Reprinted, with permission, from: *Internal Medicine on Call,* 3rd ed. Haist SA, Robbins JB [eds]. McGraw-Hill, New York, 2001.)

Materials

Commercial kits are usually available that contain all the materials necessary. A technician from the hematology lab or BMT facility is necessary to ensure delivery and processing of specimens.

Procedure

1. Explain the procedure to the patient and/or the legally responsible surrogate in detail, and obtain informed consent.
2. Usually local anesthesia is all that is required; however, in extremely anxious patients, premedication with an anxiolytic or sedative such as diazepam (Valium) or midazolam (Versed) or an analgesic is reasonable.
3. Bone marrow can be obtained from numerous sites: sternum, the anterior or posterior iliac crest. The posterior iliac crest is the safest and the site of choice (described here). Position the patient on either the abdomen or on the side opposite the side from which the biopsy specimen is to be taken.
4. Identify the posterior iliac crest by palpation and mark the desired biopsy site with indelible ink.
5. Use sterile gloves, mask, and gowns, and follow strict aseptic technique.
6. Prep the site with povidone-iodine solution and allow to dry. Wipe the site free of povidone-iodine using alcohol. Drape the surrounding areas.
7. Use 1% lidocaine intradermally to raise a skin wheal with a 25–26-gauge needle; then use a 22-gauge needle to infiltrate the deeper tissues until the periosteum is reached. Advance the needle just through the periosteum and infiltrate lidocaine subperiosteally. Infiltrate an area approximately 2 cm in diameter, using repeated periosteal punctures.
8. Use a #11 scalpel blade to make a 2–3-mm skin incision over the biopsy site.

9. Insert the bone marrow biopsy needle through the skin incision and advance with a rotating motion and gentle pressure until the periosteum is reached. Once it is firmly seated on the periosteum, advance the needle through the outer table of bone into the marrow cavity with the same rotating motion and gentle pressure. Generally, a slight change in the resistance to needle advancement signals entry into the marrow cavity. At this point, advance the needle 2–3 mm.

10. Remove the stylet from the biopsy needle, and attach a 10-mL syringe to the hub of the biopsy needle. Withdraw the plunger on the syringe briskly, and aspirate 1–2 mL of marrow into the syringe. This may cause severe, instantaneous pain, but slow withdrawal of the plunger or collection of more than 1–2 mL of marrow with each aspiration results in excessive contamination of the specimen with peripheral blood.

11. The specimen can be used to prepare coverslips for viewing under the microscope or sent for special studies (cytogenetics, cell markers, culture). Repeat aspirations may be required to obtain enough marrow for all studies needed. Certain studies may require heparin or EDTA for collection. Contact lab prior to the procedure to confirm specimen collection procedures.

12. For biopsy, replace the stylet and withdraw the needle. Reinsert the needle at a slightly different angle and location (within the area of periosteum anesthetized). Once the marrow cavity has been reentered, remove the stylet and advance 5–10 mm, using the same rotating motion with gentle pressure. Withdraw the needle several millimeters (but not outside the marrow cavity), and redirect at a slightly different angle and advance again; repeating several times results in 2–3 cm of core material entering the needle. Rotate the needle rapidly on its long axis in a clockwise and then a counterclockwise manner to sever the specimen from the marrow cavity. Withdraw the needle completely without replacing the stylet. Some physicians prefer to hold their thumb over the open end of the needle to create a negative pressure in the needle as it is withdrawn; may help prevent loss of the biopsy specimen.

13. Remove the sample by inserting a probe (provided with the biopsy needle) into the distal end of the needle and gently push the specimen the full length of the needle and **out the hub end.** Attempting to push the specimen out the distal end may damage the specimen. Most biopsy needles are tapered at the distal end, presumably allowing the specimen to expand once in the needle and preventing it from being lost when the needle is withdrawn from the patient.

14. The core biopsy specimen is usually placed in formalin. (Confirm with lab before procedure.)

15. Observe for excess bleeding and apply local pressure for several minutes. Clean the area with alcohol and apply an adhesive bandage or gauze patch. Recommend (not required unless coagulopathic) that patient assume a supine position and place a pressure pack between the bed or examining table and the biopsy site to apply pressure for 10–15 min. A patient who is stable at this point may resume normal activities.

13

Complications

Local bleeding and hematoma, retroperitoneal hematoma, pain, bone fracture, infection

CENTRAL VENOUS CATHETERIZATION

Indications

- Administration of fluids and medications (peripheral access preferred)
- Administration of hyperalimentation solutions or other hypertonic fluids (eg, amphotericin B) that damage peripheral veins
- Measurement of CVP (See Chapter 20, page 413)
- Acute dialysis or plasmapheresis (Shiley catheter)
- Insertion of a pulmonary artery catheter or transvenous pacemaker

Contraindications

- Coagulopathy dictates the use of the femoral or median basilic vein approach to minimize complications.

Background

A central venous catheter (or **"deep line"**) is a catheter introduced into the superior or inferior vena cava or one of their main branches. One technique (**Seldinger technique**) involves puncturing the vein with a small needle through which a thin guidewire is placed. The needle is withdrawn, and the intravascular appliance or a sheath through which a smaller catheter will be placed is introduced into the vein over the guidewire. Another technique involves puncturing the vein with a larger bore needle through which the intravascular catheter will fit. This section focuses on the more common Seldinger technique and placement of either a triple-lumen catheter or a sheath through which a smaller catheter (eg, a pulmonary artery catheter) can be placed. The internal jugular and subclavian approaches are commonly used; the femoral approach, although infrequently utilized, offers several advantages (see section on Femoral Vein Approach). The PICC line is designed for more long-term outpatient administration of medications and is described on page 301.

13

Materials

Commercially, trays provide all the necessary needles, wires, sheaths, dilators, suture materials, and anesthetics. If needles, guidewires, and sheaths are collected from different places, it is very important to make sure that the needle will accept the guidewire, that the sheath and dilator will pass over the guidewire, and that the appliance to be passed through the sheath will indeed fit the inside lumen of the sheath. Supplies should include the following items:

- Minor procedure and instrument tray (page 245); 1% lidocaine (mixed 1:1 with sodium bicarbonate 1 mEq/L removes the sting)
- Guidewire (usually 0.035 floppy-tipped J wire)
- Vessel dilator
- Intravascular appliance (triple-lumen catheter or a sheath through which a pulmonary artery catheter could be placed)
- Heparinized flush solution 1 mL of 1:100 U heparin in 10 mL of NS (to fill lumens prior to placement to prevent clotting during placement)
- Mask, sterile gown, gloves

Subclavian Approach (Left or Right)

The left subclavian approach affords a gentle, sweeping curve to the apex of the right ventricle (preferred site for temporary transvenous pacemaker without fluoroscopy). Hemodynamic measurements are easier from the left subclavian approach; catheters do not have to negotiate an acute angle, as is the case at the junction of the right subclavian with the right brachiocephalic vein en route to the superior vena cava. This is a common site for kinking of the line. This site has the lowest risk of infection. *Caution:* The thoracic duct is on the left side, and the dome of the pleura rises higher on the left.

Procedure

1. Use sterile technique (povidone-iodine prep, gloves, mask, and a sterile field).
2. Place the patient flat or head down (Trendelenburg position) with the head in the center or turned to the opposite side. (*Note:* The "ideal" position is controversial and based on operator preference). Placing a towel roll along the patient's spine may help.
3. Use a 25-gauge needle to make a small skin wheal 2 cm below the midclavicle with 1% lidocaine. Next, a larger needle (eg, 22-gauge) is used to anesthetize the deeper tissues as well as locate the vein.
4. Attach a large-bore, deep-line needle (a 14-gauge needle with a 16-gauge catheter at least 8–12 in. long) to a 10–20 mL syringe, and introduce it into the site of the skin wheal.
5. Advance the needle under the clavicle, aiming for a location halfway between the suprasternal notch and the base of the thyroid cartilage. The vein is encountered under the clavicle, just medial to the lateral border of the clavicular head of the sternocleidomastoid muscle. In most patients this is roughly two finger-breadths lateral to the sternal notch. Apply gentle pressure on the needle at the skin entrance site to assist in lowering the needle under the clavicle (Figure 13–6).
6. Apply back pressure as the needle is advanced deep to the clavicle, but above the first rib, and watch for a "flash" of blood.
7. Free return of blood indicates entry into the subclavian vein. Remember that occasionally the vein is punctured through *both* walls, and a flash of blood may not appear as the needle is advanced. Therefore, if a free return of blood does not occur on needle advancement, withdraw the needle slowly with intermittent pressure. A free return of blood heralds the entry of the end of the needle into the lumen. Bright red blood that forcibly enters the syringe indicates that the subclavian artery has been entered. If the arterial entry occurs, remove the needle. In the majority of patients, the surrounding tissue will tamponade any bleeding from the arterial puncture. *Note:* The artery is under the clavicle, holding pressure has little effect on bleeding.
8. **a.** If you are using an Intracath device, remove the syringe, place a finger over the needle hub, and advance the catheter an appropriate distance through the needle. Withdraw the needle to just outside the skin and snap the protective cap over the tip of the needle.
    b. For the Seldinger wire technique, advance the wire through the needle and withdraw the needle. The pulse or ECG should be monitored during wire passage because the wire can induce ventricular arrhythmias.

13

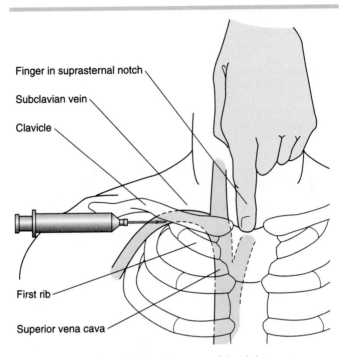

Finger in suprasternal notch

Subclavian vein

Clavicle

First rib

Superior vena cava

FIGURE 13-6. Technique for the catheterization of the subclavian vein.

13

Arrhythmias usually resolve by pulling the wire out several centimeters. Nick the skin with a No. 11 blade, and advance the dilator approximately 5 cm; remove the dilator and advance the catheter in over
the guidewire (use the brown port on the triple-lumen catheter). While
advancing either the dilator or the catheter over the wire, periodically
ensure that the wire moves freely in and out. When placing a Cordis
(multiport catheter sheath) system, advance the catheter and dilator
over the guidewire as one unit. (See Chapter 20 Pulmonary Artery
Catheter Insertion, page 418). If the wire does not move freely, it usually is kinked, and the catheter or dilator should be removed and repositioned. Maintain a grip on the guidewire at all times. Remove the
wire and attach the IV tubing. Note that the wire used to insert a single-lumen catheter is shorter than the wire supplied with the triple-
lumen catheter. This is critical when exchanging a triple-lumen for a
single-lumen catheter; use the longer triple-lumen wire and insert the
wire into the brown port. Place Shiley (hemodialysis) catheters using
the Seldinger wire technique.

9. Attach the catheter to the appropriate IV solution, and place the IV bottle
below the level of the deep-line site to ensure a good backflow of blood
into the tubing. If no backflow occurs, the catheter may be kinked or not in
the proper position.

10. Securely suture the assembly in place with 2-0 or 3-0 silk. Apply an occlusive dressing with povidone-iodine ointment.

11. Obtain a CXR immediately to verify location of the catheter tip and to R/O pneumothorax. Ideally, the catheter tip lies in the superior vena cava at its junction with the right atrium (about the 5th thoracic vertebra). Malpositioned catheters into the neck veins may only be used only for saline infusion and not for monitoring or TPN infusion.

12. Catheters that cannot be manipulated at the bedside into the chest can usually be positioned properly during the interventional radiology with fluoroscopy.

Right Internal Jugular Vein Approach

Three different sites for access to the right internal jugular vein: anterior (medial to the sternocleidomastoid muscle belly), middle (between the two heads of the sternocleidomastoid muscle belly), and posterior (lateral to the sternocleidomastoid muscle belly). The middle approach is most common and uses well-defined landmarks. The major disadvantage of the internal jugular site is patient discomfort (difficult to dress, uncomfortable when turning the head).

Procedure

1. Sterilize the site with povidone-iodine, and drape area with sterile towels. Administer local anesthesia with lidocaine in the area to be explored as noted in previous section.

2. Place the patient in the **Trendelenburg** (head down) position.

3. Use a small-bore (21-gauge) needle with syringe to locate the internal jugular vein. It may help to have a small amount of anesthetic in the syringe to inject during exploration if the patient has discomfort. Some prefer to leave this needle and syringe in the vein and place the large-bore needle directly over the smaller needle, into the vein. This is commonly called the "seeker needle" technique.

4. The internal diameter of the needle used to locate the internal jugular vein should be large enough to accommodate the passage of the guidewire (typically 22 gauge or larger).

5. Percutaneous entry should be made at the apex of the triangle formed by the two heads of the sternocleidomastoid muscle and the clavicle (Figure 13–7).

6. Direct the needle slightly lateral toward the ipsilateral nipple and enter at a 45-degree angle to the skin.

7. A notch can sometimes be palpated on the posterior surface of the clavicle; this can help locate the vein in the lateral/medial plane because the vein lies deep to this shallow notch.

8. Vein puncture is accomplished often at an unnerving depth of needle insertion and is heralded by sudden aspiration of nonpulsatile venous blood. Bedside Doppler ultrasound is available in most ORs or ICUs and can aid in localization of the internal jugular vein if the standard techniques fail.

9. Inadvertent carotid artery puncture is common if the needle is inserted medial to where it should be on the middle approach and is common with the anterior approach. With arterial puncture, the syringe fills without negative pressure because of arterial pressure, and bright red blood pulsates from the needle after the syringe is removed. In this case remove the needle and apply manual pressure for 10–15 min.

10. Follow steps 8–12 as for subclavian line (page 259) to confirm position and end procedure.

13

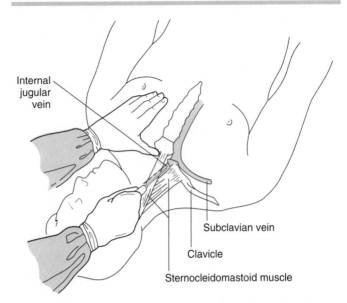

FIGURE 13-7. Technique for the catheterization of the right internal jugular vein.

Complications

Overall, a safe procedure when the small-bore needle is used to identify the vein.

- Pneumothorax may be detected when a sudden gush of air is aspirated instead of blood. A postprocedure CXR is always done to R/O pneumothorax and check line placement. Pneumothorax requires chest tube placement in virtually all cases, especially when the patient is on a ventilator or is a trauma patient. The left-sided approach is associated with higher pneumothorax risk (higher dome of the left pleura).
- Perforation of ET cuffs
- Hemothorax (vascular injury) or hydrothorax (administration of IV fluids into the pleural space)
- **Deep vein thrombosis:** Greatest risk factor for an upper extremity DVT is a history of or the presence of a subclavian or an internal jugular deep line.
- **Catheter tip embolus: Never** withdraw the catheter through the needle (can shear off the tip).
- **Air embolus: Always** keep the open end of a deep line covered with a finger. As little as 50–100 mL of air in a vein may be fatal. For suspected **air embolization, place the patient's head down and turn on left side to keep the air in the right atrium.** A STAT portable chest film will determine if air is present in the heart.

Left Internal Jugular Vein Approach

This approach is not commonly used for central lines. Better options exist and should be tried before using this approach. The procedure is similar to right internal jugular vein approach. In addition to the usual complications, this approach has unique complications, including inadvertent left brachiocephalic vein and superior vena cava puncture with intravascular wires, catheters, and sheaths and laceration of the thoracic duct with chylothorax.

External Jugular Vein Approach

This is a safe approach to central venous catheterization but technically demanding due to difficulty threading the catheter into the central venous system. This is an uncomfortable site for the patient because the dressing and IV tubing is on the neck. If the central venous system cannot be entered, this is also a site of last resort for placing a standard IV catheter ("peripheral") for the administration of routine nonsclerosing IV fluids. The external jugular vein is usually visible with the patient in the 30-degree Trendelenburg position. The vein, located in the SQ tissues, crosses the sternocleidomastoid muscle arising from just behind the angle of the jaw inferiorly where it drains into the subclavian vein just lateral to the inferior aspect of the sternocleidomastoid muscle.

Procedure

1. Place the patient in the Trendelenburg position with the head turned away from the side of insertion. Prep and drape the neck from the ear to the subclavicular area.
2. Have the patient perform the Valsalva maneuver or gently occlude the vein near its insertion into the subclavian vein to help engorge the vein.
3. At the midpoint of the vein, make a skin wheal with a 25-gauge needle and lidocaine solution. Use a 21-gauge needle to anesthetize the deeper SQ tissue and to locate the vein.
4. Remove the syringe from the needle and insert a floppy-tipped J wire into the needle. Use the guidewire with gentle pressure to negotiate the turns into the intrathoracic portion of the venous system. With difficult wire passage, have the patient turn the head slightly to help direct the wire. **Never forcibly push the wire.** As a last resort, fluoroscopy can be used to direct the wire into the superior vena cava.
5. Once a sufficient length of guidewire is passed, remove the needle.
6. Nick the skin with a No. 11 blade to accommodate the catheter; the catheter is advanced over the guidewire and the guidewire removed. Aspirate blood from the end of the catheter to confirm venous placement.
7. Follow steps 8–12 as for placement via the subclavian vein (page 259).

Complications

See Right Internal Jugular Vein Approach, page 261.

Femoral Vein Approach

This approach is safe (arterial and venous sites are easily compressible), and pneumothorax is not possible. Placement can be accomplished without interrupting cardiopulmonary resuscitation. This site can be used to place a variety of intravascular appliances, including temporary pacemakers, pulmonary artery catheters (expertise with fluoroscopy may be needed), and triple-lumen catheters. The major disadvantages are the high risk of sepsis, the immobilization it causes, and the need for fluoroscopy to ensure proper placement of pulmonary artery catheters or transvenous pacemakers.

13

Procedure

1. Place the patient in the supine position.
2. Use sterile preparation and appropriate draping. Administer local anesthesia in the area to be explored.
3. Palpate the femoral artery. Use the NAVEL technique to locate the vein (see page 250).
4. Guard the artery with the fingers of one hand.
5. Explore for the vein just medial to the operator's fingers with a needle and syringe as described previously.
6. It may be helpful to have a small amount of anesthetic in the syringe to inject with exploration.
7. Direct the needle cephalad at about a 30-degree angle and insert below the femoral crease.
8. Puncture is heralded by the return of venous, nonpulsatile blood on application of negative pressure to the syringe.
9. Advance the guidewire through the needle.
10. The guidewire should pass with ease into the vein to a depth at which the distal tip of the guidewire is always under the operator's control even when the sheath/dilator or catheter is placed over the guidewire.
11. Remove the needle once the guidewire has advanced into the femoral vein.
12. With catheter size > Fr 6, a skin incision with a No. 11 scalpel blade and the use of a vessel dilator are generally needed. The catheter can then be advanced along with the guidewire in unison into the femoral vein. Be sure always to control the distal end of the guidewire.
13. Follow steps 8–12 as for the subclavian line.

Complications

- The femoral site has the highest risk of contamination and sepsis. If an occlusive dressing can remain in place and remain free from contamination, this is a safe option.
- DVT has occurred following femoral vein catheterization. The risk for DVT increases if the catheter remains in place for prolonged periods.
- Uncontrolled retroperitoneal bleeding can occur if the iliac/common femoral artery is inadvertently punctured above the inguinal ligament.

Removal of a Central Venous Catheter (any site)

1. Turn off the IV flow.
2. Cut the retention sutures, and gently withdraw the catheter. Visually inspect the catheter to ensure it is intact.
3. Apply pressure for at least 2–3 min, and apply a sterile dressing.

CHEST TUBE PLACEMENT (CLOSED THORACOSTOMY, TUBE THORACOSTOMY)

Indications

- Pneumothorax (simple or tension)
- Hemothorax, hydrothorax, chylothorax, or empyema evacuation
- Pleurodesis for chronic recurring pneumothorax or effusion that is refractory to standard management (eg, malignant effusion)

Materials

- Chest tube (Adult: 22–24 Fr for pneumothorax, 32–38 Fr for hemothorax or pleural effusion; Newborn: 12–18 Fr, 1–2 y 14–24 Fr, 5 y 20–32, > 5 y as for adult)
- Water-seal drainage system (Pleur-Evac, etc) with connecting tubing to wall suction
- Minor procedure tray and instrument tray (see page 245)
- Silk or nylon suture (0 to 2-0)
- Petrolatum gauze (Vaseline) (optional)
- 4 × 4 gauze dressing and cloth tape
- Pulse oximeter monitoring (recommended)

Background

A chest tube is usually placed to treat an ongoing intrathoracic process that cannot be managed by simple thoracentesis (page 310). The traditional methods of chest tube placement are described. Percutaneous tube thoracostomy kits are also available based on the Seldinger technique (used for small pneumothoraces when there is no risk of ongoing air leak), but is contraindicated in significant conditions (empyema, major pneumothorax > 20%, tension pneumothorax, chronic effusion).

Procedure

> **If a patient manifests signs of a tension pneumothorax (acute shortness of breath, hypotension, distended neck veins, tachypnea, tracheal deviation) before a chest tube is placed, urgent treatment is needed. Insert a 14-gauge needle into the chest in the 2nd ICS in the midclavicular line to rapidly decompress the tension pneumothorax and proceed with chest tube insertion.**

13

1. Prior to placing the tube, review the CXR unless an emergency does not allow enough time. For a pneumothorax, choose a high anterior site (2nd, 3rd ICS, midclavicular line, or subaxillary position). Subaxillary placement is most cosmetic. Place a low lateral chest tube in the 5th or 6th ICS in the midaxillary line and direct posteriorly for fluid removal (usually corresponds to the inframammary crease.) In traumatic pneumothorax, use a low lateral site because it is usually associated with bleeding. Rarely, a loculated apical pneumothorax or effusion may require placement of an anterior tube in the 2nd ICS at the midclavicular line.

2. Choose the appropriate chest tube. Use a 24–28 Fr tube for pneumothorax and 36 Fr for fluid removal. A "**thoracic catheter**" has multiple holes and works best for nearly all purposes.

3. Prep the area with povidone-iodine solution and drape it with sterile towels. Use lidocaine (with or without epinephrine) to anesthetize the skin, intercostal muscle, and periosteum of the rib; start at the center of the rib and gently work over the top. Remember, the neurovascular bundle runs under the rib (Figure 13–8). The needle then can be gently "popped" through the pleura, and the aspiration of air or fluid confirms the correct location for the chest tube. If the procedure is elective, the patient is extremely anxious, and the patient's respiratory status is not compromised, sedation **occasionally** may be helpful.

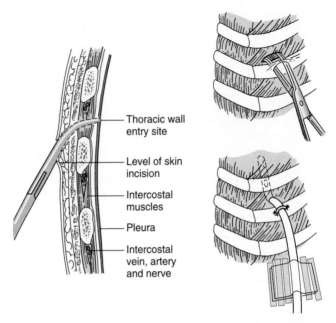

- Thoracic wall entry site
- Level of skin incision
- Intercostal muscles
- Pleura
- Intercostal vein, artery and nerve

FIGURE 13–8. Chest tube technique demonstrating the procedure for creating a subcutaneous tunnel. The skin incision is lower than the thoracic wall entry site. (Reprinted, with permission, from: Gomella TL [ed] *Neonatology: Basic Management, On-Call Problems, Diseases, Drugs,* 5th ed. McGraw-Hill, 2004.)

13

4. Make a 2–3-cm transverse incision over the center of the rib with a No. 15 or 11 scalpel blade. Use a blunt-tipped clamp to dissect over the top of the rib and create a SQ tunnel (see Figure 13–8).
5. Puncture the parietal pleura with the hemostat, and spread the opening. **Be careful not to injure the lung parenchyma with the hemostat tips.** Insert a gloved finger into the pleural cavity to gently clear any clots or adhesions and to make certain the lung is not accidentally punctured by the tube.
6. Carefully insert the tube into the desired position with a hemostat or gloved finger as a guide. Make sure all the holes in the tube are in the chest cavity. Attach the end of the tube to a water-seal or Pleur-Evac suction system. Some chest tubes are provided with sharp trocars that are used to pierce the chest wall and place the chest tube simultaneously with minimal amounts of dissection. These instruments are extremely dangerous and are usually placed in the anterior high position (ie, 2nd, 3rd, or 4th ICS).
7. Suture the tube in place. Place a heavy silk (0 or 2-0) suture through the incision next to the tube. Tie the incision together, then tie the ends around the chest tube. Make sure to wrap the suture around the tube several times. Alternatively, a purse string suture (or "U stitch") can be placed around the insertion site. Make sure all of the suction holes are in the chest cavity before the tube is secured.

8. Cover the insertion site with plain gauze. Make the dressing as airtight as possible with tape, and secure all connections in the tubing to prevent accidental loss of the water seal. Some physicians still wrap the insertion site with petroleum (Vaseline or Xeroform) gauze; however, these materials can be problematic (not water-soluble and act as foreign bodies), inhibit wound healing, and may not actually seal the site.

9. Start suction (usually –20 cm in adults, –16 cm in children) and take a portable CXR immediately to check the placement of the tube and to evaluate for residual pneumothorax or fluid.

Chest Tube Removal

1. Verify the pneumothorax or hemothorax is cleared. Check for an air leak by having the patient cough; observe the water-seal system for bubbling that indicates either a system (tubing) leak or persistent pleural air leak.

2. Take the tube off suction **but not off water seal,** and cut the retention suture. Have the patient inspire deeply and perform the Valsalva maneuver while you apply pressure with petrolatum gauze or with a sufficient amount of antibiotic ointment on 4 × 4 gauze with additional 4 × 4 gauze squares. Pull the tube rapidly while the patient performs the Valsalva maneuver and make an airtight seal with tape. Check an "upright" exhalation CXR film for pneumothorax.

Pleurodesis

1. This is performed in the setting or recurrent pneumothorax or in recurrent malignant effusion with the goal to obliterate pleural space. It is an uncomfortable procedure, and sedation with a short-acting narcotic is recommended. Sclerosing agents used include tetracycline (1 g in 100 mL NS), talc (2 g/100 mL NS), and bleomycin 60 U/100 mL NS)

2. After the chest tube is placed, 20–40 mL 1% lidocaine is injected into the tube and allowed to enter the pleural space. The tube is clamped, and the patient is moved through various positions (Trendelenburg, reverse Trendelenburg, right and left lateral decubitus positions) to allow the lidocaine to disperse.

3. Connect the syringe containing the sclerosing agent to the chest tube and release the clamp. Inject the agent and clamp the tube. Repeat the repositioning of the patient as before.

4. The tube is unclamped and connected to the Pleur-Evac device for 24–48 additional hours and then removed.

Complications

Infection, bleeding, lung damage, SQ emphysema, persistent pneumothorax/hemothorax, poor tube placement, cardiac arrhythmia

CRICOTHYROTOMY (NEEDLE AND SURGICAL)
Background

Cricothyrotomy is a emergency procedure that should be performed when obtaining an airway using endotracheal or orotracheal intubation is impossible.

Indications

- When immediate mechanical ventilation is indicated, but an endotracheal or orotracheal tube cannot be placed (eg, severe maxillofacial trauma, excessive oropharyngeal hemorrhage)

Contraindications

- Surgical cricothyrotomy is contraindicated in children < 12 y; use needle approach.

Basic Materials

- Oxygen connecting tubing, high-flow oxygen source (tank or wall)
- Bag ventilator

Needle Cricothyrotomy

- 12–14-gauge catheter-over-needle (Angiocath or other)
- 6–12-mL syringe
- 3-mm pediatric endotracheal tube adapter

Surgical Cricothyrotomy (minimum requirements)

- Minor procedure and instrument tray (page 245) plus tracheal spreader if available
- No. 5–7 tracheostomy tube (6–8 Fr endotracheal tube can be substituted)
- Tracheostomy tube adapter to connect to bag-mask ventilator

Procedures

13

Needle Cricothyrotomy

1. With the patient supine, place a roll behind the shoulders to gently hyperextend the neck.
2. Palpate the cricothyroid membrane, which resembles a notch located between the caudal end of the thyroid cartilage and the cricoid cartilage. Prep the area with povidone-iodine solution. Local anesthesia can be used if the patient is awake.
3. Mount the syringe on the 12- or 14-gauge catheter-over-needle assembly, and advance through the cricothyroid membrane at a 45-degree angle, applying back pressure on the syringe until air is aspirated.
4. Advance the catheter, and remove the needle. Attach the hub to a 3-mm endotracheal tube adapter that is connected to the oxygen tubing. Allow the oxygen to flow at 15 L/min for 1–2 s on, then 4 s off by the use of a Y-connector or a hole in the side of the tubing to turn the flow on and off.
5. The needle technique is only useful for about 45 min because the exhalation of CO_2 is suboptimal.

Surgical Cricothyrotomy

1. Follow steps 1 and 2 as for needle cricothyrotomy.
2. Make a 3–4-cm vertical skin incision through the cervical fascia and strap muscles in the midline over the cricothyroid membrane. Expose the cricothyroid membrane, and make a horizontal incision. Insert the knife handle, and rotate it 90 degrees to open the hole in the membrane. Alternatively, a hemostat or tracheal spreader can be used to dilate the opening.

3. Insert a small (5–7 mm) tracheostomy tube, inflate the balloon (if present), and secure in position with the attached cotton tapes.
4. Attach to oxygen source and ventilate. Listen to the chest for symmetrical breath sounds.
5. A surgical cricothyrotomy should be replaced with a formal tracheostomy after the patient has been stabilized and generally within 24–36 h.

Complications

Bleeding, esophageal perforation, SQ emphysema, pneumomediastinum, and pneumothorax, CO_2 retention (especially with the needle procedure)

CULDOCENTESIS

Indications

- Diagnostic technique for problems of acute abdominal pain in the female
- Evaluation of female patient with signs of hypovolemia and possible intraabdominal bleeding
- Evaluation of ascites, especially in possible cases of gynecologic malignancy

Materials

- Speculum
- Antiseptic swabs
- Povidone-iodine or chlorhexidine
- 1% lidocaine
- 18–21-gauge spinal needle
- 2 (10 mL) syringes and tenaculum

13

Procedure

1. First, perform a careful pelvic exam to document uterine position and R/O pelvic mass at risk of perforation by the culdocentesis.
2. Obtain informed consent, and prep the vagina with antiseptic, such as iodine or chlorhexidine.
3. Inject 1% lidocaine submucosally in the posterior cervical fornix prior to tenaculum application using the long needle.
4. Traction is improved by application of the tenaculum to the posterior cervical lip.
5. Connect an 18–21 gauge spinal needle to a 10-mL syringe, filled with 1 mL of air.
6. As you move the needle forward through the posterior cervical fornix, apply light pressure to the syringe until the air passes. Maintain traction on the tenaculum as you advance the spinal needle to maximize the surface area of the cul-de-sac for needle entry.
7. After intraabdominal entry, ask the patient to elevate herself on elbows to permit gravity drainage into the area of needle entry. Apply negative pressure to the syringe. Slow rotation of the needle followed by slow removal may enable a pocket of fluid to be found and aspirated.
8. If first culdocentesis attempt is not successful, the procedure can be repeated with a different angle of approach.

9. Although perforation of viscus is a possibility, the complication rate has been very low. Fresh blood that clots rapidly is probably secondary to traumatic tap, and the procedure can be repeated.

10. If blood is aspirated, it should be spun for HCT and placed into an empty glass test tube to demonstrate the presence or absence of a clot. Failure of blood to clot suggests old hemorrhage.

11. If pus is aspirated, send specimens for GC, aerobic, anaerobic, *Chlamydia, Mycoplasma,* and *Ureaplasma* cultures.

12. If a malignancy is suspected, send fluid for cytologic evaluation.

Complications

Infection, hemorrhage, air embolus, perforated viscus

DOPPLER PRESSURES
Indications

- Evaluation of peripheral vascular disease (ankle-brachial or ankle-arm index)
- Routine BP measurement in infants or critically ill adults

Materials

- Doppler flow monitor
- Conductive gel (lubricant jelly can also be used)
- BP cuff

Procedure (Ankle-Brachial or Ankle-Arm Index)

13

1. Determine the BP in each arm.
2. Measure the pressures in the popliteal arteries by placing a BP cuff on the thigh. The pressures in the dorsalis pedis arteries (on the top of the foot) and the posterior tibial arteries (behind the medial malleolus) are determined with a BP cuff on the calf.
3. Apply conductive jelly and place the Doppler probe over the artery. Inflate the BP cuff until the pulsatile flow is no longer heard. Deflate the cuff until the flow returns. This is the systolic, or Doppler, pressure. *Note:* The Doppler cannot determine the diastolic pressure, and a palpable pulse need not be present to use the Doppler.
4. The **A/B,** or **AAI index** is often computed from Doppler pressure. It is equal to the pressure in the ankle (usually the posterior tibial) divided by the systolic pressure in the arm. An A/B index of > 0.9 is usually normal, and an index of < 0.5 is usually associated with significant peripheral vascular disease.

ELECTROCARDIOGRAM

Basic ECG interpretation can be found in Chapter 19, page 383.

Indications

- Evaluation of chest pain and other cardiac conditions

Materials

- ECG machine with paper and lead electrodes
- Adhesive electrode pads

Procedure

1. Most hospitals have converted to fully automated ECG machines. It is important to become acquainted with your particular machine prior to using it. The following is a general outline.
2. Start with the patient in a comfortable, recumbent position. Explain the procedure to dispel any myths. Instruct the patient to lie as still as possible to cut down on artifacts in the tracing.
3. Plug in the ECG machine and turn it on.
4. Attach the electrodes as outlined here:
   a. **Patient Cables.** The standard ECG machine has five lead wires, one for each limb and one for the chest leads. Newer machines have six precordial electrodes, which are all placed in the proper positions prior to performing the procedure. The leads may be color-coded in the following fashion:
      - RA: White—right arm
      - LA: Black—left arm
      - RL: Green—right leg
      - LL: Red—left leg
      - C: Brown—chest
   b. **Limb Electrodes.** Newer machines use self-adhering electrode pads. Older machines use flat, rectangular plates held in place by straps that encircle the limb. Place each electrode on the limb indicated, wrist or ankle, usually on the ventral surface. In case of amputation or a cast, the lead may be placed on the shoulder or groin with minimal effect on the tracing.
   c. **Chest (Precordial) Electrodes.** Newer machines allow all leads to be placed prior to running the ECG with all pads applied at the same time. This makes locating the proper positions much quicker and easier (Figure 13–9 page 272). Older units have a suction cup chest electrode that is brown and designated by the letter "C." It is attached in sequence to each of the positions on the precordium. Precordial leads are placed as follows:
      - V_1 = 4th ICS just to the **right** of the sternal border
      - V_2 = 4th ICS just to the **left** of the sternal border
      - V_3 = midway between leads V_2 and V_4
      - V_4 = midclavicular line in the 5th ICS
      - V_5 = anterior axillary line at the same level as V_4
      - V_6 = midaxillary line at the same level as leads V_4 and V_5
5. When everything is ready, follow the directions for your particular machine to obtain the ECG tracing. It should include 12 different leads, that is, I, II, III, AVR, AVL, and V_{1-6}. Standard paper speed is at 25 mm/s.
6. Label the tracing with the patient's name, date, time, and any other useful information, such as medications, and your name. A routine 12-lead ECG should take 4–8 min.

13

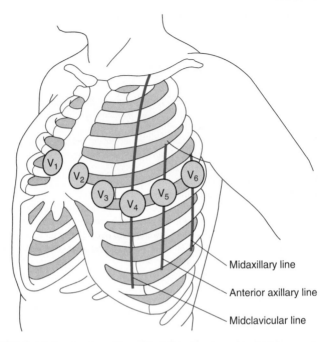

FIGURE 13–9. Location of the precordial chest leads used in obtaining a routine ECG.

13

Helpful Hints

1. The second rib inserts at the sternal angle, and therefore the second ICS is directly inferior to the sternal angle. Feel down two more ICSs and you have the fourth ICS to position V_1 and V_2.
2. Learn the color scheme for the leads; it could be very useful in an emergency. Some memory aids include
   a. Red and green go to the legs: "Christmas on the bottom" or "When driving your car you use your left leg to brake (red light) and your right leg to go (green light)."
   b. Black (left) and white (right) go to the arms: "Remember white is right and black is left."
   c. Brown is for the chest.

ENDOTRACHEAL INTUBATION

Indications

- Airway management during cardiopulmonary resuscitation
- Any indication for using mechanical ventilation (respiratory failure, coma, general anesthesia, etc)

Contraindications

- Massive maxillofacial trauma (relative)
- Fractured larynx
- Suspected cervical spinal cord injury (relative)

Materials

- Endotracheal tube of appropriate size (Table 13–3 below)
- Laryngoscope handle and blade (straight [Miller] or curved [MAC]; size No. 3 for adults, No. 1–1.5 for small children)
- 10-mL syringe, adhesive tape, benzoin
- Suction equipment (Yankauer suction)
- Malleable stylet (optional)
- Oropharyngeal airway

Procedure

1. Orotracheal intubation is most commonly used and is described here. In suspected cervical spine injury, nasotracheal intubation is preferred.
2. Any patient who is hypoxic or apneic must be ventilated prior to attempting endotracheal intubation (bag mask or mouth to mask). Avoid prolonged periods of no ventilation if the intubation is difficult. A rule of thumb is to hold your breath while attempting intubation. When you need to take a breath, so must the patient. Resume ventilation, and reattempt intubation in a minute or so.
3. Extend the laryngoscope blade to 90 degrees to verify the light is working, and check the balloon on the tube (if present) for leaks.
4. Place the patient's head in the "sniffing position" (neck extended anteriorly and the head extended posteriorly). Use suction to clear the upper airway if needed.
5. Hold the laryngoscope in the left hand, hold the mouth open with the right hand, and use the blade to push the tongue to patient's left while keeping it anterior to the blade. Advance the blade carefully toward the midline until the epiglottis is visualized. Use suction if needed.
6. If the **straight laryngoscope blade** is used, pass it under the epiglottis and **lift** upward to visualize the vocal cords (Figure 13–10, page 274). If the

TABLE 13–3
Recommended Endotracheal Tube Sizes

Patient	Internal Diameter (mm)	
Premature infant	2.5–3.0	(uncuffed)
Newborn infant	3.5	(uncuffed)
3–12 mo	4.0	(uncuffed)
1–8 y	4.0–6.0	(uncuffed)[a]
8–16 y	6.0–7.0	(cuffed)
Adult	7.0–9.0	(cuffed)

[a]Rough estimate is to measure the little finger.

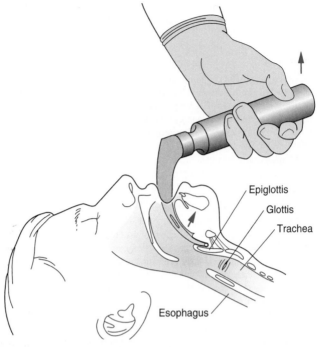

Epiglottis

Glottis

Trachea

Esophagus

FIGURE 13-10. Endotracheal intubation using a curved laryngoscope blade.

13

curved blade is used, place it anterior to the epiglottis (into the vallecula) and gently lift anteriorly. In either case, do **not** use the handle to pry the epiglottis open, but rather gently lift to expose the vocal cords.

7. While maintaining visualization of the cords, grasp the tube in your dominant hand and pass it through the cords. With more difficult intubations, the malleable stylet can be used to direct the tube.

8. In patients who may have eaten recently, gentle pressure placed over the cricoid cartilage by an assistant helps to occlude the esophagus and prevent aspiration during intubation. "Cricoid pressure" can also help visualize the vocal cords in patients whose larynx is situated more anteriorly than usual.

9. When using a cuffed tube (adult and older children), gently inflate air with a 10-mL syringe until the seal is adequate (about 5 mL). Ventilate the patient while auscultating and visualizing both sides of the chest to verify positioning. If the left side does not seem to be ventilating, it may signify that the tube has been advanced down the right mainstem bronchus. Withdraw the tube 1–2 cm, and recheck the breath sounds. Also auscultate over the stomach to ensure the tube is not mistakenly placed in the esophagus. Confirm positioning with a CXR. The tip of the endotracheal tube should be a few centimeters above the carina.

10. Tape the tube in position, and insert an oropharyngeal airway to prevent the patient from biting the tube. Consider an orogastric tube to prevent regurgitation.

Complications

Bleeding, oral or pharyngeal trauma, improper tube positioning (esophageal intubation, right mainstem bronchus), aspiration, tube obstruction or kinking

FEVER WORK-UP

Although not a standard "bedside procedure," fever work-up involves judicious use of invasive procedures. The true definition of a *fever* can vary from service to service. General guidelines to follow are a temperature > 100.4°F orally on a medical or surgical service, or a temperature ≥ 101°F rectally or 100°F orally in an infant or immunocompromised patient. When evaluating a patient for a fever, consider if the temperature is oral, rectal, tympanic, or axillary (rectal and tympanic temperatures are about 1°F higher and axillary temperatures are about 1°F lower than oral); has the patient drunk any hot or cold liquids or smoked around the time of the determination; and is the patient on any antipyretics. Also, remember the temperature is highest at about 8 PM (+ 0.5°F from 98.6°F) and lowest at about 4 AM (−1–1.5°F). Differential diagnosis of fever and fever of unknown origin are discussed in Chapter 3.

General Fever Work-Up

1. Quickly review the chart and medication record if the patient is not familiar to you.
2. Question and examine the patient to locate any obvious sources of fever.
   a. **Ears, nose, sinuses and throat:** Especially in children
   b. **Neck:** Pain with flexion
   c. **Nodes:** Adenopathy
   d. **Lungs:** Rales (crackles), rhonchi (wheezes), decreased breath sounds, or dullness to percussion. Can the patient generate an effective cough?
   e. **Heart:** A new or changing heart murmur, which may suggest endocarditis
   f. **Abdomen:** Presence or absence of bowel sounds, guarding, rigidity, tenderness, bladder fullness, or costovertebral angle tenderness
   g. **Genitourinary:** If a Foley catheter is in place, note appearance of the urine, grossly and microscopically
   h. **Rectal Exam:** Tenderness or fluctuance to suggest an abscess, or acute prostatitis
   i. **Pelvic Exam:** Especially in the postpartum patient or sexually active woman with multiple partners
   j. **Wounds:** Erythema, tenderness, swelling, or drainage from surgical sites
   k. **Extremities:** Signs of inflammation at IV sites. Look for thigh or calf tenderness and swelling.
   l. **Miscellaneous:** Consider the possibility of a drug fever (eosinophil count on the CBC may be elevated) or NG tube fever. Do all this before you begin to investigate the less common or less obvious causes of a fever.
3. **Laboratory Studies**
   a. **Basic:** CBC with diff, UA, cultures as indicated: urine, blood, sputum, wound, spinal fluid (**especially** in children less than 4–6 mon old)
   b. **Other:** Order based on clinical findings:
      (i) **Radiographic:** Chest or abdominal films, CT or ultrasound exams
      (ii) **Invasive:** LP, thoracentesis, paracentesis are more aggressive procedures that may be indicated.

13

Miscellaneous Fever Facts

1. **Causes of Fever in the Postop Patient:** Think of the "Six W's":
   a. **Wind:** Atelectasis secondary to intubation and anesthesia is the most common cause of immediate postop. To treat, have the patient sitting up and ambulating, using incentive spirometry, P&PD, etc.
   b. **Water:** UTI; may be secondary to a bladder catheter
   c. **Wound:** Infection
   d. **Walking:** Phlebitis, DVT
   e. **Wonder drugs:** Drug fever (common causes are listed on pages 38 & 39).
   f. **Woman:** Endometritis, or mastitis (common only in postpartum)
2. **Elevated White Cell Counts:** Commonly elevated secondary to catecholamine discharge after a stress such as surgery or childbirth
3. **Temperatures of 103–105°F:** In adults, think of lung or kidney infections, or bacteremia.
4. **Lethargy, Combativeness, Inappropriate Behavior:** Strongly consider doing an LP to rule out meningitis.
5. **Elderly Patients:** Can be extremely ill without many of the typical manifestations; they may be hypothermic or may deny any tenderness that could point toward any obvious source. You must be very aggressive to identify the cause.
6. **Infants and Children:** Have normally elevated baseline temperatures (up to 3 mon 99.4°F, 1 y 99.7°F, 3 y 99.0°F)

GASTROINTESTINAL INTUBATION

Indications

- GI decompression: ileus, obstruction, pancreatitis, postoperatively
- Lavage of the stomach with GI bleeding or drug overdose
- Prevention of aspiration in an obtunded patient
- Feeding a patient who is unable to swallow

Materials

- GI tube of choice (see following list)
- Lubricant jelly
- Catheter tip syringe
- Glass of water with a straw, stethoscope

Types of Gastrointestinal Tubes

1. **Nasogastric Tubes**
   a. **Levin:** A tube with a single lumen, a perforated tip, and side holes for the aspiration of gastric contents. Connect it to an intermittent suction device to prevent the stomach lining from obstructing the lumen. Sometimes it is necessary to cut off the tip to allow for the aspiration of larger pills or tablets. The size varies from 10 to 18 Fr (1 Fr unit = ⅓ mm in diameter, see pages 245 & 246).
   b. **Salem-Sump:** A double-lumen tube; the smaller tube is an air intake vent so that continuous suction can be applied. The best tube for irrigation and lavage because it will not collapse on itself. If a Salem-sump tube stops working even after it is repositioned, often a "shot" of

air from a catheter-tipped syringe in the air vent will clear the tube. Both the Salem-sump and Levin tubes have radiopaque markings.

2. **Intestinal Decompression Tubes** ("long intestinal tubes")

   a. **Cantor Tube:** A long single-lumen tube with a rubber balloon at the tip. The balloon is partially filled with mercury (5–7 mL using a tangentially directed 21-gauge needle, then the air is aspirated), which allows it to gravitate into the small bowel with the aid of peristalsis. Used for decompression when the bowel is obstructed distally.

   b. **Miller–Abbott Tube:** A long double-lumen tube with a rubber balloon at the tip. One lumen is used for aspiration; the other connects to the balloon. After the tube is in the stomach, inflate the balloon with 5–10 mL of air, inject 2–3 mL of mercury into the balloon, and then aspirate the air. Functioning and indications are essentially the same as for the Cantor tube. **Do not** tape these intestinal tubes to the patient's nose or the tube will not descend. The progress of the tube can be followed on radiography.

3. **Feeding Tubes.** Although any NG tube can be used as a feeding tube, it is preferable to place a specially designed nasoduodenal feeding tube. These are of smaller diameter (usually 8 Fr) and are more pliable and comfortable for the patient. Weighted tips tend to travel into the duodenum, which may help prevent regurgitation and aspiration. Most are supplied with stylets that facilitate positioning, especially if fluoroscopic guidance is needed. Always verify the position of the feeding tube with a radiograph prior to starting tube feeding. Commonly used tubes include the mercury-weighted varieties (**Keogh tube, Duo-Tube, Dobbhoff**), the tungsten-weighted (**Vivonex tube**), and the unweighted pediatric feeding tubes.

4. **Miscellaneous Gastrointestinal Tubes**

   a. **Sengstaken–Blakemore Tube:** A triple-lumen tube used exclusively for the control of bleeding esophageal varices by tamponade. One lumen is for gastric aspiration, one is for the gastric balloon, and the third is for the esophageal balloon. Other types include the **Linton** and **Minnesota** tubes.

   b. **Ewald Tube:** An orogastric tube used almost exclusively for gastric evacuation of blood or drug overdose. The tube is usually double lumen and large diameter (18–36 Fr).

   c. **Dennis, Baker, Leonard Tubes:** Used for intraoperative decompression of the bowel and are manually passed into the bowel at the time of laparotomy.

13

Procedure (For Nasogastric and Feeding Tubes)

1. Inform the patient of the nature of the procedure and encourage cooperation if the patient is able. Choose the nasal passage that appears most open. Have the patient sitting up if able.

2. Lubricate the distal 3–4 in. of the tube with a water-soluble jelly (K-Y Jelly or viscous lidocaine), and insert the tube gently along the floor of the nasal passageway. Maintain gentle pressure that will allow the tube to pass into the nasopharynx. Have the patient flex the neck slightly from neutral.

3. When the patient can feel the tube in the back of the throat, ask patient to swallow small amounts of water through a straw as you advance the tube 2–3 in. at a time.

4. To be sure that the tube is in the stomach, aspirate gastric contents or blow air into the tube with a catheter-tipped syringe and listen over the stomach with your stethoscope for a "pop" or "gurgle." The position of feeding tubes **must** be verified by radiography prior to institution of feedings to prevent accidental bronchial instillation of tube feedings.

5. NG tubes are attached either to low wall suction (Salem-sump type tubes with a vent) or to intermittent suction (Levin type tubes); the latter allows the tube to fall away from the gastric wall between suction cycles.

6. Feeding and pediatric feeding tubes in adults are more difficult to insert because they are more flexible. Many are provided with stylets that make their passage easier. Feeding tubes are best placed into the duodenum or jejunum in order to decrease the risk of aspiration. Administering 10 mg of metoclopramide (Reglan) IV 10 min before insertion of the tube assists in placing the tube into the duodenum. Once the feeding tube is in the stomach, the bell of the stethoscope can be placed on the right side of the patient's midabdomen. As the tube is advanced, air can be injected to confirm progression of the tube to the right, toward the duodenum. If the sound of the air becomes fainter, the tube is probably curling in the stomach. Pass the tube until a slight resistance is felt, heralding the presence of the tip of the tube at the pylorus. Holding constant pressure and slowly injecting water through the tube is often rewarded with a "give," which signifies passage through the pylorus. The tube often can be advanced far into the duodenum with this method. The duodenum usually provides constant resistance that will give with slow injection of water. Placing the patient in the right lateral decubitus position may help the tube enter the duodenum. Always confirm the location of the tube with an abdominal radiograph.

7. Tape the tube securely in place, but do not allow it to apply pressure to the ala of the nose. (*Note:* Intestinal decompression tubes should not be taped because they are allowed to pass through the intestine). Patients have been disfigured because of ischemic necrosis of the nose caused by a poorly positioned NG tube.

Complications

- Inadvertent passage into the trachea may provoke coughing or gagging in the patient.
- Aspiration
- If the patient is unable to cooperate, the tube often becomes coiled in the oral cavity.
- The tube is irritating and may cause a small amount of bleeding in the mucosa of the nose, pharynx, or stomach. The drying and irritation can be lessened by throat lozenges or antiseptic spray.
- Intracranial passage in patient with a basilar skull fracture
- Esophageal perforation
- Esophageal reflux caused by the tube-induced incompetence of the distal esophageal sphincter
- Sinusitis from edema of the nasal passages that blocks drainage from the nasal sinuses.

HEELSTICK AND FINGERSTICKS (CAPILLARY BLOOD SAMPLING)

Indication

- Used to collect blood samples from infants
- Fingerstick can also be used for small samples in older children and adults

Materials

- Alcohol swabs
- Lancet (BD Quickheel lancet, BD Genie Lancet for fingersticks that require high volume of blood). BD Genie Needle lancet for glucose determinations)
- Collection container: capillary tube, BD Microtainer tube (with Micro-Guard closure) or Caraway tubes
- Clay or other capillary tube sealer

Background

To avoid the risk of repeated venous punctures, especially in infants, assays were developed that rely on small volumes of blood. Although called "heelstick," or "fingerstick," any highly vascularized capillary bed can be used (finger pad, ear lobe, or great toe).

Heelstick Technique

1. The heel can be warmed for 5–10 min by wrapping it in a warm washcloth. Wipe the area with an alcohol swab. Use Figure 13–11A to choose the site for the puncture; these sites helps decrease risk of osteomyelitis.
2. Use a lancet, and make a quick, deep puncture so that blood flows freely (see Figure 13–11A). Automated safety lancets (BD Quick Heel Lancet in neonatal and infant sizes) for heelsticks are also available (eg, the BD Quikheel lancet) is held over the site at a 90-degree angle to the foot (Figure 13–11 B). A button activates the blade , after which the blade retracts into its casing.
3. Wipe off the first drop of blood. Gently squeeze the heel and touch a collection tube to the drop of blood. The tube should fill by capillary action and is sealed.
4. Labs can make determinations on small samples from the pediatric age group. A **Caraway tube** can hold 0.3 mL of blood. One to three Caraway tubes can be used for most routine tests. For a capillary blood gas, the blood is usually transferred to a 1-mL heparinized syringe and placed on ice. BD Microtainer tubes with Microgard closure are available in color-coded styles for specific blood determinations similar to larger Vacutainer tubes (See Table 13–8, page 317).
5. Samples should flow freely enough that the specimen can be collected in less than 2 min. Longer time periods may be affected by microclotting of the sample.
6. Wrap the site with 4×4 gauze squares, or apply an adhesive bandage.

Fingerstick Technique

1. Clean the puncture site with alcohol, and allow to air dry.
2. Remove the protective cap from the safety lancet and position over pad of finger (BD Genie lancet).

13

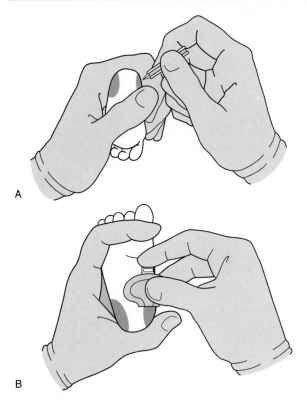

A

B

13

FIGURE 13-11. **A.** Demonstration of the preferred sites and technique of performing a heelstick in an infant. (Reprinted, with permission, from: Gomella TL [ed]
Neonatology: Basic Management, On-Call Problems, Diseases, Drugs, 5th ed.
McGraw-Hill, 2004.) **B.** The use of an automated lancet (BD Quikheel Lancet [Bec-
ton-Dickson]) for heelstick in an infant. The device is held at 90 degrees to the axis of
the foot and activated.

3. Press the white activation button with your thumb. Discard device.
4. Gently massage from base of finger to puncture site to collect sample.
    Holding hand below level of elbow will enhance blood flow. For glucose
    determinations using a device such as the Genie needle lancet, only a drop
    of blood is needed to apply to the reagent strip for glucose determination.
    A lancet style device is not necessary due to the small amount of blood
    needed.
5. Follow steps 3–6 as for heelstick.

Complications

Cellulitis at site, osteomyelitis for heelstick in infants

INTERNAL FETAL SCALP MONITORING
Indication

- To accurately assess FHR patterns during labor to screen for possible fetal distress

Contraindications

- Presence of placenta previa
- When it is otherwise impossible to identify the portion of the fetal body where application is contemplated

Materials

- Fetal scalp monitoring electrode
- Sterile vaginal lubricant or povidone-iodine spray
- Spiral electrode
- Leg plate/fetal monitor

Procedure

1. Position the patient in the dorsal lithotomy position (knees flexed and abducted), and perform an aseptic perineal prep with sterile vaginal lubricant or povidone-iodine spray.
2. Perform a manual vaginal exam, and clearly identify the fetal presenting part. The membranes **must** be ruptured prior to attachment of the spiral electrode.
3. Remove the spiral electrode from the sterile package and place the guide tube firmly against the fetal presenting part. Electrode should not be applied to fetal face, fontanels, or genitalia.
4. Advance the drive tube and electrode until the electrode contacts the presenting part. Maintaining pressure on the guide tube and drive tube, rotate the drive tube clockwise until mild resistance is met (usually one turn).
5. Press together the arms on the drive tube grip, which releases the locking device. Carefully slide the drive and guide tubes off the electrode wires while holding the locking device open.
6. Attach the spiral electrode wires to the color-coded leg plate, which is then connected to the electronic fetal monitor.

13

Complications

- Fetal or maternal hemorrhage, fetal infection (usually scalp abscess at the site of insertion)

Interpretation

- **Normal** FHR is 120–160 bpm.
- **Accelerations:** Increases in the FHR can be associated with fetal distress (usually in association with late decelerations) but are almost always a sign of fetal well-being.
- **Decelerations:** Transient falls in FHR are related to a uterine contraction and are of three types:
    1. **Early Decelerations:** Seen in normal labor, slowing of the FHR associated with the onset of the contraction and the FHR promptly returns to normal after the contraction is over. Usually caused by head compression, and occasionally by cord compression.

   2. **Late Deceleration:** Slowing of the FHR that occurs after the uterine contraction starts and the rate does not return to normal until well after the contraction is over. This type of pattern is often associated with uteroplacental insufficiency (fetal acidosis or hypoxia).

   3. **Variable Decelerations:** Irregular pattern of decelerations unassociated with contractions caused by cord compression.

- **Other Patterns:**
  1. **Beat-to-Beat Variability:** Small fluctuations in FHR 5–15 BPM over the baseline FHR usually associated with fetal well-being
  2. **Bradycardia:** Associated with maternal and fetal hypoxia, fetal heart lesions including heart block. If bradycardia persists, evaluate with scalp pH.
  3. **Tachycardia:** Often an early sign of fetal distress, seen with febrile illnesses, hypoxia, fetal thyrotoxicosis
  4. **Sinusoidal Pattern** Can be drug-induced and is seen occasionally with severe fetal anemia

INJECTION TECHNIQUES

Indications

- **Intradermal:** Most commonly used for skin testing
- **Subcutaneous:** Useful for low-volume medications such as insulin, heparin, and some vaccines
- **Intramuscular:** Administration of parenteral medications that cannot be absorbed from the SQ layer or of high volume (≤ 10 mL)

Contraindications

13

- Allergy to any components of the injectate
- Active infection or dermatitis at the injection site
- IM injections are generally contraindicated with coagulopathy

Procedures

Intradermal: (see Skin Testing, page 308)

Subcutaneous

1. Deposit the drug within the fat but above the muscle. With careful placement, nerve injury is rarely a danger.
2. Choose a site free of scarring or active infection. Injection sites include the outer surface of the upper arm, anterior surface of the thigh, and lower abdominal wall. With repeated injections (diabetics, etc) sites should be rotated.
3. 25–27 gauge ¾–1 in. needles are most commonly used; volume of medication must not exceed 5 mL. Draw up the medication, making certain to expel any air bubbles.
4. Clean site with an alcohol swab. Bunch up the skin between the thumb and forefinger so that the SQ tissue is off the underlying muscle.
5. Warn the patient that there will be "pinch" or "sting," and insert the needle firmly and rapidly at a 45-degree angle until a sudden release signifies penetration of the dermis.

6. Release the skin, and aspirate to make certain a blood vessel has not been entered and inject slowly.

7. Withdraw the needle and apply gentle pressure. Activate the automatic needle shield (eg, BD SafetyGlide shielding hypodermic needle) and discard. A dressing is not usually necessary. Apply pressure longer if there is bleeding from the site.

Intramuscular

1. Common sites include the deltoid, gluteus, and the vastus lateralis.
   - **Deltoid Muscle:** The safe zone includes only the main body of the deltoid muscle lying lateral and a few centimeters beneath the acromion. Low risk of radial nerve injury unless the needle strays into the middle or lower third of the arm.
   - **Gluteus Muscles:** This is the preferred site in children > 2 y and in adults. Draw an imaginary line from the femoral head to the posterior superior iliac spine. This site (upper outer quadrant of the buttocks) is safe for injections because it is away from the sciatic nerve and superior gluteal artery.
   - **Vastus Lateralis Muscle** (anterior thigh): A very safe site in all patients and the site of choice in infants. The only disadvantage of this site is that the firm fascia lata overlying the muscle can make needle insertion somewhat more painful.

2. A 22-gauge, 1½ in. needle is acceptable for most IM injections. Remove air bubbles from the syringe and needle. Wipe the skin with alcohol.

3. Gently stretch the skin to one side and warn the patient of a sting. Penetrate the skin at a 90-degree angle, and advance approximately 1 in. into the muscle. (Obese patients may require deeper penetration with a longer needle.)

4. Aspirate to make sure that you have not entered a vessel. Administer the medication. Gently massage the site with alcohol swab or gauze to promote absorption.

13

Complications

- Nerve and arterial injury
- Abscesses (sterile or septic). Use good technique and rotate injection sites.
- Bleeding can usually be controlled with pressure.

INTRAUTERINE PRESSURE MONITORING

Indication

- To accurately assess uterine contraction during labor

Contraindication

- Placenta previa

Materials

- Pressure catheter and introducer
- Transducer connected to fetal monitor
- Sterile gloves, vaginal lubricant, povidone-iodine spray
- 10-mL syringe, 30 mL sterile water

Procedure

1. Prime the transducer with sterile water.
2. Position the patient in the dorsal lithotomy position (knees flexed and abducted), and perform an aseptic perineal prep with sterile vaginal lubricant or povidone-iodine spray.
3. Perform a manual vaginal exam, and clearly identify the fetal presenting part. The membranes **must** be ruptured prior to insertion of catheter.
4. Remove the catheter from the sterile package, and place the guide tube through fingers around the presenting part into the uterine cavity.
5. Prime the catheter with sterile water and thread through the guide tube.
6. Attach the distal catheter to transducer and zero to air.

Complications

Infection, placental perforation if low lying

IV TECHNIQUES
Indication

- IV access for the administration of fluids, blood, or medications (Other techniques include Central Venous Catheters, page 258 and PICC lines (page 301)

Materials

- IV fluid
- Connecting tubing
- Tourniquet
- Alcohol swab
- IV cannulas (a catheter over a needle [eg, BD Insyte Autoguard shielded IV catheter, BD Angiocath Autoguard shielded IV catheter] or a butterfly style needle)
- Antiseptic ointment, dressing, and tape

Procedure

1. It helps to rip the tape into strips, attach the IV tubing to the solution, and flush the air out of the tubing before you begin.
2. The upper, nondominant extremity is the site of choice for an IV, unless the patient is being considered for placement of permanent hemodialysis access. In this instance, the upper nondominant extremity should be "saved" as the access site for hemodialysis. If the patient has previously undergone a axillary lymph node dissection (eg, some breast cancer surgeries), the IV should be started on the other side. Choose a distal vein (dorsum of the hand) so that if the vein is lost, you can reposition the IV more proximally. Figure 13–12, page 285 demonstrates some common upper extremity veins; avoid veins that cross a joint space. Also avoid the leg because of the increased risk of thrombophlebitis.
3. Apply a tourniquet above the proposed IV site. Use the techniques described in the section on venipuncture to help expose the vein (page 316). Carefully clean the site with an alcohol or povidone-iodine swab. If a large-bore IV is to be used (16 or 14), local anesthesia (lidocaine injected with a 25-gauge needle) is helpful.

13

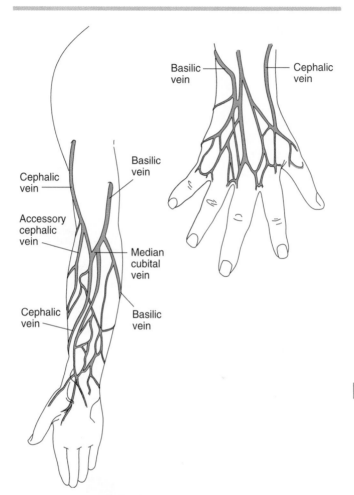

FIGURE 13-12. Principal veins of the arm used to place IV access and in venipuncture, the pattern can be highly variable. (Reprinted, with permission, from: Stillman RM [ed] *Surgery, Diagnosis, and Therapy*, Appleton & Lange, Norwalk, CT, 1989.)

4. Stabilize the vein distally with the thumb of your free hand. Using the catheter-over-needle assembly either enter the vein directly or enter the skin alongside the vein first and then stick the vein along the side at about a 20-degree angle. Direct entry and side entry IV techniques are illustrated in Figures 13–13 and 13–14. Once the vein is punctured, blood should appear in the "flash chamber." Lower the needle assembly. The next steps vary if you are using a standard catheter-over-needle device or a self-shielding device:

   a. **Standard Catheter-over-Needle** (Figure 13–13A). Advance a few more millimeters to be sure that **both** the needle **and** the tip of the catheter have entered the vein. Thread the catheter into the vein while

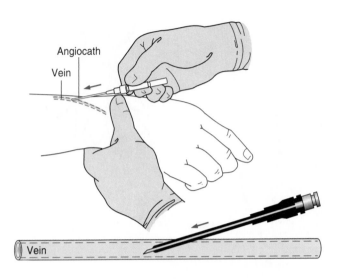

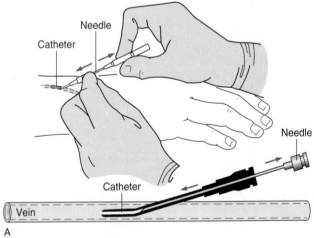

A

FIGURE 13–13A. Technique for insertion of a standard catheter-over-needle device for IV access. Stabilize the vein with gentle traction. Enter the vein; when a flash of blood is observed in the chamber, advance the entire assembly slightly to ensure that the catheter tip is in the lumen of the vein. Advance the catheter off the end of the needle, and remove the needle.

maintaining traction on the skin. Remove the tourniquet, compress the vein and stabilize the catheter hub. Connect the IV fluid.

After the flashback is seen, lower the catheter assembly to almost parallel to the skin. Advance the entire unit before attempting to thread catheter. Thread catheter into vein while maintaining traction. Next, release the tourniquet and apply pressure beyond catheter tip, making

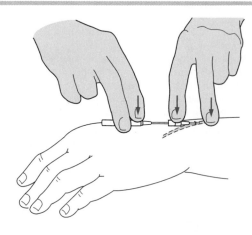

FIGURE 13–13B. When using a device such as BD Angiocath Autoguard (Becton-Dickson & Company), before pressing the autoshield button, apply digital pressure as shown to stabilize the catheter and to prevent blood from escaping after the needle is removed. Activate the self-shielding needle by pushing the white button on the needle device.

sure that digital pressure is maintained beyond the catheter tip. (Figure 13–13B). Press the white button and the needle retracts into a shield. Connect the IV line to the catheter.

5. With the IV fluid running, observe the site for signs of induration or swelling that indicate improper placement or damage to the vein. See Chapter 9 for choosing IV fluids and how to determine infusion rates.

6. Tape the IV securely in place; apply a drop of povidone-iodine or antibiotic ointment and apply a sterile dressing. Ideally, the dressing should be

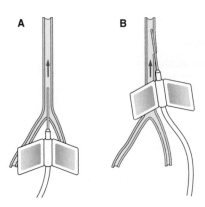

FIGURE 13–14. Example of a "butterfly" needle assembly and the two different techniques of entering a vein for intravenous access: **A** direct puncture; and **B** side entry. (Reprinted, with permission, from: Gomella TL [ed] *Neonatology: Basic Management, On-Call Problems, Diseases, Drugs,* 5th ed. McGraw-Hill, 2004.)

changed every 24–48 h to help reduce the likelihood of infection. Arm boards are also useful to help maintain an IV site.

7. **Never** reinsert the needle into the catheter because this can result in shearing the catheter.

8. **A "butterfly," or "scalp vein,"** needle can sometimes be used (see Figure 13–14). This is a small metal needle with plastic "wings" on the side. It is very useful in infants (who often have poor peripheral veins but prominent scalp veins), children, and in adults who have small, fragile veins.

9. Troubleshooting difficult IV placement

- If the veins are deep and difficult to locate, a small 3–5-mL syringe can be mounted on the catheter assembly. Proper positioning inside the vein is determined by aspiration of blood. If blood specimens are needed on a patient who also needs an IV, this technique can be used to start the IV and to collect samples at the same time.

- **Whaid's maneuver** can be attempted (*J Emerg Nurs,* 1993;19:186). Spend about 1 min using both hands to "milk" blood from the arm toward the forearm. While holding the arm compressed with both hands, place a tourniquet above the elbow. Milk the blood from the fingers to the forearm for 3–5 min. When a vein becomes prominent, wrap your hand around the patient's wrist and place the IV.

- If no extremity vein can be found, try the external jugular. Placing the patient in the head down position can help distend the vein.

- If all these fail, the next alternative is a central venous line insertion (page 258).

LUMBAR PUNCTURE

Indications

- **Diagnostic purposes:** Analysis of CSF for conditions such as meningitis, encephalitis, Guillain–Barré syndrome, staging work-up for lymphoma, others
- Measurement of CSF pressure or its changes with various maneuvers (Valsalva, etc)
- **Injection of various agents:** Contrast media for myelography, antitumor drugs, analgesics, antibiotics

Contraindications

- Increased intracranial pressure (papilledema, mass lesion)
- Infection near the puncture site
- Planned myelography or pneumoencephalography
- Coagulation disorders

Materials

- A sterile, disposable LP kit

or

- Minor procedure tray (see page 258)
- Spinal needles (21-gauge for adults, 22-gauge for children)

Background

The objective of an LP is to obtain a sample of CSF from the subarachnoid space. Specifically, during an LP the fluid is obtained from the **lumbar cistern,** the CSF located between the termination of the spinal cord (conus medullaris) and the termination of the dura mater at the coccygeal ligament. The cistern is surrounded by the subarachnoid membrane and the overlying dura. Located within the cistern are the filum terminale and the nerve roots of the cauda equina. When an LP is done, the main body of the spinal cord is avoided and the nerve roots of the cauda are simply pushed out of the way by the needle. The termination of the spinal cord in the adult is usually between L1 and L2, and in the pediatric patient between L2 and L3. The safest site for an LP is the interspace between L4 and L5. An imaginary line drawn between the iliac crests (the supracrystal plane) intersects the spine at either the L4 spinous process or the L4–L5 interspace. A spinal needle introduced between the spinous processes of L4 and L5 penetrates the layers in the following order: skin, supraspinous ligament, interspinous ligament, ligamentum flava, epidural space (contains loose areolar tissue, fat, and blood vessels), dura, "potential space," subarachnoid membrane, subarachnoid space (lumbar cistern) (Figure 13–15 below).

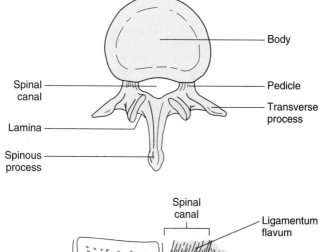

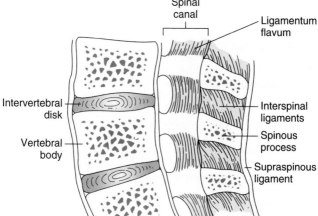

FIGURE 13–15. Basic anatomy to review before performing a lumbar puncture.

Procedure

1. Examine the fundus for evidence of papilledema, and review the CT or MRI of the head if available. Discuss the relative safety and lack of discomfort to the patient to dispel any myths. Some clinicians prefer to call the procedure a "subarachnoid analysis" rather than a spinal tap. As long as the procedure and the risks are outlined, most patients will agree to the procedure. Have the patient sign an informed consent form.

2. Place the patient in the lateral decubitus position close to the edge of the bed or table. The patient (held by an assistant, if possible) should be positioned with knees pulled up toward stomach and head flexed onto chest (Figure 13–16, page 290). This position enhances flexion of the vertebral spine and widens the interspaces between the spinous processes. Place a pillow beneath the patient's side to prevent sagging and ensure alignment of the spinal column. If the patient is obese or has arthritis or scoliosis, the sitting position, leaning forward, may be preferred.

3. Palpate the supracristal plane (see under Background) and carefully determine the location of the L4–L5 interspace.

4. Open the kit, put on sterile gloves, and prep the area with povidone-iodine solution in a circular fashion and covering several interspaces. Next, drape the patient.

5. With a 25-gauge needle and lidocaine, raise a skin wheal over the L4–L5 interspace. Anesthetize the deeper structures with a 22-gauge needle.

6. Examine the spinal needle with a stylet for defects and then insert it into the skin wheal and into the spinous ligament. Hold the needle between your index and middle fingers, with your thumb holding the stylet in place. Direct the needle cephalad at a 30–45-degree angle, in the midline and parallel to the bed (see Figure 13–16).

7. Advance through the major structures and pop into the subarachnoid space through the dura. An experienced operator can feel these layers, but an inexperienced one may need to periodically remove the stylet to look for return of fluid. It is important to always replace the stylet prior to advancing the spinal needle. The needle may be withdrawn, however, with the stylet removed. This technique may be useful if the needle has passed through the back wall of the canal. Direct the bevel of the needle parallel to the long axis of the body so that the dural fibers are separated rather than sheared. This method helps cut down on "spinal headaches."

8. If no fluid returns, it is sometimes helpful to rotate the needle slightly. If still no fluid appears, and you think that you are within the subarachnoid space, inject 1 mL of air because it is not uncommon for a piece of tissue to clog the needle. **Never** inject saline or distilled water. If no air returns and if spinal fluid cannot be aspirated, the bevel of the needle probably lies in the epidural space; advance it with the stylet in place.

9. When fluid returns, attach a manometer and stopcock and measure the pressure. Normal opening pressure is 70–180 mm water in the lateral position. Increased pressure may be due to a tense patient, CHF, ascites, subarachnoid hemorrhage, infection, or a space-occupying lesion. Decreased pressure may be due to needle position or obstructed flow (you may need to leave the needle in for a myelogram because if it is moved, the subarachnoid space may be lost).

10. Collect 0.5–2.0-mL samples in serial, labeled containers. Send them to the lab in this order:

13

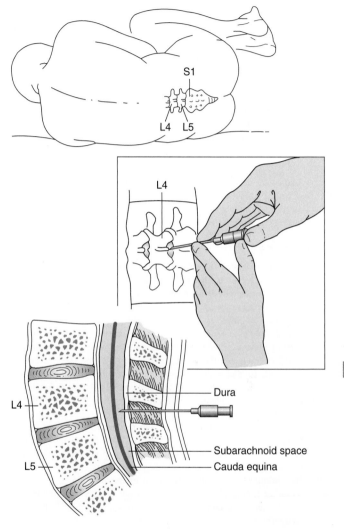

FIGURE 13–16. When performing a lumbar puncture, place the patient in the lateral decubitus position, and locate the L4–L5 interspace. Control the spinal needle with two hands, and enter the subarachnoid space.

- **First tube for bacteriology:** Gram's stain, routine C&S, AFB, and fungal cultures and stains
- **Second tube for glucose and protein:** Additionally, if MS is suspected, order electrophoresis to detect oligoclonal banding and assay for myelin basic protein.
- **Third tube for cell count:** CBC with diff

- **Fourth tube for special studies as clinically indicated:** VDRL (neurosyphilis), CIEP (counterimmunoelectrophoresis) for bacterial antigens such as *H. influenzae, S. Pneumoniae, N. meningitidis*), PCR assay for tuberculous meningitis or herpes simplex encephalitis (allows rapid diagnosis). If *Cryptococcus neoformans* is suspected (most common cause of meningitis in AIDS patients), India ink preparation and cryptococcal antigen (latex agglutination test).
- *Note:* Some clinicians prefer to send the first and last tubes for CBC because this procedure permits a better differentiation between a **subarachnoid hemorrhage** and a **traumatic tap.** In a traumatic tap, the number of RBCs in the first tube should be much higher than in the last tube. In a subarachnoid hemorrhage, the cell counts should be equal, and **xanthochromia** of the fluid should be present, indicating the presence of old blood.

11. Withdraw the needle, and place a dry, sterile dressing over the site.
12. Instruct the patient to remain recumbent for 6–12 h, and encourage an increased fluid intake to help prevent "spinal headaches."
13. Interpret the results based on Table 13–4, page 293.

Complications

- **Spinal headache:** The most common complication (about 20%), appears within the first 24 h after. It is relieved when the patient is lying down and is aggravated when the patient sits up. It is characterized by a severe throbbing pain in the occipital region and can last a week. It is thought to be caused by intracranial traction caused by the acute volume depletion of CSF and by persistent leakage from the puncture site. To help prevent spinal headaches, keep the patient recumbent for 6–12 h, encourage the intake of fluids, use the smallest needle possible, and keep the bevel of the needle parallel to the long axis of the body to help prevent a persistent CSF leak. If the headache persists, a blood patch (peripheral blood injected into the epidural space, usually performed by anesthesia service) may be needed to seal the leak.
- **Trauma to nerve roots or to the conus medullaris:** Much less frequent (some anatomic variation does exist, but it is very rare for the cord to end below L3). If the patient suddenly complains of paresthesia (numbness or shooting pains in the legs), stop the procedure.
- **Herniation of either the cerebellum or the medulla:** Occurs rarely, during or after a spinal tap, usually in a patient with increased intracranial pressure. This complication can often be reversed medically if it is recognized early.
- **Meningitis**
- **Bleeding** in the subarachnoid/subdural space can occur with resulting paralysis especially if the patient is receiving anticoagulants or has severe liver disease with a coagulopathy.

ORTHOSTATIC BLOOD PRESSURE MEASUREMENT
Indication

- Assessment of volume depletion

Materials

- BP cuff and stethoscope

TABLE 13-4
Differential Diagnosis of Cerebrospinal Fluid

Condition	Color	Opening Pressure (mm H$_2$O)	Protein (mg/100 mL)	Glucose (mg/100 mL)	Cells (#/mm^3)
NORMAL					
Adult	Clear	70–180	15–45	45–80	0–5 lymphocytes
Newborn	Clear	70–180	20–120	2/3 serum	40–60 lymphocytes
INFECTIOUS					
Viral infection ("aseptic meningitis")	Clear or opalescent	Normal or slightly increased	Normal or slightly increased	Normal	10–500 lymphocytes PMNs early
Bacterial infection	Opalescent yellow, may clot	Increased	50–10,000	Decreased, usually <20	25–10,000 PMNs
Granulomatous infection (TB, fungal)	Clear or opalescent	Often increased	Increased, but usually <500	Decreased, usually <20–40	10–500 lymphocytes

(continued)

13

TABLE 13-4
(Continued)

Condition	Color	Opening Pressure (mm H₂O)	Protein (mg/100 mL)	Glucose (mg/100 mL)	Cells (#/mm³)
NEUROLOGIC					
Guillain–Barré Syndrome	Clear or Cloudy	Normal	Markedly increased	Normal	Normal or increased lymphocytes
Multiple sclerosis	Clear	Normal	Normal or increased	Normal	0–20 lymphocytes
Pseudotumor cerebri	Clear	Increased	Normal	Normal	Normal
MISCELLANEOUS					
Neoplasm	Clear or xanthochromic	Increased	Normal or increased	Normal or decreased	Normal or increased lymphocytes

(continued)

13

TABLE 13–4
(Continued)

Condition	Color	Opening Pressure (mm H₂O)	Protein (mg/100 mL)	Glucose (mg/100 mL)	Cells (#/mm³)
Traumatic tap	Bloody, no xanthochromia	Normal	Normal	Sl increased	RBC = peripheral blood; less RBC in tube 4 than in tube 1
Subarachnoid hemorrhage	Bloody or xanthochromic after 2–8 h	Usually increased	Increased	Normal	WBC/RBC ratio same as blood, RBC in tube 4

WBC = white blood cell; RBC = red blood cell; PMNs = polymorphonuclear neutrophils.

13

295

es in BP and pulse when a patient moves from supine to the upright
on are very sensitive guides for detecting early volume depletion. Even
e a person becomes overtly tachycardic or hypotensive because of volume loss, the demonstration of orthostatic hypotension aids in the diagnosis.

2. Have the patient assume a supine position for 5–10 min. Determine the BP
   and pulse.
3. Then have the patient stand up. If the patient is unable to stand, have the
   patient sit at the bedside with legs dangling.
4. After about 1 min, determine the BP and pulse again.
5. A drop in systolic BP greater than 10 mm Hg or an increase in pulse rate
   greater than 20 (16 in the elderly) suggests **volume depletion.** A change in
   heart rate is more sensitive and occurs with a lesser degree of volume depletion. Other causes of a drop in BP with body position change (usually without
   an increase in heart rate) include peripheral neuropathies, surgical sympathectomy, diabetes, and medications (prazosin, hydralazine, or reserpine).

PELVIC EXAMINATION

Indications

- Part of a complete physical examination in the female
- Used to assist in the diagnosis of diseases and conditions of the female
  genital tract

Materials

- Gloves
- Vaginal speculum and lubricant
- Slides, fixative (Pap smear aerosol spray, etc), cotton swabs, endocervi-
  cal brush and cervical spatula prepared for a Pap smear

Materials for Other Diagnostic Tests

- Culture media to test for gonorrhea, *Chlamydia,* herpes
- Sterile cotton swabs
- Plain glass slides
- KOH
- NS solutions, as needed

Procedure

1. The pelvic exam should be carried out in a comfortable fashion for both
   the patient and physician. A female assistant **must** be present for the procedure. The patient should be draped appropriately with her feet placed in the
   stirrups on the examining table. Prepare a low stool, a good light source,
   and all needed supplies before the exam begins. In unusual situations examinations are conducted on a stretcher or bed; raise the patients buttocks
   on one or two pillows to elevate the perineum off the mattress.
2. Inform the patient of each move in advance. Glove hands before proceeding.
3. **General inspection:**
   a. Observe the skin of the perineum for swelling, ulcers, condylomata
      (venereal warts), or color changes.

13

    b. Separate the labia to examine the clitoris and vestibule. Multiple clear vesicles on an erythematous base on the labia suggest herpes.

    c. Observe the urethral meatus for developmental abnormalities, discharge, neoplasm, and abscess of Bartholin's gland at the 4 or 8 o'clock positions.

    d. Inspect the vaginal orifice for discharge, or protrusion of the walls (cystocele, rectocele, urethral prolapse).

    e. Note the condition of the hymen.

4. Speculum examination:

    a. Use a speculum moistened with warm water **not** with lubricant (lubricant will interfere with Pap tests and slide studies). Check the temperature of the speculum on the patient's leg to see if the speculum is comfortable.

    b. Because the anterior wall of the vagina is close to the urethra and bladder, do not exert pressure in this area. Pressure should be placed on the posterior surface of the vagina. With the speculum directed at a 45-degree angle to the floor, spread the labia and insert the speculum fully, pressing posteriorly. The cervix should pop into view with some manipulation as the speculum is opened.

    c. Inspect the cervix and vagina for color, lacerations, growths, nabothian cysts, and evidence of atrophy.

    d. Inspect the cervical os for size, shape, color, discharge.

    e. Inspect the vagina for secretions and obtain specimens for a Pap smear, other smear, or culture (see tests for vaginal infections and Pap smear in item 7).

    f. Inspect the vaginal wall; rotate the speculum as you draw it out to see the entire canal.

5. Bimanual examination:

    a. For this part, stand up. It is best to use whichever hand is comfortable to do the internal vaginal exam. Remove the glove from the hand that will examine the abdomen.

    b. Place lubricant on the first and second gloved fingers, and then, keeping pressure on the posterior fornix, introduce them into the vagina.

    c. Palpate the tissue at 5 and 7 o'clock between the first and second fingers and the thumb to rule out any abnormality of Bartholin's gland. Likewise, palpate the urethra and paraurethral (Skene's) gland.

    d. Place the examining fingers on the posterior wall of the vagina to further open the introitus. Ask the patient to bear down. Look for evidence of prolapse, rectocele, or cystocele.

    e. Palpate the cervix. Note the size, shape, consistency, and motility, and test for tenderness (the **"chandelier" sign**) or cervical motion tenderness, which is suggestive of PID or ruptured ectopic pregnancy.

    f. With your fingers in the vagina posterior to the cervix and your hand on the abdomen placed just above the symphysis, force the corpus of the uterus between the two examining hands. Note size, shape, consistency, position, and motility.

    g. Move the fingers in the vagina to one or the other fornix, and place the hand on the abdomen in a more lateral position to bring the adnexal areas under examination. Palpate the ovaries, if possible, for any masses, consistency, and motility. Unless the fallopian tubes are diseased, they usually are not palpable.

13

6. **Rectovaginal examination:**
   a. Insert your index finger into the vagina, and place the well-lubricated middle finger in the rectum.
   b. Palpate the posterior surface of the uterus and the broad ligament for nodularity, tenderness, or other masses. Examine the uterosacral and rectovaginal septum. Nodularity here may represent endometriosis.
   c. It may also be helpful to do a test for occult blood if a stool specimen is available.

7. **Papanicolaou (Pap) smear:**
   The Pap smear is helpful in the early detection of cervical intraepithelial neoplasia and carcinoma. Endometrial carcinoma is occasionally identified on routine Pap smears. It is recommended that low-risk patients have routine Pap smears done every 2–3 y, but only after three annual Pap smears are negative. High-risk patients such as those exposed to in utero DES; patients with HPV infections, history of HIV infection; history of cervical dysplasia or cervical intraepithelial neoplasia; more than two sexual partners in the patient's lifetime; and intercourse prior to age 20 should obtain an annual Pap smear.
   a. With the unlubricated speculum in place, use a wooden cervical spatula to obtain a scraping from the squamocolumnar junction. Rotate the spatula 360 degrees around the external os. Smear on a frosted slide that has the patient's name written on it in pencil. Fix the slide either in a bottle of fixative or with commercially available spray fixative. The slide must be fixed within 10 s or a drying artifact may occur.
   b. Next, obtain a specimen from the endocervical canal using a cotton swab or commercial available endocervical brush and prepare the slide as described in part a.
   c. Using a wooden spatula, an additional specimen should be obtained from the posterior/lateral vaginal pool of fluid and smeared on a slide.
   d. Complete the appropriate lab slips. Forewarn the patient that she may experience some spotty vaginal bleeding following the Pap smear.

8. **Tests for cervical/vaginal infections:**
   a. **GC and *Chlamydia* culture:** Use a sterile cotton swab to obtain a specimen from the endocervical canal and plate it out on **Thayer–Martin** medium for GC. *Chlamydia* testing varies but can include DNA probe, EIA or DFA testing.
   b. **Vaginal saline (wet) prep:** Helpful in the diagnosis of *Trichomonas vaginalis* or bacterial vaginosis. Mix a drop of discharge with a drop of NS on a glass slide and cover with a coverslip. Observe the slide while still warm to see the flagellated, motile trichomonads. Bacterial vaginosis is most often caused by *Gardnerella vaginalis* and can be diagnosed by the presence of "clue cells," which represent polymorphonuclear white cells dotted with the *G. vaginalis* bacteria, a vaginal pH of > 4.5, and a fishy amine odor with addition of KOH to the secretions. Alternatively, these can be seen by using a hanging drop of saline and a concave slide. *Lactobacillus* are normally the predominant bacteria in the vagina in the absence of specific infection and the normal pH is usually < 4.5.
   c. **Potassium hydroxide prep:** If a thick, white, curdy discharge is present, the patient may have a *Candida albicans* (monilial) yeast infec-

tion. Prepare a slide with one drop of discharge and one drop of aqueous 10% KOH solution. The KOH dissolves the epithelial cells and debris and facilitates viewing of the hyphae and mycelia of the fungus that causes the infection.

d. **Gram's stain:** Material can easily be stained in the usual fashion (Chapter 7, page 118). Gram-negative intracellular diplococci (so-called GNIDs) are pathognomonic of *Neisseria gonorrhoeae.* The most commonly found bacteria in Gram's stains are large gram-positive rods (lactobacilli), which are normal vaginal flora.

e. **Herpes cultures:** A routine Pap smear of the cervix or a Pap smear of the herpetic lesion (multiple, clear vesicles on a painful, erythematous base) may demonstrate herpes inclusion bodies. A herpes culture may be done by taking a viral culture swab of the suspicious lesion or of the endocervix.

PERICARDIOCENTESIS

Indications

- Emergency treatment of cardiac tamponade
- Diagnose cause of pericardial effusion

Contraindications

- Minimal pericardial effusion (< 200 mL)
- After CABG due to risk of injury to grafts
- Uncorrected coagulopathy

Materials

- Electrocardiogram machine
- Prepackaged pericardiocentesis kit **or** procedure and instrument tray (page 245) with pericardiocentesis needle or 16–18-gauge needle 10 cm long

Background

Cardiac tamponade results in decreased cardiac output, increased right atrial filling pressures, and a pronounced pulsus paradoxus.

Procedure

1. If time permits, use sterile prep and draping with gown, mask, and gloves.
2. Draining the pericardium can be approached either through the left paraxiphoid or the left parasternal 4th ICS. The paraxiphoid is safer, more commonly used, and described here (Figure 13–17, page 300).
3. Anesthetize the insertion site with lidocaine. Connect the needle with an alligator clip to a chest lead (brown) on the ECG machine. Attach the limb leads, and monitor the machine.
4. Insert the pericardiocentesis needle just to the left of the xiphoid and directed upward 45 degrees toward the left shoulder.
5. Aspirate while advancing the needle until the pericardium is punctured and the effusion is tapped. If the ventricular wall is felt, withdraw the needle

13

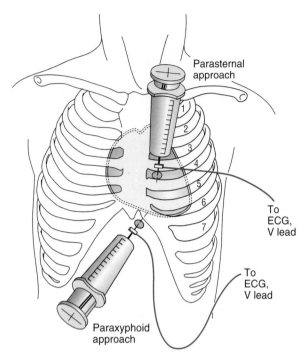

FIGURE 13–17. Techniques for pericardiocentesis. The paraxiphoid approach is the most popular.

slightly. Additionally, if the needle contacts the myocardium, pronounced ST segment elevation will be noted on the ECG.

6. If performed for cardiac tamponade, removal of as little as 50 mL of fluid dramatically improves BP and decreases right atrial pressure.

7. Blood from a bloody pericardial effusion is usually defibrinated and will not clot, whereas blood from the ventricle will clot.

8. Send fluid for HCT, cell count, or cytology if indicated.

   • **Serous fluid:** Consistent with CHF, bacterial infection, TB, hypoalbuminemia, or viral pericarditis

   • **Bloody fluid (HCT > 10%):** May result from trauma; be iatrogenic; or due to MI, uremia, coagulopathy, or malignancy (lymphoma, leukemia, breast, lung most common)

9. **If continuous drainage is necessary, use a guidewire to place a 16-gauge IV catheter and connect to a closed drainage system.**

Complications

Arrhythmia, ventricular puncture, lung injury

PERIPHERALLY INSERTED CENTRAL CATHETER (PICC LINE)
Indications

- Home infusion of hypertonic or irritating solutions and drugs
- Long-term infusion of medications (antibiotics, chemotherapeutics)
- TPN
- Repetitive venous blood sampling

Contraindications

- Infection over placement site
- Failure to identify veins in an arm with a tourniquet in place

Materials

- PICC catheter kit (contains most items necessary including the silastic long arm line, eg, Introsyte Autoguard system)
- Tourniquet, sterile gloves, mask, sterile gown, heparin flush, 10-mL syringes

Background

Installation of a PICC allows for central venous access through a peripheral vein. Typically, a long-arm catheter is placed into the basilic or cephalic vein (See Figure 13–12) and is threaded into the subclavian vein/superior vena cava. PICCs are useful for long-term home infusion therapies. The design of PICC catheters can vary, and the operator should be familiar with the features of the device (attached hub or detachable hub designs).

13

Procedure

1. Explain the procedure to the patient and then obtain informed consent. Position the patient in a sitting or reclining position with the elbow extended and the arm in a dependent position. The arm should be externally rotated.
2. Using a measuring tape, determine the length of the catheter required. Measure from the extremity vein insertion site to the subclavian vein.
3. Wear mask, gown, protective eyewear, and sterile gloves. Prep and drape the skin in the standard fashion. Set up an adjacent sterile working area.
4. Anesthetize the skin at the proposed area of insertion. Apply a tourniquet above the proposed IV site.
5. Trim the catheter to the appropriate length. Most PICC lines have an attached hub, and the distal end of the catheter is cut to the proper length. Flush with heparinized saline.
6. Insert the catheter and introducer needle (usually 14-gauge) into the chosen arm vein as detailed in the section on IV Techniques (page 284). Once the catheter is in the vein, push the white button on the Introsyte device to shield the needle. Discard the needle assembly.
7. Place the PICC line in the catheter and advance (use a forceps if provided by the manufacturer of the kit to advance the PICC line). Remove the tourniquet and gradually advance the catheter the requisite length. Remove the inner stiffening wire slowly once the catheter has been adequately advanced.

8. Peel away the introducer catheter. Attach the Luer-lock, and flush the catheter again with heparin solution. Attempt to also aspirate blood to verify patency.

9. Attach the provided securing wings, and suture in place. Apply a sterile dressing over the insertion site.

10. Confirm placement in the central circulation with a chest radiograph. Always document the type of PICC, the length inserted, and the site of its radiologically confirmed placement.

11. If vein cannulation is difficult, a surgical cutdown may be necessary to cannulate the vein. If the catheter will not advance, fluoroscopy may be helpful.

12. Instruct the patient on the maintenance of the PICC. The PICC should be flushed with heparinized saline after each use. Dressing changes should be performed at least every 7 d under sterile conditions. Patient must be instructed to evaluate the PICC site for signs and symptoms of infection. Patient must also be instructed to come to the ER for evaluation of any fevers.

13. For venous samples, a specimen of at least the catheter volume (1–3 mL) must first be withdrawn and then discarded. The PICC must always be flushed with heparinized saline after each blood draw.

PICC Removal

1. Position the patient's arm at a 90-degree angle to the body. Remove the dressing and gently pull the PICC out.

2. Apply pressure to site for 2–3 min. Always measure the length of the catheter and check prior documentation to ensure that the PICC line has been removed in its entirety. If a piece of a catheter is left behind, an emergency interventional radiology consult is in order.

Complications

13

Site bleeding, clotted catheter, subclavian thrombosis, infection, broken catheter (leakage or embolization), arrhythmia (catheter inserted too far)

PERITONEAL LAVAGE

Indications

- **Diagnostic peritoneal lavage (DPL)** is used in the evaluation of intraabdominal trauma (bleeding, perforation) (*Note:* Spiral CT of the abdomen has largely replaced this as an initial screening for intraabdominal trauma in the emergency setting.)
- Acute peritoneal dialysis and the treatment of severe pancreatitis

Contraindications

- None are absolute. Relative contraindications include multiple abdominal procedures, pregnancy, known retroperitoneal injury (high false-positive rates) cirrhosis, morbid obesity and any coagulopathy.

Materials

- Prepackaged DPL or peritoneal dialysis tray

Procedure

1. A Foley catheter and an NG or orogastric tube **must** be in place. Prep the abdomen from above the umbilicus to the pubis.

2. The site of choice is in the midline 1–2 cm below the umbilicus. Avoid the site of old surgical scars (danger of adherent bowel). If a subumbilical scar or pelvic fracture is present, a supraumbilical approach is recommended.

3. Infiltrate the skin with lidocaine with epinephrine. Incise the skin in the midline vertically, and expose the fascia.

4. Either pick up the fascia and incise it, or puncture it with the trocar and peritoneal catheter. Caution is needed to avoid puncturing any organs. Use one hand to hold the catheter near the skin and to control the insertion while using the other hand to apply pressure to the end of the catheter. After entering the peritoneal cavity, remove the trocar and direct the catheter inferiorly into the pelvis.

5. During a diagnostic lavage, gross blood indicates a positive tap. If no blood is encountered, instill 10 mL/kg (about 1 L in adults) of RL or NS into the abdominal cavity.

6. Gently agitate the abdomen to distribute the fluid and after 5 min, drain off as much fluid as possible into a bag on the floor. (Minimum fluid for a valid analysis is 200 mL in an adult.) If the drainage is slow, try instilling additional fluid, carefully repositioning the catheter.

7. Send the fluid for analysis (amylase, bile, bacteria, hematocrit, cell count). See Table 13–5 below for interpretation.

8. Remove the catheter and suture the skin. If the catheter is inserted for pancreatitis or peritoneal dialysis, suture the catheter in place.

9. A negative DPL does not rule out retroperitoneal trauma. A false-positive DPL can be caused by a pelvic fracture or bleeding induced by the procedure (eg, laceration of an omental vessel).

13

TABLE 13–5
Criteria for Evaluation of Peritoneal Lavage Fluid

Positive	>20 mL gross blood on free aspiration (10 mL in children)
	≥100,000 RBC/mL
	≥500 WBC/mL (if obtained >3 h after the injury)
	≥175 units amylase/dL
	Bacteria on Gram's stain
	Bile (by inspection or chemical determination of bilirubin content)
	Food particles (microscopic analysis of strained or spun specimen)
Intermediate	Pink fluid on free aspiration
	50,000–100,000 RBC/mL in blunt trauma
	100–500 WBC/mL
	75–175 units amylase/dL
Negative	Clear aspirate
	≤ 100 WBC/μL
	≤75 units amylase/dL

Source: Reprinted, with permission, from: Way, L., Doherty GM (eds): *Current Surgical Diagnosis and Treatment,* 11th ed. McGraw-Hill, 2003.
RBC = red blood cells; WBC = white blood cells.

Complications

Infection/peritonitis or superficial wound infection, bleeding, perforated viscus (bladder, bowel)

PERITONEAL (ABDOMINAL) PARACENTESIS
Indications

- To determine the cause of ascites
- To determine if intraabdominal bleeding is present or if a viscus has ruptured (DPL is considered a more accurate test. See preceding procedure.)
- Therapeutic removal of fluid when distention is pronounced or respiratory distress is associated with it (acute treatment only)

Contraindications

- Abnormal coagulation factors
- Bowel obstruction, pregnancy
- Uncertainty if distention is due to peritoneal fluid or to a cystic structure (ultrasound can usually differentiate)

Materials

- Minor procedure tray (see page 245)
- Catheter-over-needle assembly (Angiocath Autoguard, Insyte Autoguard 18–20-gauge with a 1½-in. needle)
- 20–60-mL syringe
- Sterile specimen containers

13 Procedure

Peritoneal paracentesis is surgical puncture of the peritoneal cavity for the aspiration of fluid. Ascites is indicated by abdominal distention, shifting dullness, and a palpable fluid wave.

1. Explain the procedure and have the patient sign an informed consent form. Have the patient empty the bladder, or place a Foley catheter if voiding is impossible or if significant mental status changes are present.
2. The entry site is usually the midline 3–4 cm below the umbilicus. Avoid old surgical scars because the bowel may be adhering to the abdominal wall. Alternatively, the entry site can be in the left or right lower quadrant midway between the umbilicus and the anterior superior iliac spine or in the patient's flank, depending on the percussion of the fluid wave (Figure 13–18, page 305). Avoid the rectus abdominus due to bleeding potential.
3. Prep and drape the area and raise a skin wheal with the lidocaine over the entry site.
4. A Z track technique will help limit persistent leakage of peritoneal fluid after the tap. Manually retract the skin caudally and release traction on the skin when the peritoneum is entered. With the catheter mounted on the syringe, go through the anesthetized area while aspirating. There is resistance as the fascia is entered. When you get free return of fluid, leave the catheter in place, remove the needle or activate the self-shielding mecha-

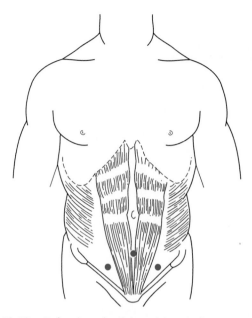

FIGURE 13-18. Preferred sites for abdominal (peritoneal) paracentesis. Be sure to avoid old surgical scars.

nism. Begin to aspirate; reposition the catheter because of abutting bowel as needed.

5. Aspirate the amount of fluid needed for tests (20–30 mL). If the tap is therapeutic, 10–15 L can be safely removed. The removal of a large volume can be facilitated by the use of vacuum container bottles (500 mL–1 L) supplied at most hospitals. Tubing is first connected to the catheter and then to the vacuum container bottles.
6. Apply a sterile 4 × 4 gauze square, and apply pressure with tape.
7. Depending on the clinical picture of the patient, send samples for cell count including differential, total protein, albumin, amylase, LDH, glucose, cytology, culture and stains.

Complications

Peritonitis, perforated viscus (bowel, bladder), hemorrhage, precipitation of hepatic coma if patient has severe liver disease, oliguria, hypotension

Diagnosis of Ascitic Fluid

A differential diagnosis is in Chapter 3, page 35. The older classification of ascitic fluid as either transudative or exudative is no longer used. The cause of ascites is more likely to be found by determining the serum-to-ascites albumin gradient. See Table 13–6, page 306 to interpret the results of ascitic fluid analysis.

TABLE 13–6
Differential Diagnosis of Ascitic Fluid

Albumin Gradient:
  Serum Alb – Ascites Alb = X
    if $X > 1.1$ g/dL, then portal hypertension
    if $X < 1.1$ g/dL, then not from portal hypertension
Total Protein: < 1.0 g/dL, high risk for spontaneous bacterial peritonitis
Cell Count: absolute neutrophil count > 250/μL, presume infected
Bacterial culture: Blood culture bottles 85% sensitivity
                    Routine cultures 50% sensitivity
Bacterial Peritonitis: Spontaneous versus secondary
  Secondary: (1) polymicrobial; (2) total protein > 1.0 g/dL;
              (3) LDH > normal serum value; (4) glucose < 50 mg/dL
Food Fibers: Found in most cases of perforated viscus.
Cytology: Bizarre cells with large nuclei may represent reactive
              mesothelial cells and *not* a malignancy. Malignant cells
              suggest a tumor.

Source: Reprinted with permission. From: Haist SA, Robbins JB (eds.) *Internal Medicine on Call,* 3rd ed. McGraw-Hill, 2002.

PULMONARY ARTERY CATHETERIZATION

(See Chapter 20, page 418)

PULSUS PARADOXUS MEASUREMENT (PARADOXICAL PULSE)

(See also Chapter 20, page 410)

Indication

- Used in the evaluation of cardiac tamponade and other diseases (eg, the severity of asthma)

Materials

- BP cuff and stethoscope

Background

Pulsus paradoxus is an exaggeration of the normal inspiratory drop in arterial pressure. Inspiration decreases intrathoracic pressure. The result is increased right atrial and right ventricular filling with an increase in right ventricular output. Because the pulmonary vascular bed also distends, these changes lead to a delay in left ventricular filling and subsequently a decreased left ventricular output. This drop in systolic BP is usually < 10 mm Hg. In the case of cardiac compression (eg, acute asthma or pericardial tamponade), the right side of the heart fills more with inspiration and decreases the left ventricular volume to even greater degree as a result of compression of the pericardial sac. This exaggerated decrease in left ventricular output drops the systolic pressure > 10 mm Hg. See Figure 20–1 (page 410) for a graphic representation of a paradoxical pulse.

Procedure

1. A simple, **qualitative method** involves palpating the radial pulse, which "disappears" on normal inspiration.
2. A more precise **quantitative method** requires measuring the systolic BP at end-exhalation during tidal breathing.
3. Then determine the systolic BP at end-inspiration during tidal breathing.
4. The difference in systolic pressure between end-exhalation and end-inspiration should be < 10 mm Hg. If not, a so-called paradox exists.
5. Differential diagnosis includes pericardial effusion, cardiac tamponade, pericarditis, COPD, bronchial asthma, restrictive cardiomyopathies, hemorrhagic shock, massive PE, tricuspid stenosis and mitral stenosis.

SKIN BIOPSY

Indications

- Any skin lesion or eruption for which the diagnosis is unclear
- Any refractory skin condition

Contraindications

- Any skin lesion that is suspected to be a malignancy (eg, melanoma) should be referred to a plastic surgeon or dermatologist for excisional biopsy rather than a punch biopsy.

Materials

- 2-, 3-, 4-, or 5-mm skin punch
- Minor procedure tray (page 245)
- Curved iris scissors and fine-toothed forceps (Ordinary forceps may distort a small biopsy specimen and should not be used.)
- Specimen bottle containing 10% formalin
- Suturing materials (3-0 or 4-0 nylon)

13

Procedure

1. If more than one lesion is present, choose one that is well developed and representative of the dermatosis. For patients with vesiculobullous disease, an early edematous lesion should be chosen rather than a vesicle. Avoid lesions that are excoriated or infected.
2. Mark the area to be biopsied with a skin-marking pen. Inject the lidocaine to form a skin wheal over the site of the biopsy.
3. After putting on sterile gloves and preparing a sterile field, take the punch biopsy specimen. First, immobilize the skin with the fingers of one hand, applying pressure perpendicular to the skin wrinkle lines with the skin punch. Core out a cylinder of skin by twirling the punch between the fingers of the other hand. As the punch enters into the SQ fat, resistance will lessen. At this point, the punch should be removed. The core of tissue usually pops up slightly and can be cut at the level of the SQ fat with curved iris scissors without using forceps. If a tissue core does not pop up, it may be elevated by use of a hypodermic needle or fine-toothed forceps. Be sure to include a portion of the SQ fat in the specimen.
4. Place the specimen in the specimen container.

5. Hemostasis can be achieved by pressure with the gauze pad.
6. Defects from 1.5- and 2-mm punches usually do not require suturing and heal with very minimal scarring. Punch defects that are 2–4 mm can generally be closed with a single suture.
7. A dry dressing should be applied and removed the following day.
8. Sutures can be removed as early as 3 d from the face and 7–10 d from other areas.

Complications

Infection (unusual); hemorrhage (usually controlled by simple application of pressure); keloid formation, especially in a patient with a prior history of keloid formation

SKIN TESTING
Indications

- Screening for current or past infectious agent (TB, coccidioidomycosis, etc)
- Screening for immune competency (so-called anergy screen) in debilitated patients

Materials

- Appropriate antigen (usually 0.1 mL) (eg, 5 TU PPD)
- A small, short needle (25-, 26-, or 27-gauge)
- 1-mL syringe
- Alcohol swab

13

Procedure

1. Skin tests for **delayed type hypersensitivity (type IV, tuberculin)** are the most commonly administered and interpreted. Delayed hypersensitivity (so called because a lag time of 24–48 h is required for a reaction) is caused by the activation of sensitized lymphocytes after contact with an antigen. The inflammatory reaction results from direct cytotoxicity and the release of lymphokines. Allergy tests (immediate wheal and flare) are rarely performed by the student or house officer.
2. The most commonly used site is the flexor surface of the forearm, approximately 4 in. below the elbow crease.
3. Prep the area with alcohol. With the bevel of the 27-gauge needle up, introduce the needle into the upper layers of skin, but **not** into the subcutis. Inject 0.1 mL of antigen such as the PPD. The goal is to inject the antigen intradermally. If done properly, you will raise a discrete white bleb, approximately 10 mm in diameter (known as the **Mantoux test**). The bleb should disappear soon, and no dressing is needed. If a bleb is not raised, move to another area and repeat the injection.
4. Mark the test site with a pen, and if multiple tests are being administered, identify each one. Also, document the site in the patient's chart.
5. To interpret the skin test, examine the injection site at 48–72 h. If nonreactive, check again at 72 h. **Measure the area of induration (the firm raised area), not the erythematous area.** Use a ballpoint pen held at ap-

proximately a 30-degree angle and bring it lightly toward the raised area. Where the pen touches is the area of induration. Measure two diameters and take the average.

6. It is important to check the PPD and other tests at intervals. If the patient develops a severe reaction to the skin test, apply hydrocortisone cream to prevent skin sloughing.

Specific Skin Tests

TST (Tuberculin Skin Testing):   Routine TST in low-risk individuals is not currently recommended. High-risk individuals should undergo periodic TST (CXR findings suspicious for TB, recent contact of known or suspected TB cases, [includes health care workers], high-risk immigrants [from Asia, Africa, Middle East, Latin America], medically underserved (IV drug abusers, alcoholics, homeless), chronically institutionalized, and HIV-infected or others that are immunosuppressed.

The **Mantoux test** is the standard technique for TST and relies on the intradermal injection of **PPD.** The **tine test** for TB is no longer recommended by the CDC. The PPD comes in three tuberculin unit "strengths": 1 TU ("first"), 5 TU ("intermediate"), and 250 TU ("second"). 1 TU is used if the patient is expected to be hypersensitive (history of a positive skin test); 5 TU is the standard initial screening test. A patient who has a negative response to a 5-TU test dose may react to the 250-TU solution. A patient who does not respond to the 250-TU is considered nonreactive to PPD. A patient may not react if he or she has not been exposed to the antigen or if the patient is anergic and unable to respond to any antigen challenge. A positive TST indicates the presence of *Mycobacterium tuberculosis* infection, either active or past (dormant) and an intact cell-mediated immunity.

Interpretation of a positive PPD test is based on the clinical scenario. **Patients who have been previously immunized with percutaneous BCG may give a false-positive PPD, usually 10 mm or less.**

- 0–5 mm induration: Negative response

- ≥ 5 mm: Considered positive in contacts of known TB cases, CXR findings consistent with TB infection, HIV infection or in patients who are immunosuppressed, occasionally in non-TB mycobacterial infection due to cross reactivity

- ≥ 10 mm induration: Considered positive in patients with chronic diseases (diabetics, alcoholics, IV drug abusers, other chronic diseases), homeless, immigrants from known TB regions, children < 4 y

- > 15 mm induration: Positive in individuals who are healthy and otherwise do not meet the preceding risk categories

Anergy Screen (Anergy Battery):   An anergy screen is based on the assumption that a patient has been exposed in the past to certain common antigens and a healthy patient is able to mount a reaction to them. To perform the screen, antigens such as mumps, or *Candida* are generally applied, and the results are read just like the PPD test (a reaction of > 5 mm induration is considered a positive test and indicates intact cellular immunity). Anergy screens are sometimes used to evaluate a patient's immunologic status and in the following specific situations: If you suspect a patient is PPD-positive, and the patient does not react to the test, do an anergy screen along with the PPD test to see if the patient has **any** cellular immune response.

THORACENTESIS
Indications

- Determining the cause of a pleural effusion
- Therapeutically removing pleural fluid in the event of respiratory distress
- Aspirating small pneumothoraces where the risk of recurrence is small (ie, postoperative without lung injury)
- Instilling sclerosing compounds (eg, tetracycline) to obliterate the pleural space

Contraindications

- None are absolute (pneumothorax, hemothorax, or any major respiratory impairment on the contralateral side, or coagulopathy)

Materials

- Prepackaged thoracentesis kit with either needle or catheter (preferred)

or

- Minor procedure tray (page 245)
- 20–60-mL syringe, 20- or 22-gauge needle 1½-in. needle, three-way stopcock
- Specimen containers

Procedure

Thoracentesis is the surgical puncture of the chest wall to aspirate fluid or air from the pleural cavity. The area of pleural effusion is dull to percussion with decreased breath sounds. Pleural fluid causes blunting of the costophrenic angles on CXR. Blunting usually indicates that at least 300 mL of fluid is present. If you suspect that less than 300 mL of fluid is present or you suspect that the fluid is loculated (trapped and not free-flowing), a lateral decubitus film is helpful. Loculated effusions do not layer out. Thoracentesis can be done safely on fluid visualized on lateral decubitus film if at least 10 mm of fluid is measurable on the decubitus x-ray. Ultrasound may also be used to localize a small or loculated effusion.

1. Explain the procedure, and have the patient sign an informed consent form. Have the patient sit up comfortably, preferably leaning forward slightly on a bedside tray table. Ask the patient to practice increasing intrathoracic pressure using the Valsalva maneuver or by humming.
2. The usual site for thoracentesis is the posterior lateral aspect of the back superior to the diaphragm but inferior to the top of the fluid level. Confirm the site by counting the ribs based on the CXR and percussing out the fluid level. Avoid going below the 8th ICS because of the risk of peritoneal perforation.
3. Use sterile technique, including gloves, povidone-iodine prep, and drapes. Thoracentesis kits come with an adherent drape with a hole in it.

4. Make a skin wheal over the proposed site with a 25-gauge needle and lido-caine. Change to a 22-gauge, 1½-in. needle and infiltrate up and over the rib (Figure 13–19); try to anesthetize the deeper structures and the pleura. During this time, you should be aspirating back for pleural fluid. Once fluid returns, note the depth of the needle and mark it with a hemostat. This gives you an approximate depth. Remove the needle.

5. Use a hemostat to measure the 14–18-gauge thoracentesis needle to the same depth as the first needle. Penetrate through the anesthetized area with the thoracentesis needle. **Make sure that you "march" over the top of the rib** to avoid the neurovascular bundle that runs below the rib (see Figure 13–19). With the three-way stopcock attached, advance the thoracentesis catheter through the needle, withdraw the needle from the chest, and place the protective needle cover over the end of the needle to prevent injury to the catheter. Next, aspirate the amount of pleural fluid needed. Turn the stopcock, and evacuate the fluid through the tubing. **Never remove more than 1000–1500 mL per tap!** This may result in hypotension or the devel-opment of pulmonary edema due to reexpansion of compressed alveoli.

6. Have the patient hum or do the Valsalva maneuver as you withdraw the catheter. This maneuver increases intrathoracic pressure and decreases the chances of a pneumothorax. Place a sterile dressing over the site.

7. Obtain a CXR to evaluate the fluid level and to rule out a pneumothorax. An expiratory film is preferred because it is superior in identifying a small pneumothorax.

8. Distribute specimens in containers, label slips, and send them to the lab. Always order pH, specific gravity, protein, LDH, cell count and differen-tial, glucose, Gram's stain and cultures, acid-fast cultures and smears, and fungal cultures and smears. Optional lab studies are cytology if you sus-pect a malignancy, amylase if you suspect an effusion secondary to pancre-

13

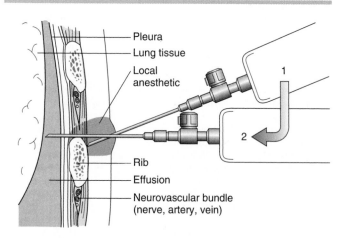

FIGURE 13–19. When performing a thoracentesis, the needle is passed over the top of the rib to avoid the neurovascular bundle.

atitis (usually on the left) or esophageal perforation, and a Sudan stain and triglycerides (> 110 mg/dL) if a chylothorax is suspected.

Complications

- Pneumothorax, hemothorax, infection, pulmonary laceration, hypotension, hypoxia due to V/Q mismatch in the newly aerated lung segment

Differential Diagnosis of Pleural Fluid

For a more complete differential, see Chapter 3. A **transudate** suggests nephrosis, CHF, cirrhosis; an **exudate,** infection (pneumonia, TB), malignancy, empyema, peritoneal dialysis, pancreatitis, chylothorax. See Table 13–7, below for the differential diagnosis.

TABLE 13–7
Differential Diagnosis of Pleural Fluid

Lab Value	Transudate	Exudate
Appearance	Clear yellow	Clear or turbid
Specific gravity	<1.016	>1.016
Absolute protein	<3 g/100 mL	>3 g/100 mL
Protein (pleural to serum ratio)	<0.5	>0.5
LDH (pleural to serum ratio)	<0.6	>0.6
Absolute LDH	<200 IU	>200 IU
Glucose (serum to pleural ratio)	<1	>1
Fibrinogen (clot)	No	Yes
WBC (pleural)	Very low	>2500/mm^3
Differential (pleural)		PMNs early, monocytes later

OTHER SELECTED TESTS

Cytology: Bizarre cells with large nuclei may represent reactive mesothelial cells and not a malignancy. Malignant cells suggest a tumor.
pH: Generally >7.3. If between 7.2 and 7.3, suspect TB or malignancy or both. If <7.2, suspect empyema.
Glucose: Normal pleural fluid glucose is ⅔ serum glucose. Pleural fluid glucose is much lower than serum glucose in effusions due to rheumatoid arthritis (0–16 mg/100 mL); low <40 mg/100 mL in empyema.
Triglycerides and positive Sudan stain: Chylothorax.

LDH = lactate dehydrogenase; WBC = white blood cells; RBC = red blood cells; PMNs = polymorphonuclear neutrophils; TB = tuberculosis.

URINARY TRACT PROCEDURES

Bladder Catheterization

Indications

- Relieving urinary retention
- Collect an uncontaminated urine specimen for diagnostic purposes
- Monitoring urinary output in critically ill patients
- Performing bladder tests (cystogram, cystometrogram)

Contraindications

- Urethral disruption, often associated with pelvic fracture
- Acute prostatitis (relative contraindication)

Materials

- Prepackaged bladder catheter tray (may or may not include a Foley catheter)
- Catheter of choice (Figure 13–20 below):

Foley: Balloon at the tip to keep it in the bladder. Use a 16–18 Fr for adults (the higher the number, the larger the diameter). Irrigation catheters ("three-way Foley") should be larger (20–22 Fr).

Coudé (pronounced "COO-DAY"): An elbow-tipped catheter useful in males with prostatic hypertrophy (the catheter is passed with the tip pointing to 12 o'clock).

Red rubber catheter (Robinson): Plain rubber or latex catheter without a balloon, usually used for "in-and-out catheterization" in which urine is removed but the catheter is not left indwelling.

13

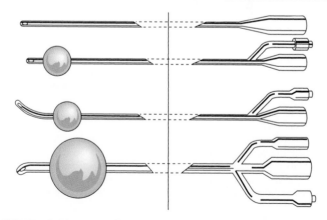

FIGURE 13–20. Types of bladder catheters include (from the top) the straight "Robinson" or red rubber catheter, Foley catheter with standard 5-mL balloon, the Coudé catheter, and "three-way" irrigating catheter with 30-mL balloon. Catheters have been shortened for illustrative purposes.

Procedure

1. Use strict aseptic technique.
2. Have the patient lie supine in a well-lighted area; females with knees flexed wide and heels together to get adequate exposure of the meatus.
3. Get all the materials ready before you attempt to insert the catheter. Open the kit, and put on the gloves. Open the prep solution, and soak the cotton balls. Apply the sterile drapes.
4. Inflate and deflate the balloon of the Foley catheter to ensure its proper function. Coat the end of the catheter with lubricant jelly.
5. In females, use one gloved hand to prep the urethral meatus in a pubis-toward-anus direction; hold the labia apart with the other gloved hand. With uncircumcised males, retract the foreskin to prep the glans; use a gloved hand to hold the penis still.
6. The hand used to hold the penis or labia should not touch the catheter to insert it; a disposable forceps in the kit can be used to insert it. Or the forceps can be used to prep, then the gloved hand can insert the catheter.
7. In the male, **stretch** the penis upward perpendicular to the body to eliminate any internal folds in the urethra that might lead to a false passage. Use **steady, gentle** pressure to advance the catheter. The bulbous urethra is the most likely part to tear. Any significant resistance encountered may represent a stricture and requires urologic consultation. In males with BPH, a Coudé tip catheter may facilitate passage. Some tricks used to get a catheter to pass in a male are to make sure that the penis is well stretched and to instill 30–50 mL of sterile water-based surgical lubricant (K-Y jelly) into the urethra with a catheter-tipped syringe prior to passage of the catheter. Viscous lidocaine jelly for urologic use can help lubricate and relieve the discomfort of difficult catheter placement. Allow at least 5 min after instillation of the lidocaine jelly for the anesthetic effect to take place.
8. In both males and females, insert the catheter to the hilt of the drainage end. In males, compress the penis toward the pubis. These maneuvers ensure that the balloon inflates in the bladder and not in the urethra. Inflate the balloon with 5–10 mL of sterile water or, occasionally, air. After inflation, pull the catheter back so that the balloon comes to rest on the bladder neck. There should be good urine return when the catheter is in place. If a large amount of lubricant jelly was placed into the urethra, the catheter may need to be flushed with sterile saline to clear the excess lubricant. A catheter that will not irrigate is probably **in the urethra, not the bladder.**
9. In uncircumcised males, reposition the foreskin to prevent massive edema of the glans after the catheter is inserted.
10. Catheters in females can be taped to the leg. In males, the catheter should be taped to the abdominal wall to decrease stress on the posterior urethra and help prevent stricture formation. The catheter is usually attached to a gravity drainage bag or some device for measuring the amount of urine. Many new kits come with the catheter already secured to the drainage bag. These systems are considered "closed" and should not be opened if at all possible.

"In-and-Out" Catheterized Urine

1. If urine is needed for analysis or for culture and sensitivity, especially in a female patient, a so-called in-and-out catheterization can be done. This is

also useful for measuring residual urine in males or females. The incidence of inducing infection with this procedure is about 3%.

2. The procedure is identical to that described for bladder catheterization. The main difference is that a red rubber catheter (no balloon) is often used and is removed immediately after the specimen is collected.

Clean-Catch Urine Specimen

1. A clean-catch urine is useful for routine urinalysis, is usually good for culturing urine from males, but is only fair for culturing urine from females because of the potential for contamination.

2. For males:
   a. Expose the glans, clean with a povidone-iodine solution and dry it with a sterile pad.
   b. Collect a midstream urine in a sterile container after the initial flow has escaped.

3. For females:
   a. Separate the labia widely to expose the urethral meatus; keep the labia spread throughout the procedure.
   b. Cleanse the urethral meatus with povidone-iodine solution from front to back, and rinse with sterile water.
   c. Catch the midstream portion of the urine in a sterile container.

Percutaneous Suprapubic Bladder Aspiration

Indications

(Used most frequently in young children)
- When urine cannot be obtained by a less invasive method
- In the presence of urethral abnormalities
- In the presence of a refractory UTI

13

Contraindications

- If the child has voided within the last hour, or if the bladder cannot be percussed

Procedure

1. This procedure is almost exclusively limited to the very young pediatric patient (usually < 6 mon).

2. Immobilize the child. Do not attempt this procedure if the child has voided within the last hour.

3. Palpate the bladder above the pubic symphysis (the bladder sticks out high above the pubis in a young child when it is full). Some suggest occluding the urethra by holding the penis in a male and by inserting a finger in the rectum to exert pressure in the female. Percuss out the limits of the bladder.

4. Obtain a 20-mL syringe with a 23- or 25-gauge, 1½-in. needle. Prep with povidone-iodine and alcohol 0.5–1.5 cm above the pubis. Anesthesia is not routinely used.

5. Insert the needle perpendicular to the skin in the midline; maintain negative pressure on the downstroke and on withdrawal until urine is obtained (Figure 13–21).

6. If no urine is obtained, wait at least 1 h before reattempting the procedure.

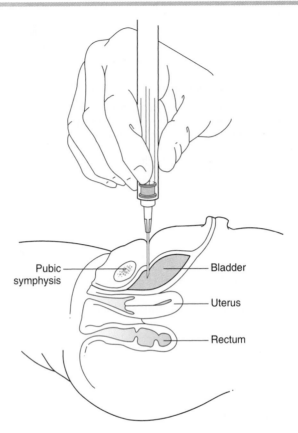

FIGURE 13–21.   The technique and anatomic structures in suprapubic bladder as-piration. (Reprinted, with permission, from: Gomella TL [ed] *Neonatology: Basic Management, On-Call Problems, Diseases, Drugs,* 5th ed. McGraw-Hill, 2004.)

VENIPUNCTURE

Indications

- Venipuncture (**phlebotomy**) is the puncture of a vein to obtain a sample of venous blood for analysis.

Materials

- A tourniquet (a 1½-in. Penrose drain or BP cuff are acceptable replacements)
- Alcohol prep pad, gauze pad, and adhesive bandage
- Proper specimen tubes for desired studies (red top, purple top, etc) (Table 13–8, page 318)
- Appropriate-sized syringe for volume of blood needed (5 mL, 10 mL, etc), or a Vacutainer tube and appropriate needle and Vacutainer holder.

TABLE 13-8
Tube Guide for Venipuncture Using the Vacutainer System (from Becton, Dickson & Company)

Vacutainer Tubes	Vacutainer Hemogard Closure	Additive	Number or Inversions at Blood Collection (Invert gently, do not shake)	Laboratory Use
Black/red marbled ("Tiger Top")	Gold	Clot activator and gel for serum separation	5	SST brand tube for serum demonstrations in chemistry. Tube inversions ensure mixing of clot activator with blood and clotting within 30 min
Green/red marbled	Light green	Lithium heparin and gel for plasma separation	8	PST brand tube for plasma determinations in chemistry. Tube inversions prevent clotting
Red	Red	None	0	For serum determinations in chemistry, serology, and blood banking.
Yellow/black marbled	Orange	Thrombin	8	For stat serum determinations in chemistry. Tube inversions prevent clotting, usually in less than 5 min
Royal blue	Royal blue	Sodium heparin Na EDTA None	8 8 0	For trace element, toxicology, and nutrient determinations. Special stopper formulation offers the lowest verified levels of trace elements available. (See package insert)

13

(continued)

TABLE 13–8
(Continued)

Vacutainer Tubes	Vacutainer Hemogard Closure	Additive	Number or Inversions at Blood Collection (Invert gently, do not shake)	Laboratory Use
Green	Green	Sodium heparin	8	For plasma determinations in chemistry. Tube inversions prevent clotting
		Lithium heparin	8	
		Ammonium heparin	8	
Gray	Gray	Potassium oxalate/ Sodium fluoride	8	For glucose determinations. Tube inversions ensure proper mixing of additive and blood. Oxalate and heparin, anticoagulants, will give serum samples that are serum
		Sodium fluoride	8	
		Lithium iodoacetate	8	
			8	
Brown	Brown	Sodium heparin	8	For lead determinations. This tube is certified to contain less than .01 μ/mL (ppm) lead. Tube inversions prevent clotting
Yellow	Yellow	Sodium polyanetholesulfonate (SPS)	8	For blood culture specimen collections in microbiology. Tube inversions prevent clotting.

(continued)

13

318

TABLE 13-8
(Continued)

Vacutainer Tubes	Vacutainer Hemogard Closure	Additive	Number or Inversions at Blood Collection (Invert gently, do not shake)	Laboratory Use
Lavender	Lavender	Liquid EDTA Freeze-dried Na EDTA	8 8	For whole blood hematology determinations. Tube inversions prevent clotting
Light blue	Light blue	0.105 M sodium citrate (3.2%) 0.129 M sodium citrate (3.8%)	8 8	For coagulation determinations on plasma specimens. Tube inversions prevent clotting. *Note:* Certain tests require chilled specimens. Follow recommended procedures for collection and transport of specimen

EDTA = ethylene diamine tetraacetic acid.

13

BD Eclipse blood collection system includes a manually activated needle shield.

- A 20–22-gauge needle (Larger needles are uncomfortable, and smaller ones can cause hemolysis or clotting; the higher the gauge number, the smaller the needle, see Figure 13–1A.)

Procedure

Blood cultures, IV techniques, and arterial punctures are discussed in other sections of the chapter.

1. Collect the necessary materials before you begin, including extras in case there is a problem.
2. The common sites for routine venipuncture are the veins of the antecubital fossa (see Figure 13–12, page 285). Alternative sites include the dorsum of the hand, the forearm, the saphenous vein near the medial malleolus, or the external jugular vein. If peripheral sites are unacceptable, use the femoral vein. **Never draw a blood sample proximal to an IV site due to** the high concentration of IV fluid in the veins.
3. Apply the tourniquet at least 2–3 in. above the venipuncture site. Have the patient make a fist to help engorge the vein. If veins are difficult to locate, try gently slapping/flicking the vein to cause reflex dilation, hang the extremity in a dependent position, wrapping the extremity in a warm wet towel, substituting a BP cuff for the standard tourniquet, or applying nitroglycerin paste below and over the area may help dilate the veins.
4. Swab the site with the alcohol prep pad, and allow the alcohol to evaporate.
5. The **Vacutainer system** has become the standard means of collecting blood for analysis. Screw 20–22-gauge Vacutainer needle on the Vacutainer cup, and rotate the safety shield back. The Eclipse needle system (Becton Dickinson) has a shield to cover the end of the needle that is manually activated after the sample is collected. Remove the protective needle cap.
6. Keep the needle bevel up, and puncture the skin alongside the vein. After the needle is through the skin, use the thumb of your free hand to stabilize the vein and prevent it from rolling. Enter the vein on the side at about a 30-degree angle. An alternative technique is to enter both the skin and vein in one stick. This maneuver requires practice because the vein is often punctured through and through.
7. Advance the appropriate collection tube (See Table 13-8, page 317) onto the needle inside the Vacutainer cup. The vacuum inside the tube automatically collects the sample. If you hold the Vacutainer steady, several tubes can be collected in this fashion.
8. After the blood is collected, remove the tourniquet, withdraw the needle, and apply firm pressure with the alcohol swab or sterile gauze for 2–3 min. The BD Eclipse needle allows rapid one-handed reshielding of the needle tip. Elevation of the extremity is helpful for limiting hematoma. Bending the arm actually increases the size of the venipuncture site and should be discouraged.
9. If no peripheral veins can be located, puncture of the **femoral vein** can be attempted. Locate the femoral artery. The mnemonic of lateral to medial structures in the groin is **NAVEL: N**erve, **A**rtery, **V**ein, **E**mpty space, **L**ymphatic. The femoral vein should be just medial to the femoral artery.

After prepping the skin, insert the needle perpendicular to the skin, and gently aspirate. The vein should be about 1-1½ in. below the skin.

Apply firm pressure after the collection of the sample; hematomas are frequent complications of femoral venipunctures. Should you accidentally enter the femoral artery, it is acceptable to collect the sample. Apply pressure for a longer period (5 min) if the artery is entered.

10. In children and the elderly with fragile veins, a butterfly (21–25 gauge) can be used to obtain a sample (see Figure 13–14).A syringe can be attached or a needleless Vacutainer system can be used.

PAIN MANAGEMENT

Defining Pain and Educating the Patient
Classification of Pain
Adverse Physiologic Effects of Pain
Assessing Pain

Practical Pain Management (Acute vs
    Chronic)
Patient-Controlled Analgesia

DEFINING PAIN AND EDUCATING THE PATIENT

The International Association for the Study of Pain defines pain as: An "unpleasant sensory and emotional experience associated with actual or potential tissue damage." Pain is the most common symptom that brings patients to see a physician, and it is frequently the first alert of an ongoing pathologic process. It is critically important, whenever possible, to inform the patient beforehand about the nature and the degree of pain to be expected during their hospital stay. Pain control options during and after hospitalization should be made clear, thus patients will have realistic expectations.

CLASSIFICATION OF PAIN

Somatic Pain

A well-localized constant, achy area in skin and subcutaneous tissues and a bit less well-localized in bone, connective tissues, blood vessels, and muscles. Examples of somatic pain include incisional pain, bone fractures, bony metastases, osteo/rheumatoid arthritis, and peripheral vascular disease.

Visceral Pain

This type of pain is poorly localized, crampy, diffuse, and deep, and originates from an internal organ or a cavity lining. Examples of visceral pain include bladder distention or spasms, intestinal distention, inflammatory bowel disease, hiatal hernia, organ metastasis, and pericarditis.

Neuropathic Pain

This electric-shock-like, lancinating, shooting pain may originate from an injury to a peripheral nerve, the spinal cord, or the brain, and it is poorly localized. Examples of this type of pain include diabetic neuropathy, radiculopathy, postherpetic neuralgia, phantom limb pain, and tumor-related nerve compression.

ADVERSE PHYSIOLOGIC EFFECTS OF PAIN

Table 14–1, page 324 shows adverse effects of pain as they relate to specific organ systems.

ASSESSING PAIN

Always keeping in mind the multiple facets of this assessment: the physiologic, emotional, and psychologic aspect. A good physician may want to ask appropriate questions regarding the patients' discomfort. A detailed history is almost always pertinent in supplying information regarding the patients' pain.

TABLE 14–1
Adverse Physiologic Sequelae of Pain

Organ System	Adverse Effect
RESPIRATORY	
Increased skeletal muscle tension	Hypoxia, hypercapnia
Decreased total lung compliance	Ventilation–perfusion abnormality, atelectasis, pneumonitis
ENDOCRINE	
Increased adrenocorticotropic hormone	Protein catabolism, lipolysis, hyperglycemia
Decreased insulin, decreased testosterone	Decreased protein anabolism, decreased sex drive
Increased aldosterone, increased antidiuretic hormone	Salt and water retention, congestive heart failure, edema
Increased catecholamines	Vasoconstriction, hypertension
Increased angiotensin II	Increased myocardial contractility
CARDIOVASCULAR	
Increased myocardial work	Dysrhythmias, angina, ischemia
IMMUNOLOGIC	
Lymphopenia, depression of reticuloendothelial system leukocytosis	Decreased immune function, increased susceptibility to infection
Reduced killer T-cell cytotoxicity	
COAGULATION EFFECTS	
Increased platelet adhesiveness, diminished fibrinolysis	Increased incidence of thromboembolic phenomena
Activation of coagulation cascade	
GASTROINTESTINAL	
Increased sphincter tone	Ileus
Decreased smooth muscle tone	
GENITOURINARY	
Increased sphincter tone	Urinary retention
Decreased smooth muscle tone	

14

Information about what makes the pain better, and what makes it worse is as important as how long the pain lasts; is it constant or intermittent? Does it have any precipitating factors? Does the pain radiate to a specific extremity or is it referred from an internal source? An example of a pain radiating to a limb is lower back pain with associated right or left leg radiation. An example of referred pain is a ureteral calculus referring pain to the ipsilateral testicle. Are there any accompanying symptoms such as nausea, vomiting or headache?

In addition to a thorough physical exam, a number of pain assessment instruments and rating scales can be used to further stratify the patients' level of pain.

Visual Analogue Scales

These are often referred to as the "fifth vital sign". Patients are asked to indicate on a visual scale the intensity of their pain with these scales being particularly useful for assessing pain management interventions. Examples of commonly used visual scales are shown in Figure 14–1 below.

McGill Pain Questionnaire: The MPQ (Malzack RR: The McGill Pain Questionnaire: Major properties and scoring methods. *Pain* 1975; 1:227–299) is a checklist of words describing symptoms. Scores are then analyzed in various dimensions (sensory and affective) to identify the quality of pain. This tool can be used in the detailed management of pain syndromes.

Psychologic Evaluation: A psychologic evaluation is indicated if medical work-up fails to reveal any apparent cause for the patients' pain. *The Minnesota Multiple Personality Inventory* (Hathway SR and McKinley JC: MMPI. University of Minnesota Press, Minneapolis, 1989) and Beck Depression Inventory (Beck AT, Steer RA: Internal consistencies of the original and revised Beck Depression Inventory. *J Clin Psychol* 1984;40(6):1365–1367) are two frequently used tools for evaluating chronic pain and depression. These questionnaires not only determine the patient's psychologic status but may also evaluate his or her behavior and response to pain and its management.

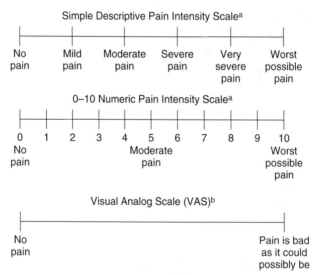

FIGURE 14–1.   Various scales used to determine pain intensity. The patient is asked to indicate where on the scale they would rate their pain level. (Reprinted, with permission, from: *Clinical Practice Guidelines Number 9: Management of Cancer Pain,* Rockville, MD, US Department of Health and Human Services ACHPR Publication 94-0592.)

Electromyography and Nerve Conduction Testing: This method differentiates between neurogenic and myogenic causes and confirms diagnosis of nerve entrapment, neural trauma, and polyneuropathies.

Thermography: Normally, heat from body surfaces is emitted in the form of infrared energy; this emission is symmetrical in homologous areas. Neurogenic pathophysiologic changes result in asymmetry. This infrared energy can be measured and displayed; hyperemission indicates an acute stage and hypoemission a chronic stage.

Diagnostic and Therapeutic Neural Blockade: Neural blockade with local anesthetics can be used to diagnose and manage both acute and chronic pain.

PAIN MANAGEMENT (ACUTE VS CHRONIC)

The goal of pain management is to provide the patient adequate relief with minimum side effects (eg, drowsiness). Always begin therapy with the lowest dose of any medicine that provides significant relief.

Pain management can be generally divided into:

- Pharmacologic
- Nonpharmacologic
- Combinations according to the patient response and compliance

Pharmacologic

The World Health Organization has made specific recommendations concerning pain management. These principles apply primarily to cancer pain but can be used in any clinical setting. Start at step 1 and advance to the next level based on patient's response.

Step 1: Nonopioid agents (NSAIDs, acetaminophen, aspirin, COX-2 inhibitors, etc)
Step 2: Weak opioids (codeine, oxycodone) or opioid-like agents

- Use concurrently with level one agents (ie, oxycodone, hydrocodone combinations)
- Weak opioids as single agents (immediate release codeine, propoxyphene)
- Opioid agonist/antagonists (pentazocine, butorphanol)
- Other agents such as ketorolac or tramadol

Step 3: Strong opioids. Controlled-release oxycodone, morphine, or fentanyl
Step 4: There may be a fourth step in which a multimodal approach is warranted.(ie, neurolysis)

Specific pharmacologic agents are reviewed in the following section and in Table 14–2. Additional pharmacologic information can be found in Chapter 22. Supplements can enhance the effects of analgesics and allow dose reduction of some agents.

Nonopioid Analgesics: A multimodal approach may involve pharmacologic and nonpharmacologic venues of treatment. Aspirin, acetaminophen, and NSAIDs are the principle nonopioid analgesics used to treat mild and moderate pain. NSAIDs are primarily cyclooxygenase inhibitors that prevent prostaglandin-mediated amplification of chemical and mechanical irritants of the sensory pathways. Short-term (maximum 5 d of use) perioperative use of ketorolac (Toradol) can reduce pain medication requirement. **Side effects:** Possible hepatotoxicity (large dose of acetaminophen); stomach upset, nausea, dyspepsia,

TABLE 14-2
List of Commonly Used Analgesic Agents

Generic and (Brand) Names	Dose range/ Interval (Adults)	Dose range/ Interval (Children)	Indications	Contra-indications	Comments
Acetaminophen (Tylenol)	650–1000 mg/ q4–6h and PRN; max 4000 mg/d	10–15 mg/kg q4h	Mild/moderate pain. Use in aspirin-sensitive patients	Caution in liver disease, or history of alcohol abuse	No peripheral antiinflammatory effects, unlike NSAIDs
Tramadol	50–100mg/ q4–6h; daily max 400mg/d	Not recommended under age 16	Moderate/ moderately severe pain	Caution if used with hypnotics, centrally acting analgesics, opioids, or psychotropic drugs or acute intoxication with alcohol	Risk of nausea, dizziness, seizure risk in patients on SSRIs, tricyclics, MAO inhibitors, neuroleptics and history of seizures; seizure risk increased >400 mg/d
SALICYLATES—ACETYLATES					
Aspirin	650–975 mg daily q4h; max. 4000 mg	10–15 mg/kg 1 q4h	Mild/moderate pain	Do not use in children < 12 w/viral illness because of risk of Reyes syndrome	Risk of GI bleeding, ulcers, perforation, platelet dysfunction. Must be discontinued for 7–10 days if patient is to undergo surgery

(continued)

14

327

TABLE 14–2
(Continued)

Generic and (Brand) Names	Dose range/ Interval (Adults)	Dose range/ Interval (Children)	Indications	Contra-indications	Comments
SALICYLATES—NONACETYLATED					
Choline magnesium trisalicylate (Trilisate)	1000–1500 mg bid; daily max 2000–3000 mg	25 mg/kg bid	Long-term management of OA, RA; acute pain of shoulder or knee	Sensitivity to nonacetylated salicylates	Useful in patients with bony metastases and those who are allergic to ASA. The drug has minimal antiplatelet activity.
Diflunisal (Dolobid)	1000 mg initial, followed by 500 mg q12h; 1500 mg/d max	Not recommended under age 12	Acute and long-term mild to moderate pain; OA, RA	Hypersensitivity to aspirin or other NSAIDs	Potential for life-threatening (NSAID) hypersensitivity syndrome; disrupts platelet function with high doses; Reyes syndrome
Salsalate (Disalcid)	500 mg q4h; daily max. varies	Not indicated	Pain related to OA, RA, other rheumatic disorders	Hypersensitivity or allergy to salicylate	Minimal antiplatelet activity; useful in patients with bony metastases and those who are allergic to ASA

(continued)

TABLE 14-2
(Continued)

Generic and (Brand) Names	Dose range/ Interval (Adults)	Dose range/ Interval (Children)	Indications	Contra- indications	Comments
NONSELECTIVE NSAIDs					
Ibuprofen (Advil, Motrin, Nu-prin, Medi-prin, Rufen)	600–800 mg q6–8hr; daily max. 2400	10 mg/kg q4–8h	Mild/moderate pain, fever in children, RA, OA, other pain	Hypersensitivity to aspirin or other NSAIDs; severe kidney disease	Increases risk of GI bleeding, ulcers, perforation, platelet dysfunction
Indomethacin (Indocin)	25 mg q8–12h; daily max. 100 mg	Not indicated for pediatric use	Mild/severe acute pain, OA, RA, other rheumatic disorders	Hypersensitivity to aspirin or other NSAIDs	Usually a second-line drug because of high incidence of GI, and CNS sensory adverse effects
Ketorolac (Toradol)	30–60 mg IM or 30 mg IV initial, 15 or 30 IV or IM q6h, also available PO	Not indicated for pediatric use	Short-term management of moderate to severe acute pain, eg, postoperative	Hypersensitivity to aspirin or other NSAIDs; GI disease; bleeding disorders; renal disorders; labor and delivery; nursing mothers	Increases risk of renal failure in dehydrated patients; may cause fluid retention, CHF. Treatment should be limited to 5 d max.

(continued)

14

329

TABLE 14-2
(Continued)

Generic and (Brand) Names	Dose range/ Interval (Adults)	Dose range/ Interval (Children)	Indications	Contra-indications	Comments
NONSELECTIVE NSAIDs					
Nabumentone (Relafen)	1000–2000 mg/day q12–24h; daily max. 2000 mg	Not indicated for pediatric use	Signs/symptoms of OA, RA, ankylosing spondylitis	Hypersensitivity to aspirin or other NSAIDs	Has increased risk of GI bleeding, ulcers and perforation like any other NSAIDs
Naproxen (Aleve, Anaprox, Naprosyn)	550 mg initial, 250 subsequent q6–8h; daily max. 1250–1375 (depends on formulation)	5 mg q12h	Acute/chronic pain of OA, RA, other rheumatic type disorders	Hypersensitivity to aspirin or other NSAIDs	Risk of GI bleeding, ulcers and perforation
Oxoprozin (Daypro)	600–1200 mg q24h; daily max 1800 mg	Not indicated for pediatric use	Acute and long-term management of OA, RA	Hypersensitivity to aspirin or other NSAIDs	Increased NSAID related. Risk of GI bleeding, ulcers, perforation
Piroxicam (Feldene)	20mg/day, q12-24h; daily max. 20 mg	Not indicated for pediatric use	Acute and long-term management of OA, RA	Hypersensitivity to aspirin or other NSAIDs	Increases risk of GI bleeding, ulcers, perforation; steady-state blood levels are reached in 7–12 d

(continued)

TABLE 14-2
(Continued)

Generic and (Brand) Names	Dose range/ Interval (Adults)	Dose range/ Interval (Children)	Indications	Contra- indications	Comments
COX-2 SELECTIVE NSAIDs					
Celecoxib (Celebrex)	100–200 mg q12–24h; 400 mg daily max. acute pain 400 mg initially followed by 200 mg dose for break-through pain	Not indicated for pediatric use	Signs/symptoms of OA, RA; also used to reduce number of polyps in patients with familial adenomatous polyposis	Hypersensitivity to aspirin or other NSAIDs	Less risk of GI bleeding/ulceration than nonselective NSAIDs; may alter use with renal function; caution in patients with a history of allergy to sulfonamides
Rofecoxib (Vioxx)	12.5–50 mg q24h; daily max 50 mg; 50 mg cannot be given for more than 5 d	Not indicated for pediatric use	Signs/symptoms of OA, RA	Hypersensitivity to aspirin or other NSAIDs	Less risk of GI bleeding/ulceration than nonselective NSAIDs; may alter use with renal function, cause dose-dependent peripheral edema and increased BP; use w/caution in patients at risk for cardiovascular problems

(continued)

14

TABLE 14-2
(Continued)

Generic and (Brand) Names	Dose range/ Interval (Adults)	Dose range/ Interval (Children)	Indications	Contra- indications	Comments
COX-2 SELECTIVE NSAIDs					
Valdecoxib (Bextra)	10–40 mg q12–24h, depending on indication	Not indicated for pediatric use	Signs/symptoms of OA, RA; other pain	Hypersensitivity to aspirin or other NSAIDs	Less risk of GI bleeding/ulceration than nonselective NSAIDs. May affect renal function; and use w/caution in patients with history of allergy to sulfonamides
Carisoprodol (Soma)	350 mg q8h and hs	Not indicated	Acute, painful musculoskeletal conditions; does not directly relax tense skeletal muscles	Acute intermittent porphyria; sensitivity to related compounds	Caution in patients with altered kidney/liver function it has potential for abuse
Cyclobenza- prine HCl (Flexeril)	20–40 mg/day q6–8h; daily max. 60 mg	Not indicated	Muscle spasm associated with acute painful musculoskeletal conditions	Use of MAO inhibitors; acute MI; heart disorders; hyperthyroidism	Enhances the effects of alcohol, barbiturates, and other CNS depressants

(continued)

TABLE 14-2
(Continued)

Generic and (Brand) Names	Dose range/ Interval (Adults)	Dose range/ Interval (Children)	Indications	Contra-indications	Comments
OPIOID ANALGESICS					
Codeine	15–60 mg q4–6h; daily max. varies	1 y old; 0.5 mg/kg q4–6h	Mild to moderate pain	Hypersensitivity to codeine	Drug effects may be exaggerated in head injury; may obscure its clinical course, caution with liver/kidney disease. May cause significant respiratory depression; patients should be monitored judiciously either with pulse oxymetry or respiratory checks or both
Hydromorphone (Dilaudid)	Start tabs 2–4 mg q4–6h; liquid 2.5–10 mL q3–6h; daily max. varies	Not indicated	Moderate to severe pain	Impaired respiration	Caution in head injury, abdominal conditions and decrease dose with older patients. Significant respiratory depression may occur, monitor respiration carefully
Meperidine (Demerol, Mepergan)	Tabs/syrup: 50–150 mg q3–4h; daily max. 600 mg	Tabs/syrup: 0.5–1 mg/lb q3–4h	Moderate to severe pain	Do *not* use concomitantly with MAO inhibitors. Avoid its use in elderly and renal disease.	Caution in head injury, abdominal conditions, sickle cell disease, impaired respiration; may cause seizures, psychosis, anxiety, delirium, toxic metabolites; normeperidine can accumulate, especially in renal insufficiency and the elderly

(continued)

14

333

TABLE 14-2
(Continued)

Generic and (Brand) Names	Dose range/ Interval (Adults)	Dose range/ Interval (Children)	Indications	Contra-indications	Comments
OPIOID ANALGESICS					
Methadone (Dolophine)	Tabs/soln 2.5–10 mg q4h	Not indicated	Severe acute/chronic pain; Heroin withdrawal	Hypersensitivity to methadone	Caution in head injury, abdominal conditions, or concomitant use of other CNS depressants
Morphine immediate release (MSIR, Roxanol)	Oral forms given only after establishing daily opioid requirement; ½ daily requirement is given q12h	Some forms may be used in children; most are not indicated	Moderate to severe pain with opioids are needed for more than a few days	Respiratory depression, severe asthma, paralytic ileus	Use with caution in head injury, abdominal conditions, renal disease, use of other CNS depressants, and older patients. Respiratory depression precautions.
Morphine sustained release (Kadian, MS Contin, Oramorph SR, Avinza)	Used more often than immediate release; given only after establishing daily opioid requirement	Some forms may be used in children; most are not indicated	Moderate to severe pain	Respiratory depression, severe asthma, paralytic ileus	Caution in head injury, abdominal conditions, renal disease, use of other CNS depressants, and older patients. Respiratory depression precautions.

(continued)

14

TABLE 14-2
(Continued)

Generic and (Brand) Names	Dose range/ Interval (Adults)	Dose range/ Interval (Children)	Indications	Contra-indications	Comments
OPIOID ANALGESICS					
Oxycodone immediate release (OxyIR, Roxicodone)	Regimen can be individualized based on opioid/nonopioid requirements	Dosage forms should be adjusted for weight	Moderate to severe pain	Respiratory depression, severe asthma, paralytic ileus	Caution in head injury, abdominal conditions, renal disease, use of other CNS depressants
Oxycodone sustained release (OxyContin)	Regimen can be individualized based on opioid/nonopioid requirements	Not indicated < age 18	Moderate to severe pain	Respiratory depression, severe asthma, paralytic ileus	Caution in head injury, abdominal conditions, renal disease, use of other CNS depressants
Propoxyphene (Darvon)	100 mg q4h	Not indicated	Mild to moderate pain w/wo fever	Suicidal or addiction-prone patients; do not use with alcohol; hypersensitivity to propoxyphene	Propoxyphene metabolites may accumulate. Overdose may cause seizures. Drug carries risk of renal toxicity.

(continued)

14

335

TABLE 14-2
(Continued)

Generic and (Brand) Names	Dose range/ Interval (Adults)	Dose range/ Interval (Children)	Indications	Contra-indications	Comments
COMBINATION ANALGESICS					
Codeine/aceta-minophen (Tylenol w/ codeine)	15–60 mg/300–100 mg on varying sched-ule; daily max. 360/4000 mg; elixir form is available as well	Not indicated < age 3 years	Tabs for mild to moderately severe pain; elixir for mild to moderate pain	Hypersensitivity to any component	Use with caution in head injury, abdominal conditions and older patients.
Hydrocodone/ acetaminophen (Hydrocet, Lorcet, Lortab, Vicodine)	1–2 (mg/500 mg) caps 2 4–6h; daily max. 8 caps	Not indicated	Moderate to moderately severe pain	Hypersensitivity to hydrocodone or acetaminophen	Caution in head injury, abdominal conditions, respiratory depression may ensue, monitor respiratory function closely
Oxycodone/ acetamino-phen (Percocet, Roxicet, Tylox)	11 (5 mg/325 mg) tab q6h; daily max. varies	Not indicated	Moderate to moderately severe pain	Hypersensitivity to oxycodone or acetaminophen	Caution in head injury, abdominal conditions and elderly population

(continued)

14

TABLE 14-2
(Continued)

COMBINATION ANALGESICS

Generic and (Brand) Names	Dose range/ Interval (Adults)	Dose range/ Interval (Children)	Indications	Contra-indications	Comments
Propoxyphen/ acetaminophen (Darvocet)	100 mg/650 mg q4h; propoxy-phene daily max 600 mg	Not indicated	Mild to moderate pain w/wo fever	Hypersensitivity to propoxyphene or acetaminophen	Caution in head injury, abdominal conditions and impaired hepatic or renal functions
Pentazocine/ aspirin (Talwin)	2 (12.5 mg/325 mg) caplets q6–8h; daily max varies 30 mg IM/IV q3–4h; IM max 60 mg; IV max 30 mg	Not recom-mended < age 12	Moderate pain	Hypersensitivity to pentazocine or acetaminophen	Potential for abuse. Caution in head injury, abdominal conditions, may cause respiratory depression, renal/hepatic disorders and risk of Reyes syndrome. Subcutaneous injections may cause severe tissue damage
Hydrocodone/ ibuprofen (Vicoprofen)	1 (7.5 mg/200 mg) tablet q4–6h; max 4 tabs/d	Not recom-mended < age 16	Best for short-term (< 10 d) of mod-erate to severe acute pain treatment	Hypersensitivity to hydrocodone, ibuprofen, aspirin or other NSAIDs	Increases risk of anaphylactic reaction; poss-ible GI ulceration, bleeding, perforation; caution in head injury, abdominal con-ditions. Can cause respiratory depression

14

OA = osteoarthritis; RA = rheumatoid arthritis; NSAID = nonsteroidal antiinflammatories; SSRI = selective serotonin inhibitors; MAO = monoamine oxidase; GI = gastrointestinal; CHF = congestive heart failure; CNS = central nervous system; MI = myocardial infarction ulceration of gastric mucosa, dizziness, platelet dysfunction, exacerbation of bronchospasm, and acute renal insufficiency (aspirin and NSAIDs).

Opioids: These drugs attach to opioid receptors, which are responsible for their analgesic. **Side effects:** In the acute pain setting nausea/vomiting are the most common side effects and usually resolve with time or antiemetics. In the chronic pain setting, constipation is the most common side effect, and this unfortunately persists until treatment cessation. Other side effects may include sedation, miosis and dizziness with smaller doses, whereas larger doses may precipitate respiratory depression, apnea, circulatory arrest, comma, and death. These more serious side effects may require supplemental oxygen therapy, in addition to pulse oximetry monitoring and closer patient supervision. Opioids can be taken orally, parenterally, or neuroaxillary (intrathecal/epidural). They are available in short- (q4h) and long-duration forms (eg, q12h, q24h). Opioids can also be given as a patient-controlled analgesia IV (PCA) (see page 339). Comparison of different opioids can be found in Table 14–2.

Antidepressants: These drugs work well as adjuncts usually and are an appropriate consideration mostly with chronic pain associated with diabetic neuropathy, postherpetic neuralgia, and chemotherapy. **Side effects:** Antimuscarinic effects (dry mouth, impaired visual accommodation, urinary retention), antihistaminic (sedation), and alpha-adrenergic blockage (orthostatic hypotension), can all be present as side effects.

Neuroleptics: These agents may be useful in patients with agitation and psychologic symptomatology. **Side effects:** Their side effects include extrapyramidal and neuroleptic drug symptoms; mask-like facies, festinating gait, cogwheel rigidity (bradykinesia). These side effects may be treated with either benztropine or diphenhydramine.

Anticonvulsants: These medications act by suppressing spontaneous neural discharge. **Side effects:** Anticonvulsants side effects include bone marrow depression, hepatotoxicity, possible ataxia, dizziness, confusion, and sedation (at higher doses).

Corticosteroids: These are antiinflammatory agents. **Side effects:** Corticosteroids may cause hyperglycemia, and increased tendency to infection, peptic ulcer, osteoporosis, HTN, myopathies, and Cushing's syndrome.

Local Anesthetics: Local anesthetics bind to sodium channels, exerting their effect on the cellular level. Their effect is usually localized to the area where the drug is injected. **Side effects:** These drugs have relatively few side effects and safety profiles. Allergic reactions may occur but usually result from the PABA-like preservatives incorporated in the solution and not the local anesthetics themselves. Toxicity may occur if any of these agents are overdosed. Toxic levels of local anesthetics may precipitate tonic–clonic seizures, respiratory arrest, and subsequently cardiovascular collapse.

Benzodiazepines: Used to treat anxiety and muscle spasms associated mostly with acute pain. **Side effects:** These drugs have no analgesic effects and must be used with caution because of abuse potential.

Nerve Blocks or Neurolysis: Destruction of the nerve. **Side effects:** Permanent nerve damage

Nonpharmacologic

Physical Therapy: Heat and cold can provide pain relief by alleviating muscle spasm. Heat decreases joint stiffness and increases blood flow; cold vasoconstricts and reduces tissue edema.

Osteopathic or Chiropractic Treatment(s):   This physical manipulation is intended to relax soft tissues, increase range of motion, and alleviate pain. It may be done as biweekly or monthly treatments and is best for chronic pain. However, it can be used acutely to minimize musculoskeletal-type pain.

Radiation: This modality may be beneficial in treatment of cancer pain (ie, bony metastasis).

Psychologic Intervention: Using cognitive therapy, behavioral therapy, or biofeedback relaxation technique and hypnosis. Pain is often associated with depression especially when it becomes chronic.

Acupuncture: Needles are inserted into discrete anatomically defined points or meridians and stimulated by mild electric current. This method of treatment is believed to release endogenous opioids.

Electrical Stimulation of the Nervous System: Analgesia is achieved using various methods of treatment. The three methods are:

1. Transcutaneous electrical stimulation (TENS) with electrodes applied to skin.
2. Spinal cord stimulators: These devices involve inserting electrodes connected to an external generator into the epidural space. This is done under general anesthesia and the patient is awakened half-way through the procedure in the lateral recumbent position. The device is tested asking the patient specific questions and adjusting the programming accordingly. Then the patient is put to sleep again so the surgeon can close the skin.
3. Intracerebral stimulation with electrodes implanted in the periaqueductal or periventricular area.

14

PATIENT-CONTROLLED ANALGESIA (PCA)

Most commonly used after surgery, PCA allows the patient to self-administer doses of narcotics via an IV pump. The patient treats the pain as soon as he or she feels it coming on, thus avoiding the peak and trough of a narcotic dosing regimen that may lead to extremes of pain or have the potential of oversedation. The pain management team can titrate the dose of the drug as required using a computerized system that controls the total dose and the interval between each dose with or without a continuous basal infusion. PCA duration varies, based on procedure and patient response (eg, gyn 1–2 d, bowel 2–5 d, thoracotomy 4–6 d). Reduce dose in elderly ($1/3$–$2/3$), and consider discontinuation of PCA when patients are able to take analgesics PO.

PCA Ordering Parameters

Table 14–3, page 340 shows examples of PCA orders.

- **Dose:** Number of milliliters (typically morphine concentration or its equivalent) given on activation of button by patient
- **Lockout:** Minimum interval of time in minutes between PCA doses

TABLE 14–3
Illustrative PCA Orders

Typical Procedure	Dose (mL)	Lockout (min)	Hourly Max (mL)	Basal
Somewhat painful (lower abdominal, incisions, minor orthopedic, gynecologic or plastics procedures)	1	6	10	None
Fairly painful (upper abdominal incisions)	1–1.5	6	10–15	None. Nursing PRN bollus 2–3 mL q1–2 PRN
Very painful (thoracotomy, total knee replacement, shoulder joint repairs)	1–2.0	6	10–20	None Nursing PRN bolus 2–4 mL q1–2 PRN

- **Hourly Max:** Maximum volume (mL) that machine will administer in an hour
- **Basal Rate:** Continuous infusion rate may be programmed in addition to the bolus dosing, however, not recommended unless a qualified person from the anesthesiology department's pain team has evaluated the patient. Basal infusions increase the risk of significant respiratory depression and should be monitored more closely with hourly respiratory checks.
- **Nursing PRN Bolus:** Number of milliliters the nurses can administer at their own discretion in addition to PCA dose for breakthrough pain.

PCA Opiod Concentrations at Equipotent Levels

Drug	Dose
Morphine	1.0 mg/mL
Meperidine[a]	10 mg/mL
Hydromorphone	0.2 mg/mL
Fentanyl	10–15 μc/mL

[a]Use only if a patient has allergies to other medications secondary to its greater side effects profile (ie, seizure from metabolites).

PCA in Renal Failure (nonencephalopathic patient):

Use fentanyl or hydromorphone only, avoiding morphine and meperidine because of their renal excretion.

1. Load with fentanyl 25 mcg or hydromorphone 0.5 mcg IV in PACU and repeat every 5–10 min until patient is comfortable.
2. Maintenance: PCA dose 1 mL; lockout 6 min; hourly max 3–5 mL

IMAGING STUDIES

X-Ray Preparations
Common X-Ray Studies: Noncontrast
Common X-Ray Studies: Contrast
Ultrasound
Computed Tomography (CT) Scans
Spiral (Helical) CT Scan

Magnetic Resonance Imaging (MRI)
Nuclear Scans
Positron Emission Tomography (PET)
    Scans
How to Read a Chest X-Ray

X-RAY PREPARATIONS

In general, follow this principle: plain films studies should be obtained before studies that require oral contrast. Each hospital has its own guidelines for patient x-ray preps. Consult the radiology department prior to ordering. Examinations that require no specific bowel preparation include routine chest x-rays, flat and upright abdominal films, T-tube cholangiograms, cystograms, C-spines, skull series, extremity films, CT scan of the head or chest, and many others.

Studies that usually require such preps as enemas, laxatives, oral contrast agents, or those that require that the patient be NPO prior to the examination include oral cholecystogram, upper GI series, SBFT, barium enema, IVP, and many others.

COMMON X-RAY STUDIES: NONCONTRAST

Chest

Chest X-Ray (Routine):   Includes PA and lateral chest films. Used in the evaluation of pulmonary, cardiac and mediastinal diseases, and traumatic injury. See page 351 on How to Read a Chest X-Ray.

Expiratory Chest: Used to help visualize a small pneumothorax

Lateral Decubitus Chest: Allows small amounts of pleural effusion or suspected subpulmonary effusion to layer out and permits diagnosis of as little as 175 mL of pleural fluid

Lordotic Chest: Allows better visualization of apices and lesions of the right and left upper lobes. Often used in the evaluation of TB

Portable Chest and AP Films: Cannot be used to accurately evaluate heart size or widened mediastinum but can be used to detect effusions, pneumonia, edema, and to verify line or tube placement

Rib Details: Special views that more clearly delineate rib pathology; useful when plain chest radiogram or bone scan suggests fractures or other metastatic lesions.

Abdominal

Abdominal Decubitus: Used in debilitated patients instead of an upright abdominal film. The left side should be down to find free air outlining the liver and right lateral gutter.

Acute Abdominal Series ("obstruction series"): Includes a flat and upright abdominal (KUB) and chest x-ray. Good for initial evaluation of an acute abdomen (See KUB.)

Cross-Table Lateral Abdominal: Used in debilitated patients to look for free air

KUB, Supine and Erect: Short for "kidneys, ureter, and bladder" and also known as **"flat and upright abdominal," "scout film,"** or **"flat plate."** Useful when the patient complains of abdominal pain or distension, and for initial evaluation of the urinary tract (80% of kidney stones and 20% of gallstones are visualized on these films). To read, look for calcifications, foreign bodies, the gas pattern, psoas shadows, renal and liver shadows, flank stripes, the vertebral bodies, and pelvic bones. On the upright, look for air–fluid levels of an adynamic ileus or mechanical obstruction and for free air under the diaphragm, which suggests a perforated viscus or recent surgery; however, the upright chest x-ray (especially the lateral view) is often best to spot a pneumoperitoneum.

Other Noncontrast X-Rays

C-Spine: Usually includes PA, lateral, and oblique films. Useful for the evaluation of trauma, neck pain, and neurologic evaluation of the upper extremities. All seven cervical vertebrae must be seen for this study to be acceptable.

DEXA: Measures bone mineral density at a variety of sites (femur/lumbar spine); used in the diagnosis and monitoring of response to treatment of osteoporosis

Mammography: Detects cancers greater than 5 mm in size. Two forms equal in diagnostic quality:

- **Screen film.** Produces standard black and white x-ray via a specially designed mammographic machine; 3–5× smaller radiation dose
- **Digital mammography.** Digital images may improve the resolution over film techniques

Sinus Films (Paranasal Sinus Radiographs): Used to evaluate sinus trauma, sinusitis, neoplasms, or congenital disorders

Skull Films: Used to detect fractures and aid in the identification of pituitary tumors or congenital anomalies; not generally as useful as other imaging studies

Vertebral Radiography: Used to evaluate fractures, dislocations, subluxations, disk disease, and the effects of arthritic and metabolic disorders of the spine

COMMON X-RAY STUDIES: CONTRAST

An agent, such as barium or Gastrografin, or an IV contrast agent is used for these studies. If a GI tract fistula or perforation is suspected, inform the radiologist because this may affect the choice of contrast agent (ie, water-soluble contrast [eg, Gastrografin] instead of barium). Standard IV contrast media are ionic, potentially nephrotoxic, and may be associated with rare contrast reaction when administered systemically (see following section). The use of nonionic contrast media may limit these side effects.

Ionic Contrast Media

- Oral cholecystographic agents: Telepaque etc
- GI contrast agents: Barium sulfate—Baro-CAT, Tomocat, etc
- Injection:

  Diatrizoate meglumine: Hypaque Meglumine, Urovist Meglumine, Angiovist, etc
  Diatrizoate sodium: Hypaque Sodium, Urovist Sodium, etc
  Gadopentetate dimeglumine: Magnevist, etc
  Iodamide meglumine: Renovue, etc
  Iothalamate meglumine: Conray, etc
  Iothalamate sodium: Angio Conray, etc
  Diatrizoate meglumine and diatrizoate sodium: Angiovist, Hypaque-M, etc

- Not for intravascular use, for instillation into cavities:

  Diatrizoate meglumine, Cystografin, etc
  Diatrizoate meglumine and diatrizoate sodium Gastrografin, etc
  Diatrizoate sodium: Oral or rectal (Hypaque sodium oral)
  Iothalamate meglumine: Cysto-Conray urogenital
  Diatrizoate meglumine and iodipamide meglumine
  Sinografin intrauterine instillation

Nonionic Contrast Media

Injectable: Iohexol: Omnipaque; Iopamidol: Isovue; Ioversol: Optiray; Metrizamide: Amipaque

    Contrast reactions to IV agents may occur; severe reaction occurs 1/1000 and death due to anaphylaxis 1/40,000. Reactions include hives, bronchospasm, or pulmonary edema. (Premedication with steroids may not prevent a reaction.) Vagal reactions (hypotension and bradycardia) are another adverse effect. A history of asthma is a risk factor, and a previous reaction to contrast does not necessarily preclude using IV contrast (allergy to seafood or iodine is no longer considered an important risk factor). Premedication with two doses of PO methylprednisolone, once at 12 h prior and then 2 h prior to IV contrast, is effective in reducing the incidence of reactions. Alternatively, use of new and more expensive (up to 10× the cost) nonionic contrast agents, lessens pain and cardiovascular effects, with a possible overall decrease in adverse reactions.

Angiography: A rapid series of films obtained after a bolus contrast injection via percutaneous catheter. Used to image the aorta, major arteries and branches, tumors, and venous drainage via late "run-off" films. Helical CT scans are now capable of generating angiographic images.

- **DSA.** This is the latest enhancement of this study, allows reverse negative views and requires less contrast load
- **Cardiac angiography.** Definitive study for diagnosis and assessment of severity of CAD. Significant (> 70% occlusion) stenotic lesions seen: 30% involve single vessels, 30% involve two, and 40%, three vessels.
- **Cerebral angiography.** Evaluation of intra- and extracranial vascular disease, atherosclerosis, aneurysms, and A-V malformations. Not used for detection of cerebral structural lesions (use MRI or CT instead)
- **Pulmonary angiography.** Visualization of emboli, intrinsic or extrinsic vascular abnormalities, A-V malformations, and bleeding due to tumors.

15

Most accurate diagnostic procedure for PE but only used if helical CT or lung V/Q scan is not diagnostic

Barium Enema (BE): Examining the colon and rectum. Indications include diarrhea, crampy abdominal pain, heme-positive stools, change in bowel habits, and unexplained weight loss

- **Air-contrast BE.** Done with the "double contrast" technique (air and barium) to better delineate the mucosa. More likely to show polyps than standard BE
- **Gastrografin enema.** Similar to the barium enema, but water-soluble contrast is used (clears colon more quickly than barium). If the Gastrografin leaks from the GI tract, it is less irritating to the peritoneum (does not cause "barium peritonitis"). Therapeutic in the evaluation of severe obstipation or colonic volvulus, can identify postop anastomotic leak

Barium Swallow (Esophagogram): Evaluating the swallowing mechanism and investigating esophageal lesions or abnormal peristalsis

Cystogram: Bladder filled with and emptied with a catheter in place. Used to evaluate bladder filling defects (tumors, diverticula) and bladder perforation. Can also be done using CT scanning (see also VCUG)

Enteroclysis: Selective intubation of the proximal jejunum and rapid infusion of contrast. Better than an SBFT in evaluating polyps or obstruction (adhesions, internal hernia, etc). May be used to evaluate small-bowel sources of chronic bleeding after negative upper and lower endoscopy

ERCP: Contrast endoscopically injected into the ampulla of Vater to visualize the common bile and pancreatic ducts in evaluating obstruction, stones, and ductal pattern

ExU or IVP: Contrast study of the kidneys and ureters. Limited usefulness for evaluating bladder abnormalities. Indications include flank pain, kidney stones, hematuria, UTI, trauma, and malignancy. Bowel prep helpful but not essential. Verify recent creatinine level. Becoming largely replaced by CT urogram. **Nephrotomograms** often included with cuts of the kidney to further define the three-dimensional location or nature of renal lesions or stones

15

Fistulogram (Sinogram): Injection of water-soluble contrast media into any wound or body opening to determine the connection of the wound or opening with other structures

HSG: Evaluating uterine anomalies (congenital, fibroids, adhesions) or tubal abnormalities (occlusion or adhesion) often as part of infertility evaluation. Contraindicated during menses, undiagnosed vaginal bleeding, acute PID, or if pregnancy suspected. Patient in pelvic exam position, speculum placed and uterine os cannulated; then contrast injected

Lymphangiography. Iodinated oil injected to opacify lymphatics of the leg, inguinal, pelvic, and retroperitoneal areas. Used to test the integrity of the lymphatic system or evaluate for metastatic tumors (testicular, etc) or lymphoma

Myelogram: Evaluating the subarachnoid space for tumors, herniated disks, or other cause of nerve root injury. Using LP technique, contrast injected in the subarachnoid space

OCG: Oral contrast given for visualizing gallbladder; generally replaced by ultrasound evaluation

Percutaneous Nephrostogram: In the management of renal obstruction, percutaneous placement through the renal parenchyma and into the collecting system to relieve and or evaluate the level and cause of obstruction

PTHC: Visualizing biliary tree in a patient unable to concentrate the contrast medium (bilirubin > 3 mg/100 mL). Percutaneous needle inserted into a dilated biliary duct; contrast injected.

RPG: Contrast material injected into the ureters through a cystoscope. Indications include allergy to IV contrast medium, a kidney or ureter that cannot be visualized on an IVP, filling defects in the collecting system, renal mass, and ureteral obstruction

RUG: Demonstrates traumatic disruption of the urethra and urethral strictures

SBFT: Usually done after a UGI series. Delayed films show the jejunum and ileum. Used in the work-up of diarrhea, abdominal cramps, malabsorption, and UGI bleeding

T-Tube Cholangiogram: Contrast injection into T-tube placed in the common bile duct for drainage after gallbladder and common bile duct surgery. To evaluate the degree of swelling, look for residual stones, and evaluate patency of bile duct drainage

UGI Series: Includes the esophagogram plus the stomach and duodenum. Useful for visualizing ulcers, masses, hiatal hernias, and in the evaluation of heme-positive stools and upper abdominal pain

VCUG: Bladder filled with contrast through a catheter, then catheter is removed, and the patient allowed to void. Used for diagnosis of vesicoureteral reflux and urethral valves and in the evaluation of UTI

Venography, Peripheral: Contrast medium slowly injected into a small foot or ankle vein to evaluate patency of deep veins of leg and calf. Look for a filling defect or outline of a thrombus. Noninvasive exams for DVT, such as Doppler ultrasound and compression ultrasound; highly sensitive (> 90%) for proximal thrombi and have largely replaced contrast venography.

ULTRASOUND   `15`

Abdominal: Gallbladder (95% sensitivity in diagnosing stones), cholecystitis, biliary tree obstruction, pancreas (pseudo-cyst, tumor, pancreatitis), aorta (aneurysm), kidneys (obstruction, tumor, cyst), abscesses, ascites

Echocardiograms

- **M-mode.** Valve mobility, chamber size, pericardial effusions, septal size
- **Two-dimensional.** Valvular vegetations, septal defects, wall motion, chamber size, pericardial effusion, valve motion, wall thickness
- **Doppler.** Cross-valvular pressure gradients, blood flow patterns, and valve orifice areas in the work-up of cardiac valvular disease

Endovaginal: Most useful in the diagnosis of gynecologic pathology (uterus, ovaries)

Pelvic (A full bladder is desirable)

- **Pregnancy.** Fetal dating (biparietal diameters); diagnosis of multiple gestations; determination of intrauterine growth retardation, hydrocephalus, and hydronephrosis; localization of the placenta

- **Gynecology.** Ovarian and uterine masses (tumors, cysts, fibroids, etc.), ectopic pregnancy, abscesses

Thyroid: Evaluate thyroid nodules (cyst versus solid) and direct biopsies. Ultrasound alone cannot usually differentiate benign from malignant lesions.

Transrectal: Most useful in the diagnosis of rectal wall and prostate pathology, directing prostate biopsies, drain abscesses

Other Ultrasound Uses: Testicular (identify and characterize masses, eg, hydrocele versus tumor), intraoperative, determine bladder emptying

COMPUTED TOMOGRAPHY (CT) SCANS

Computerized tomography (also called CAT for computerized axial tomography) can be performed with or without IV contrast. A dilute oral contrast agent administered prior to abdominal or pelvic scans helps delineate the bowel. IV contrast is used to provide vascular and tissue enhancement for some CT scans; a current creatinine level should be available to determine suitability of IV contrast administration. Virtually any body part can be scanned depending on the indications, but CT is most helpful in evaluating the brain, lung, mediastinum, retroperitoneum (pancreas, kidney, nodes, aorta), and liver, and to a lesser extent in the pelvis, colon, or bone. CT scans allow for the use of density measurements (also known as **Hounsfield units**) to differentiate cysts, lipomas, hemochromatosis, vascular ("enhancing") and avascular ("nonenhancing") lesions. In Hounsfield units, bone is +1000, water is 0, fat is −1000, and other tissues fall within this scale, depending on the machine settings. Metal and barium can cause distortion of the image.

Abdomen: Images all intraabdominal and retroperitoneal organs and defines disease processes. Good accuracy with abscesses, but ultrasound may show smaller collections adjacent to the liver, spleen, or bladder. Surgical clips or barium in the gut may cause artifacts. IV contrast usually given, so check creatinine level; when using a water-soluble medium (Tomocat, others) to visualize the gut, the patient must receive an oral contrast beforehand.

Chest: Able to find 40% more nodules than whole lung tomograms, which demonstrate 20% more nodules than plain chest x-ray. Although calcification is suggestive of benign disease (eg, granuloma), no definite density value can reliably separate malignant from benign lesions. Useful in differentiating hilar adenopathy from vascular structures seen on plain chest x-ray; useful for interstitial lung disease

Head: Evaluation of tumors, subdural and epidural hematomas, atrioventricular (A-V) malformations, hydrocephalus, and sinus and temporal bone pathology. Initial test of choice for trauma; may be superior to MRI in detecting hemorrhage within first 24–48 h

Mediastinum: Masses, nodes, ectopic parathyroids

Neck: Work-up of neck masses, abscesses, and other diseases of the throat and trachea

Pelvis: Staging and diagnosis of bladder, prostate, rectal, and gynecologic carcinoma; diagnosis of appendicitis, diverticulitis, and complications of pregnancy

Retroperitoneum: Useful for evaluating pancreatitis and its complications; pancreatic masses; nodal metastasis from colon, prostate, renal, or testicular tumors; adrenal masses (> 3 cm suggestive of carcinoma); psoas masses; aortic aneurysms, retroperitoneal hemorrhage

Spine: MRI generally preferred over CT. However, rare conditions, contraindication to MRI, or artifact from metal may make the CT the preferred test.

SPIRAL (HELICAL) CT SCAN

Spiral CT can be used for any type of CT imaging and minimizes motion artifact and allows for capturing a bolus of contrast at peak levels in the region being scanned. Standard CT is too slow to capture this peak flow. Newer scanners (multidetector CT units) obtain multiple (4, 8, or 16) spiral scans at one time and provide higher resolution images compared with older units. These contrast-enhanced scans allow detailed 3-D reconstruction and angiographic evaluations. Bony structures can also be visualized and do not require contrast. The term *spiral/helical* is derived from the fact that the tube spins around the patient while the table moves. Spiral CT can compensate for "streak" artifact due to implanted metallic devices. Examples for uses of this technology include diagnosis of PE, pretransplant angiography, evaluation of flank pain and determination of kidney stones (largely replacing emergency IVP), and rapid evaluation of trauma.

MAGNETIC RESONANCE IMAGING (MRI)
How It Works

Certain key concepts are essential to interpreting studies generated by this technology. MRI uses measurements of the magnetic movements of atomic nuclei to delineate tissues. Specifically, when nuclei, such as hydrogen, are placed in a strong magnetic field, they resonate and emit radio signals when pulsed with radio waves. A defined sequence of magnetic pulses and interval pauses produces measured changes in the tissue's magnetic vectors, which results in an MRI image. T1, or longitudinal relaxation time, is the measurement of magnetic vector changes in the z axis during the relaxation pause. T2, or transverse relaxation time, is the magnetic vector changes in the x-y plane.

Each tissue, normal or pathologic, has a unique T1 and T2 for a given MRI field strength. In general T1 > T2. T1 = 0.1–2 s and T2 = 0.03–0.6 s. The inherent tissue differences between various T1's and T2's give the visual contrast seen between tissues on the MRI image. An image is **T1-weighted** if it depends on the differences in T1 measurements for visual contrast, or **T2-weighted** if the image depends on T2 measurements.

The oldest most common pulse sequence is called spin echo (SE). Partial saturation (PS) and inversion recovery (IR) are variations of the traditional SE sequence. Many sequences now use a gradient echo technique to obtain tissue contrast that is similar to that obtained with older SE methods. Available MRI views are transverse, sagittal, oblique, and coronal.

How to Read an MRI

SE T1-Weighted Images: Provide good anatomic planes due to the wide variances of T1 values among normal tissues.

- Brightest (high signal intensity): Fat
- Dark or black: Pathologic tissues, tumor or inflammation, fluid collections

15

- Black (low signal intensity): Respiratory tract, GI tract, calcified bone and tissues, blood vessels, heart chambers, and pericardial effusions

SE T2-Weighted Images: Pathology prolongs T2 measurements, and normal tissues have a very small range of T2 values. T2-weighted images provide the best detection of pathology and a decreased visualization of normal tissue anatomy. Tumor surrounded by fat may be lost on T2 imaging.

- Brightest : Fat and fluid collections
- Bright : Pheochromocytomas

When to Use MRI

In general, MRI provides superior soft tissue contrast compared with CT imaging. MRI is superior to CT for imaging of brain, spinal cord, musculoskeletal soft tissues, and areas of high CT bony artifact. However, spiral CT may now have overcome some of these disadvantages.

Advantages

- No ionizing radiation
- Display of vascular anatomy without contrast
- Visualization of linear structures: Spine and spinal cord, aorta, and cava
- Visualization of posterior fossa and other hard to see CT areas
- High-contrast soft tissue images

Disadvantages

- Claustrophobia due to confining magnet; **open** MRI scaners may obviate this problem
- Longer scanning time resulting in motion artifacts
- Unable to scan critically ill patients requiring life support equipment
- Metallic foreign bodies: Pacemakers, shrapnel, CNS vascular clips, metallic eye fragments, and cochlear implants are contraindications

MRI Contrast: Gadolinium (gadopentetic dimeglumine) is an ionic contrast agent that acts as a paramagnetic agent and enhances vessels or lesions with abnormal vascularity.

Uses of MRI

MRI is very sensitive to motion artifact; anxious or agitated patients may require sedation. Intramuscular glucagon may be used to suppress intestinal peristalsis on abdominal studies. If metallic eye fragments are possible, a screening CT of the orbits should be obtained prior to any MRI examination. It is generally contraindicated in patients with intracranial aneurysm clips, intraocular metallic fragments, and pacemakers. Dental fillings and dental prostheses have thus far not been a problem.

Abdomen: Useful for differentiating adrenal lesions, staging tumors (renal, GI, pelvic), evaluation of abdominal masses, and virtually all intraabdominal organs and retroperitoneal structures. Useful in differentiating benign adenomas from metastasis

Chest: Mediastinal masses, differentiates nodes from vessels, cardiac diseases, tumor staging, aortic dissection or aneurysm

Head: Analysis of all intracranial pathology may identify demyelinating diseases; some conditions are better evaluated by CT (see previous section), including acute trauma. **MRS** may increase the sensitivity of diagnosis of many neurologic diseases by providing a biochemical "fingerprint" of tissues in the brain. Performed in conjunction with an MRI equipped with the MRS capability. Some uses include differentiating dementias, tumors, MS, and many others.

Musculoskeletal System: Bone tumors, bone and soft tissue infections, evaluation of joint spaces (except if a prosthesis is in place), marrow disorders, aseptic necrosis of the femoral head

Pelvis: Evaluation of all pelvic organs in males and females. Differentiates endometrium from myoma and adenomyosis. Diagnosis of congenital uterine anomalies (eg, bicornuate, septate). Endorectal surface coil allows enhanced imaging of structures such as the prostate.

Spine: Diseases of the spinal column (herniated discs, tumors, etc)

NUCLEAR SCANS

The following is a listing of some of the more commonly used nuclear scans and their purposes. Most are contraindicated in pregnancy; check with your nuclear medicine department.

Adrenal Scan: Used to accurately localize a pheochromocytoma when MRI or CT is equivocal. Uses labeled **MIBG;** patient must return several days later for imaging after administration.

Bleeding Scan: Used to detect the source of GI tract bleeding.

- **Technetium-99m (^{99m}Tc) sulfur colloid scan.** Used to detect bleeding of 0.05–0.1 mL/min.
- **Technetium-99m (^{99m}Tc)-labeled red cell scan.** Same as sulfur colloid scan, but may be superior for localizing intermittent bleeding

Bone Scan: Metastatic work-ups (cancers most likely to go to bone: prostate, breast, kidney, thyroid, lung); evaluation of delayed union of fractures, osteomyelitis, avascular necrosis of the femoral head, evaluation of hip prosthesis, to distinguish pathologic from traumatic fractures

Brain Scan: Metastatic work-ups, determination of blood flow (in brain death or atherosclerotic disease), evaluation of space-occupying lesions (tumor, hematoma, abscess, [AV] malformation), and encephalitis

Cardiac Scans: Diagnosis of MI, stress testing, ejection fractions, measurement of cardiac output, diagnosis of ventricular aneurysms

- **Thallium-201 (^{201}Tl).** Examines myocardial perfusion via uptake of ^{201}Tl by normal myocardium. Normal myocardium appears hot, and ischemic or infarcted areas cold. AMI (< 12 h) seen as a hotspot, old MI (scar) seen as cold on both resting and exercise scans, and ischemia is cold on exercise scan and returns to normal after rest.
- **Technetium-99m (^{99m}Tc) pyrophosphate.** Recently damaged myocardium concentrates ^{99m}Tc pyrophosphate, producing a myocardial hotspot. Most sensitive 24–72 h after AMI
- **Technetium-99m (^{99m}Tc) ventriculogram.** ^{99m}Tc-labeled serum albumin or RBCs are used. Demonstrates abnormal wall motion, cardiac shunts, size and function of heart chambers, cardiac output, and ejection fraction. Another form of this study is the **MUGA scan,** data collection

15

from which is synchronized to ECG, and selected aspects are used to create a "moving picture" of cardiac function. May be done at rest or during exercise stress test.

Gallium Scans: Location of abscesses (5–10 d old), chronic inflammatory lesions, original lymphoma staging or follow-up for disease detection, lung cancer, melanoma, other neoplastic tissues

Hepatobiliary Scans (HIDA-Scan, BIDA-Scan): Differential diagnosis of biliary obstruction (when bilirubin > 1.5 and < 7 mg/100 mL), acute cholecystitis, diagnosis of biliary atresia; *not* good for stones unless cystic duct is completely occluded and acute cholecystitis present

Indium-111 (^{111}In) Octreotide (OctreoScan): Imaging method for tumors with somatostatin receptors (pheochromocytoma, gastrinomas, insulinomas, small-cell lung cancer)

Iodine-125 (^{125}I) Fibrinogen Scanning: Used to detect venous thrombosis in the lower extremities. After injection of the tracer, the patient is scanned several hours and for several days after. Most useful for identifying clot at or below the knees. False-positives with varicosities, cellulitis, incisions, arthritis, hematomas and with recent venography. Product availability is a problem at present.

Liver–Spleen Scan: Estimation of organ size, parenchymal diseases (hepatitis, etc), abscess, cysts, primary and secondary tumors

Lung Scan (V/Q Scan): Used along with a chest x-ray for evaluation of PE (a normal scan rules out a PE, an indeterminate scan requires further study via a pulmonary angiogram, and a clear perfusion deficit coupled with a normal ventilation scan is highly probable for a PE). V/Q scans can provide evidence of pulmonary disease, COPD, and emphysema.

Renal Scans: Agents are generally classified as functional tracers or morphologic tracers.

- **Iodine-131 (^{131}I) Hippuran.** Primarily a renal function agent; useful in renal insufficiency for evaluation of function; visualization is poor, and radiation dose can be high
- **Technetium-99m (^{99m}Tc) glucoheptonate.** Useful as a combination renal cortical imaging agent and renal function agent; primarily used to evaluate overall function, but can be used to determine vascular flow and to visualize the renal parenchyma and collecting system
- **Technetium-99m (^{99m}Tc) DMSA** (dimercaptosuccinic acid). Used only as a renal cortical imaging agent
- **Technetium-99m (^{99m}Tc) DTPA** (diethylenetriamine pentaacetic acid). Primarily a renal function agent; useful for renal blood flow studies, estimation of GFR, evaluation of the collecting system
- **Technetium-99m (^{99m}Tc) mercaptoacetyltriglycine (MAG3).** A relatively new agent, primarily a functional agent, very good imaging of the renal parenchyma can be obtained within minutes of injection and a low radiation dose. May eventually replace all other renal agents.

Strontium-89 (^{89}Sr)(Metastron): Not technically an imaging agent, but used in the palliative therapy of multiple painful bony metastasis (ie, prostate or breast cancer). Because this is a pure beta emitter, the radioactivity remains in the body, so no special precautions (other than blood and urine analysis) are needed.

SPECT Scan: **S**ingle-**p**hoton **e**mission-**c**omputed **t**omography, a technique whereby multiple nuclear images are sequentially displayed similar to a CT scan; can be applied to many nuclear scans.

Thyroid Scan: Most commonly with technetium-99m pertechnetate. Useful for evaluation of nodules (solitary cold nodules require a tissue diagnosis because 25% are cancerous). Scan patterns in correlation with lab tests may help diagnose hyperfunctioning adenomas, Plummer's and Graves' diseases, and multinodular goiters; localize ectopic thyroid tissues (especially after thyroidectomy for cancer); and identify superior mediastinal thyroid masses

POSITRON EMISSION TOMOGRAPHY (PET) SCAN

Positron emission tomography (PET) involves the injection of a positron-emitting tracer. This tracer is attached to a metabolically active molecule and accumulates in areas of increased metabolic activity. Tomographic images are obtained to localize the tracer within the body. PET scans are often obtained together with CT or MR scans—the functional information provided by the PET scan is correlated with the precise anatomic detail obtained from the CT or MR. The most commonly used PET tracer is 18-fluoro-deoxyglucose (18-FDG). Fluorine-18 decays by positron emission. As the positron is ejected from the nucleus it strikes an electron. The mutual annihilation of these two particles results in two photons that travel in exactly the opposite direction (180 degree difference). A PET scanner employs coincidence imaging of these two photons to determine the location of the original positron in the body.

The positron emitters used in PET generally have a short half-life. The half-life of ^{18}F is 110 min. This short half-life results in a low dose to the patient, but means that a cyclotron must be available to produce the agent shortly before it is to be used. There are several current clinical applications for PET imaging:

- **Cancer:** Because malignant tissue has a higher metabolic rate than benign tissue, PET tracers of glucose metabolism will be selectively concentrated in living tumor. PET is useful for detecting small foci of cancer that may be missed on standard CT or MR imaging. PET can also be used to distinguish live tumors from treated dead tissue and fibrosis. The tumors most commonly imaged with PET include colorectal cancer, lung cancer, brain cancer, breast cancer, lymphoma and melanoma.
- **Neurologic imaging:** To localize specific functions—to define functional neuroanatomy. PET has been used to localize epileptogenic foci in patients with seizures and may be useful in the diagnosis of various brain disorders, including dementia, depression, and schizophrenia.
- **Cardiac imaging:** PET can be used to define myocardial viability; PET is complementary to the anatomic information obtained from cardiac angiography and may be used in treatment planning.

15

HOW TO READ A CHEST X-RAY
Determine the Adequacy of the Film

- **Inspiration:** Diaphragm below ribs 8–10 posteriorly and 5–6 anteriorly
- **Rotation:** Clavicles are equidistant from the spinous processes
- **Penetration:** Disc spaces are seen, but bony details of spine cannot be seen

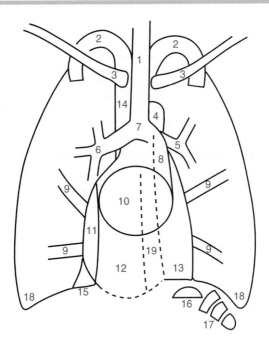

Posteroanterior Chest X-ray

1. Trachea
2. First rib
3. Clavicle
4. Aortic knob
5. Left pulmonary artery
6. Right pulmonary artery
7. Carina
8. Pulmonary trunk
9. Pulmonary veins

10. Left atrium
11. Right atrium
12. Right ventricle
13. Left ventricle
14. Superior vena cava
15. Inferior vena cava
16. Gastric air bubble
17. Splenic flexure air
18. Costophrenic angles
19. Descending aorta

FIGURE 15–1.   Structures seen on a posteroanterior (PA) chest x-ray film.

PA Film

Remember, the film is on the patient's chest and the x-rays are passing from back (posterior) to front (anterior). The structures described in the following material are shown in Figure 15–1 above.

Soft Tissues: Check for symmetry, swelling, loss of tissue planes, and subcutaneous air.

Skeletal Structures: Examine the clavicles, scapulas, vertebrae, sternum, and ribs. Look for symmetry. In a good x-ray, the clavicles are symmetrical. Check

15

for osteolytic or osteoblastic lesions, fractures, or arthritic changes. Look for rib-notching.

Diaphragm: Sides should be equal and slightly rounded, although the left may be slightly lower. Costophrenic angles should be clear and sharp. Blunting suggests scarring or fluid. It takes about 100–200 mL of pleural fluid to cause blunting. Check below the diaphragm for the gas pattern and free air. A unilateral high diaphragm suggests paralysis (either from nerve damage, trauma, or an abscess), eventration or loss of lung volume on that side because of atelectasis or pneumothorax. A flat diaphragm suggests COPD.

Mediastinum and Heart: The aortic knob should be visible and distinct. Widening of the mediastinum is seen with traumatic disruption of the thoracic aorta. In children, do not mistake the normally prominent thymus for widening. Mediastinal masses can be associated with Hodgkin's disease and other lymphomas. The trachea should be in a straight line with a sharp carina. Tracheal deviation suggests a mass (tumor), goiter, unilateral loss of lung volume (collapse), or tension pneumothorax. The heart should be less than one-half the width of the chest wall on a PA film. If greater than one-half, think of CHF or pericardial fluid.

Hilum: The left hilum should be up to 2–3 cm higher than the right. Vessels are seen here. Look for any masses, nodes, or calcifications.

Lung Fields: Note the presence of any shadows from CVP lines, NG tubes, pulmonary artery catheters, etc. The fields should be clear with normal lung markings all the way to the periphery. The vessels should taper to become almost invisible at the periphery.

Vessels in the lower lung should be larger than those in the upper lung. A reversal of this difference (called cephalization) suggests pulmonary venous hypertension and heart failure. **Kerley's B lines,** small linear densities found usually at the lateral base of the lung, are associated with CHF. Check the margins carefully; look for pleural thickening, masses, or pneumothorax. If the lungs appear hyperlucent with a relatively small heart and flattening of the diaphragms, COPD is likely. Thin plate-like linear densities are associated with atelectasis. To locate a lesion, do not forget to check a lateral film and remember the "silhouette sign." Obliteration of all or part of a heart border means the lesion is anterior in the chest and lies in the right middle lobe, lingula, or anterior segment of the upper lobe. A radiopacity that overlaps the heart but does not obliterate the heart border is posterior and lies in the lower lobes.

Examine carefully for the following:

1. Coin lesions: Causes are granulomas (50% which are usually calcified), (histoplasmosis 25%, TB 20%, coccidioidomycosis 20%, varies with locale); primary carcinoma (25%), hamartoma (< 10%), and metastatic disease (< 5%).

2. Cavitary lesions: Causes are abscess, cancer, TB, coccidioidomycosis, Wegener's granulomatosus.

3. Infiltrates: Two major types
   a. **Interstitial pattern.** "Reticular." Causes are granulomatous infections, miliary TB, coccidioidomycosis, pneumoconiosis, sarcoidosis, CHF. "Honeycombing" represents end-stage fibrosis caused by sarcoid, RA, and pneumoconiosis.

15

   b. Alveolar pattern. Diffuse, quick progression and regression. Can see either "butterfly" pattern or air bronchograms. Causes are PE, pneumonia, hemorrhage or PE associated with CHF.

Lateral Film

Examine the structures shown in Figure 15–2 below. Use this study to check for the three-dimensional location of lesions. Pay close attention to the retrosternal clear space, costophrenic angles, and the path of the aorta.

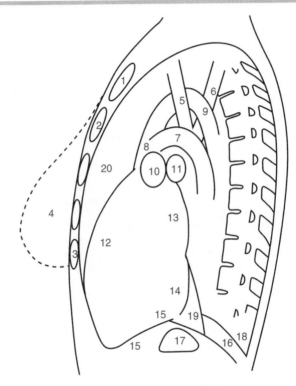

Lateral Chest X-ray

1. Manubrium	11. Left mainstem bronchus
2. Body of sternum	12. Right ventricle
3. Xiphoid process	13. Left atrium
4. Breast shadow	14. Left ventricle
5. Trachea	15. Right diaphragm
6. Scapula	16. Left diaphragm
7. Left pulmonary artery	17. Gastric air bubble
8. Ascending aorta	18. Costophrenic angles
9. Aortic arch	19. Inferior vena cava
10. Right pulmonary artery	20. Retrosternal clear space

FIGURE 15–2.   Structures seen on a lateral chest x-ray film.

INTRODUCTION TO THE OPERATING ROOM

Sterile Technique	Draping the Patient
Entering the OR	Finding Your Place
The Surgical Hand Scrub	Universal Precautions
Preparing the Patient	Latex Allergy
Gowning and Gloving	

Working in the OR can be the best or worst experience of a clinical rotation. However, familiarity with OR procedure is crucial to the success of any such experience. Preparing yourself before you get to the OR by knowing the patient thoroughly and having a basic understanding of what is planned will greatly enhance your OR experience. Don't fall into the trap of stereotyping the nurses as "cranky", the surgeons as "egotistical", and the medical students as clueless". Avoid this by learning the routine of the OR. Be alert, attentive, and, above all, patient. Soon, the routine will become second nature. Most importantly, don't be afraid to admit to the scrub nurse and the circulating nurse that you're new at this. They are usually more than happy to help you follow correct procedures.

STERILE TECHNIQUE

Members of the OR team, which includes the surgeon, assistants, students, and scrub nurse (the one who is responsible for passing the instruments and gowning the OR team), maintain a sterile field. The circulating nurse acts as a go-between between the sterile and nonsterile areas.

Sterile areas include the front of the gown to the waist, gloved hands and arms to the shoulder, draped part of the patient down to the table level, covered part of the Mayo stand, and the top of the back table where additional instruments are kept. The sides of the back table are not considered sterile, and anything that falls below the level of the patient table is considered contaminated.

ENTERING THE OR

From the moment you enter the OR, everything is geared toward maintaining a sterile field. The use of sterile technique begins in the locker room. Change into scrub clothing (remove T-shirts and tuck the scrub shirt into the pants). Be sure that the ties of the scrub pants are also tucked inside the pants. Scrub clothes may occasionally be worn on the wards, provided that they are covered by a clinic coat or some other form of gown, but you need to check your hospital or departmental requirements on this. If you do wear scrub clothing out of the OR, be sure that it is not bloodstained.

Pass into the anteroom to get your mask, cap, and shoe covers. The mask should cover your entire nose and mouth. Full hoods are necessary for men with beards. The cap must cover all of your hair. Because of universal precautions, OR staff are now required to use protective eyewear while at the operative field. While wearing glasses, use masks with adhesive at the bridge of the nose to prevent fogging. Tape the glasses to your forehead if you think they may be loose enough to fall onto the table during the operation. Do not wear nail polish, and remove any loose jewelry, watches, and rings before scrubbing. Make sure that shoelaces are tucked inside the shoe covers.

The mask does not need to be worn in the hall of the OR suite (but everything else does) at most hospitals. The mask must be worn in the OR itself, near the scrub sinks, and in the substerile room between ORs.

Find the OR where the patient is located, and assist in transport, if necessary. Introduce yourself to the intern or resident and nurse, and try to get an idea of when to begin scrubbing (usually when the first surgeon starts to scrub). If you have a pager, follow the OR procedures and remove the pager if you are going to scrub into the case.

THE SURGICAL HAND SCRUB

The purpose of a surgical hand scrub is to decrease the bacterial flora of the skin by mechanically cleansing the arms and hands before the operation. Key points to remember: (1) If contamination occurs during the scrub, it is necessary to start over, and (2) In emergency situations exceptions are made to the time allowed for scrubbing (as in obstetrics, when the baby is brought out from the delivery room and the student is still scrubbing!). Caps and masks should be properly positioned before the start of the scrub.

Povidone-Iodine (Betadine) Hand Scrub

Scrubbing technique depends somewhat on local custom. Some ORs want a timed scrub in which the duration of scrubbing is determined by watching the clock. Other ORs use an "anatomic" scrub in which the duration of scrubbing is determined by counting strokes. Either is acceptable, and you should find out what the custom is at your institution.

Timed Scrub

1. Perform a general prewash, with surgical soap and water, up to 2 in. above the elbows.
2. Use disposable brushes if available. Aseptically open one brush and place it on the ledge above the sink for the second half of the scrub. Open another brush and begin the scrub with Betadine. Use the nail cleaner to clean under all fingernails.
3. Scrub both arms during the first 5 min. Start at the fingertips and end 2 in. above the elbows; pay close attention to the fingernails and interdigital spaces. Discard the brush and rinse from fingertips to elbows.
4. Take the second brush and repeat step 3. Always start at the fingertips and work up to the elbows.
5. Always allow water to drip off the elbows by keeping the hands above the level of the elbows.
6. Move into the OR to dry your hands and arms (back into the room to push the door open).
7. Scrubbing times:
   a. Ten minutes at the start of the day or with no previous scrub within the last 12 h and on all orthopedic cases.
   b. Five minutes with a previous scrub or between cases if you have not been out of the OR working with other patients

16

Chlorhexidine (Hibiclens) 6-Min Hand Scrub (Timed)

1. Wet your hands and forearms to the elbows with water.
2. Dispense about 5 mL of Hibiclens into your cupped hands and spread it over both hands and arms to the elbows.
3. Scrub vigorously for 3 min without adding water. Use a sponge or brush for scrubbing, and pay particular attention to fingernails, cuticles, and interdigital spaces.
4. Rinse thoroughly with running water.
5. Dispense another 5 mL of Hibiclens into your cupped hands.
6. Wash for an additional 3 min. There is no need to use a brush or sponge at this point. Rinse thoroughly. Move into the OR back first to dry your hands.

Anatomic Scrub

1. Perform a general prewash, with surgical soap and water, up to 2 in. above the elbows.
2. Use disposable brushes if available. Aseptically open one brush and place it on the ledge above the sink for the second half of the scrub. Open another brush and begin the scrub with Betadine. Use the nail cleaner to clean under all fingernails.
3. Each surface is to be scrubbed vigorously 10 times. Start with each finger (each of which has four surfaces), proceeding to the hand, the forearm, and the arm above the elbow. After finishing one extremity, do the other from fingers to above the elbow. Be sure to include all parts of your hand, especially the interdigital spaces.
4. Rinse both arms thoroughly.
5. Now rescrub each extremity, this time not going above the elbow. This is done in a similar fashion, 10 times on each surface from fingers to elbow.
6. Rinse thoroughly and proceed into the OR.

PREPARING THE PATIENT

The exact technique may vary in different medical centers, but the patient prep involves mechanically cleansing the patient's skin in the region of the surgical site to reduce bacterial flora. Ask the intern or resident to guide you through the procedure the first time, and consider doing it yourself thereafter. It is always better to prep a wider area than you think necessary. For example, for a midline laparotomy, the patient is prepped from nipples to pubis, and from the flank at table level on one side to the table level on the other side.

Materials

Usually, a small prep table is present containing the following: gloves, towels, Betadine or other scrub soap (optional), Betadine or other paint solution, 4 × 4 gauze squares or sponges, ring forceps (optional).

Technique

1. Patient prep is usually done before putting on the sterile gown. Don a pair of gloves, and scrub the area designated by the intern or resident for 4–6 min. Use the 4 × 4s (or sponges) and the soap solution. This is generally done three times with a gauze or sponge in each hand for a total of 4–6 min. At many centers, this traditional wound scrubbing is no longer per-

formed routinely and is used only in specific circumstances, such as, contaminated wounds.

2. Drape the area with a towel, and then gently pat the area dry if the wound was scrubbed. Taking care not to contaminate the area, gently peel off the towel from one side, being careful not to allow the towel to fall back on the prepped area. Also be careful not to contaminate your own arms, so that you do not have to rescrub before gowning.

3. Use 4 × 4s or sponges to paint the exposed area with the Betadine or other provided solution, using the proposed incision site as the center. Move circumferentially away from the incision site. Never bring the 4 × 4s back to the center after they have painted more peripheral areas. This is done as a series of concentric circles. Some centers will only "paint" and not "scrub" with the soap solution. Some surgeons want the paint dried with a towel at the end, and others like to leave it "wet." Check with the resident or attending physician before you start, to find out exactly what is wanted.

4. When you are finished with the prep, remove your gloves in a sterile manner and proceed to get your gown on.

GOWNING AND GLOVING

1. If you have just completed the hand scrub, back into the room to push the door open; keep your hands above your elbows.

2. Ask the scrub nurse for a towel. Do not be impatient because the scrub nurse is often very busy. Stick out one hand, palm up and well away from the body. The nurse will drape the towel over your hand.

3. Bend at the waist to maintain sterility of the towel. It should never touch your clothing.

4. With one-half of the towel, dry one arm, beginning at the fingers; change hands and dry the other arm with the remaining half of the towel. Never go back to the forearm or hands after drying your elbows.

5. Drop the towel in the hamper. Again, remember to keep your hands above your elbows.

6. Ask for a gown and hold your arms out straight. The scrub nurse will place the gown on you, and the circulator will tie the back for you.

7. The nurse will usually hold out a right glove with the palm toward you. Push your hand through the glove. Gloves come in different sizes—small (5½–6½), medium (7–7½), and large (8–8½)—and different materials: standard latex gloves, hypoallergenic (powder-free), reinforced (orthopedic), and latex-free. Ask the resident or scrub nurse for guidance on the type of glove to request. It is good form to ask the circulating nurse to open your gloves before you actually begin to scrub.

8. Repeat the procedure with the left glove. It is easier if you use two fingers of your gloved right hand to help hold the left glove open.

9. Visually inspect the gloves for any holes. Double gloving is becoming common place due to increased awareness of universal precautions and may be mandatory based on the procedure to be performed.

10. Give the scrub nurse the long string of your front gown-tie. Hold the other string yourself and turn around in place. Tie the strings.

11. The nurse may offer you a damp sponge to clean the powder off the gloves (the powder has been implicated in some postoperative complications, eg, adhesions). This varies by locale.

16

12. Now wait patiently; stay out of the way, and keep your hands above your waist. Hold them together to prevent yourself from accidentally dropping them or touching your mask. This is one of the most difficult things for the neophyte to remember. Be attentive. The only things that are sterile are your chest to your waist in the front and your hands to the shoulders. Your back is not sterile, nor is your body below the waist. Avoid crossing your arms.

DRAPING THE PATIENT

Draping the patient is usually done by the surgeon and assistants. Watch how they do it, and consider helping at a later date. It is harder to keep sterile than it looks.

FINDING YOUR PLACE

The medical student is often the "low man or woman on the totem pole" and should stand where the senior surgeon indicates. The first thing to remember is that once you are scrubbed, you must not touch anything that is not sterile. Put your hands on the sterile field and do not move about unnecessarily. If you need to move around someone else, pass back to back. When passing by a sterile field, try to face it. When passing a nonsterile field, pass it with your back toward it. If you are observing a case and are not scrubbed in, do not go between two sterile fields, and stay about 1 ft away from all sterile fields to avoid contamination (and condemnation!). When not scrubbed in, it often helps to keep your hands behind your back, being careful not to back into the instrument table.

When scrubbed, do not drop your hands below your waist or the table level. Do not grab at anything that falls off the side of the table—it is considered contaminated. If something falls, you can quietly inform the circulating nurse. Do not reach for anything on the scrub nurse's small instrument stand (the Mayo stand). You may ask for the instrument to be given to you.

If someone says that you have contaminated a glove, light handle, or anything else, do not move and do not complain or disagree. Remember that the focus of the OR is maintaining a sterile field, so if anyone says, "You're contaminated," accept the statement and change gloves, gown, or whatever is needed. If a glove alone is contaminated, hold the hand out away from the sterile field, fingers extended and palms up, and a circulating nurse will pull the glove off. The same is true if a needle sticks you or if a glove tears. Tell the surgeon and scrub nurse that you have experienced a needlestick and are contaminated and change gloves.

If you have to change your gown, step away from the table. The circulator will remove first the gown and then the gloves. This procedure prevents the contaminated inside of the gown from passing over the hands. Regown and reglove without scrubbing again.

Always be aware of "sharps" on the field. When passing a potentially injurious instrument, always make the other members of the team aware that you are passing a sharp (ie, "needle back," "knife back," etc). Attempt to learn the names and functions of the common instruments. A knowledgeable student may be more likely to actively participate in the case.

At the end of the case (once the dressing is on the wound), you may remove the gown and gloves but not the mask, cap, or shoe covers. To protect yourself, remove your gown first, and remove your own gloves last. This keeps your hands clean of any blood or fluids that got onto your gown during the procedure.

16

Assist in the transfer of the patient to the postoperative recovery room. Postop orders and a brief operative note are written immediately.

See Chapter 2 on how to write postop notes and orders. It is good form to offer to write the postop note and orders if you are comfortable with the process. Due to governmental regulations that affect attending physicians at teaching hospitals, the attending must often write the note him- or herself. At the very least, the attending of record will annotate an "attestation" to your note saying that the surgeon was "personally present during the critical portions of the procedure."

UNIVERSAL PRECAUTIONS

All operating room personnel are at risk for infection with blood-borne agents responsible for such diseases as AIDS and hepatitis. To reduce the incidence of such transmission, a set of guidelines called universal precautions has been developed by the CDC. The underlying principle is that, because patients cannot be routinely tested for HIV and are rarely tested preoperatively for transmissible diseases such as hepatitis, the safest policy is to treat all patients as though they are infected with an infectious agent. This approach ensures evenhanded treatment of all patients and the safest work environment for those who are exposed to the blood of others.

Minimizing the risks to all who are in the OR requires constant vigilance. Movements must be coordinated among surgeon, assistant, and technician. Fingers are never used to pick up needles; this is done only with another instrument. Fingers and hands should not be used as retractors. Two people should never be holding the same sharp instrument. Placing a sharp instrument down or handing it to another member of the team is always preceded by a verbal warning that notifies the recipient that a sharp object is about to be passed. Protective eyewear must be worn by all members of the operating team.

The practice of "double gloving" is often reserved for cases in which the patient is known to carry a transmissible agent. This technique definitely reduces the incidence of blood–skin contact, especially in light of the extraordinarily high incidence of unrecognized glove perforations. Until puncture-resistant gloves are developed, this is the best approach we have.

LATEX ALLERGY

Individuals with certain medical conditions or occupations that are heavily exposed to products containing natural rubber latex may became sensitized to it and develop allergic reactions. Up to 7% of health care workers can have allergic reactions. Certain conditions (ie, spina bifida, cerebral palsy) predispose patients to an 18–40% incidence of allergy. Reactions can vary from mild rash and itching to anaphylaxis and death. Latex products are found in a surprisingly wide array of products, from gloves and drapes, to IV tubing and syringes. Occasionally patients will have documented latex allergy. Hospitals have latex allergy protocols, and hospitals maintain an inventory of latex-free products that should be used in these cases (see also page 244).

17

SUTURING TECHNIQUES AND WOUND CARE

Wound Healing	Suturing Patterns
Vacuum-Assisted Closure	Surgical Knots
Suture Materials	Suture Removal
Suturing Procedure	Tissue Adhesives

WOUND HEALING

The process of wound healing is generally divided into four stages: inflammation, fibroblast proliferation, contraction, and remodeling. There are three different types of wound healing: primary intent (routine primary suturing, stapling, or gluing) epithelialization occurs in 24–48 h; secondary intent (the wound is not closed with suture, closes by spontaneous contraction and epithelialization at a rate of 1 mm/day), most often used for wounds that are infected and packed open; and tertiary intent (also called delayed primary closure), the wound is left open for a time and then sutured at a later date, (used often with grossly contaminated wounds).

VACUUM-ASSISTED CLOSURE

This method is used for healing both acute and chronic wounds and implements continuous negative pressure distributed over the wound surface. The system consists of a soft sponge cut to fit and occupy the volume of the wound, a plastic tube imbedded in the center of the sponge and extending out of the wound to a controlled suction pump, and a gas- and fluid-impermeable plastic outer film that adheres to the back of the sponge and the surrounding normal skin. It provides "active" removal of extracellular debris (exudate). Clinically, soft tissue defects heal faster when subatmospheric pressure is applied. The applications are extensive, including wounds resulting from pressure, trauma, infection, IV extravasation, arterial and venous insufficiency, and skin grafting.

SUTURE MATERIALS (SEE TABLE 17–1, PAGE 362)

Suture materials can be broadly defined as absorbable and nonabsorbable. **Absorbable sutures** can be thought of as temporary and include plain gut; chromic gut; and synthetic materials such as polyglactin 910 (Vicryl), polyglycolic acid (Dexon), and polyglecaprone (Monocryl). These are resorbed by the body when left internally after a variable period. Polydioxanone (PDS) is a long-lasting absorbable suture. **Nonabsorbable sutures** can be thought of as "permanent" unless they are removed; these include silk, stainless steel wire, polypropylene (Prolene), and nylon.

The size of a suture is defined by the number of zeros. The more zeros in the number, the smaller the suture. For example, a 5-0 suture (00000) is much smaller than a 2-0 (00) suture. Most sutures come prepackaged and mounted

TABLE 17–1
Common Suture Materials

ABSORBABLE

Suture (Brand Names)	Description	Tensile Strength[a]	Absorbed[b]	Common Uses
Fast catgut	Twisted/fast absorption	3–5 d	30 d	Facial lacerations in children
Plain catgut	Twisted/rapidly absorbable	7–10 d	70 d	Vessel ligation, subcutaneous tissues
Chromic catgut	Twisted/absorbable	10–14 d	90 d	Mucosa
Polyglycolic acid (Dexon)	Braided/absorbable	14–21 d	60–90 d	GI, subcutaneous tissues
Polyglactin 910 (Vicryl Rapide)	Braided/absorbable	5 d	42 d	Skin repair needing rapid absorption
Polyglactin 910 (Vicryl)	Braided/absorbable	21 d	56–70 d	Bowel, deep tissue
Poliglecaprone 25 (Monocryl)	Monofilament/absorbable	7–14 d	91–119 d	Skin, bowel
Polydioxanone (PDS)	Monofilament/absorbable	28 d	6 mon	Fascia, vessel anastomosis
Polyglyconate (Maxon)	Braided/absorbable	28 d	6 mon	GI, muscle, fascia
Panacryl	Braided/absorbable	>6 mon	>24 mon	Fascia, tendons

(continued)

17

TABLE 17-1
(Continued)

NONABSORBABLE

Suture (Brand Names)	Description	Common Uses
Nylon (Dermalon, Ethilon)	Monofilament	Skin, drains
Nylon (Nurolon)	Braided	Tendon repair
Polyester (Ethibond, Tycron)	Braided	Cardiac, tendon
Polypropylene (Prolene)	Monofilament	Vessel, fascia, skin
Silk		GI, vessel ligation, drains
Stainless steel	Monofilament	Fascia, sternum

[a]When suture looses approximately 50% strength.
[b]Approximate.

17

on needles ("swaged on"). **Cutting needles** are used for tough tissues such as skin, and tapered needles are used for more delicate tissues such as the intestine. The most common needle for skin closure is the 3/8 in. circle cutting needle.

SUTURING PROCEDURE

The following guidelines cover the repair of lacerations in the emergency setting. Similar principles hold true for closure of wounds in the operating room. The choice of appropriate suture material is based on many factors, including location, extent of the laceration, strength of the tissues, and preference of the physician.

- **Face:** 5-0 and 6-0 nylon or polypropylene where cosmetic concerns are important
- **Scalp:** 3-0 nylon or polypropylene
- **Trunk or extremities:** 4-0 or 5-0 nylon or polypropylene
- Use 3-0 and 4-0 absorbable sutures such as Dexon or Vicryl to approximate deep tissues. Skin is usually best closed by using interrupted sutures placed with good approximation with a minimum amount of tension or by a running subcuticular suture. Tissue adhesives may be used selectively (see page 371). Suture patterns are discussed in the next section. Suture marks ("tracks") are the result of excessive tension on the tissue or leaving the sutures in for too long. Thus, the length of time and the technique used are probably more important in determining the final result than is the type of suture used in most cases.

1. Remove all foreign materials and devitalized tissues by sharp excision (debridement). Clean the wound with plain saline (antiseptic solutions used on wound cleansing should be discouraged because they can be toxic to viable cells). A useful technique involves irrigation with at least 200 mL of saline through a 35-mL syringe and a 19-gauge needle. Anesthesia may be necessary before any of this is done. If all the debris is not removed, traumatic "tattooing" of the skin may result.
2. In general, do not suture infected or contaminated wounds, lacerations more than 6–12 h old (24 h on the face), missile wounds, and human or animal bites without surgical consultation.
3. Anesthetize the wound by infiltrating it with an agent such as 0.5% or 1% lidocaine (Xylocaine). The maximum safe dosage is 4.5 mg/kg (about 28 mL of a 1% solution in an adult). Lidocaine and the other local anesthetic agents are available with epinephrine (1:100,000 or 1:200,000) added to produce local vasoconstriction that prolongs the anesthetic effect and helps decrease systemic side effects and bleeding. Epinephrine should be used with caution, particularly in patients with a history of hypertension, and should not be used on the digits, toes, or penis. 1 mL of 1:10 $NaHCO_3$ can be mixed with 9 mL of lidocaine to help minimize the discomfort of the injection. Commonly used local anesthetics are compared in Table 17–2, page 365.
4. When using local anesthetics, always aspirate before injecting to prevent intravascular injection of the drug. Anesthetize with a 26–30-

17

TABLE 17-2
Local Anesthetic Comparison Chart for Commonly Used Injectable Agents

Agent	Proprietary Names	Onset	Duration	Maximum Dose mg/kg	Maximum Dose Volume in 70-kg Adult[a]
Bupivacaine	Marcaine, Sensoricaine	7–30 min	5–7 h	3	70 mL of 0.25% solution
Lidocaine	Xylocaine, Anestacon	5–30 min	2 h	4	28 mL of 1% solution
Lidocaine with epinephrine (1:200,000)		5–30 min	2–3 h	7	50 mL of 1% solution
Mepivacaine	Carbocaine	5–30 min	2–3 h	7	50 mL of 1% solution
Procaine	Novocaine	Rapid	30 min–1 h	10–15	70–105 mL of 1% solution

[a]To calculate the maximum dose if the patient is not a 70-kg adult, use the fact that a 1% solution has 10 mg of drug per milliliter.

17

365

gauge needle. Symptoms of toxicity from local anesthetics includes twitching, restlessness, drowsiness, light-headedness, and seizures.

5. Close the wound using one of the suturing patterns discussed in the next section. To decrease trauma, use fine-toothed forceps (Adson or Brown-Adson) with gentle pressure to handle the skin edges. The toothed forceps are *less damaging* to the skin than other forceps with flat surfaces that may crush the tissue.

6. Cover the wound and keep it dry for at least 24–48 h. Dry gauze or Steri-Strips are sufficient. On the face, simply covering with antibiotic ointment is often used, especially around the eyes or mouth. After that time, *epithelialization is complete* in healthy patients with uninfected wounds and the patient may shower and wet the wound without increasing the risk of infection.

7. Finally, keep tetanus and antibacterial prophylaxis in mind, particularly for contaminated wounds (Table 17–3, below).

SUTURING PATTERNS

Opinions vary greatly on the ideal technique for skin closure. The following are the common techniques used for approximation of skin. Critical to any suturing technique is making certain that the edges of the wound closely approximate without overlapping or inversion and that there is no tension. Remember "approximation without strangulation" or eversion of the skin edges gives the best results (Figure 17–1). Figures 17–2 through 17–6 illustrate the commonly used suturing patterns. These include the simple interrupted suture (Figure 17–2), running (locked or unlocked) suture (Figure 17–3), vertical mattress suture (Figure 17–4), horizontal mattress suture (Figure 17–5), and subcuticular suture (Figure 17–6).

TABLE 17–3
Tetanus Prophylaxis

History of Absorbed Tetanus Toxoid Immunization	Clean, Minor Wounds		All Other Wounds[a]	
	Td[b]	TIG[c]	Td[b]	TIG[c]
Unknown or <3 doses	Yes	No	Yes	Yes
<3 doses[d]	No[e]	No	No[f]	No

[a]Such as, but not limited to, wounds contaminated with dirt, feces, soil, saliva, etc; puncture wounds; avulsions; and wounds resulting from missiles, crushing, burns, and frostbite.
[b]Td = tetanus–diphtheria toxoid (adult type), 0.5 mL IM.
• For children <7 y of age, DPT (DT, if pertussis vaccine is contraindicated) is preferred to tetanus toxoid alone.
• For persons >7 years of age, Td is preferred to tetanus toxoid alone.
• DT = diphtheria-tetanus toxoid (pediatric), used for those who cannot receive pertussis.
[c]TIG = tetanus immune globulin, 250 U IM.
[d]If only three doses of fluid toxoid have been received, then a fourth dose of toxoid, preferably an absorbed toxoid, should be given.
[e]Yes, if >10 y since last dose.
[f]Yes, if >5 y since last dose.
Source: Based on guidelines from the Centers for Disease Control and reported in MMWR.

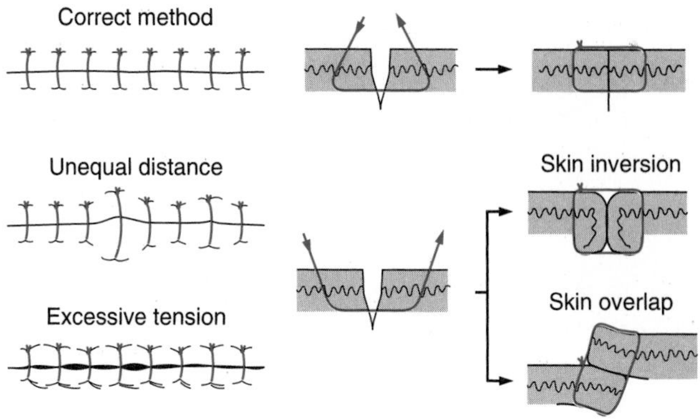

Correct method

Unequal distance

Skin inversion

Excessive tension

Skin overlap

FIGURE 17–1. Proper method for simple interrupted suturing of a skin wound compared to incorrect techniques that result in poor scars from skin overlap, skin inversion, or necrosis of the skin edges because of excessive tension.

SURGICAL KNOTS

There are three basic knot-tying techniques: the one handed and two-handed ties and the instrument tie. The most advanced knot-tying technique is a one-handed tie, not recommended for the medical student or junior resident. The two-handed tie is easier to learn than the one-handed tie, although one-handed ties may be more useful in certain situations (eg, with deep cavities or where speed is essential). Instrument ties are more useful for closing skin and for emergency room laceration repair. Figure 17–9 , page 375, shows the technique for tying a two-

17

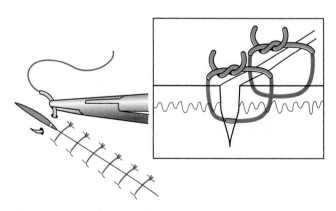

FIGURE 17–2. Simple interrupted suture. "Bites" are taken through the thickness of the skin, and the width of each stitch should equal the distance between sutures to avoid inverting the skin edges.

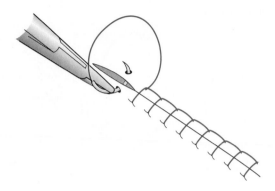

FIGURE 17–3. Continuous running suture. It allows rapid closure, but depends on only two knots for security and may not allow precise approximation of the skin edges. "Locking" each stitch, as shown, may increase scarring.

handed square knot, the standard surgical knot that should be learned first. Figure 17–7 page 371 & 372 shows the technique for the one-handed tie. Figure 17–8, pages 373 & 374, shows the technique for an instrument tie.

SUTURE REMOVAL

The longer a permanent suture material is left in place in the skin, the more scarring it will produce. Using a topical antibiotic (Polysporin, others) ointment on the wound is helpful in decreasing suture tract epithelialization. This epithe-

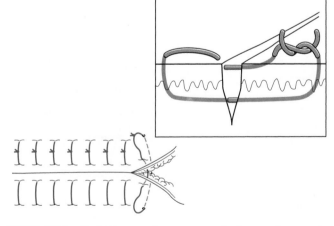

FIGURE 17–4. Vertical interrupted mattress suture. It allows precise approximation of the skin edges with little tension, but may result in more scarring than a simple stitch. The needle is placed in the skin in a "far, far, near, near" sequence.

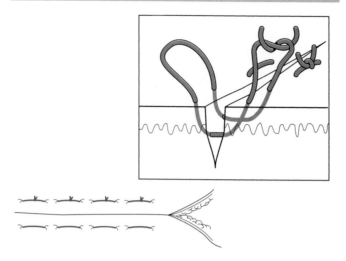

FIGURE 17-5. Horizontal interrupted mattress suture. This is an everting stitch that is more frequently used in fascia than in skin. It is often used in calloused skin such as the palms and soles.

lialization results from crusting around the suture that increases suture marks and subsequent scarring. Sutures can be safely removed when a wound has developed sufficient tensile strength. Situations vary greatly, but general guidelines for removing sutures from different areas of the body are: face and neck, 3–5 d; scalp and body, 5–7 d; and extremities, 7–12 d. Any suture material or skin clips can be removed earlier if they have been reinforced with a deep absorbable suture or with the application of Steri-Strips after the suture is removed. Steri-Strips will stay in place more securely if tincture of benzoin (spray or solution) is applied to the skin and allowed to dry before the Steri-Strips are applied. The length of time absorbable sutures remain in tissues is shown in Table 17–1.

Suture Removal Procedure

1. Gently clear away any dried blood with saline and gauze. Verify that the wound is sufficiently healed to allow suture removal. Use a forceps to gently elevate the knot off the skin. This can be uncomfortable for the patient.
2. Cut the suture as close to the skin as possible so that a minimal amount of "dirty suture" is dragged through the wound. When removing continuous sutures, cut and pull out each section individually. Never pull a knot through the skin. Often the suture material is pulled tight to the skin and it is difficult to remove the stitch with thick scissors. A No. 11 blade scalpel, with knife blade pointed up, is helpful in this situation.
3. The use of skin staples is commonplace in the OR because of the rapidity of closure and the nonreactive nature of the steel staples. These are typically removed 3–5 d after surgery (abdominal incisions) as shown in Fig-

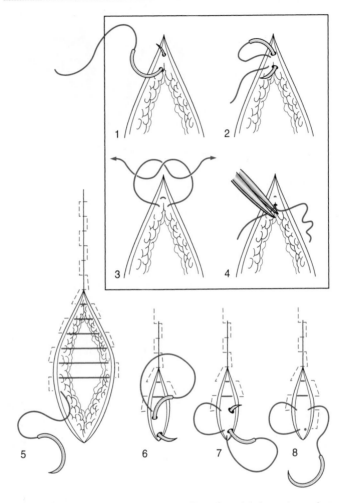

17

FIGURE 17-6. Subcuticular closure is usually performed with continuous, horizontally applied intradermal sutures. These are ideal for linear cosmetic closures since they eliminate possible cross-hatching deformities. If nonabsorbable suture material (eg, 5-0 or 6-0 Prolene) is used, the knot is placed on the skin and pulled taut. If absorbable (5-0 or 6-0 Dexon or Vicryl) is used, the knot is usually buried as shown.

ure 17–10. Because these are removed fairly quickly, reinforce the incision with Steri-Strips and benzoin. When removing skin staples, make sure that the staple is completely reformed (see Figure 17–10) before pulling it out of the skin to decrease patient discomfort. Before removal, verify that the wound is epithelialized and there is no sign of infection or wound leakage. If the wound gaps or if there is a discharge as the staples are removed, do

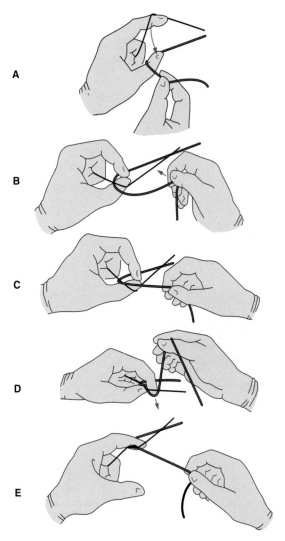

FIGURE 17-7.   Technique for tying the two-handed square knot. Suture ends are uncrossed as step a begins. (continued on next page).

not continue the removal procedure until the wound is evaluated by a senior physician.

TISSUE ADHESIVES

Octyl cyanoacrylate (Dermabond, Ethicon) and *n*-butyl-2-cyanoacrylate (Indermil, US Surgical/Davis and Geck) are topical skin adhesives (similar to cyano-

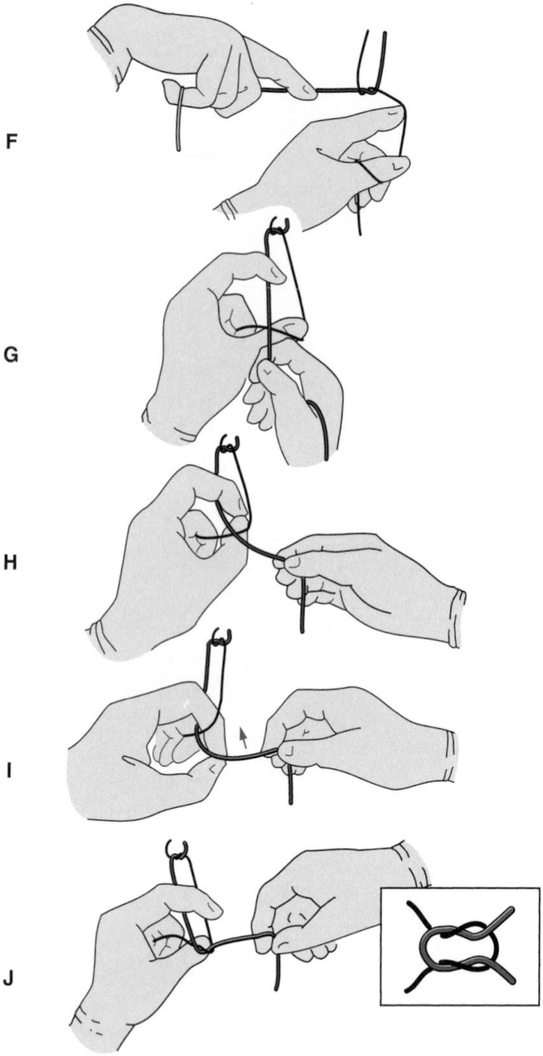

FIGURE 17-7. (contd.) The two-handed square knot (continued from previous page). Hands must be crossed at the end of the first loop tie (step F) to give a flat knot; hands are not crossed at the end of the second loop tie (step J).

acrylate glue) that hold wound edges together. These are useful in the closure of topical skin incisions and lacerations in areas of low skin tension that are simple, thoroughly cleansed, and have easily approximated skin edges. They can be used in conjunction with, but not in place of, deep dermal stitches. These are particularly useful in young children, for whom suture removal may be a problem. The

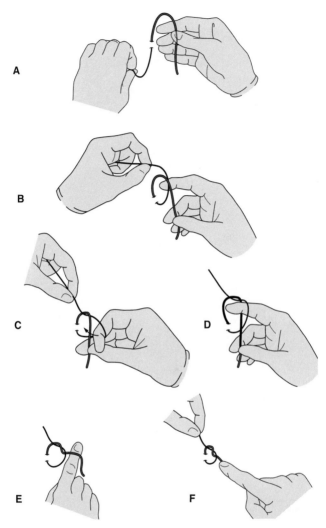

FIGURE 17–8. One handed tie. The right hand sets up the loop and manipulates the working strand. (continued next page)

17

wound should be nonmucosal on the face, torso, or extremity. They are recommended for wounds < 8 cm with minimal tension (skin gap < 0.5 cm) and for stabilizing wounds after early suture removal to minimize suture marks. Tissue adhesives should not be used for puncture wounds, bites or wounds that need debridement, or in regions subjected to frequent movement (ie, joints). The patient may shower for brief periods with this type of closure.

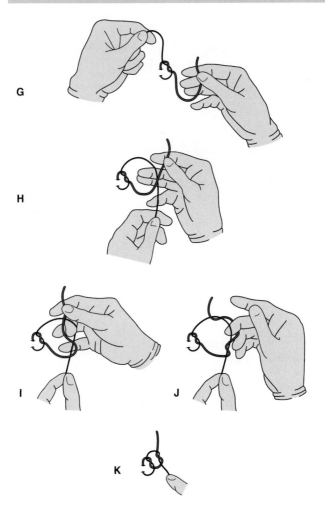

G

H

I   **J**

K

17   **FIGURE 17–8B.**   One handed not continued. (contd.)

1. Gently approximate the wound edges with fingers or a forceps and place a small coating of the glue directly on the wound. Dermabond uses a direct contact applicator tip; Indermil has a noncontact application tip.
2. After 2–3 min, the glue has dried, and an additional one or two coats may be applied. The glue will shed in approximately 5–10 d.
3. Once the glue is in place and stable, it is not necessary to use any topical medication or ointment. If the adhesive remains tacky, too much glue has been applied.

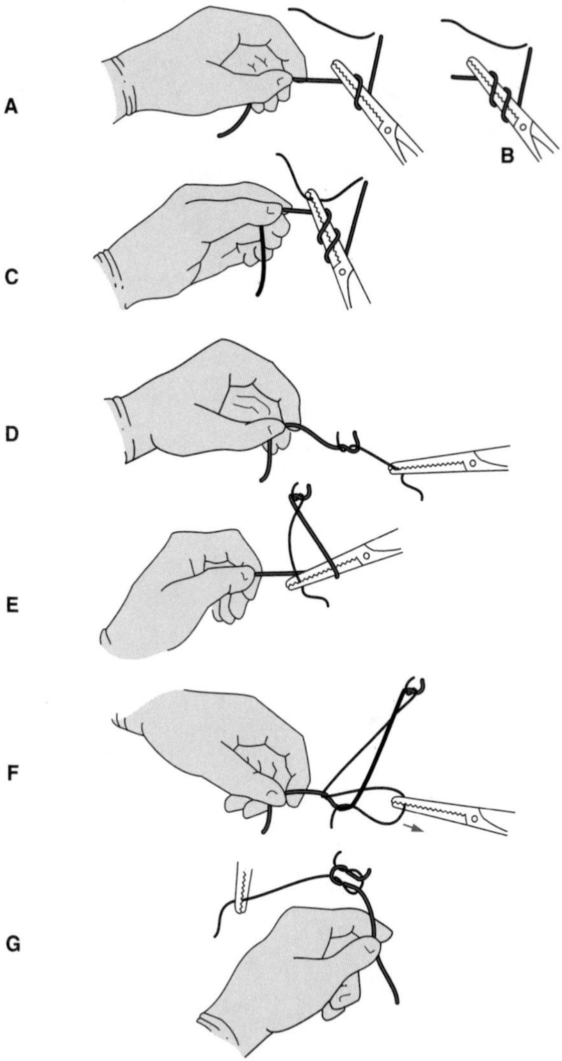

FIGURE 17–9. The instrument tie. Begin with either a single or double (illustrated) looping of the lower end of the suture around the needle holder. The first loop is laid flat without crossing the hands. Hands must be crossed after the second loop tie (step G) to produce a flat square knot.

17

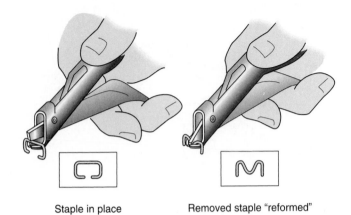

Staple in place   Removed staple "reformed"

FIGURE 17-10. Removal of skin staples. The staple removal instrument is passed beneath the staple and completely closed. Be sure that the staple is completely "reformed" before removal to decrease patient discomfort. (Courtesy of Ethicon, Inc.)

17

RESPIRATORY CARE

Respiratory Therapy
Pulmonary Function Tests (PFTs)
Differential Diagnosis of PFTs
Oxygen Supplements

Bronchopulmonary Hygiene
Topical Medications
Metered-Dose Inhalers

RESPIRATORY THERAPY

Respiratory therapy is a vital component of health care. The objective is the treatment and care of all types of patients with cardiopulmonary diseases. Functions of the respiratory therapist include emergency care, ventilatory support, airway management, oxygen therapy, humidity and aerosol therapies, chest physiotherapy, physiologic monitoring, and pulmonary diagnostics.

PULMONARY FUNCTION TESTS (PFTS)

PFTs are useful in diagnosing a variety of pulmonary disorders. Common PFTs include spirometry, lung volume determinations, and diffusing capacity. Important measures include the FVC and the FEV_1. Spirometry may identify obstructive airway diseases such as asthma or emphysema when the ratio of FEV_1/FVC is < 70%, or restrictive lung diseases such as sarcoidosis or ankylosing spondylitis when both the FVC and FEV_1 are reduced.

Spirometry may also be an important part of a preoperative evaluation. Spirograms can be obtained before and after the administration of bronchodilators if they are not contraindicated (ie, history of intolerance). Bronchodilator responsiveness will help in predicting the response to treatment and in identifying asthma.

Lung volumes commonly determined by helium dilution must be ordered to definitively diagnose restrictive lung disease. This is usually indicated by TLC < 80% of predicted normal. Diffusion capacity is important in the diagnosis of interstitial lung disease or pulmonary vascular disease, where it is reduced. It is also frequently followed to determine the response to therapy in interstitial diseases.

Obstructive pulmonary diseases include asthma, chronic bronchitis, emphysema, and bronchiectasis. Restrictive pulmonary disease includes interstitial pulmonary diseases, diseases of the chest wall, and neuromuscular disorders. Interstitial disease may be due to inflammatory conditions [usual interstitial pneumonitis (UIP)], inhalation of organic dusts (hypersensitivity pneumonitis), inhalation of inorganic dusts (asbestosis), or systemic disorders with lung involvement (sarcoidosis).

Normal PFT values vary with age, sex, race, and body size. Normal values for a given patient are established from studies of normal populations and are provided along with the results. ABG should be included in all PFTs. Typical volumes and capacities are illustrated in Figure 18–1, page 378.

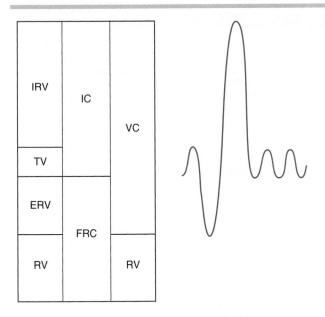

VC = vital capacity   ERV = expiratory reserve volume
RV = residual volume   IRV = inspiratory reserve volume
FRC = functional residual capacity   IC = inspiratory capacity
TV = tidal volume

FIGURE 18–1.   Lung volumes in the interpretation of pulmonary function tests.

- **Tidal Volume (TV).** Volume of air moved during a normal breath on quiet respiration
- **Forced Vital Capacity (FVC):** Maximum volume of air that can be forcibly expired after full inspiration
- **Functional Residual Capacity (FRC).** Volume of air in the lungs after a normal tidal expiration (FRC = reserve volume + expiratory reserve volume)
- **Total Lung Capacity (TLC).** Volume of air in the lungs after maximal inspiration
- **Forced Expired Volume in 1 Second (FEV$_1$).** Measured after maximum inspiration, the volume of air that can be expelled in 1 s
- **Vital Capacity (VC).** Maximum volume of air that can be exhaled from the lungs after a maximal inspiration
- **Residual Volume (RV).** The volume of air remaining in the lungs at the end of a maximal exhalation

DIFFERENTIAL DIAGNOSIS OF PFTS

Table 18–1 shows the differential diagnosis of various PFT patterns. When interpreting PFTs, remember that some patients may have combined restrictive and obstructive diseases such as emphysema and asbestosis.

TABLE 18–1
Differential Diagnosis of Pulmonary Function Tests

Test	Restrictive Disease	Obstructive Disease
FVC	↓	N or ↓
TLC	↓	↑
FEV$_1$/FVC	N or ↑	↓
FEV$_1$	↓	↓

OBSTRUCTIVE AIRWAYS DISEASE (COPD)

Test	Normal	Mild	Moderate	Severe
FEV$_1$ (% of VC)	>75	60–75	40–60	<40
RV (% of predicted)	80–120	120–150	150–175	>200

RESTRICTIVE LUNG DISEASE

Test	Normal	Mild–Moderate	Severe	
FVC (% of predicted)	>80	60–80	50–60	<50
FEV$_1$ (% of VC)	>75	>75	>75	>75
RV (% of predicted)	80–120	80–120	70–80	70

N = normal; ↑ = increased; ↓ = decreased; FVC = forced vital capacity; TLC = total lung capacity; RV/FRC = residual volume/functional residual capacity; FEV$_1$ = forced expiratory volume in 1s; VC = vital capacity.

OXYGEN SUPPLEMENTS

Table 18–2, page 380 describes various methods of oxygen supplementation. To bring the percentage RH of the inspired gas up to room humidity (30–40% RH) when using the nasal cannula, simple oxygen mask, partial rebreathing mask, or nonrebreathing mask, the bubble-diffuser humidifier is the device of choice.

BRONCHOPULMONARY HYGIENE

The following is a listing of the modalities available through the respiratory care or nursing services of most hospitals. All are designed to help patients with their bronchopulmonary hygiene, more commonly referred to as "pulmonary toilet." Bronchopulmonary hygiene is defined as maintenance of clear airways and removal of secretions from the tracheobronchial tree. This is important for routine postoperative surgical patients, medical patients with obstructive pulmonary diseases, or any patient with excessive respiratory secretions.

Aerosol (Nebulizer) Therapy

Aerosolized medications such as bronchodilators and mucolytic agents can be delivered via nebulizer for spontaneously breathing, awake patients or intubated patients.

18

TABLE 18–2
Various Methods of Oxygen and Humidity Supplementation

Device	O_2 Range	L/min	F_iO_2	Uses
Nasal cannula	Low	1–6	0.24–0.5	COPD, general oxygen needs
Simple face mask	Medium	6–8	0.5–0.6	General oxygen needs
Partial rebreathing face mask	High	8–12	0.6–0.7	High oxygen emergency needs
Nonrebreathing face mask	High	8–12	0.7–0.95	High oxygen emergency needs
Venturi mask	Low–medium	—	0.24–0.50	COPD (can specify exact F_iO_2)

Note: F_iO_2 may vary with fluctuations in the patient's minute ventilation when using a nasal cannula. This is not true when using the Venturi mask because it is a "high-flow oxygen enrichment system" that supplies three times the patient's minute ventilation, thus providing an exact F_iO_2.
COPD = chronic obstructive pulmonary disease; F_iO_2 = fraction of inspired oxygen.

Indications
- Treatment of COPD, acute asthma, CF, and bronchiectasis
- Help in inducing sputum for diagnostic tests

Goals
- Relief of bronchospasm
- Help in decreasing the viscosity and in clearing of secretions

To Order: Specify the following:
- Frequency
- Heated or cool mist
- Medications: In sterile water or NS
- F_iO_2
- *Example.* Albuterol 2.5 mg in 3 mL of sterile saline, F_iO_2 0.28.

Chest Physiotherapy

18

This technique uses percussion and postural drainage (P&PD) along with coughing and deep breathing exercises (TC&DB). P&PD is performed by positioning the patient so that the involved lobes of the lung are placed in a dependent drainage position and then using a cupped hand or vibrator to percuss the chest wall. Nasotracheal (NT) suctioning is quite uncomfortable for the patient but is still useful in the appropriate clinical setting in the absence of significant coagulopathy.

Indications
- Treatment of pneumonia, atelectasis, and diseases resulting in weak or ineffective coughing

To Order
1. **P&PD:** Specify the following:

    - Frequency
    - Segments or lobes involved (RUL, etc)
    - Duration
    - Drainage only

2. **TC&DB:** Ordered on a timed schedule or as needed

    - *Example.* P&PD qid of RUL and RML 5 min/lobe or TC&DB q4h

Incentive Spirometry

This method encourages patients to make a maximal and sustained inspiratory effort to help reinflate the lungs or prevent atelectasis.

Indications
- Treatment of patients at risk for developing postoperative pulmonary complications
- Treatment and prevention of atelectasis, especially in postoperative setting

Goals: Set for the patient depending on the device available:

- Lighting lights
- Moving "Ping-Pong-like" balls

To Order: Specify the following:

- Frequency (eg, 10 min q1–2h while awake or 10 repetitions q1h while awake)
- Device (if you have a preference)
- *Example.* Incentive spirometry 10 repetitions every hour while awake

TOPICAL MEDICATIONS

The following agents can be added to aerosol therapy to prevent or treat pulmonary complications caused by bronchoconstriction, mucosal congestion, or inspissated secretions. Remember, even though these are primarily topical agents, some systemic absorption can often occur.

Acetylcysteine (Mucomyst):   A mucolytic agent useful for treating retained mucoid secretions; inspissated secretions; and impacted mucoid plugs seen in diseases such as COPD, CF, and pneumonia. A bronchodilator should be given along with Mucomyst. *Usual Adult Dosage.* 1–3 mL of 20% acetylcysteine in 3 mL albuterol

Albuterol (Ventolin, Proventil):   A short-acting selective bronchodilator with principally beta-2 activity; can cause tachycardia. Onset 15 min. Peak effect at 0.5–1 h, duration 3–5 h. *Usual Adult Dosage.* 2.5 mg in 3 mL NS q4h

Levalbuterol (Xopenex):   "L" isomer of the short-acting albuterol; more expensive but this form causes less tachycardia. Onset 15 min. Peak effect at 0.5–1 h, duration 3–5 h; *Usual Adult Dosage.* 0.63–1.25 mg in 3 mL NS q6h

Racemic Epinephrine: Contains both "D" and "L" forms of epinephrine. Alpha effects cause mucosal vasoconstriction to reduce mucosal engorgement,

18

and bronchodilation lessens the risk of hypoxemia. Most useful for laryngotracheobronchitis and immediately after extubation in children. *Usual Adult Dosage.* 0.125–0.5 mL (3–10 mg) in 2.5 mL NS

Ipratropium Bromide (Atrovent): A parasympatholytic agent that causes bronchodilation and decreases secretions with "drying" of the respiratory mucosa. This is minimally absorbed and rarely results in tachycardia. Onset 45 min, duration 4–6 h; *Usual Adult Dosage.* 0.5 mg in 3 mL NS qid

Atropine: A parasympatholytic agent; causes bronchodilation and decreases secretions with "drying" of the respiratory mucosa. Readily absorbed and, therefore has cardiac effects (tachycardia); *Usual Adult Dosage.* 0.025–0.05 mg/kg of a 1% solution

METERED-DOSE INHALERS

(See Chapter 22 for additional prescribing information). All bronchodilating agents can be effectively delivered by metered-dose inhaler as long as proper technique is used. For these devices to be successful, in-patients must be well trained or have the assistance of a nurse or respiratory therapist. Albuterol and ipratropium bromide (Atrovent) can each be delivered two puffs q4h. A combination bronchodilator (Combivent) containing the equivalent of one puff of each is also available and provides synergistic bronchodilatation.

18

19

BASIC ECG READING

INTRODUCTION

The formal procedure for obtaining an ECG is given in Chapter 13, page 270. Every ECG should be approached in a systematic, stepwise fashion. Many automated ECG machines can give a preliminary interpretation of a tracing; however, all automated interpretations require analysis and sign-off by a physician. Determine each of the following:

- **Standardization.** With the ECG machine set on 1 mV, a 10-mm standardization mark (0.1 mV/mm) is evident (Figure 19–1).
- **Axis.** If the QRS is upright (more positive than negative) in leads I and aVF, the axis is normal. The normal axis range is –30 degrees to +105 degrees.
- **Intervals.** Determine the PR, QRS, and QT intervals (Figure 19–2). Intervals are measured in the limb leads. The PR should be 0.12–0.20 s, and the QRS, < 0.12 s. The QT interval increases with decreasing heart rate, usually < 0.44 s. The QT interval usually does not exceed one half of the RR interval (the distance between two R waves).
- **Rate.** Count the number of QRS cycles in a 6-s strip and multiply it by 10 to roughly estimate the rate. If the rhythm is regular you can be more exact in determining the rate by dividing 300 by the number of 0.20-s intervals (usually depicted by darker shading) and then extrapolating for any fraction of a 0.20-s segment.
- **Rhythm.** Determine whether each QRS is preceded by a P wave, look for variation in the PR interval and RR interval (the duration between two QRS cycles), and look for ectopic beats.
- **Hypertrophy.** One way to determine LVH is to calculate the sum of the S wave in V_1 or V_2 plus the R wave in V_5 or V_6. A sum > 35 indicates LVH. Some other criteria for LVH are R > 11 mm in aVL or R in I + S in III > 25 mm.
- **Infarction or Ischemia.** Check for ST-segment elevation or depression, Q waves, inverted T waves, or poor R-wave progression in the precordial leads. A more detailed discussion of these categories is presented in the section on Myocardial Infarction.

19

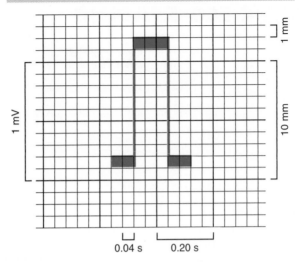

FIGURE 19–1. Examples of a 10-mm standardization mark and time marks and standard electrocardiogram paper running at 25 mm/s.

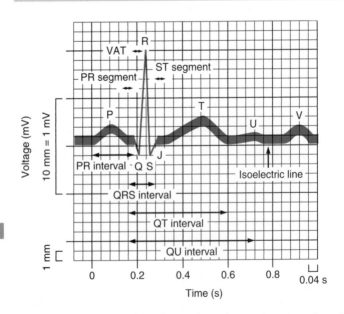

FIGURE 19–2. Diagram of the electrocardiographic complexes, intervals, and segments. The U wave is normally not well seen.

19

BASIC INFORMATION

Equipment

Bipolar Leads

- Lead I: Left arm to right arm
- Lead II: Left leg to right arm
- Lead III: Left leg to left arm

Precordial Leads: V_1 to V_6 across the chest (see Figure 13–9, page 272).

ECG Paper: With the ECG machine set at 25 mm/s, each small box represents 0.04 s and each large box 0.2 s (see Figure 19–1). Most ECG machines automatically print a standardization mark.

Normal ECG Complex

Note: A small amplitude in the Q, R, or S wave is represented by a lowercase letter; a large amplitude by an uppercase letter. The pattern shown in Figure 19–2 could also be noted as qRs.

- **P Wave.** Caused by depolarization of the atria. With normal sinus rhythm, the P wave is upright in leads I, II, aVF, V_4, V_5, and V_6 and inverted in aVR.
- **QRS Complex.** Represents ventricular depolarization
- **Q Wave.** The first negative deflection of the QRS complex (not always present and, if present, may be pathologic). To be significant, the Q wave should be > 25% the QRS complex.
- **R Wave.** The first positive deflection (R) is the positive deflection that sometimes occurs after the S wave.
- **S Wave.** The negative deflection following the R wave
- **T Wave.** Caused by repolarization of the ventricles and follows the QRS complex, normally upright in leads I, II, V_3, V_4, V_5, and V_6 and inverted in aVR

AXIS DEVIATION

The term *axis,* which represents the sum of the vectors of the electrical depolarization of the ventricles, gives some idea of the electrical orientation of the heart in the body. In a healthy person, the axis is downward and to the left, as shown in Figure 19–3. The QRS axis is midway between two leads that have QRS complexes of equal amplitude, or the axis is 90 degrees to the lead in which the QRS is isoelectric, that is, the amplitude of the R wave equals the amplitude of the S wave.

- **Normal Axis.** QRS positive in I and aVF (0–90 degrees). Normal axis is actually –30 to 105 degrees
- **LAD.** QRS positive in I and negative in aVF, –30 to –90 degrees
- **RAD.** QRS negative in I and positive in aVF, +105 to +180 degrees
- **Extreme Right Axis Deviation.** QRS negative in I and negative in aVF, +180 to +270 or –90 to –180 degrees

19

Clinical Correlations

- **RAD.** Seen with RVH, RBBB, COPD, and acute PE (a sudden change in axis toward the right), as well as in healthy individuals (occasionally)
- **LAD.** Seen with LVH, LAHB (–45 to –90 degrees), LBBB, and in some healthy individuals

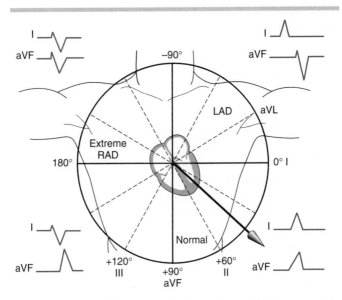

FIGURE 19–3. Graphic representation of "axis deviation." Electrocardiographic representations of each type of axis are shown in each quadrant. The large arrow is the normal axis.

HEART RATE

Bradycardia: Heart rate < 60 bpm

Tachycardia: Heart rate > 100 bpm

Rate Determination: Figure 19–4, below.

- **Method 1.** Note the 3-s marks along the top or bottom of the ECG paper (15 large squares). The approximate rate equals the number of cycles (ie, QRSs) in a 6-s strip × 10.

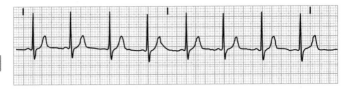

FIGURE 19–4. Sample strip for rapid rate determination (see text for procedure). Estimating the rate by counting the number of beats (eight) in the two 3-s intervals. The rate would be 8 × 10, or 80 bpm (method 1).Using method 2, each beat is separated from another beat by four 0.20-s intervals, so you divide 300 by 4, and the rate is 75 bpm. Because the beats are separated by exactly four beats you do not need to extrapolate.

19

- **Method 2** (for regular rhythms). Count the number of large squares (0.2-s boxes) between two successive cycles. The rate is equal to 300 divided by the number of squares. Extrapolate if the QRS complex does not fall exactly on the 0.2-s marks (eg, if each QRS complex is separated by 2.4 0.20-s segments, the rate is 120 bpm. The rate between two 0.20-s segments is 150 bpm, and between three 0.20-s segments is 100 bpm. Each of the five smaller 0.04-s marks between the second and third 0.20 mark would be 10 bpm (150–100 = 50 ÷ 5), and because the rate was three of the 0.04-s marks from the third 0.20-s segment the rate would be 100 + 30, or 130 bpm. Remember that the number of beats per minute for each 0.04-s mark will vary depending on which two 0.20 marks they are associated with (eg, between the fifth and sixth 0.20-s mark each 0.04 mark is 2 bpm).

RHYTHM

Sinus Rhythms

Normal: Each QRS preceded by a P wave (which is positive in II and negative in aVR) with a regular PR and RR interval and a rate between 60 and 100 bpm (Figure 19–5 below)

Sinus Tachycardia: Normal sinus rhythm with a heart rate > 100 bpm and < 180 bpm (Figure 19–6, page 388)
   Clinical Correlations. Anxiety, exertion, pain, fever, hypoxia, hypotension, increased sympathetic tone (secondary to drugs with adrenergic effects [eg, epinephrine]), anticholinergic effect (eg, atropine), PE, COPD, AMI, CHF, hyperthyroidism, and others

Sinus Bradycardia: Normal sinus rhythm with a heart rate < 60 bpm (Figure 19–7, page 388)
   Clinical Correlations. Well-trained athlete, normal variant, secondary to medications (eg, beta-blockers, digitalis, clonidine, nondihydropyridine calcium channel blockers [verapamil or diltiazem]), hypothyroidism, hypothermia, sick sinus syndrome (tachy–brady syndrome), and others.
   Treatment

- If asymptomatic (good urine output, adequate BP, and normal sensorium), no therapy needed.
- If hypotensive or disoriented: See Chapter 21, page 475

Sinus Arrhythmia: Normal sinus rhythm with a somewhat irregular heart rate. Inspiration causes a slight increase in rate; expiration decreases the rate. Normal variation between inspiration and expiration is 10% or less.

19

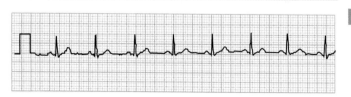

FIGURE 19–5.   Normal sinus rhythm.

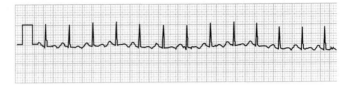

FIGURE 19–6.   Sinus tachycardia. The rate is 120–130 bpm.

Atrial Arrhythmias

PAC: Ectopic atrial focus firing prematurely followed by a normal QRS (Figure 19–8, page 389). The compensatory pause following the PAC is partial; the RR interval between beats 4 and 6 is less than between beats 1 and 3 or 6 and 8.

Clinical Correlations. Usually not of clinical significance; can be caused by stress, caffeine, and myocardial disease

PAT: A run of three or more consecutive PACs. The heart rate is usually between 140 and 250 bpm. The P wave may not be visible, but the RR interval is very regular (Figure 19–9, page 389).

Clinical Correlations. Can be seen in healthy individuals but also occurs with a variety of heart diseases. Symptoms include palpitations, light-headedness, and syncope.

Treatment

- **Increase Vagal Tone.** Valsalva maneuver or carotid massage
- **Medical Treatment.** Can include adenosine, verapamil, digoxin, edrophonium, or beta-blockers (propranolol, metoprolol, and esmolol). Verapamil and beta-blockers should be used cautiously at the same time because asystole can occur.
- **Cardioversion with Synchronized DC Shock.** Particularly in the hemodynamically unstable patient (see Chapter 21, page 483)

MAT: Multifocal atrial tachycardia is an atrial arrhythmia that originates from ectopic atrial foci. It is characterized by varying P-wave morphology and PR interval and is irregular (Figure 19–10).

Clinical Correlations. Most commonly associated with COPD, also seen in elderly patients, CHF, diabetes, or use of theophylline. Antiarrhythmics are often ineffective. Treat the underlying disease.

19

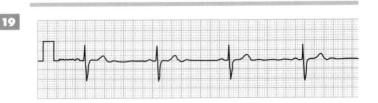

FIGURE 19–7.   Sinus bradycardia. The rate is approximately 38 bpm.

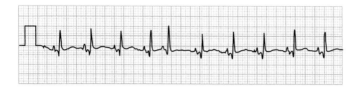

FIGURE 19–8. Premature atrial contraction (PAC). The fifth beat is a PAC.

AFib: Irregularly irregular rhythm with no discernible P waves. The ventricular rate usually varies between 100 and 180 bpm (Figure 19–11, page 390). The ventricular response may be < 100 bpm if the patient is taking digoxin, verapamil, or a beta-blocker or has AV nodal disease.

Clinical Correlations. Seen in some healthy individuals but commonly associated with organic heart disease (CAD, hypertensive heart disease, or rheumatic mitral valve disease), thyrotoxicosis, alcohol abuse, pericarditis, PE, and postoperatively.

Treatment

- **Pharmacologic Therapy.** IV adenosine, verapamil, diltiazem, digoxin, and beta-blockers (propranolol, metoprolol, and esmolol) can be used to slow down the ventricular response, and quinidine, procainamide, propafenone, ibutilide, and amiodarone can be used to maintain or convert to sinus rhythm (see individual agents in Chapter 21, Emergencies, page 469)
- **DC-Synchronized Cardioversion.** Indicated if associated with increased myocardial ischemia, hypotension, or pulmonary edema (see Chapter 21, page 483)

Atrial Flutter: Characterized by sawtooth flutter waves with an atrial rate between 250 and 350 bpm; the rate may be regular or irregular depending on whether the atrial impulses are conducted through the AV node at a regular interval or at a variable interval (Figure 19–12, page 391).

Example: One ventricular contraction (QRS) for every two flutter waves = 2:1 flutter.

Clinical Correlations. Seen with valvular heart disease, pericarditis, ischemic heart disease, pulmonary disease including PE, and alcohol abuse.

Treatment. Do *not* use quinidine or procainamide (atrial conduction may decrease to the point where 1:1 atrial:ventricular conduction can occur and the ven-

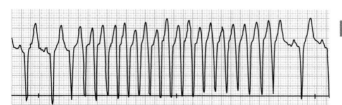

19

FIGURE 19–9. Paroxysmal atrial tachycardia.

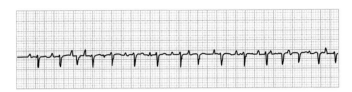

FIGURE 19–10.   Multifocal atrial tachycardia.

tricular rate will increase and hemodynamic compromise can occur), otherwise, similar to treatment of atrial fibrillation. Ibutilide (a new class III antiarrhythmic) is very effective.

Nodal Rhythm

AV Junctional or Nodal Rhythm: Rhythm originates in the AV node. Often associated with retrograde P waves that may precede or follow the QRS. If the P wave is present, it is negative in lead II and positive in aVR (just the opposite of normal sinus rhythm) (Figure 19–13). Three or more premature junctional beats in a row constitute a junctional tachycardia, which has the same clinical significance as PAT.

Ventricular Arrhythmias

PVC: As implied by the name, a premature beat arising in the ventricle. P waves may be present but have no relation to the QRS of the PVC. The QRS is usually > 0.12 s with an LBB pattern. A compensatory pause follows a PVC that is usually longer than after a PAC (Figure 19–14, page 391). The RR interval between beats 1 and 3 is equal to that between beats 3 and 5. Thus, the pause following the PVC (the fourth beat) is fully compensatory. The following patterns are recognized:

- **Bigeminy.** One normal sinus beat followed by one PVC in an alternating fashion (Figure 19–15, page 391)
- **Trigeminy.** Sequence of two normal beats followed by one PVC
- **Unifocal PVCs.** Arise from one site in the ventricle. Each has the same configuration in a single lead. (See Figure 19–14.)
- **Multifocal PVCs.** Arise from different sites; therefore, have different shapes (Figure 19–16, page 392)

19

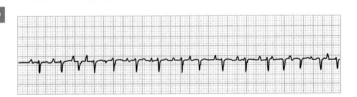

FIGURE 19–11.   Atrial fibrillation.

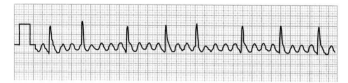

FIGURE 19–12.   Atrial flutter with atrioventricular (AV) block (3:1 to 5:1 conduction).

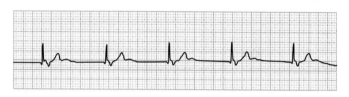

FIGURE 19–13.   Junctional rhythm with retrograde P waves (inverted) following the QRS complex.

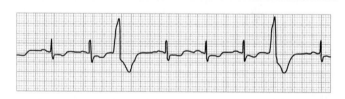

FIGURE 19–14.   Premature ventricular contractions (PVCs). The fourth and eighth beats are PVCs.

19

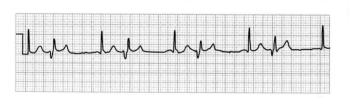

FIGURE 19–15.   Ventricular bigeminy.

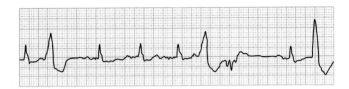

FIGURE 19–16. Multifocal PVCs. The second, sixth, seventh, and ninth beats are PVCs. Only the second and sixth PVCs have the same morphology.

Clinical Correlations. PVCs occur in healthy persons and with excessive caffeine ingestion, anemia, anxiety, organic heart disease (ischemic, valvular, or hypertensive), secondary to medications (epinephrine and isoproterenol; from toxic level of digitalis and theophylline), or predisposing metabolic abnormalities (hypoxia, hypokalemia, acidosis, alkalosis, or hypomagnesemia)

Criteria for Treatment. No treatment is necessary if no underlying cardiac disease is present and if the patient is asymptomatic. In the setting of an AMI:

- \> 5 PVCs in 1 min (some clinicians would treat any PVC associated with an MI or injury pattern on ECG)
- PVCs in couplets (two in a row)
- Numerous multifocal PVCs
- PVC that falls on the preceding T wave (R on T)

Treatment. See also Chapter 21, page 469.

- **Beta-blockers.** For symptomatic individuals without heart disease.
- **Lidocaine.** Most commonly used; other antiarrhythmics include procainamide, and amiodarone.
- Treatment of aggravating cause often sufficient (eg, treat hypoxia, hypokalemia, hyperkalemia, hypomagnesemia alkalosis or acidosis).

Ventricular Tachycardia: By definition, three or more PVCs in a row (Figure 19–17 below). A wide QRS usually with an LBBB pattern (vs. narrow complex seen with supraventricular tachycardia). May occur as a short paroxysm or a sustained run with rate 120—250 bpm. Can be life-threatening because of hypotension and tendency to degenerate into ventricular fibrillation. Treatment of nonsustained ventricular tachycardia is controversial.

19

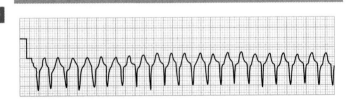

FIGURE 19–17. Ventricular tachycardia.

Clinical Correlations. See the previous section on PVCs. Patients with ventricular aneurysm are more susceptible to developing ventricular arrhythmias, especially in the presence of cardiac disease.

Treatment. See Chapter 21, page 478.

Ventricular Fibrillation: Erratic electrical activity from the ventricles, which fibrillate or twitch asynchronously. No cardiac output occurs with this rhythm (Figure 19–18 below).

Clinical Correlations. One of two patterns seen with cardiac arrest (the other would be asystole or flat line)

Treatment. See Chapter 21, page 472.

Heart Blocks

First-Degree Block: PR interval > 0.2 s (or five small boxes). Usually not clinically significant (Figure 19–19). Drugs such as beta-blockers, digitalis, and calcium channel blockers (especially verapamil) can cause first-degree block.

Second-Degree Block

Mobitz Type I (Wenckebach). Progressive prolongation of the PR interval until the P wave is blocked and not followed by a QRS complex (Figure 19–20 page 394). May occur as a 2:1, 3:2, or 4:3 block. The ratio of the atrial:ventricular beats can vary. With a 4:3 block, every fourth P wave is not followed by a QRS.

Clinical Correlations. Seen with acute myocardial ischemia such as inferior MI, ASDs, valvular heart disease, rheumatic fever, or digitalis or propranolol toxicity. Can be transient. May progress to life-threatening bradycardia (rare)

Treatment. Usually expectant; if bradycardia occurs: atropine, isoproterenol, or a pacemaker

Mobitz Type II. A series of P waves with conducted QRS complexes followed by a nonconducted P wave. The PR interval for the conducted beats remains constant. May occur as a 2:1, 3:2, or 4:3 block. The ratio of the atrial:ventricular beats can vary. With a 4:3 block, every fourth P wave is not followed by a QRS. (*Note:* AV block that is 2:1 can be either Mobitz type I or type II and may be difficult to differentiate. In general, Mobitz I has a prolonged PR with a narrow QRS; Mobitz II has a normal PR interval with an LBB pattern [wide QRS]).

Clinical Correlations. Implies severe conduction system disease that can progress to complete heart block. May be seen in acute anterior MI and cardiomyopathies.

Treatment. Use of a temporary cardiac pacemaker, particularly when associated with an acute anterior MI

19

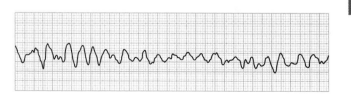

FIGURE 19–18. Ventricular fibrillation.

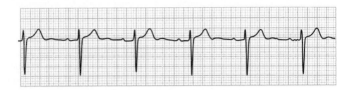

FIGURE 19–19.   First-degree AV block. The PR interval is 0.26 s.

Third-Degree Block: Complete AV block with independent atrial and ventricular rates. The ventricular rate is usually 20–40 bpm (Figure 19–21, page 395).

Clinical Correlations. May occur as the result of degenerative changes in the conduction system in the elderly, from digitalis toxicity, transiently with an acute inferior MI (ischemia of the AV junction), and after acute anterior MI (higher probability of mortality than after inferior MI); can result in syncope or CHF.

Treatment. Usually requires placement of a temporary or permanent pacemaker.

BBB: Complete BBB is present when the QRS complex is > 0.12 s (or three small boxes on the ECG strip). Look at leads I, V_1, and V_6. Degenerative changes and ischemic heart disease the most common causes.

RBBB: The RSR pattern seen in V_1 and or V_2. Also a wide S in leads I and V_6 (Figure 19–22, page 395)

Clinical Correlations. May be seen in healthy persons but usually associated with diseases affecting the right side of the heart (pulmonary hypertension, ASD, or ischemia); sudden onset is associated with PE or acute exacerbation of COPD.

LBBB: The RR′ in leads I and/or V_6. The QRS complex may actually be more slurred than double-peaked as in the RBBB. A wide S wave is seen in V_1 (Figure 19–23, page 396).

Clinical Correlations. Associated with organic heart disease (hypertensive, valvular, and ischemic) as well as severe aortic stenosis. Development of a new LBBB after an AMI may be an indication for inserting a temporary cardiac pacemaker.

19

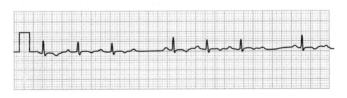

FIGURE 19–20.   Second-degree AV block, Mobitz type I (Wenckebach), with 4:3 conduction.

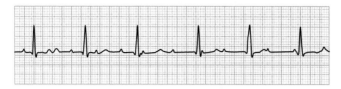

FIGURE 19–21. Third-degree AV block (complete heart block). The atrial rate is 100 bpm; the ventricular rate is 57 bpm.

CARDIAC HYPERTROPHY

Atrial Hypertrophy

P wave > 2.5 mm in height and > 0.12 s wide (three small boxes on the ECG paper)

RAE: Tall, slender, peaked P waves in leads II, III, aVF (may also be seen in V_1 and V_2)(Figure 19–24)

Clinical Correlations. Seen with chronic diffuse pulmonary disease, pulmonary hypertension, and congenital heart disease (ASD).

LAE: Notched P wave ("P mitral pattern") seen in leads I and II. A wide (0.11 s or greater), slurred biphasic P in V_1 with a wider terminal than initial component (negative deflection) (Figure 19–25, page 396)

Clinical Correlations. Seen with mitral stenosis or mitral regurgitation or secondary to LVH with hypertensive cardiovascular disease

Ventricular Hypertrophy

RVH: Tall R wave in V_1 (R wave > S wave in V_1), persistent S waves in V_5 and V_6, progressively smaller R wave from V_1 to V_6, slightly widened QRS intervals (Figure 19–26, page 397), and strain pattern with ST-segment depression and T-wave inversion in V_1 to V_3. May also see a pattern of small R waves with relatively large S waves in V_1 to V_6. Invariably right axis deviation (> 105 degrees) is present.

Clinical Correlations. Associated with mitral stenosis, chronic diffuse pulmonary disease, chronic recurrent PE, congenital heart disease (eg, tetralogy of Fallot), and biventricular hypertrophy (VH and RVH, with LVH findings often predominating).

LVH: Voltage criteria (> age 35 y): S wave in V_1 or V_2 plus the R wave in V_5 or V_6 > 5 mm, or R wave in aVL > 1 mm or R wave in I + S wave in III > 5 mm,

19

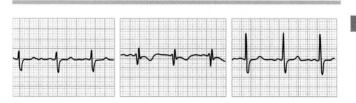

FIGURE 19–22. Leads I, V_1, and V_6 demonstrate the right bundle branch block (RBBB) pattern.

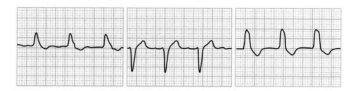

FIGURE 19–23. Leads I, V_1, and V_6 demonstrate the left bundle branch block (LBBB) pattern.

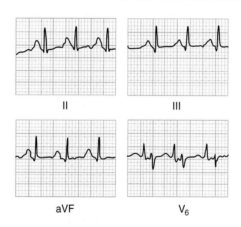

II

III

aVF

V_6

FIGURE 19–24. Right atrial enlargement, leads II, III, aVF, and V_1. Note the tall P waves in II, III, and aVF and the tall slender P waves in V_1.

19

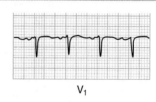

V_1

FIGURE 19–25. Left atrial enlargement.

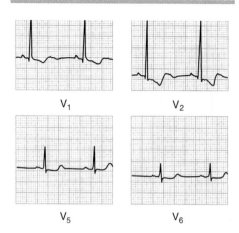

FIGURE 19–26. Right ventricular hypertrophy, leads V_1, V_2, V_5, and V_6. Note the tall R waves in V_1 and V_2, greater than the R waves in V_5 and V_6.

or an R wave in V_5 or V_6 > 26 mm. The QRS complex may be >.10 s wide in V_5 or V_6. ST-depression and T-wave inversion in the anterolateral leads (I, aVL, V_5 or V_6) suggest LVH with strain (Figure 19–27, page 398).

Clinical Correlations. HTN, aortic stenosis or insufficiency, long-standing CAD, and some forms of congenital heart disease

MYOCARDIAL INFARCTION

(See also Chapter 21, page 479.)

Myocardial Ischemia: Inadequate oxygen supply to the myocardium because of blockage or spasm of the coronary arteries. The ECG can show ST-segment depression (subendocardial ischemia) (Figure 19–28, page 398), ST elevation (transmural ischemia) (Figure 19–29 page 398), or symmetrically inverted ("flipped") T waves (Figure 19–30, page 399) in the area of ischemia (eg, inferior ischemia in II, III, and F; anterior ischemia in V_1 to V_6; lateral ischemia in I, aVL; anterolateral ischemia in I, aVL, V_5, and V_6; anteroseptal ischemia in V_1, V_2, V_3, and V_4.

MI: Refers to myocardial necrosis caused by severe ischemia. Can be transmural (ST elevation early, T-wave inversion, and Q waves late) or subendocardial (ST depression and T-wave inversion without evidence of Q waves). Table 19–1, page 399 outlines the localization of MIs.

- **Acute Injury Phase (transmural).** Hyperacute T waves, then ST-segment elevation. Hyperacute T waves return to normal in minutes to hours. ST elevation usually regresses after hours to days. Persistent ST elevation suggests a left ventricular aneurysm.
- **Evolving Phase (transmural).** Hours to days after an MI. Deep T-wave inversion occurs and then replaces ST-segment elevation, and the T wave may return to normal.

19

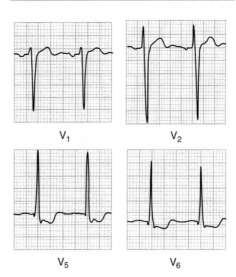

FIGURE 19–27. Left ventricular hypertrophy, leads V_1, V_2, V_5, and V_6. The S wave in the V_2 + R wave in V_5 is 55 mm. Note the ST changes and T-wave inversion in V_5 and V_6, suggesting "strain."

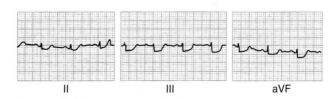

FIGURE 19–28. ST-segment depression in leads II, III, and aVF in a patient with acute inferior subendocardial ischemia/infarction.

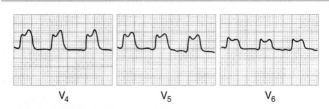

FIGURE 19–29. ST elevation in leads V_4, V_5, and V_6 in a patient with acute anterolateral transmural ischemia/infarction.

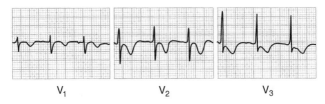

V₁   V₂   V₃

FIGURE 19–30. Inverted T waves.

- **Q Waves (transmural).** Hours to days after a transmural MI. A Q wave is the initial negative deflection of the QRS complex. A "significant" Q wave is 0.04 s in duration and > 25% the height of the R wave (Figure 19–31, page 400). May regress to normal after years.

ELECTROLYTE AND DRUG EFFECTS

Electrolytes

Hyperkalemia: Narrow, symmetrical, diffuse, peaked T waves. With severe hyperkalemia, PR prolongation occurs, the P wave flattens and is lost, and the QRS widens and can progress to ventricular fibrillation (Figure 19–32, page 400).

Hypokalemia: ST-segment depression with the appearance of U waves (a positive deflection after the T wave) (Figure 19–33, page 401)

Hypercalcemia: Short QT interval

TABLE 19–1
Localization of Transmural Myocardial Infarction on ECG

Location of MI	Presence of Q Wave or ST-Segment Elevation	Reciprocal ST Depression
Anterior	V₁ to V₆ (or poor R-wave progression in leads V₁ to V₆)ᵃ	II, III, aVF
Lateral	I, aVL, V₅, V₆	V₁, V₃
Inferior	II, III, aVF	I, aVL, possibly anterior leads
Posterior	Abnormally tall R and T waves in V₁ to V₃	V₁ to V₃
Subendocardial	No abnormal Q wave. ST-segment depression in the anterior, lateral, or inferior leads	

ᵃNormally in V₁ to V₆, the R-wave amplitude gradually increases and the S wave decreases with a "biphasic" QRS (R = S) in V₃ or V₄. With an anterior MI, there will be a loss of R-wave voltage (instead of Q waves) and the biphasic QRS will appear more laterally in V₄ to V₆, hence the term *poor R-wave progression.*

19

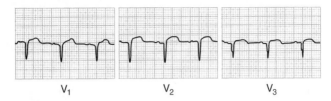

FIGURE 19–31.   Q waves in leads V_1, V_2, and V_3 in a patient with an acute anteroseptal transmural myocardial infarction. Note the ST elevation in helping to determine the acute nature of the infarction.

Hypocalcemia: Prolonged QT interval

Drugs

Digitalis Effect: Downsloping ST segment

Digitalis Toxicity
- **Arrhythmias.** PVCs, bigeminy, trigeminy, ventricular tachycardia, ventricular fibrillation, PAT, nodal rhythms, and sinus bradycardia.
- **Conduction Abnormalities.** First-degree, second-degree, and third-degree heart blocks

Quinidine and Procainamide: With toxic levels, prolonged QT, flattened T wave, and QRS widening

MISCELLANEOUS ECG CHANGES

Pericarditis: Diffuse ST elevation concave upward and/or diffuse PR depression and/or diffuse T-wave inversion (Figure 19–34, page 401)
   Clinical Correlations. Idiopathic, viral as well as other infections, including bacterial, fungal, and TB, AMI, collagen–vascular diseases, uremia, cancer, Dressler's syndrome, and postpericardiotomy syndrome

Hypothermia: Sinus bradycardia, AV junctional rhythm, or ventricular fibrillation common. Classically, **J point** (the end of the QRS complex and the beginning of the ST segment) elevation and an intraventricular conduction delay and a prolonged QT interval possible (Figure 19–35, page 401)

19

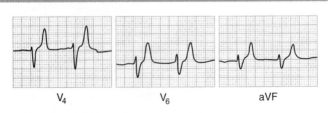

FIGURE 19–32.   Diffuse tall T waves in leads V_4, V_6 and aVF with widened QRS and junctional rhythm (loss of P waves), secondary to hyperkalemia.

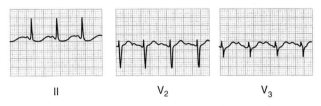

FIGURE 19–33.   Leads II, V_2, and V_3 in a patient with hypokalemia. A U wave is easily seen in V_2 and V_3, but difficult to distinguish from the T wave in II.

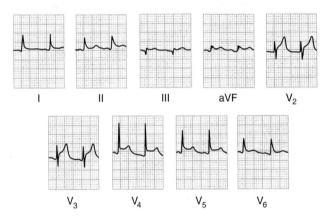

FIGURE 19–34.   Acute pericarditis.

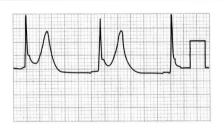

FIGURE 19–35.   Sinus bradycardia, J-point elevation with ST-segment elevation and prolonged QT interval (0.56 s) in a patient with hypothermia.

19

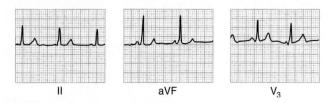

FIGURE 19–36. Short PR interval and delta waves in leads II, aVF, and V₃ in a patient with Wolff-Parkinson–White syndrome.

WPW Syndrome: A preexcitation syndrome caused by conduction from the SA node to the ventricle through an accessory pathway that bypasses the AV node. Classically, a short PR interval occurs along with a delta wave (a delay in the initial deflection of the QRS complex). Clinically, these patients commonly have tachyarrhythmias, such as atrial fibrillation (Figure 19–36 above).

CRITICAL CARE

MANAGEMENT OF THE CRITICALLY ILL PATIENT

Patients admitted to the ICU typically have multisystem disease, traumatic injuries, or are under intensive treatment regimens to avoid or manage end-organ dysfunctions. Despite vast advancements in knowledge, the interactions *between dysfunctional organ systems* remain complicated and are often overwhelming to the junior house officer. Physicians must systematically focus on each organ system and evaluate its real-time functional status as well as its interactions within the host. A thorough approach allows the physician to integrate organ system therapies into a treatment strategy for the patient as a whole. This chapter describes a system-by-system approach to evaluating, analyzing, integrating, and treating critically ill patients as well as some commonly encountered critical care complications.

One of the most important aspects of caring for the critically ill patient is performing a thorough daily physical exam. A methodical, detail-oriented examination of the ICU patient often identifies problems that, if acted on early, will markedly alter the patients' recovery. In other words, being **proactive,** not **reactive,** may prove to be the difference between the critically ill patient surviving the illness or not.

ICU PROGRESS NOTE

The ICU progress note is a concise, systematic, well-organized means of documenting the patient's major problems, the events over the past 24 h, the physical exam, pertinent laboratory data, and the treatment plan (see Sample ICU Progress Note). Although the information may be found elsewhere in the chart, the physician's interpretation of data and events, assessment, and treatment plan communicate the medical decision-making process to those who read the chart. A simple, organized approach to the daily progress note includes:

A. Outline of the patient's problem list and/or injury summary
   1. Active problems, major inactive problems and significant allergies
   2. Significant past medical or surgical history relevant to the present illness
   3. List hospital day, posttrauma day, postoperative day, etc.

B. Outline of events and procedures over the past 24 h
C. List of current medications including analgesic and sedation regimens
D.. Sequential, system-specific physical exam and pertinent flow sheet data

    1. **CNS:** Central nervous system functioning or other neurologic assessment and sedation level (Modified Ramsay Sedation scale, Richmond Agitation Scale, etc)

    2. **CV:** Cardiovascular function, including indicators of systemic perfusion, measured BPs, and calculated pulmonary artery catheter data

    3. **Pulm:** Pulmonary function, including mechanical ventilator settings, and ABG values

    4. **GI/Nut:** GI function and nutritional status

    5. **F/E/R:** Fluids, electrolytes, and renal function

    6. **Heme/ID:** Hematologic function, including CBC, coagulation values; infectious disease status (recent culture data, antibiotic regimen, treatment duration)

    7. **Prophylaxis:** Therapies to prevent complications, such as DVT, ethanol withdrawal, stress gastritis, etc

E. Other relevant laboratory or radiographic data
F. Assessment and plan for the next 24 h

Sample ICU Progress Note

(written for a trauma patient)

Date: January 21, 2004

PROBLEM LIST:

- S/P MVC (PTD # 3)
- L pulmonary contusion
- L hemopneumothorax S/P L chest tube
- Grade 4 splenic injury S/P splenectomy (POD #2)
- Acute renal failure
- ARDS
- PMHx: Hypertension/gout
- Allergies: Morphine

EVENTS OF PAST 24 HOURS:

- Increasing FiO_2 and PEEP
- Renal consult
- L subclavian vein cordis/Swan–Ganz catheter placement
- Nasojejunal feeding tube placed

MEDICATIONS:

- Dopamine gtt
- Fentanyl gtt
- Lorazepam gtt
- Vaccines given (POD # 1)

EXAM AND FLOW SHEET DATA:

CNS: Intubated, sedated (RAS –2), moves all 4 extremities
- Atraumatic head

20

- Pupils equal and reactive
- EOM intact
- Neck immobilized

CV: RRR w/o murmurs
- No JVD
- 2+ capillary refill
- Toes warm
- Minimal peripheral edema
- P 150 (sinus tach), BP 110/65, PAP 45/20, PCWP 14, CO 3.7, CI 2.5, EDVI 89

Pulm: Coarse BS bilaterally
- L chest tube in place
- Ventilator setting: SIMV rate 16/4; FIO_2 75%; PEEP 12; PS 10
- ABG: 7.38/42/78/19/–3

GI/Nut: Midline incision healing well
- Soft, nontender, nondistended
- + Bowel sounds
- Nasojejunal feeding tube in stomach
- Tube feedings started (20 mL/h)

F/E/R: LR
- Electrolytes wnl
- BUN 48
- Cr 1.9
- Total I/O: 3400/2210
- UO 45 mL/h

Heme/ID: WBC 17.5
- Hgb 9.4
- HCT 30
- Coags wnl
- Blood cultures $(–) \times 2$
- Vancomycin (D # 2/7)

Prophylaxis: SCDs on LE
- Heparin 5000 U SQ q12h
- Famotidine 20 mg IV q12h

ASSESSMENT AND PLAN:

- *CNS*: Stable neuro exam; sedation level adequate; continue fentanyl and lorazepam gtt while on ventilator; wean narcotics as ventilator dependence improves
- *CV:* Hemodynamically stable, however, continues to require intermittent fluid challenge to maintain BP; this may be the cause of acute renal failure; will continue IV fluids and wait for capillary leak to cease; will wean dopamine gtt as tolerated
- *Pulm:* Worsening FIO_2 and PEEP requirements overnight; likely ARDS complicated by pulmonary contusion; will obtain CXR this AM and wean FIO_2/increase PEEP as tolerated by BP and CO; continue L chest tube to suction; will DC when ventilatory status improves

20

- *GI / Nut:* S/P splenectomy; ileus continues; will continue trophic tube feedings
- *F/E/R:* Acute renal failure continues; will proceed with renal ultrasound to R/O postrenal cause; no significant renal toxic drugs currently given
- *Heme/ID:* S/P splenectomy; HCT stable; postsplenectomy vaccines given; will expect mild leukocytosis and thrombocytosis
- *Prophylaxis:* Continue as prescribed

Signature,_____

(See Abbreviations list at the beginning of the book for definitions of abbreviations.)

ROUTINE MONITORING

Critically ill patients require continuous monitoring of basic physiologic parameters to identify perturbations. Such perturbations should then prompt a timely clinical adjustment in order to improve the patient's outcome:

1. **Continuous ECG:** Allows use of computerized arrhythmia detection systems; rapid, continuous access enables prompt assessment of cardiac rhythm to ensure proper treatment; increases the likelihood of successful resuscitation.
2. **Blood Pressure:** Intermittent (sphygmomanometer) or continuous (intravascular) assessment of BPs (ie, systolic / diastolic/mean arterial/central venous pressures, etc); allows tracking of treatments and minute-to-minute titration of vasoactive drugs; continuous, intravascular methods are warranted in patients with significant hemodynamic instability.
3. **Pulse Oximetry:** Continuous, quantitative arterial O_2 saturation (Sao_2); ensures adequate oxygenation of systemic arterial blood for tissue delivery and utilization.
4. **Temperature:** Critically ill patients are at high risk for thermoregulatory disorders due to their pathophysiology (ie, fluid resuscitation, burns, sepsis, etc); continuous measurements in the esophagus (esophageal probe) or central venous blood compartment (pulmonary artery catheter) are accurate methods for monitoring core body temperature; changes in temperature should prompt investigation.
5. **Capnography:** Allows continuous measurement of expired CO_2; changes warrant further investigation as they imply a change in clinical status (ie, hypoventilation, overfeeding, fever, sepsis, etc).

TRANSPORTING CRITICALLY ILL PATIENTS

Murphy's law dictates "Whatever may go wrong, will go wrong"; this is especially true during the transport of critically ill patients. Adherence to "common sense" guidelines will help to minimize potential adverse events:

1. **Always Remember:** *Maintain the patient's airway;* if airway concerns exist, intubate the patient *prior* to transport.
2. Transport only stable patients (unless the role for transport is to provide a life-saving intervention).

20

3. Pay attention to IV catheters/pumps and their attachments to each other; loss of IV access in a critically ill patient is dangerous.
4. Ensure the patient has sufficient transportable O_2, IV fluids, medications, etc.
5. Be certain enough assistance is available to safely transport the patient and the many machines; make sure the destination is prepared for the patient's arrival and transfer will be expeditious.
6. Expect the unexpected; have personnel, equipment, and supplies available that could make the difference in a crisis situation.

CENTRAL NERVOUS SYSTEM

Severe acute illness often results in altered mental status (AMS). AMS may manifest a spectrum of disability from simple, mild delirium to complex, life-threatening coma. The precise CNS pathophysiology of AMS states remains unknown; however, false neurotransmitters, excess catecholamines, alterations in ion fluxes, and deranged cerebral blood flow all appear to play a role.

Critically ill patients are often intubated. Medications must be administered to the intubated patient to provide sedation and analgesia. Inadequate sedation and pain control have well known adverse sequelae (ie, increased catabolism, tachycardia and higher myocardial oxygen consumption, immunosuppression, hypercoagulability, severe anxiety, etc), so great care must be taken in finding the proper balance of medications.

When acute agitation occurs, *life-threatening pathology* (ie, inadequate blood flow or nutrient availability to the brain) *should be ruled out first*. Assessment of vital signs, blood glucose concentration, and oxygenation/ventilation status must be performed prior to administering CNS-altering medications.

Benzodiazepines are potent inducers of sedation, amnesia, muscle relaxation, and anxiolysis. These properties make this class of drug ideal for short- to intermediate-term use in this patient population. Great care should be taken to choose a drug that will not accumulate in the patient's system if end-organ dysfunction is present:

- **Lorazepam:** Good intermediate-duration benzodiazepine; metabolized by the liver with inactive metabolite excreted in the urine; very potent but has a long time to peak-effect (ie, ideal agent for longer-term sedation)
- **Midazolam:** Shorter-onset, shorter-acting benzodiazepine; metabolism altered by calcium channel blockers, erythromycin, and triazole antifungals

Either agent should be used and titrated to achieve a sedation level according to published scales (ie, Modified Ramsay Scale, Richmond Agitation Scale, etc). The **Ramsey Sedation scale** is:

1. Anxious and agitated or restless or both
2. Cooperative, oriented and tranquil
3. Responding to commands only
4. Brisk response to light glabellar tap
5. Sluggish response to light glabellar tap
6. No response to light glabellar tap.

20

If over medication occurs (ie, inadvertent overadministration, accumulation of metabolites), cessation of the medication, preparation to institute cardiopulmonary support, and the use of flumazenil will assist to reverse the overly sedated state.

- **Propofol:** Nonbenzodiazepine, lipid-based sedative-hypnotic; little analgesic properties; extremely short onset and half-life make accumulation unlikely (ie, ultra-short-term drug); expensive; longer-term use has adverse financial and infectious consequences. One approach is to initiate at 10 mcg/kg/min and adjust by increments of 10–20 mcg/kg/min q5–15 min to achieve desired level of sedation (dosing > 50 mcg/kg/min should be reconsidered). To discontinue, wean the infusion by 25% q10–15 min, then D/C when conscious.
- **Haloperidol:** Short-term treatment of agitation especially with components of delirium; however, use is not without potential adverse electrocardiographic consequences (ie, prolongation of QT interval); use should be discontinued if the QT interval increases by > 50 % of baseline or exceeds 450 ms

Critically ill patients may also have acute pain requirements due to recent surgeries or prehospital trauma. Opioid narcotic agents are best suited for acute pain control.

- **Morphine:** IV opioid narcotic; commonly used (low cost, ease of use)
- **Fentanyl:** Newer, synthetic opioid; more potent and shorter acting than morphine; less histamine release than morphine (ie, less potential for drug-induced hypotension)

These opioids may be administered as continuous infusions, intermittent boluses, or as part of patient-controlled analgesia (PCA) regimen. Because narcotics may produce respiratory depression, careful titration is necessary, especially when narcotics are combined with benzodiazepines. Epidural anesthesia provides good local analgesic properties with less need for IV narcotics, which should yield less respiratory compromise.

Many critically ill patients will require long-term sedation and analgesia. Mid- to long-acting medications provide the best means of achieving this goal. Current data suggest, however, that interruption of on-going sedation to allow the patient to awaken on a daily basis leads to decreased mechanical ventilation days and ICU length of stay.

Neuromuscular paralysis is rarely necessary, but may be used in patients with severe respiratory failure and the inability to properly oxygenate or ventilate. Eliminating the muscular elastic recoil of the chest wall and ventilator dyssynchrony may improve pulmonary compliance and ventilation/oxygenation ability.

CARDIOVASCULAR SYSTEM

Cardiovascular instability remains one of the most common problems encountered in ICU patients. Understanding the approach to evaluating the cardiovascular system is essential. As before, a thorough physical exam must begin your assessment of the patient.

20

Inspection: Jugular Venous Distention (JVD)

- Neck vein visualization (with the patient sitting at a 45-degree angle) implies a central venous pressure (CVP) of > 12–15 mm Hg
- JVD *plus* systemic hypotension suggests *life-threatening pathology*:

1. Tension pneumothorax
2. Pericardial tamponade
3. Severe cardiac dysfunction

Inspection: Precordial Contusion (ie, Bruising)

- Associated with blunt trauma from a steering wheel; injury pattern implies possible myocardial contusion. *Treatment:* continuous ECG monitoring; correction of arrhythmias (most common: sinus tachycardia). Transthoracic echocardiography should be performed if arrhythmias occur to identify anatomic heart injury and/or pericardial effusion

Inspection: Extremity Perfusion

- Check extremities for **perfusion** (ie, pulse, color, temperature, and capillary refill)
- *Note:* Pay special attention to sites distal to:
  - Long bone fractures
  - Joint dislocations
  - Indwelling arterial catheters

Blood Pressure (BP)

Over the short term, BP is considered adequate if renal perfusion is maintained (usually mean arterial pressure (MAP) > 70 mm Hg in young, previously healthy individuals). Premorbid medical problems and aging, however, may alter this somewhat.

Note: If the cuff is too small for the arm (ie, the patient is obese), the measured systolic BP will be 10–15 mm Hg higher than the actual pressure.

Systolic Hypertension: Systolic BP > 140 mm Hg with normal diastolic BP. In the acute setting, due to:

- Increased cardiac output
- Thyrotoxicosis
- Generalized response to stress
- Anemia
- Pain and/or anxiety

Diastolic Hypertension: Diastolic BP > 90 mm Hg. Isolated diastolic BP hypertension associated with:

- Intrinsic renal disease
- Endocrine disorders
- Renovascular hypertension
- Neurologic disorders

Treatment: HTN is a concern following an AMI, subarachnoid hemorrhage, or vascular anastomosis (esp. carotid artery surgery). Ideally, the systolic BP is maintained between 130–160 mm Hg in critically ill patients. A systolic BP > 180 mm Hg usually requires *immediate treatment.* Several drugs are commonly used to treat acute HTN in the ICU setting; nitroprusside, hydralazine, labetalol, esmolol, or nitroglycerin. Rapid, easily reversible beta-blockade (ie, esmolol) should be used with nitroprusside in treating HTN associated with a ruptured aortic aneurysm or blunt traumatic aortic injury. The emergency management of

20

hypertension is discussed in Chapter 21 and the specific antihypertensive agents are discussed more fully in Chapter 22.

Mean Arterial Pressure (MAP)

Calculated as DBP + [(SBP – DBP)/3]

Pulse Pressure (SBP – DBP)

Wide Pulse Pressure: (> 40 mm Hg) associated with:

- Thyrotoxicosis
- Arterial venous fistula
- Aortic insufficiency

Narrow Pulse Pressure: (< 25 mm Hg) associated with:

- Significant tachycardia
- Early hypovolemic shock
- Pericarditis
- Pericardial effusion or tamponade
- Ascites
- Aortic stenosis

Paradoxical Pulse: Systolic BP changes during the respiratory cycle as a function of changes in intrathoracic pressures (see Chapter 13 for the technique for measuring the paradoxical pulse). Normally, systolic BP falls 6–10 mm Hg with inspiration. If this variation occurs over a wider negative inspiratory range (> 10 mm Hg), the patient is said to have a paradoxical pulse (Figure 20–1 below). Associated conditions include:

- Pericardial tamponade
- Asthma and COPD
- Ruptured diaphragm
- Pneumothorax

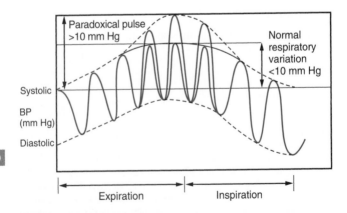

FIGURE 20–1.   The paradoxical pulse.

Auscultation: Heart Murmurs

The presence of a premorbid cardiac murmur and, more importantly, the interval development of a new cardiac murmur are important in the care of the critically ill patient. All new murmurs should be characterized by intensity, location, and variation with position and respiration as well as whether they are systolic or diastolic. In general, diastolic murmurs are usually pathologic (see Chapter 1 for more information on heart murmurs).

Systolic Murmurs: Abrupt onset of a new systolic heart murmur may be caused by:

1. **Papillary muscle dysfunction/injury:** Usually occurs following AMI; characterized by low-grade (II/V) apical pansystolic murmur; diagnosis is made by either cardiac catheterization or by echocardiography.
2. **Intraventricular septal rupture:** Indicated by abrupt appearance of loud systolic murmur usually following an AMI; usually accompanied by massive pulmonary edema; may require emergency cardiac catheterization and operative repair.

Diastolic Murmurs: The major concern of the sudden appearance of a diastolic murmur in the acutely ill or injured patient is bacterial endocarditis; more common long-term ICU patients. Foreign bodies (ie, central venous and hyperalimentation lines, pulmonary artery catheters, etc) contribute to the increasing incidence of bacterial endocarditis.

1. **Gallop:** Defined as three sequential heart sounds in which the first two beats of the triplet are closer together than the third (resulting in a sound that resembles the gallop of a horse). A newly occurring gallop may herald the onset of one or more of the following:

    - AMI
    - Anemia
    - Severe CHF
    - Mitral regurgitation secondary to injury of the papillary muscle

2. **Pericardial friction rub:** Described as the sound of two pieces of leather rubbing together; frequently high-pitched and intermittent. Common following open heart surgery and in this setting does not necessarily indicate pathologic changes. Development of a pericardial friction rub should lead to the suspicion of:

    - Pericarditis
    - Pericardial effusion
    - MI near the surface of the pericardium

CARDIOVASCULAR PHYSIOLOGY
Definitions

Cardiac Output (CO):   Volume of blood pumped by the heart each minute (mL/min); calculated as heart rate (HR; bpm) stroke volume (SV; mL/beat); approximately 3.5–5.5 L/min (adult). HR is measured directly; SV depends on the following:

Preload: Initial length of myocardial muscle fibers is proportional to the left ventricular end-diastolic volume (LVEDV), which is governed by the volume of

20

blood remaining in the left ventricle after each beat. As LVEDV increases, the stretch on myocardial muscle fibers increases. Furthermore (Panel 1, Figure 20–2 below), as the LVEDV increases (ie, stretch), the energy of contraction increases proportionally until an optimal tension develops (Starling's law; Panel 2, Figure 20–2); when the myocardial muscle fiber is overstretched, the contractile strength decreases.

Afterload: Resistance to ventricular ejection; measured clinically by aortic BP and calculation of systemic vascular resistance (SVR).

Contractility: Ability of heart to alter its contractile force and velocity independent of fiber length (ie, the intrinsic strength of the individual muscle fiber

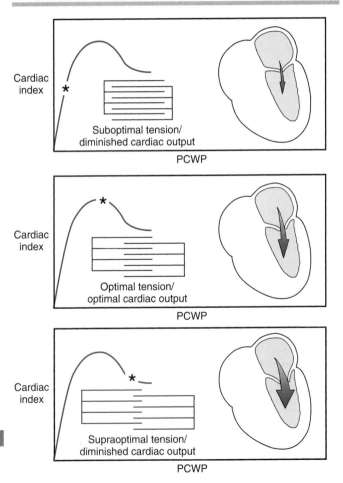

FIGURE 20–2. Representation of Starling's law. PCWP = pulmonary capillary wedge pressure.

cells). Contractility may be increased by stimulation of beta-receptors in the heart (see following section).

Cardiac Index (CI): Used to standardize CO based on body size; calculated as CO/(patient's body surface area); normal CI $\cong$ 2.8 – 3.2 L/min/m^2; CI < 2.5 L/min/m^2 may require pharmacologic interventions if it is insufficient for the patients circulatory needs.

Review of the Sympathetic Nervous System Influence on the Cardiovascular System

CO and its determinants (ie, preload, afterload, and contractility) are all influenced by the sympathetic nervous system (SNS). The SNS releases catecholamines (predominantly epinephrine and norepinephrine), which bind to end-organ receptors and exert a physiologic response. Adrenergic receptors are divided into two major classes: alpha (α) and beta (β). End-organ function after receptor activation is summarized in Table 20–1 below.

Adrenergic receptors are important because many of the cardiovascular drugs used in the ICU act through their sympathomimetic properties. Such drugs have a specific receptor affinity (ie, α versus β) and consequently differ in their end-organ effects. For example, drugs that act on the α_1 receptors are called "vasopressors" because they cause nonspecific systemic vasoconstriction. Conversely, drugs that act on β_1 receptor are called "inotropes" because they provide an increase in myocardial contractility and heart rate.

Because each drug exerts receptor-specific effects, their use provides differential activation of receptors and ultimately end-organ effects. Through tailoring pharmacologic support, the physician is able to provide the necessary cardiovascular assistance to critically ill patients. Commonly used sympathomimetics and their relative receptor affinities are listed in Table 20–2, page 414. A guide to administration of these agents appears in Table 20–11, page 459.

CENTRAL VENOUS PRESSURE (CVP)

The CVP catheter is one of two major devices used for cardiovascular instrumentation. The other, the pulmonary artery catheter (a.k.a., PA catheter, Swan–Ganz catheter, or right-heart catheter), is considered in the next section.

TABLE 20–1
Adrenergic Receptors and Their Actions on the Cardiovascular System

Receptor	Location	Action
Alpha (α)$_1$	Peripheral arterioles	Vasoconstriction (increased SVR)
Beta (β)$_1$	Myocardium	Increased contractility
	SA node	Increased heart rate
Beta (β)$_2$	Peripheral arterioles	Vasodilatation (decreased SVR)
	Bronchiolar smooth muscle	Bronchodilatation

SVR = systemic vascular resistance; SA = sinoatrial

20

TABLE 20–2
Relative Actions of Sympathomimetic Drugs on Adrenergic Receptors

Drug	Effect on			
	α	β_1	β_2	D
Phenylephrine	++++	0	0	
Norepinephrine	++++	++	0	
Epinephrine	++++	++++	++	
Dobutamine	+	++++	++	
Isoproterenol	0	++++	+++	
Dopamine (mcg/kg/min) 10–20	5–10			1–5

Key: + = Relative effect; 0 = no clinically significant effect; D=dopaminergic receptors.

For CVP monitoring, a 14-gauge IV catheter is inserted into the central venous circulation via the internal jugular or subclavian vein (see Chapter 13, page 258). A pressure transducer and monitor connected to the catheter provide the measurements. A CXR is required to confirm the position of the catheter in the superior vena cava. The zero point for the transducer is usually 5 cm below the sternal notch in the midaxillary line.

The CVP reading reflects right atrial pressures, and by association, right ventricular filling pressure. This filling pressure, or preload, is one determinant in the ability of the heart to pump blood (see Preload section). More importantly are the relative changes that take place in the patient's CVP as the fluid or cardiac status changes. Therefore, serial readings are recorded and compared over time with other physiologic measurements. The general implications of CVP readings are listed in Table 20–3 below.

TABLE 20–3
Interpretation of CVP Measurements

Reading (mm Hg)	General Description	Clinical Implications
< 3	Low	Intravenous fluids may be administered
3–10	Midrange	Probable clinical euvolemia
>10	High	Suspect fluid overload, CHF, CP, COPD, tension PTX

CVP = central venous pressure; CHF = congestive heart failure; CP = cor pulmonale; COPD = chronic obstructive pulmonary disease; PTX = pneumothorax.

CVP Limitations

1. CVP does not *entirely* reflect total blood volume or left ventricular function.
2. CVP will be altered by:

    - Changes in pulmonary artery resistance
    - Changes in compliance of the right ventricle
    - Intrathoracic pressures (ie, mechanical ventilation)

3. An accurate clinical picture may be limited by conditions that radically change intrathoracic pressure:

    - Positive pressure ventilation, especially when high PEEP is used
    - Pneumothorax, hemothorax, hydrothorax, or tension pneumothorax
    - Presence of intrathoracic tumors

4. CVP may be normal in the face of sepsis or hypovolemia when accompanied by compromised myocardial function
5. Occult left ventricular failure may occur in the presence of normal CVP
6. Patients with COPD may require an elevated CVP to optimize their cardiac output
7. PA catheter readings are more accurate than CVP with regard to a patient's fluid and cardiac status

Technical Tips Regarding CVP Measurements

- CVP readings are inaccurate if they do not fluctuate with respiration
- If appropriate, remove the patient from the ventilator when taking a CVP reading
- To ensure comparable readings, have the patient positioned in the same manner for each measurement
- Flatten the bed and use the same zero point for the transducer (5 cm below the sternal notch in the midaxillary line)

PULMONARY ARTERY CATHETERS

The pulmonary artery (a.k.a., PA, Swan–Ganz, or right-heart) catheter is a device that allows the direct measurement of central cardiovascular pressures, which, after the appropriate calculations are performed, then yield important circulatory parameters useful in the treatment of acutely ill patients. The catheter is placed in a central vein (usually the subclavian or internal jugular) and then passes into the right atrium, across the tricuspid valve, into the right ventricle, through the pulmonic valve with the distal end subsequently "floated" into the pulmonary artery (Figure 20–3, page 416). The PA catheter then allows the measurement of the pulmonary artery pressure (PAP), the pulmonary artery occlusion pressure (PAOP, also known as the pulmonary capillary wedge pressure, PCWP), and the CVP. Intravascular volume status, vascular tone (both pulmonary and systemic), and the heart's pumping ability (cardiac output) are all then calculated. Newer technology also allows for the continuous monitoring of mixed venous oxygen saturation (Svo_2), measurement of the right ventricular ejection fraction (REF), and the right ventricular end-diastolic volume index (RVEDVI).

20

  Key point: The data obtained with a PA catheter are only as good as the initial setup and the *actual* measurements obtained (ie, pressures). If the pressure measurements are in error *or* if patient data (height, weight, etc) are incorrectly entered into the system, the subsequent calculations will be *incorrect*.

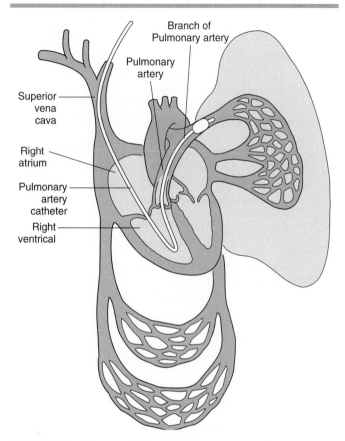

FIGURE 20–3.   Relative positioning of the pulmonary artery catheter.

Indications

Common clinical conditions requiring PA catheter monitoring include:

- Acute heart failure
- Shock states
- Complex circulatory and fluid conditions (massive resuscitation)
- Diagnosis of pericardial tamponade
- Complicated MI
- Intraoperative management in high-risk cardiac patients (ie, aneurysm repair, elderly patient undergoing major surgery)

20

Catheter Description

The PA catheter generally consists of three (or four) lumens and a thermistor at the tip (Figure 20–4, page 417); markings are typically in 10-cm increments; the catheter is radiopaque.

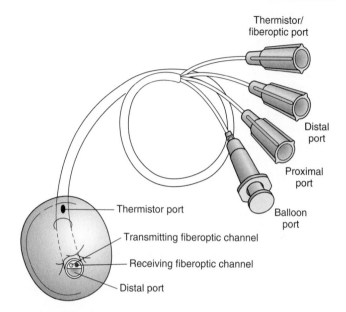

FIGURE 20-4. An example of a pulmonary artery catheter. This one features an oximetric measuring feature (see text for a complete description).

Lumens
- **Balloon port:** Usually a square white port; route to inflate the balloon at the tip of the catheter; inflation of the balloon requires between 1.0–1.5 mL of air
- **Proximal port:** Approximately 30 cm proximal to the tip; lies in the superior vena cava; may be used for fluid administration when not used for determinations of CVP and CO
- **Distal port:** Lies in the PA beyond the balloon; this port is attached to a pressure transducer for continuous PAP tracings and intermittent PAOP measurement

Thermistor: Temperature sensor that provides continuous core temperature measurement as well as measurements used in the thermal dilution CO techniques (see page 427)

Modifications of Pulmonary Artery Catheter: Several modifications of the original PA catheter allow for additional functions and measurement capabilities:

- **Pacing PA catheters:** Extra ports (approximately 19 cm from the tip) through which pacing wires are passed into the right ventricle; other models contain electrodes along the surface of the catheter; capable of pacing both the right atrium and ventricle
- **Oximetric PA catheter:** Standard PA catheter ports with fiberoptic components; emit light impulses to and from distal end of catheter; light im-

20

pulses are then reflected back by hemoglobin and measured; allows continuous O_2 saturation monitoring (see Figure 20–4)

- **Right ventricular ejection catheter:** Determines right ventricular ejection fraction (REF), which is then used to calculate the RVEDVI (best indicator of preload)

Contraindications for PA Catheter Use: There are *no* absolute contraindications if a PA catheter is needed to treat a patient in a critical care setting. Patients with LBBB may experience complete heart block (may require temporary pacemaker placement); frequent manipulation may increase the risk of infection (similarly to other IV catheters).

Materials: There are many versions of the flow-directed, balloon-tipped PA catheter (see generic representation in Figure 20–4). A PA catheter introducer insertion kit provides the introducer sheath (cordis catheter), flexible J-tip guidewire, vessel dilator, catheter contamination shield, and various other items needed to insert the catheter (Figure 20–5 below). The monitoring system (ie, transducers, tubing, stopcocks) and pressurized flush system are usually set up by the nursing staff and should be operational prior to catheter insertion.

Pulmonary Artery Catheterization Procedure

1. Informed consent is usually *required* because these catheters are usually placed in very ill patients. Subsequently, the patient's medical decision maker should grant consent.
2. The patient should be in the ICU with continuous ECG and hemodynamic monitoring. Emergency resuscitation medications must be on hand in the event of a refractory arrhythmia.
3. Choose a site (usually dictated by patient variables and operator experience). In a patient who may receive thrombolytic therapy or who has a coagulopathy, femoral and internal jugular veins are better routes due to their

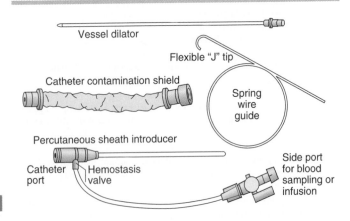

FIGURE 20–5.   Additional items used for pulmonary artery catheter placement. (Reprinted, with permission, from: Chesnutt MS, et al [eds]: *Office & Bedside Procedures.* Originally published by Appleton & Lange. Copyright © 1992 by the McGraw-Hill Companies, Inc.)

compressibility if a complication occurs. The easiest sites to "float" the PA catheter are the right internal jugular and the left subclavian vein. *Rationale:* The PA catheter is packaged in a coiled position; these sites lend to the natural curve of the catheter as it assists in placement.

4. The insertion site should be widely prepped with a topical antiinfective agent. Povidone-iodine or chlorhexidine solutions are the most commonly used antiinfectives. *Important:* Antiinfective agents must *fully dry on the skin* to be effective.

5. Full draping of the patient (not just the immediate site) is needed because of the length of the tubing and guidewire. Use a strict sterile approach with gown, gloves, and mask. Strict attention to sterile technique will decrease the rate of line infections more than six-fold.

6. With the patient in Trendelenburg position, cannulate the central vein (see Central Venous Catheterization, Chapter 13, page 258). Pass the flexible end of the J-wire (standard size: 45 cm long) into the vein through the needle. In general, **never** push a guidewire where it does not want to go and always keep one hand on the guidewire while it is in the patient (make sure the flexible tip end is passed because the stiff end may perforate the blood vessel).

7. Mount the introducer sheath on the vessel dilator. Pass the dilator/sheath unit over the wire. Make a *full-thickness skin nick* at the wire entry site (No. 11 blade provided in the set).

8. Pass the vessel dilator/sheath unit into the vessel using strict Seldinger technique (Figure 20–6). A gentle, slight twisting motion may be necessary. Slowly remove the guidewire and the vessel dilator. Catheter sheaths have a hemostatic valve mechanism to prevent air from entering the central system and blood from escaping (place a finger over the end of the sheath if no valve is present); however, the side port does not, so it should be capped or clamped. Mount a syringe on the side port and aspirate blood to confirm intravascular positioning of the sheath; flush with sterile saline after confirmation.

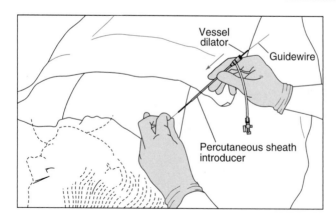

FIGURE 20–6. The introducer sheath and the vessel dilator are passed into the vessel. (Reprinted, with permission, from: Chesnutt MS, et al [eds]: *Office & Bedside Procedures.* Originally published by Appleton & Lange. Copyright © 1992 by the McGraw-Hill Companies, Inc.)

9. Prepare the PA catheter (attach to the monitor, flush lumens with sterile saline). Set the level of the pressure transducer to the middle of the patient's chest (approximately the level of the left atrium), then zero the monitor. Check balloon function and gently wave the catheter to ensure that an appropriate waveform is present on the monitor. *Note:* Never fill the balloon with fluid; use only air. The volume is typically 1.0–1.5 mL (dependent on the size of the PA catheter). Next, place the catheter through the contamination shield.

10. The prepared catheter (fluid-filled, fully monitored with contamination sheath in place) may now be inserted into the sheath (Figure 20–7). Once you have advanced approximately 15–20 cm, gently inflate the balloon with 1.0–1.5 mL of air using the volume-limiting syringe provided with the set. If you encounter resistance to full inflation, the balloon may not have yet cleared the sheath ($\cong$ 20 cm) or that it may be extravascular.

11. Once the balloon is inflated, advance the catheter to the level of the right atrium under the guidance of the pressure waveform and the ECG. Monitor the waveform and ECG at all times while advancing the balloon catheter. Figure 20–8B, page 421 displays the normal pressures encountered as the catheter is advanced. *Important:* Always advance the catheter with the balloon inflated. **Never** advance the catheter with the balloon deflated. Conversely, Always withdraw the PA catheter with the balloon deflated.

12. Positioning of the PA catheter in the right atrium is probably best determined by watching for the characteristic waveform on the monitor (see Figure 20–8). The right atrium is generally located approximately 30 cm from the right internal jugular or subclavian vein insertion site and approximately 35–40 cm from the left subclavian vein insertion site.

13. An abrupt change in the pressure tracing occurs as the catheter enters the right ventricle (see Figure 20–8B). There is generally little ectopy on entry into the right ventricle; however, as the catheter advances into the right ventricular outflow tract, PVCs may occur.

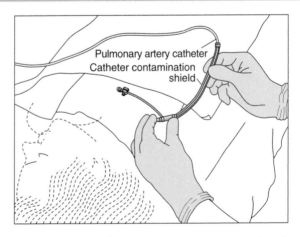

20

FIGURE 20–7. The fluid-filled pulmonary artery catheter is passed into the introducer sheath. (Reprinted, with permission, from: Chesnutt MS, et al [eds]: *Office & Bedside Procedures.* Originally published by Appleton & Lange. Copyright © 1992 by the McGraw-Hill Companies, Inc.)

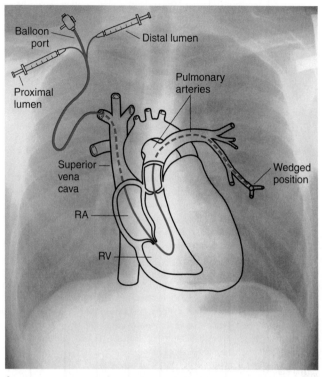

A

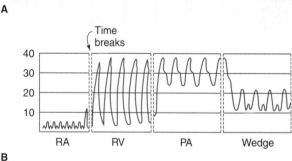

B

FIGURE 20–8. Positioning and pressure waveforms seen as the pulmonary artery catheter is advanced.

14. Steadily advance the catheter until the ectopy disappears and the pulmonary artery tracing is obtained (see Figure 20–8 above). If this does not occur (by the time 60 cm is reached), deflate the balloon, withdraw the catheter to 20 cm, and make another attempt with the balloon inflated after slightly rotating the catheter.

20

15. Once in the pulmonary artery, obtain the PCWP after advancing the catheter another 10–15 cm. The catheter's final position should be such that the PCWP is obtained with full balloon inflation *and* the PAP tracing is present with the balloon deflated. In the "ideal position," transition from PAP to PCWP (and vice versa) occurs within three or fewer heart beats. In an adult, the typical length to the pulmonary artery position is 45–60 cm. Table 20–4 below shows normal PA catheter measurements important for patient evaluation and treatment.

16. Once the position is acceptable, lock the contamination shield onto the sheath. This allows readjustment of the catheter should this be necessary after the sterile field is taken down. Suture the sheath to the patient (using 3-0 nylon or 2-0 silk on a cutting needle), secure the catheter in place and dress the surgical site according to your institution's practice. Connect catheters to the ports on the sheath. Inflow port on the sheath may be used for IV fluid and medication administration.

17. Obtain a CXR to document the catheter's present position as well as to rule out a pneumothorax or other complication from central venous catheterization. A properly positioned catheter should lie just beyond the vertebral bodies in the nonwedged position.

18. **Common problems:** Catheter placement is more difficult if severe PA hypertension is present. If there is significant cardiac enlargement, particularly dilation of the right heart structures, the catheter may coil in its path to the RV outflow tract (fluoroscopy may be required for correct positioning). Furthermore, under these conditions, the PA catheter may have difficulty holding its proper position. Placement of the catheter in the pulmonary artery may also be difficult in the setting of a low cardiac output state because the balloon-tipped catheter depends on blood flow to carry it through the right heart chambers.

TABLE 20–4
Normal Pulmonary Artery and Cardiac Performance Measurements

Parameter	Range
Right atrial pressure	1–7 mm Hg
Right ventricular pressure	
Systolic	15–25 mm Hg
Diastolic	0–8 mm Hg
PAP	
Systolic	15–25 mm Hg
Diastolic	8–15 mm Hg
Mean	10–20 mm Hg
PAOP ("wedge pressure")	6–12 mm Hg
Cardiac output	3.5–5.5 L/min
Cardiac index	2.8–3.2 L/min/m^2
Mixed venous O_2 saturation	65–85%

PAP = pulmonary artery pressure; PAOP = pulmonary artery occlusion pressure.

20

19. Cardiac output may be measured by thermal dilution (ie, Fick's equation). Connect the thermistor to the cardiac output computer and then rapidly inject fluid (usually 10 mL of ice-cooled NS) through the right atrial port. The computer displays a curve, and the CO is calculated from the area under the thermal dilution curve. Repeat two more times. If all of these values are approximately the same, then average the readings and record. Newer continuous CO-monitoring PA catheters are available in some units. Normal values for CO and CI are listed in Table 20–4.

Complications of PA Catheters

1. Most complications occur in the course of PA catheterization and are related to central vein cannulation: Arterial puncture with subsequent bleeding problems, placement of the wire or catheter in the extravascular space, and pneumothorax/hemothorax.

2. Arrhythmias are another common complication, with transient **PVCs** being the most frequent. PVCs occur when the catheter is advanced into the right ventricular outflow tract. If a patient with a PA catheter suddenly develops frequent PVCs, deflate the balloon and pull back the catheter to prepare for another attempt.

3. VT and VF are *rare* occurrences. If they continue after the catheter has been withdrawn, institute standard ACLS protocols and treat the patient accordingly (See Chapter 21, page 472).

4. Transient RBBB occurs occasionally as the catheter passes through the right ventricular outflow tract. In a patient with preexisting LBBB, this may result in complete heart block. In this setting, some form of backup pacing should be readily available. Complete heart block has been reported but occurs rarely.

5. Pulmonary infarcts and PA rupture are serious but infrequent complications of PA catheters and are usually secondary to an "overwedge" or peripheral placement of the catheter. The patient should be placed affected-lung-down, intubated (if not already done), and the ET tube placed into the unaffected mainstem bronchi to protect the airway. Emergent thoracic surgery consultation is then warranted.

6. Most complications and problems tend to increase with the time the catheter is in place. The risk of bacteremia and spontaneous bacterial endocarditis (SBE) are significant in severely ill patients receiving chronic instrumentation. In the setting of unexplained fever, the PA catheter and sheath should always be removed and cultured. The catheter and sheath should be replaced at a different site if a pulmonary catheter is still indicated.

PA Catheter Measurements

PA Pressure: Measured when the PA catheter is in its resting position (balloon deflated). Measurements include pulmonary systolic arterial pressure (PAS), mean arterial pressure (MAP), and diastolic (PAD) arterial pressure.

Pulmonary Artery Occlusion Pressure (PAOP):   (a.k.a., the "pulmonary capillary wedge pressure," "PCWP", or "wedge pressure"). This measured parameter is a reflection of the left atrial pressure and is measured when the balloon at the tip of the PA catheter is slowly inflated with air to occlude a branch of the PA.

20

Important: The balloon must be *fully deflated* when not in active use to avoid pulmonary infarction.

In the absence of mitral valvular disease, PAOP correlates closely with the left atrial pressure (LAP) and with the left ventricular end-diastolic pressure (LVEDP). This correlation exists because of the unobstructed continuity between the pulmonary artery and the left side of the heart. As a result of this continuity, the PAOP may never be greater than the PAD. If the LVEDP increases, this should be reflected by an increase in PAOP, which, in turn, increases the PAD. Therefore, *if a PA catheter monitor shows a wedge pressure higher than the PAD pressure, a technical error must exist.*

Left Ventricular End-Diastolic Pressure: LVEDP is a measure of preload and is used to guide fluid resuscitation to optimize cardiac output. Recall that to optimize stroke volume on the Starling curve, the preload must be adequate to stretch the wall of the left ventricle (see Figure 20–2). Hypovolemia results in too little tension on the muscle fibers and therefore a decreased SV and CO. Conversely, too much preload stretches beyond the point of maximum tension and causes a decrease in CO. Clinically, the LVEDP and PAOP are used to keep preload in an optimum range. The normal PAOP varies between 6 and 12 mm Hg, but may be higher for different disease states and for preexisting cardiac disease leading to decreased chamber compliance.

Right Ventricular Ejection Fraction (REF)/Right Ventricular End-Diastolic Volume Index (RVEDVI): A rapid-response thermistor and the CO computer are used to calculate the REF. Once REF and CO are known, the RVEDVI may be calculated. The RVEDVI is another measure of preload, and it allows for a more accurate assessment of volume status regardless of pulmonary disease. For example, a patient with severe ARDS may have markedly elevated peak inspiratory pressures. Although the CVP and PAOP may be falsely elevated, the RVEDVI is calculating a volume, not a pressure, thus allowing for a determination of volume status across a wide variety of clinical situations. The normal range for EDVI is 80–120 mL, but as with any value based on calculations, it must be viewed with caution if the proper conditions are not met (ie, bad data in → bad data out).

Differential Diagnosis of PA Catheter Abnormalities

Table 20–4, page 422 shows normal PA pressures and cardiovascular performance measurements (see also Figure 20–8). Perturbations of these values indicate a disease process. The broad differential diagnoses based on these alterations are shown in Table 20–5, page 425.

Clinical Applications

The PA catheter allows the clinician to approximate the patient's volume status and myocardial performance. As stated earlier, myocardial performance, or CO, depends on HR and SV. SV is, in turn, dependent on preload, afterload, and contractility.

Heart Rate: HR, in addition to SV, determines the CO (ie, CO = HR × SV). The body increases HR to increase CO in the face of inadequate tissue perfusion. Hence, tachycardia is an additional indicator of O_2 debt (ie, delivery/demand deficit). Tachycardia > 120 bpm increases myocardial O_2 demand significantly and should be promptly treated. The PA catheter allows for the es-

TABLE 20–5
Differential Diagnosis by Category Based on Perturbations in Hemodynamic Parameters[a]

Diagnosis	Systemic Blood Pressure	CVP	CO	PAOP/LVEDP	PAP	PVR	SVR
Cardiogenic shock	↓	↑	↓	↑	↑	↑	↑
Cardiac tamponade	↓	↑	↓	↑	↑	—	↑
Pulmonary embolism	↓	↑	↓	— or ↓	↑	↑	↑
Hypovolemic shock	↓	↓	↓	↓	↓	↓	↑
Neurogenic shock	↓	↓	↓	↓	↓	↓	↓
Septic shock	↓	↓	↑	↓	↓	↓	↓

[a]These are the trends usually seen with the conditions noted. Clinical variables (medications, secondary conditions, etc) may vary these trends somewhat. **Highlighted areas** denote major differences between subgroups.
CVP = central venous pressure; CO = cardiac output; PAOP = pulmonary artery occlusion pressure; LVEDP = left ventricular end-diastolic pressure; PAP = pulmonary artery pressure; PVR = peripheral vascular resistance; SVR = systemic vascular resistance.
↑ = usually increased; ↓ = usually decreased; — = usually unchanged.

20

tablishment of adequate myocardial filling pressures such that the HR may be clinically manipulated to maximize CO. In a patient with adequate filling pressures, slow HR (< 80 bpm), and a low CO, drugs that speed up the heart (called "chronotropes") may be used to increase CO. Alternatively, tachycardia > 120 bpm with an adequate PAOP may be pharmacologically slowed to decrease the strain on the heart.

Preload (Stroke Volume):   Indicated by the PAOP or EDVI, a reflection of left ventricular end-diastolic volume. In simple terms, preload is the amount of blood in the heart prior to contraction. Consequently, preload represents the stretch placed on the individual myocardial cell. When the PAOP is optimized, myocardial performance is optimized according to the Starling curve.

1. **Clinical implications in a healthy heart.** A low PAOP or EDVI means suboptimal myocardial muscle stretch. CO may be increased first by the administration of fluids. The result is an increase in LVEDV, an increase in myocardial muscle tension, and improved myocardial performance.
2. **Clinical implications in a failing heart.** Long-standing myocardial disease may shift the Starling curve to the right. Consequently, a significantly elevated PAOP may be required to optimize myocardial performance. It is common for patients who have just undergone heart valve replacement to require a PAOP of 20–25 mm Hg to optimize cardiac output (due to decreased compliance of the postoperative heart muscle). Patients with a recent MI may similarly require a PAOP of 16–18 mm Hg to optimize output.

Afterload: This is defined as the resistance to ventricular ejection and is measured clinically by the calculation of systemic vascular resistance (SVR). A normal SVR = 900 – 1200 dynes/s/cm³.

$$SVR = \frac{(MAP - CVP) \times 80}{Cardiac\ output\ (L\ /\ min)}$$

1. **Indications for afterload reduction.**
   - Significant mitral regurgitation

An increased PAOP coincident with elevated SVR/decreased CI

2. **Treatment.** Nitroprusside infusion with continuous hemodynamic monitoring.

Contractility: The ability of the heart to alter its contractile force and velocity *independent* of fiber length. This aspect is difficult to directly measure clinically but may be estimated through surrogate markers. Correctable metabolic causes for depressed contractility include:

- Hypoxia
- Acidosis (pH < 7.3)
- Hypophosphatemia
- Adrenal insufficiency
- Hypothermia

Improving contractility may be achieved by adding adrenergic agonists. Digoxin may also improve myocardial contractility; however, ensure normal levels of serum potassium prior to the administration of the drug.

DETERMINATIONS OF CARDIAC OUTPUT

Methods available to determine CO include thermal dilution, A–V o_2 difference calculation, and continuous CO measurements.

Thermal Dilution Technique

This technique requires the use of a PA catheter. A measured amount of saline (usually 10 mL) at a known temperature is injected into the proximal port of the PA catheter, and a temperature-sensitive thermistor located at the distal end of the pulmonary artery senses the temperature change in the surrounding blood. The CO computer then creates a curve over time, integrating the magnitude and rate of change in temperature. Utilizing the Fick equation, CO is then calculated as the area under the curve.

Arteriovenous Oxygen (A–Vo$_2$) Difference

A reasonable estimate of CO may be made on the basis of A–Vo$_2$ difference. A–Vo$_2$ difference is calculated as the oxygen content of arterial blood drawn from a peripheral artery minus the oxygen content of mixed venous blood drawn from the distal lumen of a PA catheter (Table 20–6, below).

$$A - Vo_2 \text{ difference} = \text{Arterial } O_2 \text{ content} - \text{Mixed venous } O_2 \text{ content}$$

Concept: The A–Vo$_2$ difference measures the extraction of oxygen by the tissues during a single transit time through the circulation. Thus, the A–Vo$_2$ difference is a function of (1) Pao$_2$, (2) hemoglobin concentration, (3) CO, and (4) tissue O$_2$ consumption.

- **If cardiac output is low:** Transit time is long and the tissues extract large amounts of oxygen during a single circulation time. Thus, the oxygen content of mixed venous blood is low and the A–Vo$_2$ difference is large
- **If cardiac output is high:** Conversely, circulation time is shorter and the amount of oxygen extracted is lower. As a result, the A–Vo$_2$ difference is low.

Calculations: Because the A–Vo$_2$ difference is inversely proportional to CO, the following approximations may be made:

TABLE 20–6
Estimate of Cardiac Index Based on A–Vo$_2$ Difference

A–Vo$_2$ Difference (Vol %)	Cardiac Index (L/min/m^2)
> 6	< 2
4–5	3–4
< 3	> 5

A–Vo$_2$ difference = Arterial o_2 content – Mixed venous O_2 content;
Cardiac index = Cardiac output/Body surface area.

20

1. **Determining Oxygen Content.** To calculate the A–Vo$_2$ difference, the oxygen content of both arterial and mixed venous blood must determined. Oxygen content per se describes the amount of O$_2$ the blood is able to carry, thus:

$$\text{Oxygen content (mL O}_2 \text{ / dL blood)} =$$
$$\text{Oxygen bound to Hgb} + \text{Oxygen dissolved in plasma}$$

so:

$$\text{Arterial O}_2 \text{ content (Cao}_2) = (\text{Sao}_2 \times [\text{Hgb}] \times 1.39 + (0.0031 \times \text{Pao}_2)$$

where: Sao$_2$ = arterial O$_2$ saturation; [Hgb] = hemoglobin content (g/dL); Pao$_2$ = arterial partial pressure of O$_2$ (mm Hg). The normal O$_2$ content of arterial blood is 16–20 mL of O$_2$/100 mL of blood. The constant 1.39 is the O$_2$-binding capacity of Hgb (mL of O$_2$/g of Hgb), and 0.0031 is the number of mL of O$_2$ dissolved in 100 mL of plasma per mm Hg of Pao$_2$. This clearly demonstrates that only a *small* percentage of O$_2$ is dissolved in plasma and that the vast majority is carried by hemoglobin. This is very important when evaluating the O$_2$ carrying capacity of blood.

Similarly:

$$\text{Venous O}_2 \text{ content (Cvo}_2) = \text{Svo}_2 \times [\text{Hgb}] \times 1.39 + (0.0031 \times \text{Pvo}_2)$$

where: Svo$_2$ = mixed venous O$_2$ saturation; Pvo$_2$ = peripheral venous partial pressure of O$_2$ (mm Hg)

Assuming that the amount of O$_2$ dissolved blood in plasma is small, then:

$$\text{A} - \text{Vo}_2 \text{ difference} = \text{Cao}_2 - \text{Cvo}_2 = 1.39 \times \text{Hgb} (\text{Sao}_2 - \text{Svo}_2)$$

2. **Calculation of A–Vo$_2$ Difference.**

   - Obtain [Hgb] through standard laboratory means
   - Determine the peripheral Sao$_2$ from heparinized arterial blood or from a reliable pulse oximeter
   - Determine the Svo$_2$ from a heparinized mixed venous blood sample from the distal lumen of a PA catheter or from an oximetric Svo$_2$ monitor (see the following discussion)
   - Calculate the A–Vo$_2$ difference according to the preceding formula
   - Determine the CI based on the data contained in Table 20–6

Continuous Svo$_2$ Monitoring

20

Oximetric PA catheters house fiberoptic channels that allow direct measurement of mixed venous Hgb saturation (Svo$_2$). These fiberoptics carry light impulses that are reflected by Hgb according to its O$_2$ saturation. An optical microprocessor then displays a continuous graph of Svo$_2$ measurements. Calibration is periodically confirmed by ABGs measured from heparinized blood drawn from the oximetric catheter's **distal port.**

Clinical Application

- Follow trends in the O_2 supply/demand balance
- A decrease in $S\bar{v}o_2$ is the best indicator of decreased peripheral O_2 delivery. This is an early sign of organ dysfunction and should allow the problem to be corrected before hemodynamic compromise occurs.
- Fix the underlying cause. Treatment interventions (ie, transfusions, fluid administration, inotropic drug use, etc) may be assessed by following $S\bar{v}o_2$ changes long before other hemodynamic parameters are adversely affected.
- Clinically, $S\bar{v}o_2$ values between 65% and 85% represent adequate tissue O_2 delivery and extraction. This *generally* implies appropriate perfusion of peripheral tissues.
- $S\bar{v}o_2$ of < 60% should prompt an *immediate* assessment of O_2 delivery. As O_2 delivery falls, $S\bar{v}o_2$ falls proportionally because there is less O_2 for the tissues to extract
- Conversely, if $S\bar{v}o_2$ is < 60% *and* O_2 delivery is unchanged, unrecognized conditions causing increased O_2 demand should be identified.

In summary, a decline of $S\bar{v}o_2$ must prompt a review of the parameters describing O_2 delivery (ie, CO, [Hgb], Sao_2) and consumption ($Sao_2 - S\bar{v}o_2$). The specific remedy for these declines of $S\bar{v}o_2$ includes:

- Supplemental O_2 and/or ventilatory support for Sao_2 < 90%
- Optimization of myocardial performance for decreased CO
- RBC transfusion for low Hgb states
- Identification and treatment of conditions leading to increased metabolic demands (ie, unrecognized seizures, shivering, excessive mobilization, and large tissue defects) as these produce a significant increase in O_2 demand (Figure 20–9 below)
- Inaccurate readings of $S\bar{v}o_2$ may occur as a result of fibrin buildup on the tip of the catheter, fiberoptic fracture (rare), or impingement of the tip of the catheter on the vessel wall. Overall, however, these catheters are extremely accurate and sensitive (with daily calibration and catheter maintenance)

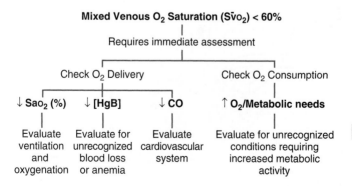

FIGURE 20–9. Algorithm for assessment of decreased $S\bar{v}o_2$.

Continuous Cardiac Output Measurement

New technology allows the CO to be measured continually. The specially designed PA catheter emits small pulses of energy that heat the surrounding blood. The CO computer then calculates the CO based on the magnitude and the rate of temperature change (with the Fick equation). This continuous measurement, as well as its many calculated derivatives, is intermittently updated and displayed on the device.

Continuous Sao$_2$ Monitoring (Pulse Oximeter)

The same fiberoptic technology used to measure mixed venous O$_2$ saturation is also used to measure arterial O$_2$ saturation (Sao$_2$). A light-emitting external probe is placed around a well-perfused appendage such as a digit, earlobe, lip, or bridge of the nose. The light is transmitted through the appendage to be reflected by Hbg according to its O$_2$ saturation (recall that the Hbg molecule absorbs different wavelengths of light at different O$_2$ saturations). The oximeter, in addition to calculating Hgb O$_2$ saturation, may also determine the pulse rate and is referred to as the "pulse oximeter." An Sao$_2$ of < 90% implies inadequate oxygenation and under most circumstances requires immediate intervention. *One exception* would be a patient with severe COPD who may have a normal O$_2$ saturation in the upper 80% range. Conversely, an Sao$_2$ > 90% does not necessarily imply adequate O$_2$ delivery (see following section). Pulse oximeter is not useful in the setting of smoke inhalation and CO poisoning because the Hgb molecule has a higher affinity for CO than for O$_2$.

CLINICAL PULMONARY PHYSIOLOGY

The goal of treating any critically ill patient is to optimize oxygenation, ventilation, and tissue perfusion. Pulmonary and cardiovascular physiologies are intimately interwoven to achieve this goal. Optimizing cardiovascular function carries little benefit if there is no O$_2$ for the Hgb to transport (ie, low Sao$_2$). Basic pulmonary physiology concepts include (Figure 20–10 below):

Ventilation: Mechanical movement of air into and out of the respiratory system; primarily results in excretion of CO$_2$

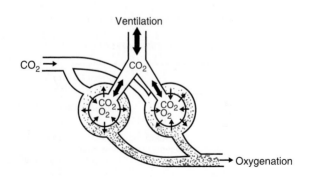

FIGURE 20–10.   Ventilation and oxygenation in typical alveoli.

Oxygenation: Diffusion of O_2 from the alveoli into the pulmonary capillary blood for systemic distribution

Ventilation

Several parameters, such as volumes and capacities, are important in assessing the adequacy of ventilation. Spirometry provides both dynamic information (ie, ability to move air into and out of the lungs) as well as static volume measurements. The lung volume subdivisions and capacities are shown on a spirometric graph (Figure 20–11 below).

Lung Volumes: Total lung capacity (TLC), or the amount of gas in the lung at full inspiration, comprises four basic lung volumes:

1. **Inspiratory reserve volume (IRV):** The volume of gas that may be maximally inspired beyond the standard, resting tidal volume breath
2. **Tidal volume (TV):** The volume of inspired gas during a normal breath; approximately 6–8 mL/kg in resting, healthy adults
3. **Expiratory reserve volume (ERV):** The volume of gas that may be maximally expired beyond the amount expired at the end of a normal tidal volume breath
4. **Residual volume (RV):** The volume of gas that remains in the lung after a maximal expiratory effort

Lung Capacity: The sum of two or more of these lung volumes make up four divisions called lung capacities (See Figure 20–11).

1. **Vital capacity (VC):** The volume of gas expired after a maximal inspiration followed by maximal expiration (VC = ERV + TV + IRV). VC is frequently used in determining whether a patient may successfully be weaned from the ventilator (normal VC ≅ 65 – 75 mL/kg; VC < 15 mL/kg is an indication for continued ventilatory support)
2. **Inspiratory capacity (IC):** The volume of gas expired from maximal inspiration to the end of a normal, resting TV (**IC = TV + IRV**)

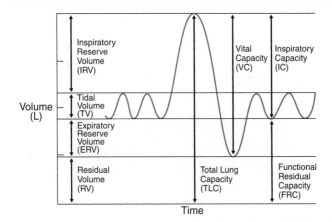

FIGURE 20–11. Spirometric graph with volumes and capacities of the lung.

3. **Functional residual capacity (FRC):** The amount of gas remaining in the lung following a normal TV expiration (FRC = ERV + RV); acts as a buffer against extreme changes in alveolar Po_2 and consequent dramatic changes in arterial Po_2 with each breath

Clinical Implications

These volumes and capacities are important factors in assessing ventilation because they may change under different conditions (ie, atelectasis, obstruction, consolidation, small airway collapse, etc). For example, as the ERV decreases with small airway collapse the FRC is similarly decreased (Figure 20–12 below). These alterations in lung volumes consequently affect respiratory reserve and the patient's ability to ventilate and oxygenate. The contributing factors and the point at which they influence such volume changes must be understood to optimize support.

Critical Closing Volume (CCV): The minimum volume and pressure of gas necessary to prevent small airways from collapsing during expiration. When collapse occurs, blood is shunted around nonventilated alveoli. This decreases the available surface area for gas exchange. The CCV is greatly affected by lung compliance. Therefore, different minimum volumes and pressures may be required to prevent collapse under varying lung conditions as compliance changes. If the CCV is > the FRC (air in the lung after tidal expiration), collapse tends to occur at a higher proportion of airways (see Figure 20–12 below).

One method to overcome the CCV is to increase the amount of positive end-expiratory pressure (PEEP) in the lung (see section on PEEP for discussion, page 440). The effect of PEEP is to increase FRC by minimizing small airway collapse at the end of expiration. This improves alveolar ventilation, decreases shunting, and ultimately improves oxygenation (Figure 20–13).

Lung Compliance: Expresses the *change* in lung volume and the *change* in pressure required to produce such a volume change (Figure 20–14). May be measured at the bedside and is a reflection of FRC and CCV.

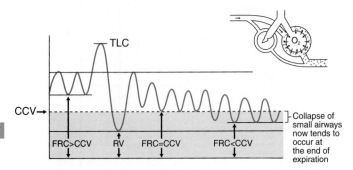

FIGURE 20–12.   Functional residual capacity (FRC) and critical closing volume (CCV). TLC = total lung capacity, RV = residual volume.

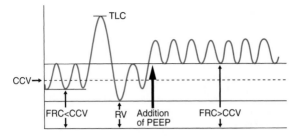

FIGURE 20–13. The effect of positive end-expiratory pressure (PEEP) is to increase the functional residual capacity (FRC). CCV = critical closing volume, TLC = total lung capacity, RV = residual volume.

$$\text{Lung compliance} = \frac{\Delta V}{\Delta P}$$

Dynamic Compliance: Determined by measuring the tidal volume and dividing it by the peak inspiratory pressure.

$$\text{Dynamic compliance} = \frac{TV}{PIP - PEEP}$$

$$\text{Normal} \cong \; > 80\text{--}100 \text{ mL/cm H}_2\text{O}$$
where: TV = tidal volume; PIP = peak inspiratory pressure

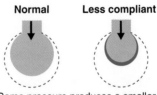

Same pressure produces a smaller
volume in the less compliant lung.

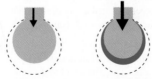

Increasing positive pressure maintains
volume in the less compliant lung.

FIGURE 20–14. Concept of pulmonary compliance.

20

Static Compliance: Similar to dynamic compliance, except that *static* PIP is substituted for PIP. *Static* peak pressure (a.k.a., plateau pressure) is measured by occluding the exhalation port at the beginning of exhalation (no flow = static pressure).

Comparing *dynamic* with *static* compliance may indicate the type of processes causing changes in the elasticity of the lung. *Dynamic* compliance is affected by both elasticity and airway resistance. *Static* compliance, in contrast, is not affected by airway resistance because there *is no flow*.

1. Reduction in dynamic compliance *without* a change in static compliance indicates an airway resistance problem (ie, obstruction, bronchospasm, or collapse of the small airways)
2. Reduction in *both* static and dynamic compliance indicates a decrease in lung elasticity (ie, pulmonary edema, atelectasis, or excessive PEEP)

Oxygenation

Oxygenation is the process of transporting oxygen from the alveolus across the capillary membrane into the pulmonary circulation and subsequently distributing that oxygen to the body's tissues. To assess the patient's ability to properly oxygenate, the following should be considered:

Arterial Hgb Content (g/dL): Obtained by standard laboratory measurements

- Measurement of systemic arterial O_2 saturation (Sao_2) (See page 430 for details.)
- Calculation of oxygen carrying capacity (Cao_2) and oxygen delivery (Do_2)
- Calculation of alveolar-to-arterial (A–a) gradient and right-to-left shunt fraction (Qs/Qt)

Oxygen Carrying Capacity: The ability of the blood to carry O_2 to the periphery is dependent on the O_2 content (Cao_2). The Cao_2 is directly influenced by Hgb concentration and the saturation of Hgb with O_2 (Sao_2) (ie, $Cao_2 = Sao_2 \times 1.39$ [Hgb])

Oxygen Delivery: Delivery of O_2 to the tissue depends on the Cao_2 and the CO.

$$O_2 \text{ delivery } (Do_2; \text{ mL } O_2 \text{ / min}) =$$
$$Cao_2 \times CO = Sao_2 \times (1.39 \text{ [Hgb]}) \times CO \text{ (L / min)}$$

These variables are measured with a PA catheter, pulse oximeter, and measured Hgb concentration. Normal Do_2 is around 800 mL of O_2/min, with an average normal O_2 uptake of 250 mL of O_2/min.

Note: This equation simplifies O_2 delivery to three parameters: CO, Sao_2, and [Hgb]. Pao_2 has been omitted due to the *vanishingly small role* it plays with regard to Cao_2 of blood (Remember its contribution is *0.0031 × Pao_2*).

Alveolar-to-Arterial (A–a) Gradient: This calculation is performed to assess the ability of the patient's lungs to adequately oxygenate. Many factors influence this, and the calculation is used as a tool to determine the cause of hypoxemia. To calculate:

1. Place the patient on 100% O_2 ($Fio_2 = 1.0$) for 20 min and obtain a peripheral ABG measurement to determine the partial pressure of O_2 (Pao_2).

20

2. Calculate the alveolar partial pressure of O_2 (P_{AO_2}). After breathing 100% oxygen for 20 min, the only gases remaining within the alveoli (other than O_2) oxygen are H_2O and excreted CO_2 from tissue metabolism (ie, the N_2 has been "washed out"). Thus, the P_{AO_2} within the alveoli is calculated as:

$$[\text{Barometric pressure} - H_2O \text{ partial pressure} - CO_2 \text{ partial pressure}] \times$$
$$F_{IO_2} = [PB - P_{H_2O} - P_{CO_2}] \times F_{IO_2}$$
$$= [760 \text{ torr} - 47 \text{ torr} - 40 \text{ torr}] \times F_{IO_2} = 673 \text{ torr} \times F_{IO_2}$$

Since the patient is breathing 100% O_2, ($F_{IO_2} = 1.0$), the equation simplifies to:

$$P_{AO_2} = 673 \text{ torr} \times F_{IO_2} = 673 \text{ torr} \times 1.0 = 673 \text{ torr}$$

3. Calculate: A–a gradient

$$P_{AO_2} - Pa_{O_2} = 673 \text{ torr} - Pa_{O_2} \times 0.8$$

where: $0.8 \cong$ respiratory quotient (constant)

Rule: The larger the A–a gradient, the more serious the degree of oxygenation compromise; A–a gradient > 400 torr indicates severe respiratory distress resulting from a process interfering with oxygen diffusion capacity; normal A–a gradient $\cong 20 - 65$ torr.

Shunt Fraction: The shunt fraction (normal < 5%) reflects the portion of CO that traverses the heart from the right to the left without increasing O_2 content (ie, $\cong 5\%$ of pulmonary capillary blood leaves the lung without being oxygenated). In an ideal state, the volume of lung ventilation equals the volume of pulmonary capillary blood flow (Figure 20–15 below). Alterations in these ventilation–perfusion relationships result from two causes:

- Relative obstruction of alveolar ventilation
- Relative obstruction of pulmonary blood flow

1. Perfusion greater than ventilation: A common scenario is that of *pulmonary consolidation* due to infection or secretions (Figure 20–16, page 436). Alveolus (A) receives no ventilation because of bronchiolar obstruction (B), yet normal pulmonary capillary perfusion continues (ie, a complete pulmonary A–V shunt exists with respect to that alveolus).

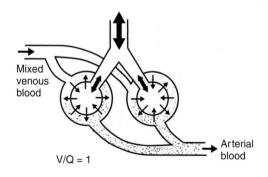

Mixed venous blood

Arterial blood

V/Q = 1

FIGURE 20–15. Ventilation–perfusion ($\dot{V}/\dot{Q}$) ratio·

20

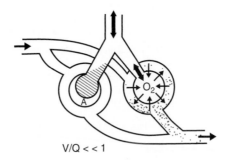

$$V/Q << 1$$

FIGURE 20–16.   Perfusion greater than ventilation.

2. **Ventilation greater than perfusion:** Impairment of pulmonary blood flow to the alveolar level occurs in the case of the postoperative lung surgery patient or one who has had a pulmonary embolism (Figure 20–17 below). Uniform ventilation continues to alveoli (A) and (B), but no blood flow passes alveolus (A). This situation increases the ventilated physiologic dead space *and* increases the shunt equation.

3. **Compensation mechanism:** Figure 20–18 represents the compensatory changes that occur when an alveolus is partially occluded. Blood flow is preferentially shunted to more efficiently ventilated alveolar units.

Principle: Recognize that at any given time, gradations of each of these situations will exist *simultaneously* within the lung (remember that the normal shunt fraction is $\cong$ 5%). Therefore, alterations in either ventilation or perfusion may seriously affect oxygenation.

1. **Decreased lung-to-blood transfer.** Associated factors include:

   - Pulmonary edema
   - ARDS
   - Bronchial secretions
   - Atelectasis

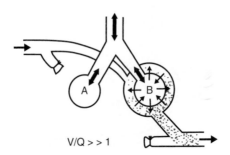

$$V/Q >> 1$$

FIGURE 20–17.   Ventilation greater than perfusion. Alveolus (**A**) receives no ventilation because of bronchiolar obstruction (**B**), yet normal pulmonary capillary perfusion continues.

20

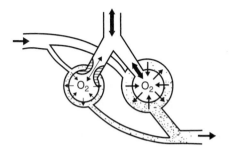

FIGURE 20–18. Compensation for ventilation–perfusion mismatching.

- Pneumonia
- Pneumonitis

2. **Decreased perfusion.** Associated factors include:

- Massive PE
- Continued micro-pulmonary embolization
- Postoperative changes

Calculation of the Shunt Fraction: In mathematical terms, Q = flow. Qt = the total CO in a system, and Qs = amount of flow through the pulmonary shunt. By definition, Qs (Figure 20–19 below) represents that portion of the total CO (Qt) that does not participate in gas exchange (ie, the volume of blood shunted past nonventilated alveoli). Thus:

$$\text{Shunt fraction (\%)} = \frac{\text{Qs (\%)}}{\text{Qt}} = \frac{C_{CO_2} - C_{aO_2} \times 100}{C_{CO_2} - C_{vO_2}}$$

where: C_{CO_2} = alveolar capillary O_2 content (mL/100 mL); C_{aO_2} = arterial O_2 content (mL/100mL); and C_{vO_2} = pulmonary mixed venous O_2 content (mL/100 mL)

With an F_{IO_2} = 100%, the O_2 oxygen content of capillary blood (C_{CO_2}), sys-

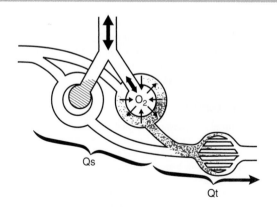

20

FIGURE 20–19. Representation of the shunt fraction.

temic arterial blood (CaO_2), and pulmonary mixed venous blood (CvO_2) is calculated as follows:

Using the alveolar PO_2 (PAO_2) from the alveolar–arterial gradient calculation, we obtain

$$CcO_2 = [Hgb] \times (1.39) \times (1.0) + [PAO_2 \times (0.0031)]$$

Using the SaO_2 and PaO_2 from ABG analysis, we obtain

$$CaO_2 = [Hgb] \times (1.39) \times (SaO_2) + [PaO_2 \times (0.0031)]$$

and finally, using the SvO_2 and PvO_2 from a mixed venous blood sample

$$CvO_2 = [Hgb] \times (1.39) \times (SvO_2) + [PvO_2 \times (0.0031)]$$

INDICATIONS FOR INTUBATION

The decision to intubate a patient to provide mechanical ventilatory support is often a difficult and stress-provoking process for clinicians. The primary objective of mechanical ventilation is to decrease the patients' work of breathing and reverse life-threatening hypoxia and hypercapnia. A recent point-prevalence study demonstrated the most common indications for intubation and mechanical ventilation were respiratory failure (66%), coma (15%), acute exacerbation of COPD (13%), and neuromuscular disorders (5%). The following basic checklist may be used to determine the need for respiratory support:

- **Inability to adequately ventilate** (ie, airway obstruction, severe chest trauma, excessive sedation, neuromuscular disease, paralyzed or fatigued respiratory muscles, etc)
- **Inability to adequately oxygenate** (ie, pneumonia, asthma/COPD, pulmonary embolism (PE), pulmonary edema, ARDS, etc)
- **Excessive work of breathing** (ie, severe bronchospasm, airway obstruction, etc)
- **Airway protection** (ie, unconsciousness, altered mental status, massive resuscitation, facial or head trauma, etc)

These basic indications should be used in conjunction with clinical judgment in the final decision regarding mechanical ventilation. The decision to intubate a patient who is clinically decompensating, if made in a timely fashion, may turn an otherwise chaotic intubation into a controlled, elective procedure. Diagnostic factors important in determining impending respiratory collapse of the adult patient are listed in Table 20–7, page 439.

SECURING THE AIRWAY

An essential treatment component of respiratory failure is securing and maintaining a patent airway (See Chapter 21). Briefly, the airway may be kept open by the chin-lift or jaw-thrust maneuver; however, these must be done with great care in the trauma patient if there is a suspicion of a cervical spine injury. Nasopharyngeal or oropharyngeal airways also assist in keeping the tongue from obstructing the oropharynx. Definitive airway management includes oral or nasal endotracheal intubation. Longer-term options include:

20

TABLE 20–7
Indicators of Impending Respiratory Failure Necessitating Intubation and Mechanical Ventilation

Condition	Normal Range (adults)
Respiratory impairment	
Tachypnea > 30 breaths/min	10–20 breaths/min
Dyspnea	
Neurologic impairment	
Loss of gag reflex	
Altered mental status (ie, patient is unable to protect airway against aspiration)	
Gas exchange impairment	
$Paco_2$ > 60 mm Hg	35–45 mm Hg
Pao_2 < 70 mm Hg (on 50% mask)	80–100 mm Hg (on room air)
Sao_2 < 90%	

- Tracheostomy should be considered in patients for whom long-term intubation is anticipated and in those patients with severe maxillofacial injuries. This is an elective procedure (as opposed to cricothyroidotomy). Improved patient comfort and oral hygiene, ease of secretion removal, and a more secure airway prove tracheostomy is a worthwhile procedure.
- Cricothyroidotomy is an *emergency procedure* when other attempts such as securing the airway have failed. Extend the neck (if possible); midline incision with No. 11 blade; puncture cricothyroid membrane with knife and rotate 90 degrees; keep finger in the cricothyroidotomy site; place a 6-cm ETT or cricoid tube into cricothyroidotomy site; confirm placement. Revision to a definitive airway should be performed when possible
- *Complications:* Esophageal intubation; pneumothorax; pneumomediastinum; recurrent laryngeal nerve injury; hemorrhage; tracheal stenosis (may be avoided by keeping cuff pressures < 25 mm Hg); ET tube dislodgement/self-extubation (life-threatening problem; use restraints liberally); unexplained tidal volume loss (check circuit; check ET tube cuff)

MECHANICAL VENTILATORS

Ventilator Classifications

Although newer ventilator modes combine many of the qualities of these classes, it is conceptually advantageous to discuss the types separately:

Volume Limited: A preset volume of air is delivered regardless of the opposing airway pressures; most common class of ventilator used (*Note:* A pressure limit setting usually allows for the modulation of excessive pressure to prevent "volutrauma").

Pressure Limited: These ventilators deliver a volume of air until a preset pressure is reached; mostly used in neonatal units (*Note:* Not generally used to ventilate adult patients because changes in airway pressure brought about by changes in lung and chest wall compliance may result in wide ranges of minute ventila-

20

tion). This technique is reserved for patients who fail to respond to traditional volume modes of ventilation.

High-Frequency Ventilation: Rapid oscillations of breath (60–1200 cycles/min) used with or without the bulk delivery of gases to the lung. Several forms of this type of ventilation exist, including high-frequency jet ventilation, high-frequency positive pressure ventilation, high-frequency oscillation, and high-frequency percussive ventilation.

To understand the components of mechanical ventilation that may be manipulated to bring about physiologic and anatomic changes, the following properties of ventilator mechanics must be understood:

Pressure Support (PS): The ventilator provides a preset level of positive pressure *only* during the inspiratory phase to augment spontaneous respirations (the positive pressure is turned *off* during expiration). This enables the patient to use their respiratory muscles and decreases the potential for atrophy.

Positive End-Expiratory Pressure (PEEP): The ventilator maintains positive airway pressure at the end of expiration even though net airflow is zero. PEEP increases alveolar ventilation by preventing small airway collapse, thereby improving lung compliance and maintaining/increasing FRC. PEEP also is often used prophylactically against postoperative atelectasis and has become a standard maneuver to treat pulmonary edema. Increasing levels of PEEP are typically used to decrease the FIO_2 in an attempt to limit oxygen toxicity. One disadvantage of PEEP, however, is that it may decrease CO by decreasing LVEDV and should be used cautiously in patients at risk for myocardial ischemia.

Ventilator Modes (Figure 20–20, page 441)

Controlled Ventilation (CV): The patient receives *only* ventilator-delivered breaths at a set rate (ie, patient cannot initiate a breath on his own). This mode was used in the past on patients who were intentionally paralyzed by drugs due to extreme illness or trauma.

Assist-Controlled Ventilation (AC): The patient gets a full mechanical tidal volume each time the patient attempts an inspiratory effort. The respiratory frequency is determined by the patient, although a backup rate is set to ensure minimum minute ventilation.

- *Advantages:* The patient may easily increase minute ventilation even if the patient is weak and has a poor inspiratory effort
- *Disadvantage:* Predisposition to hyperventilation if patient becomes agitated or has an altered respiratory drive because of neurologic injury. Agitation may also lead to "breath stacking," in which the ventilator delivers a second tidal volume before completing the expiratory phase of the first breath. Fortunately, this is rarely a clinical problem because the patient often feels more comfortable and consequently less agitated because of the decreased work of breathing on AC.

20

Synchronous Intermittent Mandatory Ventilation (SIMV): The ventilator delivers a set number of breaths each minute *and* allows the patient to supplement ventilation with the patient's own inspiratory efforts between machine breaths. This allows the patient to use her respiratory muscles and prevent atrophy. As the ventilator rate progressively is decreased, the patient assumes more and more the work of breathing. The ventilator also senses when the patient is taking a sponta-

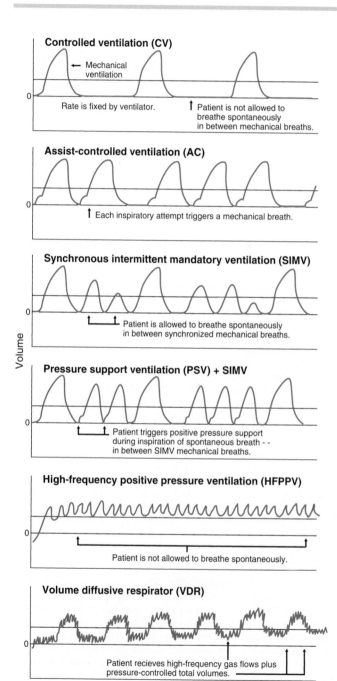

FIGURE 20–20. Representation of different ventilator modes.

20

neous breath and *will not* deliver the mandatory tidal volume until after the patient's own cycle is completed. This was developed to prevent the patient's working against the ventilator or receiving a double tidal volume (ie, a mechanical tidal volume superimposed on top of a spontaneous breath). **When combined with PS and PEEP,** this mode is the most commonly used type of ventilatory support.

Pressure Support Ventilation (PSV) plus SIMV: A preset level of positive pressure is turned on only during the inspiratory phase and is turned off during expiration. The patient controls the rate and inspiratory time while augmenting tidal volume and inspiratory flow. The higher the pressure support, the less work the patient expends to take a breath. Thus, PSV is comfortable because the patient has more control of his ventilation. PSV serves as an ideal weaning mode because the pressure may be turned down slowly, with changes as small as 1 cm H_2O. This allows the patient to assume the workload of breathing in small increments. PSV is often integrated with SIMV as a backup to ensure minimum minute ventilation.

Pressure-Regulated Volume Control (PRVC): This mode of ventilation is used in the setting of increased airway pressures. A microprocessor in the ventilator adjusts the pressure as needed to achieve the proper tidal volume. Because the pressure is constantly changing, the net peak airway pressures are less. As the patient's condition improves, less pressure is necessary to achieve a preset tidal volume. Conversely, as the patient's condition worsens, more pressure is delivered to ensure the set tidal volume. This method is one of the preferred modes in critically ill patients who manifest acute lung injury (ALI) or ARDS and PIP of > 35 mm Hg.

Continuous Positive Airway Pressure (CPAP): Positive pressure is maintained throughout inspiration and expiration without mechanical assistance during ventilation. This is equivalent to PS plus PEEP at a constant pressure level. The patient does all the breathing on her own. This mode is often used as a last step before extubation. A CPAP trial may be performed at room air or at F_{IO_2} of 40%.

High-Frequency Positive Pressure Ventilation (HFPPV): The physiologic explanation of HFPPV remains complex; suffice to say this method combines low-volume (subanatomic dead space) and rapid-sequence (> 60 breaths/min) ventilation to increase FRC and gas exchange ability. Despite the marked reduction in bulk gas flow rates, oxygenation and CO_2 exchange are still maintained. HFPPV may be ideally suited to treat such conditions as bronchopleural fistulas, to provide ventilation during operations requiring a minimum of lung movement, to have a less adverse effect on circulatory parameters or to allow similar or improved gas exchange at lower peak airway pressures.

Volumetric Diffusive Respirator (VDR): This ventilator combines the attributes of pressure control ventilation (set rate with tidal volume dependent on set peak inspiratory pressure and lung compliance) with HFPPV (to optimize oxygenation). This particular method, also known as high-frequency percussive ventilation (HFPV), has been used mostly in the burn population due to its incredible ability to mobilize pulmonary secretions secondary to inhalational injury. As with HFPPV, the technical aspects of the VDR are too detailed to be described here; look for this method to gain more exposure as its utility in other patient populations is assessed.

20

VENTILATOR MANAGEMENT
Ventilator Orders

Once the decision has been made to place a patient on a ventilator, the patient must be intubated with an appropriate endotracheal tube (see Chapter 13, page 272). The following is a sample of typical initial ventilator settings for an adult:

- Mode (ie, AC, SIMV)
- FIO_2 30–100%
- Rate 8–12/min
- Tidal volume 6–8 mL/kg
- Pressure support (level depends on the clinical situation)
- PEEP (5 cm H_2O or higher, if needed)

Ventilator Setting Changes

Five basic respiratory parameters (FIO_2, minute ventilation, PS, PEEP, I/E ratio) may be changed to improve ventilation, oxygenation, and/or compliance. Furthermore, attention to the proper use of these factors will help to prevent ventilator induced lung injury.

1. **FIO_2:** Initially, choose an FIO_2 that ensures adequate arterial O_2 saturation ($SaO_2 > 90\%$). Increasing the level of PEEP is often a helpful means of decreasing the FIO_2 requirement while maintaining adequate oxygenation. Once adequate oxygenation is established, the FIO_2 is decreased to avoid oxygen toxicity (avoid $FIO_2 > 60\%$)
   a. **Oxygen toxicity:** Damage to lungs occurs if the intraalveolar O_2 concentration is $> 60\%$ (injury actually occurs after a few hours if $FIO_2 = 1.0$). The mechanism probably involves generation of reactive O_2 species that oxidize the cell membranes. Oxygen toxicity has not been documented if FIO_2 is maintained $< 60\%$.
   b. **Nitric oxide (NO):** NO has been used for its potent pulmonary vascular relaxation properties. Although it will dilate pulmonary blood vessels and improve ventilation–perfusion mismatches, the use of NO has never been shown to improve mortality rates or shorten mechanical ventilator time in adult patients with severe ARDS.
2. **Minute volume:** Adjust to maintain PCO_2 within a normal range (35–45 mm Hg). Usually done by increasing tidal volume and/or respiratory rate. Once a tidal volume is chosen, set the respiratory rate ($\cong$ 8–16 breaths/min) to allow adequate minute ventilation
3. **Pressure support:** After the patient's respiratory pattern is established on SIMV, PS may be added initially at a level of 5–8 cm H_2O. PS may then be turned up to a level that allows the patient to breathe at a comfortable respiratory rate (ie, < 30 breaths/min). Depending on the overall stability and mental status of the patient, the number of SIMV backup breaths may be turned down to allow the patient to assume more control of ventilation. PS *rarely* needs to be > 35 cm H_2O
4. **PEEP:** "Extrinsic PEEP" supplied by the ventilator is added to decrease FIO_2 while maintaining PaO_2. PEEP $\cong$ 5 cm H_2O is considered physiologic. If the patient continues to deteriorate, PEEP is added in 2–3-cm increments until oxygenation is improved. In acute lung injury, the PEEP where lung compli-

20

ance is optimized ranges from 12–16 cm H_2O. Serial measurements of compliance are necessary to confirm improvement in pulmonary mechanics

High-Dose PEEP: If additional PEEP is required, a PA catheter is essential to monitor CO, Svo_2, PA pressures, and shunt fraction. Static pulmonary compliance and Sao_2 are also followed. At high levels of PEEP, intrathoracic pressure increases to a point that venous return is impaired. Thus, LVEDV decreases, which leads to a **drop in CO** (this point defines the maximum level of PEEP); this level may vary considerably from patient to patient or for the same patient over time.

5. **Inspiratory–expiratory (I/E) ratio:** The normal I/E ratio is 1:2 or 1:3. In patients with obstructive respiratory diseases, longer expiratory times allow full exhalation and guard against "breath stacking" (auto PEEP) or "intrinsic PEEP." By reversing the I/E ratio (ie, 2:1 or 3:1), a.k.a., "inverse ratio ventilation," distension and progressive recruitment of alveoli occurs, which leads to improved oxygenation. There may also be a favorable redistribution of pulmonary tissue edema fluid. This technique is used in patients with severe consolidating lung diseases in an attempt to improve oxygenation by increasing mean airway pressure. This beneficial effect on oxygenation is lost if "breath stacking" occurs (ie, breath stacking or intrinsic PEEP is detrimental to gas exchange).

PEEP Side Effects

- Falsely elevated PAOP (PCWP)
- Decreased cardiac output
- Barotrauma/volutrauma (leading to pneumothorax, alveolar rupture, etc)
- High peak airway pressures (> 45 cm H_2O)

Ventilator Weaning

Prior to weaning the patient from the ventilator, the patient's pulmonary mechanics and oxygenation should be assessed (Table 20–8 below). Additionally, the major problem that required the patient be placed on mechanical ventilation must have been corrected.

TABLE 20–8
Criteria for Extubation from Mechanical Ventilation

Parameter	Value
Pulmonary mechanics	
Vital capacity	> 10–15 mL/kg
Resting minute ventilation (tidal volume × rate)	> 10 L/min
Spontaneous respiratory rate	< 33 breaths/min
Lung compliance	> 100 mL/cm H_2O
(Negative) Inspiratory force (NIF)	> −25 cm H_2O
Oxygenation	
A–a gradient	< 300–500 mm Hg
Shunt fraction	< 15%
Po_2 (on 40% Fio_2)	> 70 mm Hg
Pco_2	< 45 mm Hg

Pulmonary Mechanics: These data provide useful information regarding a patient's ability to perform the work of respiration. Routine pulmonary mechanics consist of:

- Vital capacity
- Tidal volume
- Spontaneous respiratory rate
- Lung compliance

Inspiratory Force: The maximum negative pressure that may be exerted against a completely closed airway (ie, a function of respiratory muscle strength). An inspiratory force between 0 and −25 cm H_2O indicates that the patient is incapable of generating adequate inspiratory effort for successful extubation.

Weaning Modes: Modern respirators are designed to facilitate weaning. Once the preceding criteria have been met, a ventilator mode appropriate to the clinical situation may be selected. SIMV and PSV are considered weaning modes because the patient is allowed to assume more of the workload of breathing as mechanical support is reduced.

Order of Weaning: The following steps are taken routinely to wean the patient from the ventilator:

1. Sequentially reduce F_{IO_2} by 10% until 50% is reached; use pulse oximetry (Sao_2) to assist in weaning because it reduces the number of ABGs needed. F_{IO_2} may be steadily decreased as long as $Sao_2 > 90–92\%$ or $Pao_2 > 70$ mm Hg.
2. Sequentially reduce the IMV rate to a level of 4–8 breaths/min. Add PS to maintain adequate minute volume; ABGs as well as capnography are used to monitor for hypercarbia.
3. Sequentially reduce PEEP in 2–3-cm H_2O increments while maintaining $Sao_2 > 90\%$ until a level of 5 cm H_2O is achieved.
4. Sequentially reduce PS by 2–3-cm H_2O increments while maintaining minute ventilation (goal: 5–10 cm H_2O); monitor respiratory rate, work of breathing, and Pco_2.

Essential Tips in Ventilator Management

- Avoid changing more than one ventilator parameter at a time
- $Po_2 < 60$ mm Hg or $Sao_2 < 90\%$ = return to previous levels of respiratory support
- Po_2 60–70 mm Hg or $Sao_2 \cong 90$–92 % = hold at the current level of respiratory support
- $Po_2 > 70$ mm Hg or $Sao_2 > 93\%$ = continue systematic weaning

Checklist for Extubation
- Correction of primary problem that triggered intubation and mechanical ventilation (ie, successfully treated pneumonia, returned hemodynamic stability, etc)
- Level of consciousness stable or improved
- Stable vital signs
- Pulmonary mechanics and oxygenation meet acceptable criteria (see Table 20–8, page 444)

20

Extubation Trials: Once weaning has achieved minimal ventilatory settings, various trials off mechanical support may be attempted while the patient is still intubated:

1. CPAP trials (with 5 cm H_2O positive pressure) remain the most commonly used method; CPAP trial with an FIO_2 at 21% (room air) or 40% should result in a PaO_2 of > 50 mm Hg or 70 mm Hg, respectively
2. T-piece trials, which provide only humidified air with no pressure, are also occasionally used but may be unnecessarily stressful to the patient due to the lack of pressure support or CPAP.

CPAP trials are thought to be more physiologic because positive pressure partially counterbalances the added resistance encountered by breathing through a long, narrow ET tube. These trials may vary in duration from 30 min to several hours and are used primarily as the last test prior to extubation. Patients *without COPD* usually are tested with an extubation trial with: IMV rate 4, FIO_2 30%, PEEP 5 cm H_2O. The ventilator remains at the bedside in case respiratory support needs to be restarted.

Extubation: A patient who is able to maintain a PO_2 > 70 mm Hg, a PCO_2 < 45 mm Hg, and a respiratory rate < 25 breaths/min for 1–2 h on a T-piece or CPAP trial is ready for extubation.

1. Disconnect the ET tube from the ventilator or T-piece.
2. Suction the ET tube and oral pharynx.
3. Have the patient take a deep breath while you deflate the ET tube balloon.
4. As the patient expires forcefully, remove the tube and suction any secretions.
5. Apply a nasal cannula with O_2 flow at 2–4 L/min.
6. Check postextubation ABG to ensure adequate ventilation and oxygenation.

NUTRITION IN THE ICU

The nutritional support of the critically ill patient is crucial to patient survival. Restoring the patient to an anabolic state will hasten recovery and avoid complications. Protocols for nutritional support are covered in Chapters 11 and 12. Remember the following two rules:

1. The "2-day" rule applies to most patients. If you do not think the critically ill patient will take nutrition for 2 days because of postoperative ileus, intubation, etc, be sure to make arrangements for nutritional support.
2. "If the gut works, use it." That is, do not use parenteral nutrition if the GI tract is functioning properly. Enteral nutrition (ie, oral, NG tube, jejunostomy tube) should be used in all patients with a functioning intestinal tract. Enteral feeding is reviewed in Chapter 11.

COMPLICATIONS IN CRITICAL CARE
Acute Respiratory Distress Syndrome (ARDS)

ARDS, also called "wet lung" or "shock lung," is defined as respiratory failure associated with acute pulmonary injury and is manifested by marked respiratory distress and hypoxia. Pulmonary capillaries become more permeable, resulting in pulmonary edema in the setting of low to normal PA pressures. Clinical criteria ARDS include:

- PaO_2: FIO_2 ratio of < 200
- Diffuse bilateral infiltrates on CXR

20

- Pulmonary artery occlusion pressure (ie, PAOP or "wedge pressure") < 18 mm Hg
- Lack of an alternative clinical explanation for pulmonary findings

Causes: The causes of ARDS are multifactorial and include anything that could activate the systemic inflammatory response syndrome (SIRS). These include, but are not limited to:

- Severe head injury
- Severe trauma with prolonged hypotension
- Massive fluid resuscitation
- Sepsis
- Severe pancreatitis
- Severe burns
- Severe chest trauma/pulmonary contusion
- Aspiration, chemical pneumonitis, or inhalational injury

Three primary mechanisms of the final common pathway of SIRS-induced lung injury include:

1. **Increased pulmonary vascular resistance:** Pulmonary edema is caused by a dramatic increase in pulmonary capillary hydrostatic pressure. This increase forces fluid across the capillary membrane and results first in interstitial and then alveolar edema.
2. **Permeability edema:** Circulating toxic substances (interleukin -1, TNFα, etc) within the bloodstream may cause the pulmonary capillary membrane to become leaky and allow extravasation of protein into the interstitial space. This extravasation increases the interstitial hydrostatic pressure and eventually results in injury to the alveolar membrane. At this point, fluid and protein migrate into the alveolar space and directly impede oxygen exchange. Several factors have been implicated as mediators to this increased capillary–alveolar permeability, including prostaglandins and oxygen radicals.
3. **Injury to the alveolar membrane:** Conditions promoting direct toxicity to the alveolar membrane include:

- Smoke inhalation
- High doses of oxygen (> 60% FIO_2)
- Aspiration

Treatment: Primary efforts are directed at treating the underlying condition while providing sufficient pulmonary support. Currently, no specific therapy is available for ARDS except prevention.

1. **Aggressive ventilatory support:** Use PEEP to **maintain the** FIO_2 < 0.6 while maintaining a SaO_2 > 93%. Use the SaO_2, volume status, and level of PEEP to guide ventilatory management. Although some may advocate increased levels of PEEP to minimize intrapulmonary shunting (Qs/Qt), doing so may necessitate increased intravascular volume and inotropic support of the heart. Most clinicians use SaO_2 as a guide to altering PEEP levels, rather than following the specific shunt fraction.
2. **Aggressive fluid administration:** Maintain CO and peripheral perfusion; use of colloid versus crystalloid remains controversial. Many clinicians recommend the use of crystalloid (NS, RL) and PRBCs to maintain the HCT > 24 % in most patients (HCT > 30% in patients with known ischemic cardiac disease).

20

3. **Aggressive monitoring:** Use a PA catheter to guide fluid administration (by following filling pressures), and observe the effect of added PEEP on CO. Inotropic agents may be indicated if CO remains low despite adequate filling pressures. Use an arterial line to obtain arterial blood for frequent ABG determinations.
4. **Pulmonary toilet:** To manage secretions
5. **Chest x-rays:** To monitor lung improvement
6. **Watch for associated DIC, other complications related to SIRS activation**
7. **Steroids are not indicated** in the treatment of ARDS.

Upper Gastrointestinal Hemorrhage

Critically ill patients are at increased risk for GI hemorrhage secondary to stress-induced mucosal ulcerations. The development of such ulcerations is a serious, yet preventable, complication. The pathophysiology is related to diminished blood flow to the viscera during stress situations leading to alterations in the mucosal barrier to the effects of gastric acid. Head injury (**Cushing's ulcers**); mechanical ventilation; NSAID use; shock, trauma, and burns (**Curling's ulcers**); coagulopathy; or a history of peptic ulcer disease or portal HTN are a few of the risk factors.

Prophylaxis
- **Enteral feedings** (when tolerated): method of choice to protect the gastric lining
- Routine cardiovascular support of visceral perfusion
- Routine use of acid suppression methods. Meta-analysis has demonstrated that prophylaxis using H_2-blockers (ie, ranitidine, famotidine, etc) significantly reduces stress-induced GI ulcerations and clinically significant hemorrhage. Proton-pump inhibitors (ie, lansoprazole, omeprazole, etc) may be used for refractory bleeding or in patients that have side-effects to histamine blockade (ie, thrombocytopenia)
- Antacid administration (ie, Maalox, Mylanta, sucralfate, etc); in patients with renal failure, use aluminum hydroxide to avoid magnesium-containing antacids and resultant aluminum toxicity

Treatment of Ulceration
1. Early endoscopy is indicated in upper GI bleeding
2. A visible (bleeding) vessel warrants endoscopic or operative intervention.
3. Diffuse gastritis is best treated initially with aggressive acid suppression and empiric treatment for *H. pylori.*
4. Persistent bleeding from gastritis may warrant total gastrectomy.

Shock

Shock is defined as hypotension leading to delivery or utilization of O_2 and nutrients at the tissue level insufficient to meet metabolic needs. If uncorrected, shock leads to cellular dysfunction that then produces organ failure and ultimately death. The causes of shock are multifactorial; however, treatment of shock is always directed at *correcting the underlying problem.* Endogenous compensatory mechanisms directed at reversing hypotension and shock include the release of catecholamines, cortisol, and activation of the renin/angiotensin/aldosterone axis.

The morbidity and mortality of shock are related to the cause but probably more to the *degree and time of circulatory compromise.* With the causes identified and corrected, the organism is resuscitated to restore tissue perfusion and reverse the sequelae of shock. The most common causes of shock include:

20

Hypovolemic Shock: Caused by inadequate circulating blood volume (at least 20% loss) caused by severe fluid depletion (dehydration) or acute hemorrhage. Compensation includes low CO, low PAOP, and elevated PVR as a result of reflex vasoconstriction (Table 20–9 below lists the current classification and physiologic changes associated with hypovolemic shock).

Treatment:

1. Control the source of intravascular volume loss.
2. Rapidly replete intravascular volume with:
   a. PRBCs
   b. Isotonic crystalloid fluids (NS, RL): Due to equilibration with the interstitial space, the 3:1 (crystalloid:volume loss) rule must be considered.
   c. Colloid solutions (albumin, hetastarch, etc)

Cardiogenic Shock: Caused by primary heart failure either from intrinsic cardiac abnormalities (ie, severe valvular disease, acute myocardial infarction, coronary ischemia, arrhythmias, etc) or extrinsic processes (ie, tension pneumothorax, pericardial tamponade, PE, etc). Compensation includes low CO, high PAOP, and elevated PVR.

Treatment: Directed at improving cardiac performance

1. Optimize preload (filling pressures).
2. Decrease afterload (vasodilation with nitroglycerin, nitroprusside, etc).
3. Improve cardiac contractility (dobutamine).
4. Resolve extrinsic processes (if necessary).
5. Consider mechanical support (intraaortic balloon counterpulsation) if other measures fail.

Septic Shock: Caused by intravascular fluid loss (ie, extravascular fluid sequestration–"third spacing") due to systemic infection or some other initiator of

TABLE 20–9
Physiologic Changes Associated with Degree of Hemorrhagic Shock

	Class I	Class II	Class III	Class IV
Blood loss (%)	< 15	15–30	30–40	> 40
Blood loss (mL)[a]	< 750	750–1500	1500–2000	> 2000
Mental status	—	Anxiety	Confusion	Lethargy
Heart rate	—	Mild ↑	Moderate ↑↑	Severe ↑↑↑
Blood pressure				
systolic	—	—	↓	↓↓
diastolic	—	↑	↓	↓↓
Respiratory rate (breaths/min)	—	Mild ↑	Moderate ↑↑	Severe ↑↑↑
Urine output	—	Mild ↓	Oliguria	Anuria

[a]Based on 70 kg adult — = No significant change; ↑ = increased; ↓ = decreased.

20

the **SIRS** response. Compensation includes hyperdynamic CO (until late stages), low PAOP, and low PVR.

Treatment:

1. Treat the cause of sepsis ("source control—parenteral antibiotics, abscess drainage, etc) or SIRS activation.
2. Administer fluids to replace intravascular losses (usually one to two times the circulating blood volume).
3. Increase PVR (pressors, eg, norepinephrine, phenylephrine, etc).
4. Provide inotropic support to the heart (as needed); may need a PA catheter to guide fluids and pressor administration.

Neurogenic Shock: Caused by loss of sympathetic vascular tone (ie, due to a high thoracic or cervical cord injury) producing an increase in vascular capacitance. Compensation includes low CO, low PAOP, and low PVR.

Treatment:

1. Optimize filling pressures by IV fluid administration.
2. Increase PVR (pressors, eg, norepinephrine, phenylephrine, etc).
3. Keep fluids and ambient room temperature warm because these patients lose the ability to thermoregulate.

All forms of shock require therapies to improve the delivery of O_2 to the tissue level. Optimization of oxygen carrying capacity of blood (Sao_2, [Hgb]) and providing adequate CO are the mainstays of treatment. Recent studies suggest [Hgb] $\cong$ 7–9 gm/dL are satisfactory and were associated with decreased mortality in critically ill patients unless they had known ischemic heart disease (where [Hgb] $\cong$ 10–12 g/dL was optimal). In this cooperative study, previous transfusion practices of maintaining all patients at a goal [Hgb] $\cong$ 9–10 g/dL were associated with higher 30-d mortality rate unless the patient had a concurrent AMI or unstable angina pectoris.

Acute Renal Failure (ARF)

ARF is the sudden development of renal insufficiency that results in retention of nitrogenous wastes (BUN, creatinine) and variable effects on fluid balance. Diverse opinion persists as to the magnitude of BUN or creatinine elevations required to diagnose ARF (see Chapter 6). In general, oliguria/anuria and progressive azotemia are the final common pathway of a number of pathologic processes that constitute ARF, which occurs in approximately 5% of ICU admissions. Although multiple causes exist, ARF is usually divided into prerenal, renal, and postrenal causes (see Chapter 6). Despite the cause, once ARF is recognized, the primary goal is to *treat the underlying cause.*

Critically ill patients often require radiographic imaging with IV contrast materials. A recent study in well-hydrated patients with baseline creatinine > twice normal suggests that the use of *N*-acetylcysteine 24 h before and after the administration of contrast will likely prevent contrast-induced nephropathy. With this new therapy, the incidence of contrast-induced nephropathy should decline over time.

Many critically ill patients are unable to receive oral nutrition or fluid and are therefore particularly susceptible to fluid and electrolyte derangements. Furthermore, sepsis and other initiators of the SIRS response lead to massive fluid shifts that may result in severe hypovolemia. The following data provide information regarding fluid status:

20

- **Urine output:** (best and simplest) minimum of 0.5 mL/kg/h for adults; 1.0 mL/kg/h for children; 2.0 mL/kg/h for infants
- **Daily weight:** Changes result from the net loss or gain of fluid
- **PA catheter data**

Acute tubular necrosis (ATN) from multiple causes (ie, nephrotoxic medications, ischemia, hypotension, etc), intravascular volume depletion, and CHF are the most common causes of renal failure in the ICU patient. The following describes the general approach to ARF in an ICU patient:

Physical Examination

1. **Vital signs:** Hypotension with or without associated tachycardia and orthostatic BP changes may be a sign of hypovolemia (prerenal).
2. **Mucous membranes:** Dry mucous membranes indicate overall fluid depletion.
3. **Lungs:** Fluid overload often manifests auscultated crackles (pulmonary edema).
4. **Abdomen:** Low urine output may result from postrenal obstruction (palpable bladder); distended abdomen may indicate an ileus with associated bowel fluid sequestration.
5. **Extremities:** Fluid overload may be evident (ie, peripheral, dependent edema).

Diagnostic Studies

1. **Laboratory results** (serum and urine electrolytes/urine eosinophils and myoglobin)
2. **Bladder catheterization:** If a catheter is in place, irrigate gently to confirm drainage.
3. **Radiographic studies:** Renal ultrasonography helps evaluate for possible postrenal obstruction. Avoid IV contrast studies if possible (ie, contrast nephropathy).

Therapeutic trials: Certain therapies may be used to differentiate prerenal from renal or postrenal azotemia (see Chapter 6). After obstruction has been ruled out, failure to respond to these measures likely indicates an intrinsic renal cause of ARF:

- Fluid challenge (rapid 1000 mL of IV 0.9% saline infusion)
- Furosemide 80 mg IV push (furosemide has little effect in ATN)
- Intravenous inotropic support

Management: As a general approach, daily fluid intake and output as well as body weight should be closely reviewed. Follow serum electrolytes, particularly potassium, closely (remove potassium from the IV fluids immediately in cases of ARF to prevent accumulation of deadly potassium levels). Otherwise, management involves correction of the underlying abnormality and supportive care.

Prerenal

1. Optimize hemodynamic status to maximize CO and renal perfusion.
2. Replete IV fluids (use PRBCs in anemic patients, otherwise, use isotonic fluids or albumin).
3. With optimal fluid status, check urine output; if still suboptimal, use inotropic support (dopamine 2–5 mcg/kg/min) to dilate renal blood vessels; a

20

PA catheter is usually needed to further monitor the patient and adjust pharmacologic support

Renal

1. Optimize fluid status and cardiovascular function (see previous section).
2. Furosemide challenge (20–40 mg IV); if no response, try mannitol 12.5–25 g IV.
3. Restrict fluids and salt (particularly potassium) if these become troublesome.
4. Treat ARF-induced metabolic acidosis with sodium bicarbonate if pH < 7.25.
5. Hemodialysis if necessary (see below).

Postrenal

1. Place and check bladder catheter for patency; replace immediately if questionable.
2. Obtain a urologic consultation; prostatic obstruction may be easily corrected with catheterization; decompression of the upper urinary tracts may require stents or percutaneous drainage.

Fortunately, most causes of ARF are reversible (see Chapter 6). Hemodialysis, however, may be necessary for the following reasons:

- Fluid overload causing respiratory compromise
- Severe metabolic acidosis
- Severe electrolyte disturbances
- Severe uremia
- Toxic accumulation of drugs

Abdominal Compartment Syndrome (ACS)

ACS is a recently recognized entity caused by massive intraperitoneal bowel edema and fluid sequestration, or from significant retroperitoneal hemorrhage causing a mass-effect. The increased intraabdominal pressure directly decreases visceral perfusion, most notably to the kidneys, which ultimately leads to organ dysfunction and respiratory compromise.

Diagnosis: Assessment of bladder pressures (> 30 mm Hg) via a Foley catheter; a tense, distended abdomen with the appropriate clinical history; increasing peak airway pressures.

Treatment: *Early* decompressive celiotomy remains the treatment of choice (allows restoration of intraabdominal pressures and hemodynamics). The abdominal fascia may be closed when the edema and organ dysfunction resolves.

Acalculous Cholecystitis

Cholecystitis in the absence of gallstones is not uncommon in the ICU patient. Although the precise cause remains unknown, it is probably related to diminished blood flow to the gallbladder and to bacterial overgrowth.

20

Diagnosis: Presenting signs are similar to those in healthy patients with cholecystitis and include right upper quadrant pain, fever, leukocytosis, and elevated liver chemistries (especially bilirubin or alkaline phosphatase). The work-up should also include a gallbladder ultrasound. A HIDA scan may be added if the ultrasound is nondiagnostic (nonvisualization of the gallbladder is highly suggestive of acalculous cholecystitis).

Treatment: Prevention of this potentially fatal condition is key. Maintain a high index of suspicion for the development in the critically ill patient. Treatment is surgical (cholecystectomy), and should be done as early as possible. If the patient is too critically ill to tolerate an operation, a percutaneous cholecystostomy tube could be placed to drain the gallbladder and allow a "cooling off" period. Interval cholecystectomy should then be performed when possible.

Acute Adrenal Insufficiency

Acute adrenal insufficiency is an increasingly *common,* yet difficult to diagnose condition in critically ill patients. The symptoms range from subtle organ dysfunction to life-threatening, pressor-refractory circulatory shock. Categories include:

Chronic Primary Adrenal Insufficiency: Due to loss of adrenal function from surgery (adrenalectomy) or from metabolic disturbances; patients will take chronic steroid replacement; home steroid medication should be continued without interruption; may need hydrocortisone 25–75 mg/d IV × 2–3 d for mild to moderate surgical stress; for severe stress, up to 300 mg/d IV may be necessary.

Chronic Secondary Adrenal Insufficiency: Due to ACTH insufficiency likely secondary to exogenous glucocorticoid administration (steroid replacement therapy) or due to pituitary failure (postsurgical); patients will take chronic steroid replacement; home medication should be continued without interruption; may need hydrocortisone 25–75 mg/d IV × 2–3 d for mild to moderate surgical stress; for severe stress, up to 300 mg/d IV may be necessary.

Acute Adrenal Crisis: Due to acute direct (adrenal hemorrhage) or indirect (pituitary hemorrhage) adrenal loss; also due to chronic primary/secondary adrenal insufficiency patients who are acutely stressed (ie, infection, trauma, burns, etc).

    Diagnosis: Evidence continues to accumulate on the incidence of acute adrenal crisis in the ICU patient population, thus, the precise definition and treatment regimens remain controversial. Random serum cortisol levels of < *25* or > *45 mcg/dL* have been suggested to predict poor outcome and increased mortality in some reports, and in others the patients' ability to respond to ACTH stimulation has been studied. Patients who fail to increase stimulated cortisol level ≅ 9 mcg/dL above baseline ("nonresponders") or patients who have a stimulated cortisol < 18 mcg/dL appear to have a worse prognosis. As with all these patients, reasonable source control must have been achieved *and* other causes have been ruled out to account for the cardiovascular collapse. Empiric steroid replacement should be started on patients:

1. With positive random cortisol levels (see preceding section, Diagnosis)
2. Who are **"nonresponders"**
3. With pressor-unresponsive shock and no known premorbid adrenal insufficiency (provided they do not have an infectious source)

    Treatment:
1. Send blood for assessment of cortisol level.
2. Start hydrocortisone 50 mg IV q8h.
3. Continue the steroid replacement for approximately 2–3 d (with a rapid taper):
    a. If the random cortisol level is < 25 mcg/dL, or

   b. If the random cortisol level is > 25 mcg/dL and clinical improvement
       was demonstrated with treatment
4. Increase the glucocorticoid dose (300–400 mcg/d) if the patient remains
    "pressor-nonresponsive."
5. Wean the steroids quickly as tolerated (once hemodynamic stability is
    achieved).

Disseminated Intravascular Coagulation (DIC)

DIC is a complex management problem that often presents in the critically ill
patient. This clinical syndrome may accompany a number of disease states, including shock syndromes, sepsis, malignancy, and some obstetric conditions. As
with many of the pathologic conditions that accompany major illness (ie, ARDS,
ARF, etc), the successful treatment of DIC depends on treating the underlying
condition.

Diagnosis: DIC is usually contemplated in critically ill patients who develop
coagulopathy and thrombocytopenia. The following list details other laboratory
findings that are caused by the effect of plasmin on fibrinogen (ie, results in increased levels of fibrin monomers and feedback stimulation of the fibrinolytic
system):

- Low fibrinogen level
- Elevated fibrin split products (FSP) level (a.k.a. fibrin degradation products)
- Elevated PT/PTT
- Characteristic microangiopathic RBC morphologies

Treatment: (controversial)
1. The most important element of therapy is to identify and treat the underly-
    ing cause (ie, sepsis source control, adequate resuscitation of associated
    shock, etc).
2. If thrombosis occurs (ie, DVT, PE), begin heparin therapy (see Chapter 22).
3. Administer FFP or cryoprecipitate to replenish fibrinogen stores.
4. If the patient is bleeding severely, despite replacement therapy with
    FFP/cryo and platelets, begin antifibrinolytic therapy with epsilon-
    aminocaproic acid (Amicar). In general, if there is no improvement after
    12 h, therapy should be stopped.

Infections

Line Sepsis: Indwelling catheters not only provide a convenient means of in-
fusing fluids and medications, they also act as a portal of entry for bacteria. With
the widespread use of indwelling intravenous catheters (ie, central venous lines),
the diagnosis of infection from the catheter itself must be considered when evaluating a febrile patient in the ICU. As a general rule, fever in a person with a
central line should be attributed to the line until proven otherwise. The most
common mechanism of line sepsis is entry of skin flora along the catheter tract.
The use of clear polyurethane dressings left in place for prolonged periods has
been associated with increased risk of infection and should be avoided. Some institutions have a policy of routine line changes over a guidewire every 3–4 d.
Little objective data support this practice; in fact, recent CDC guidelines suggest
this practice is associated with an increased rate of complications. Prevention of
line sepsis is best accomplished by meticulous aseptic technique during line

20

placement (including fully gowning, gloving, and draping) and meticulous care of the line once in place.

Diagnosis: A presumed episode of line sepsis is treated by determining whether the line is actually responsible. The catheter may be changed over a guidewire with the intracutaneous segment and tip sent for culture. The site in question should be abandoned and a new site for IV access chosen if the catheter culture is positive. Erythema is highly suggestive of catheter site infection. However, coagulase-negative Staph the most common agent, elicit little inflammation compared with other organisms such as *S aureus*. In the absence of florid sepsis, or if placement of a new line would jeopardize the ability to obtain vascular access, quantitative cultures of blood from a peripheral site and the line in question may be obtained and treatment be based on the results of these cultures.

Treatment: Short-term central venous catheters suspected of being infected are best treated by removing the line and sending it for culture to confirm the source. Empiric antimicrobial therapy may be started in the interim. If the colony count from the catheter is > 15, the result is interpreted as probable catheter infection. Antibiotics should be continued ($\cong$ 5 d) if the patient is demonstrating signs of systemic infection.

Ventilator-Associated Pneumonia (VAP): Defined as a clinical pneumonia that develops after 48 h of mechanical ventilation, VAP occurs in approximately 25% of intubated, ICU patients with an overall mortality from 20–50%. The strongest risk factor for pneumonia in the ICU population is mechanical ventilation (6–15-fold increase); however, age > 70 y, chronic lung disease, nasoenteric tubes, altered mental status, chest trauma/surgery, and frequent transportation of the patient have all been shown to be associated with an increased incidence of VAP.

Diagnosis: Includes a positive airway culture (preferably a bronchoalveolar lavage (BAL) specimen with quantitative cultures showing > 10^4 CFU/mL) plus three of the four following:

- New, persistent, or progressive pulmonary infiltrate (by CXR)
- Purulent tracheobronchial secretions
- Fever
- Leukocytosis

Treatment: Empiric therapy should be instituted when VAP is suspected and customized according to the institutions antibiogram for the particular ICU. Directed therapy may then be formulated when bacterial culture and sensitivity data becomes available. In general, antibiotic therapy should be continued for 10–14 d. Repeat BAL with cultures should be performed if the patient fails standard antibiotic therapy.

Pulmonary Embolism (PE)

PE remains a major cause of death in the United States ($\cong$ 150,000 deaths annually). DVT is known to be responsible for a majority of PE in hospitalized patients. It is estimated that about 90% of all PE originate in the femoral–iliac–pelvic veins. DVT is caused by the classical causes of thromboses **(Virchow's triad): Vessel injury, hypercoagulability, and blood stasis.**

Prevention of DVT: Prevention is especially important in "high-risk" patients (those with malignancy, obesity, previous history, age > 40 y, extensive abdominal/pelvic surgery, long bone and/or pelvic fractures, and prolonged immobilization). For patients undergoing surgery, prevention should be initiated in the

20

operating room. Intermittent compression stockings and the selected use of heparinoids have greatly reduced the incidence of DVT in the postoperative patient. *Note:* Prophylaxis against DVT is effective only when started *preoperatively* for those patients undergoing surgery.

Physical Methods. Includes leg elevation, intermittent compression devices, and *early postoperative ambulation* (**most important**).

Pharmacologic Methods

- **Heparin** 5000 U SQ q12h. Check the platelet count intermittently ($\cong$ q3d) because of risk of heparin-induced thrombocytopenia (HIT).
- **Coumadin** for chronic therapy
- **Low-molecular-weight heparins** (ie, Enoxaparin, dalteparin, etc) is now the drug of choice in our institution for high-risk patients, despite the high cost of therapy.

Diagnosis of PE

- Maintain a high index of suspicion in high-risk patients
- **Signs and symptoms:** None is diagnostic, but may include dyspnea, tachypnea, tachycardia, chest pain (usually pleuritic), and $Po_2 < 80$ mm Hg (compared with baseline)
- **Routine CXR** may show localized volume loss or Hampton's hump due to pulmonary infarction
- **Spiral CT scan:** This scan is helpful in identifying proximal PE and is considered by our institution to be the test of choice
- **Pulmonary angiogram:** The "gold standard" but it is quickly losing favor to spiral CT scan as the imaging technology improves.
- **Nuclear V/Q scan:** Is insensitive and therefore often not helpful. A normal scan effectively rules out PE, and a positive scan is sufficient evidence to treat the patient. An indeterminate scan in a symptomatic patient with a high index of suspicion necessitates angiography.

Treatment

1. **Support oxygenation.** Monitor ABGs and support as necessary (intubation may be necessary).
2. **Use IV heparin;** prevents clot propagation, decreases inflammation, and allows intrinsic fibrinolysis to lyse the clot.
   a. Bolus with 80–100 U/kg and start an IV drip at 10–15 U/kg/h. Adjust the drip to keep the PTT at 2–2.5 × control values. The half-life of heparin is 1.5 h, so check the PTT at 3–6 h after adjusting the rate of heparin administration.
   b. Monitor the platelet count because some patients may manifest "heparin-induced thrombocytopenia."
   c. Start oral warfarin (Coumadin) by day 3 of heparin therapy, to maintain a therapeutic ratio (see Chapter 22).
3. In cases of massive embolus, thrombolytic therapy (TPA) may be used in the absence of contraindications.
4. Open embolectomy, using cardiopulmonary bypass, has been effective in rare cases of massive PE.
5. In patients who cannot undergo systemic anticoagulation (those with recent surgery, stroke, GI bleeding, etc) or patients with recurrent emboli despite adequate therapy, vena caval interruption may be indicated using an percutaneous intracaval filter.

20

TABLE 20–10
Quick Reference to Common ICU Equations

Determination	Derivation	Normal
RAP–CVP	Measured	2–10 mm Hg
RSVP/RVDP	Measured	15–30/0–5 mm Hg
PAS/PAD	Measured	15–30/8–15 mm Hg
MPAP	$PAD + \dfrac{(PAS - PAD)}{3}$	11–18 mm Hg
PAOP (ie, PCWP)	Measured	5–16 mm Hg
MAP	$DBP \times \dfrac{(SBP - DBP)}{3}$	85–90 mm Hg
CO	$SV \times HR$ $\dfrac{V_{O_2} \times 10}{(1.39[Hgb]) \times (S_{AO_2} - S_{vO_2})}$	3.5–5.5 L/min
CI	CO/BSA	2.5–4.2 L/min/m^2
SVR	$\dfrac{(MAP - CVP) \times 80}{CO}$	770–1500 dynes $\times$ s/cm^5
SVRI	SVR/BSA	
PVR	$\dfrac{(MPAP - PAOP) \times 80}{CO}$	20–120 dynes $\times$ s/cm^5
PVRI	PVR/BSA	
Alveolar O$_2$ estimate (PAO$_2$)	$F_{IO_2} \times (P_{atmospheric} - P_{H_2O}) - \dfrac{(P_{aCO_2})}{0.8}$	

(continued)

20

TABLE 20–10
(Continued)

Determination	Derivation	Normal
A–a Gradient	$PAo_2 - PAo_2$	room air = 12–22 mm Hg 100% Fio_2 = 10–60 mm Hg
Cco_2 (pulmonary capillary O_2 content)	$(1.39[Hgb] \times Sco_2) + (Pco_2 \times 0.0031)$	18–24 mL O_2/dL blood
Cao_2 (arterial O_2 content)	$(1.39[Hgb] \times Sao_2) + (Pao_2 \times 0.0031)$	16–22 mL O_2/dL blood
Cvo_2 (mixed venous O_2 content)	$(1.39[Hgb] \times Svo_2) + (Pvo_2 \times 0.0031)$	12–17 mL O_2/dL blood
$C(a-v)$ O_2 (A–v O_2 difference)	$(1.39[Hgb] \times (Sao_2 - Svo_2)$	3.5–5.5 mL O_2/dL blood
O_2 carrying capacity (Cco_2)	$[Hgb] \times Sao_2 \times CO \times 10$	700–1400 mL/min delivery
O_2 consumption (Vo_2)	$(Cao_2 - Cvo_2) \times CO \times 10$	180–280 mL/min
Qs/Qt (shunt fraction)	$\dfrac{(Cco_2 - Cvo_2)}{(Cco_2 - Cvo_2)}$	0.05
ICP	Measured	0–20 mm Hg
CPP	MAP – ICP	Ideally >70 mm Hg

BSA = body surface area (m²) = height (cm)⁰·⁷¹⁸ × Weight (kg)⁰·⁴²⁷ × 74.5; RAP = right atrial pressures CVP = central venous pressure; RVSP = right ventricular systolic pressure; RVDP = right ventricular diastolic pressure; PAS = pulmonary artery systolic pressure; PAD = pulmonary artery diastolic pressure; MPAP = mean pulmonary artery pressure; PAOP = pulmonary artery occlusion pressure; PCWP = pulmonary capillary wedge pressure; MAP = mean arterial pressure; DBP = diastolic blood pressure; SBP = systolic blood pressure; CO=cardiac output; SV = stroke volume; HR = heart rate; Vo_2 = oxygen consumption; Hgb = hemoglobin concentration; Sao_2 = arterial oxygen saturation; Svo_2 = mixed venous oxygen saturation; CI = cardiac index; SVR = systemic vascular resistance; SVRI = systemic vascular resistance index; PVR = pulmonary vascular resistance; PVRI = pulmonary vascular resistance index; Fio_2 = inhaled O_2 concentration; P atmospheric = atmospheric pressure ~ 760 torr; PH_2O = water vapor pressure ~ 47 torr $Paco_2$ = partial pressure of CO_2 in arterial blood; Pao_2 = partial pressure of O_2 in arterial blood; PAo_2 = partial pressure of O_2 in alveolus; Qs = volume of shunted blood (ie, blood shunted past nonventilated alveoli which is not participating in gas exchange); Qt = total cardiac output; ICP = intracranial pressure; CPP = cerebral perfusion pressure.

20

TABLE 20-11
Guidelines for Adult Critical Care Drug Infusions

Drug	Use/Mechanism	Dose Range	Side Effects/Cautions
Amrinone (Inocor)	Inotrope and vasodilator (systemic, pulmonary coronary); used in CHF-resistant to siuretics and afterload reduction	Load: 0.75 mg/kg over 3 min Dose: 5–20 µg/kg/min (max. 10 mg/kg/d)	Adverse effects to catecholamines and digoxin; hypotension (dose-dependent); thrombocytopenia (1–2%); increase AV and ventricu;ar conduction; nausea/vomiting/abdominal pain
Diltiazem (Cardizem)	Slow calcium channel blocker; negative intropy; prolongs AV node refractory time vasodilates to lower BP without reflex tachycardia	Bolus=0.25 mg/kg over 2 min; (may give second bolus 0.35 mg/kg 15 min after initial dose) Dose 5–15 mg/hr	Hypotension: AV block; drug-induced hepatitis; flushing *Contraindications:* Wide-complex tachycardia; Wolfe–Parkinson–White syndrome; existing second third degree AV block; concurrent β-blockade
Dobutamine (Dobutrex)	Racemic mixture (L-isomer: α-agonist/D-isomer: β-agonist]; Positive inotrope/afterload reductionr fo irculatory failure after AMI, CHF, etc	Dose: 2–20 µg/kg/min Max: 40 µg/kg/min	May exacerbate ventricular arrhythmias *Contraindications:* hypertrophic cardiomyopathy

(continued)

20

459

TABLE 20–11
(Continued)

Drug	Use/Mechanism	Dose Range	Side Effects/Cautions
Dopamine (Inotropin)	Dopaminergic (0.5–2.0 μg/kg/min): renal cerebral, mesenteric vasodilation	α-agonist (10–20 μg/kg/min); predominantly vasopressor	Enhances AV conduction especially with atrial fibrillation; may exacerbate psychosis and arrhythmias
	α–β agonist (2.0–10 g/kg/min): positive inotrope and vasopressor	Max: 40 μg/kg/min	*Caution:* Urgently treat extravasated drug with phentolamine to prevent skin necrosis
Epinephrine (Adrenalin)	Nonspecific adrenergic agonist (β > α); potent bronchodilator (β₂ agonist)	Shock: 2 μg/min, then titrate Cardiac Arrest: 1 mg IV q3–5min	Increases myocardial oxygen consumption; protachyarrhythmia; splanchnic vasoconstrictor (if dose < 4 μg/min); diabetogenic; promotes hypokalemia
Esmolol (Brevibloc)	β₁-selective; very short half-life (9 min); slows AV node conduction; useful to test β-blockade in patients with potential contraindications	Load: 500 μg/kg over 1 min Dose: 50 μg/kg min; titrate by 50 μg/kg min to target HR (may need to repeat load)	Bronchospasm; pallor; nausea; flushing; bradycardia; pulmonary edema (if heart failure occurs); asystole

(continued)

TABLE 20-11
(Continued)

Drug	Use/Mechanism	Dose Range	Side Effects/Cautions
Isoproterenol (Isuprel)	Nonspecific β-agonist; potent inotrope/chronotrope for brady-cardic states	Initially: 1–4 μg/min Titrate up to 20 μg/min based on target HR	Hypotension; tachycardia; myocardial ischemia *Contraindications:* Angina/myocardial ischemia; tachycardia; digitalis-induced bradycardia
Milrinone (Primacor)	Inotrope and vasodilator (systemic, pulmonary, coronary); used in CHF	Load: 50 μg/kg over 10 min Dose: 0.375–0.75 μg/kg/min	Renal elimination; hypotension; tachycardia; aggravates atrial, ventricular arrhythmias; headache
Nicardipine (Cardene)	Calcium channel blocker; vasodilator >> negative inotrope; short halflife and rapid hepatic elimination	Dose 5 mg/h; titrate to BP goal (increase rate by 2.5 mg/h q5–15min) Max: 15 mg/h	Delayed clearance with hepatic and renal insufficiency; may worsen portal hypertension; may cause reflex tachycardia *Contraindications:* Critical aortic stenosis; will alter cyclosporin levels

(continued)

TABLE 20–11
(Continued)

Drug	Use/Mechanism	Dose Range	Side Effects/Cautions
Nitroglycerin (Tridil)	Arterial/venous vasodilator (dose-dependent); coronary vasodilator; combined with dobutamine with acute coronary syndrome	Dose: 5–10 μg/min; titrate by 10–20 μg/min q5min based on current dose and patient condition; hypotension at 200 mg/min	Headache, nausea, vomiting, dizziness *Contraindications:* Increased ICP; narrow-angle glaucoma; pericardial tamponade
Nitroprusside (Nipride)	Arterial/venous vasodilator; donates nitric oxide to interact with vascular smooth muscle >> visceral smooth muscle	Dose: 0.5–10 μg/kg/min; titrate to goal BP every few min Max: 10 μg/kg/min	Reacts with Hgb to form met-Hgb → cyanide accumulation; detoxified to thiocyanate by liver and kidney; keep met-Hgb < 10%; may shunt blood away from renal/splanchnic beds
Norepinephrine (Levophed)	Potent β₁/α-agonist (low-dose: β > α) (high-dose: α > β); use for cardiogenic/septic/neurogenic shock after volume repletion	Initial: 2 μg/min Dose: 2–20 μg/min; titrate to response Max: 40 μg/min	Peripheral A-lines may be dampened by vasoconstriction; suspect volume depletion with hypotension; treat extravasation with phentolamine May decrease splanchnic blood flow; spares cerebral, coronary blood flow

(continued)

20

TABLE 20-11
(Continued)

Drug	Use/Mechanism	Dose Range	Side Effects/Cautions
Phenylephrine (Neo-Synephrine)	Postsynaptic α–agonist; only; use for hypotension, shock, spinal anesthesia or drug-induced hypotension	Bolus: 0.1–0.5 μg IV q15min Initial: 100 μg/min; titrate to 40–200 μg/min	May cause reflex brachycardia (blocked by atropine); constricts coronary, cerebral, and pulmonary vessels Contraindications: Use reduced doses in patients taking MAO inhibitors
Vasopressin (Pitressin)	Potent vasoconstrictor; anti-diuretic; procoagulant; used for variceal hemorrhage to reduce portal pressures; emerging indications in septic shock	Dose: 0.04–0.1 units/min	Myocardial ischemia due to coronary vasoconstriction; may need to combine with nitroglycerin; hepatic/renal metabolism with renal excretion SIADH/water intoxication; abdominal cramps

^aNote: These agents must be administered in the appropriately monitored clinical setting.
CHF = congestive heart failure; AV = atrioventricular; BP = blood pressure; AMI = acute myocardial infarction; HR = heart rate; Hgb = hemoglobin; MAO = monoamine oxidase; SIADH = syndrome of inappropriate antidiuretic hormone.

20

21

EMERGENCIES

Cardiopulmonary Resuscitation
Advanced Cardiac Life Support
    and Emergency Cardiac Care*
Advanced Cardiac Life Support
    Drugs

Electrical Defibrillation
    and Cardioversion
Other Common Emergencies

CARDIOPULMONARY RESUSCITATION

Emergency cardiac care guidelines from the American Heart Association now recommend that health care providers have the following items readily available: gloves, a barrier device or bag mask, and an automated defibrillator to handle cardiac emergencies. In cardiopulmonary resuscitation, there are now **two** sets of **ABCDs:**

Primary Survey
- **A**irway: Assess and manage noninvasively.
- **B**reathing: Use positive pressure ventilations.
- **C**irculation: Perform chest compressions as needed.
- **D**efibrillation: Assess for VT/VF and defibrillate using an AED. These are also called PADs and are becoming widely available in public areas such as airports, stadiums, health clubs, and shopping malls.

Secondary Survey: Uses advanced medical techniques:

- **A**irway: Assess and manage with airway device (eg, endotracheal intubation, etc).
- **B**reathing: Verify tube function and placement, use positive pressure ventilation system through tube.
- **C**irculation: Start IV, attach ECG, use rhythm-based ACLS medications.
- **D**ifferential Diagnosis: Search for, find, and treat problems according to AHA algorithms presented in this chapter.

Adult CPR

(Victim's age ≥ 8 y)

One Rescuer
1. Determine unresponsiveness (shake and shout). If the patient is unresponsive, call for help (activate EMS system, eg, call "code," dial 911). In trauma situation do not move the victim unless in immediate danger. Roll victim on to back as a unit if lying face down. Protect the neck.

---

* The section on basic CPR and ACLS are based on guidelines from the American Heart Association and the International Liaison Committee on Resuscitation [*Circulation* 2000;**102** (Supp 1)] and the Guidelines 2000 for Cardiopulmonary Resuscitation and Emergency Cardiovascular Care by the American Heart Association in Collaboration with the International Liaison Committee on Resuscitation (ILCOR).

21

2. Kneel at the level of the victim's shoulder. Open the airway (head-tilt, chin-lift,), determine breathlessness ("**look** [chest movement], **listen** [for air escaping], **feel** [for air movement]") for no more than 10 s. In the unresponsive victim with spontaneous respiration, place the victim in the recovery position. Jaw thrust maneuver recommended as alternative for health care providers especially if neck injury is suspected. If the victim is breathing, place in the **recovery position** (see page 469).

3. If not breathing, give patient two slow ventilations (2 s/inspiration) while maintaining airway. A barrier device (face shield or mask with one-way valve) is recommended if mouth-to-mouth or mouth-to-nose contact is necessary. Ventilate 10–12 breaths/min. If unable to ventilate, reposition head and try again. If unsuccessful, perform the **foreign body obstruction airway sequence** (see page 468).

4. Check for circulation (breathing, coughing, movement). Palpate the carotid artery no more than 10 s to determine lack of a pulse. If pulse is present, perform rescue breathing: 1 ventilation every 5 s (10–12 ventilation/min).

5. If no pulse, use four cycles of 15 compressions and two ventilations (compression rate 100/min, two ventilations 1.5–2 s each). Apply compressions to lower half of sternum using the heels of both hands placed on top of each other.

6. After the four cycles (approximately 1 min of CPR), pause and check for return pulse and spontaneous respirations.

7. If no pulse or respiration, resume cycles with two ventilations, then compressions, as noted earlier.

8. Incorporate appropriate ACLS management guidelines.

Two-Rescuer Adult CPR

For laypersons

1. Second rescuer identifies him or herself. Verify that EMS has been notified. If so, second rescuer gets into position opposite first rescuer. If EMS not notified, the second rescuer does so before assisting first rescuer.

2. First rescuer continues CPR.

3. If and when first rescuer tires, second rescuer takes over one-person CPR as described in the preceding section.

For health care professionals

1. Sequence to continue from one-rescuer CPR as mentioned in previous section. Second rescuer identifies him or herself and gets into position for compressions.

2. First rescuer completes compression and ventilation cycle (15 compression and two ventilations).

3. First rescuer then checks for spontaneous pulse and breathing, states: "No pulse\.\continue CPR," then ventilate once (1.5–2 s).

4. Second rescuer resumes compressions at same rate of 80–100/min. ("1 & 2 & 3 & 4 & 5 & pause," ventilate) Ratio of five compressions to one breath. If airway is protected, do not pause for ventilations.

5. When ready to switch, rescuer doing compressions says "switch & 2 & 3 & 4 & 5 &."

6. Both rescuers change position simultaneously immediately after ventilation.

21

7. Rescuer who will perform ventilations opens airway and performs a 5-s pulse check.
8. If no pulse, give ventilation. Rescuer states "No pulse\.\continue CPR."
9. In patient with unprotected airway, cricoid pressure may be applied

Child CPR: (Victim's age 1–8 y)

1. Determine unresponsiveness, and shout for help. Activate EMS system (call code or 911).
2. Open airway (head-tilt, chin-lift; jaw thrust if neck trauma is suspected), determine breathlessness (follow "look, listen, feel" rubric as for adult). If victim is breathing, place in **recovery position** (see page 469).
3. If victim not breathing, give two ventilations (1–1.5 s). If unable to ventilate, perform the **foreign body obstruction airway sequence** (see page 468).
4. Check for circulation (breathing, coughing, movement). Palpate the carotid artery for no more than 10 s to determine presence of a pulse. If pulse is present, perform rescue breathing using pocket mask or bag mask device (20 breaths/min).
5. If no pulse, or if pulse is < 60 bpm and perfusion is poor, begin cardiac compressions at five compressions to one ventilation at rate of 100/min. Depth of compressions less than for an adult (1–1.5 in. or one third to one half the depth of chest). Use the heel of one hand at the lower half of the sternum. Pause compressions for ventilations until patient is intubated.
6. Check for return of pulse and spontaneous breathing after 20 cycles (approximately 1 min).
7. Resume cycles with one ventilation (1–1.5 s each), then resume compressions.

Infant CPR (Victim's age, ≤ 1 y)

1. Determine unresponsiveness, and shout for help. Activate EMS system (call code or 911).
2. Open airway (head-tilt, chin-lift). Do not hyperextend head; however, create adequate head-tilt to accomplish chest rise with breath. If neck trauma suspected, use jaw thrust. If victim is breathing, place in the **recovery position** (see page 469).
3. If patient is not breathing, give two ventilations (1–1.5 s) using pocket mask or bag mask device. If unable to ventilate, perform the **foreign body obstruction airway sequence** using back blows and chest thrusts as noted on page 468.
4. Check for circulation (breathing, coughing, movement). Palpate the femoral or brachial artery for no more than 10 s to determine presence of a pulse. If pulse is present, continue rescue breathing (20 breaths/min).
5. If no pulse or if pulse is < 60 bpm and perfusion is poor, begin cardiac compressions. Draw an imaginary line between the nipples and identify where this line crosses the sternum (intermammary line). The site of compression is one finger breadth below this intersection. Use a compression depth of ½–1 in., using the middle and ring fingers. Use five compressions to one ventilation (rate of compression is 100/min or 120 min for newborns).
6. Use the mnemonic: ("1 & 2 & 3 & 4 & 5 & pause, head-tilt, chin-lift, ventilate-continue compressions"). When patient is intubated, no need to pause.
7. Check for return of pulse and spontaneous breathing after 20 cycles (1 min).

21

Neonatal CPR

1. The newborn should be dried, placed head down, gently suctioned and stimulated.
2. Supplemental oxygen is useful. If baby is not breathing, ventilate 40–60 breaths/min with gentle puff of air or with bag mask.
3. Check apical pulse. If absent or if < 60 bpm and perfusion is poor, compress at a rate of 120/min. Wrap your hands around infant's chest and compress ½–¾ in. with thumbs side by side at the midsternum.
4. The compression/ventilation ratio is 3:1 for intubated newborn with two rescuers. Discontinue compressions when rate reaches 80 bpm or greater.

Foreign Body Obstructed Airway Sequence

Adult (≥ 8 y) and Child (1–8 y)

A. **Conscious victim *can* cough, speak, breath.** Do not interfere and reassure patient. Stand by and allow patient to clear partial obstruction.
B. **Conscious victim *cannot* cough, speak, breath.**
    1. Ask "Are you choking" or "Can you speak?" Observe for "universal distress signal" for choking (hands clutched at neck).
    2. Give abdominal thrusts/Heimlich maneuver. Stand behind victim. Using arms wrapped around victim, place thumb side of fist above umbilicus but below xiphoid. Give up to five subdiaphragmatic thrusts (Heimlich maneuver).
    3. Reassess victim's status, repeat Heimlich maneuvers as needed. If not improved by 1 min, activate EMS.
C. **Victim becomes unconscious.**
    1. Place in supine (face up) position. Activate EMS or if second rescuer becomes available have that person activate EMS.
    2. Open airway with tongue-jaw lift; finger sweep to clear airway, open airway (head-tilt, chin-lift).
    3. Give five abdominal thrusts/Heimlich maneuver astride victim.
D. **Victim found unconscious: Cause unknown**
    1. Determine unresponsiveness, call for help (activate EMS).
    2. Open airway (head-tilt, chin-lift), determine breathlessness (look, listen, feel).
    3. Attempt to ventilate. If unsuccessful, reposition head and reattempt.
    4. If unsuccessful:
        a. Perform up to five Heimlich maneuvers astride victim.
        b. Open mouth (tongue-jaw lift); finger sweep; open airway (head-tilt, chin-lift)
    5. Attempt to ventilate, if unsuccessful, repeat sequence until ventilations are effective.

Infant: (Victim's age, < 1 y)
Victim conscious

1. Verify airway obstruction (ineffective cough, no strong cry).
2. Hold child with head lower than body, give five back blows or five gentle abdominal thrusts. Repeat until victim becomes responsive.

Victim becomes unconscious

1. If second rescuer is available, have that person activate EMS.
2. Open airway with tongue-jaw lift, remove foreign body if visualized. Attempt to ventilate.

21

3. If still obstructed, reposition head and attempt to ventilate. Give five back blows and five abdominal thrusts. Repeat step 2 until ventilation is effective.
4. If obstruction still not relieved after 1 min, activate EMS system.

Recovery Position

Place an unconscious person who is still breathing and who has not suffered a traumatic neck injury in this position.

1. Kneel alongside the victim and straighten the legs.
2. Place victim's arm that is closest to you in the "waving goodbye" position and place the other arm across the victim's chest.
3. Grasp the far side leg above the knee and pull the thigh up toward the body. With the other hand, grasp the shoulder on the same side as the thigh.
4. Gently roll the patient toward you. Adjust the leg you are holding until both the thigh and knee are at right angles to the body. Tilt the patient's head back and use the patient's uppermost hand to support the head and maintain a head-tilt position.
5. Continue to monitor for breathing, and call for EMS.
6. If patient stops breathing, roll on back and follow basic CPR guidelines.

ADVANCED CARDIAC LIFE SUPPORT AND EMERGENCY CARDIAC CARE

ACLS includes the use of advanced airway management (See Endotracheal Intubation, Chapter 13, page 272), defibrillation, and drugs along with basic CPR. Most cardiac arrests are due to VF. ACLS protocols incorporating all these emergency cardiac care techniques are reviewed in the following algorithms. for adults:

- Universal/International ACLS algorithm (Figure 21–1)
- Comprehensive emergency cardiac care algorithm (Figure 21–2)
- Ventricular fibrillation and pulseless VT algorithm (Figure 21–3)
- Pulseless electrical activity (PEA) algorithm (Figure 21–4)
- Asystole: The silent heart algorithm (Figure 21–5)
- Bradycardia algorithm (Figure 21–6)
- Tachycardia overview algorithm (Figure 21–7)
- Narrow-complex SVT algorithm (Figure 21–8)
- Stable VT algorithm (Figure 21–9)
- Acute coronary syndromes algorithm (Figure 21–10)
- Acute pulmonary edema, hypotension, and shock (Figure 21–11)

Advanced Cardiac Life Support Drugs

The most commonly used agents are listed on the inside covers for rapid reference.

Adenosine (Adenocard)   Uses: First drug for narrow-complex PSVT (not for AF or VT) **Supplied:** 2 mg/mL in 2-mL vial **Dose:** *Adults* initial 6 mg rapid IVP over 1–3 s followed by NS bolus of 20 mL, then elevate extremity. Repeat 12 mg in 1–2 min PRN. A third dose of 12 mg in 1–2 min PRN. *Peds.* 0.1 mg/kg rapid IV push with ECG monitoring. Follow with > 5 mL NS flush. May double (0.2 mg/kg) for second dose. Max: first dose: 6 mg; second dose: 12 mg; single dose: 12 mg

Amiodarone   Uses: Life-threatening atrial and ventricular tachydysrhythmias refractory to first-line agents **Supplied:** 50 mg/mL in 3-mL vial **Dose:** *Adults.* Max cumulative dose: 2.2 g IV/24 h. Breakthrough VF/VT. 150 mg IV PRN. Pulseless VF/VT. 300 mg IV push; may supplement with 150 mg followed by infusion of 1mg/min for 6 hours, then 0.5

21

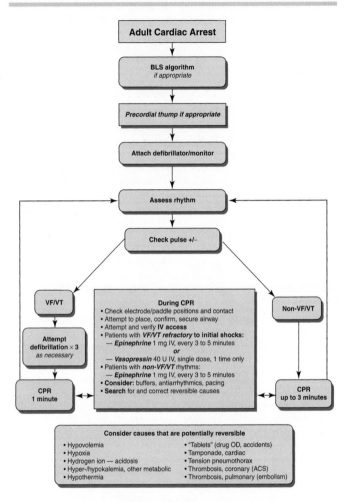

FIGURE 21–1 Universal/international ACLS algorithm. VF = ventricular fibrillation; VT = ventricular tachycardia; BLS = basic life support. (Reproduced, with permission, from *Circulation* 2000;**102** supplement 1, part 6.)

mg/min *Peds. Refractory pulseless VT, VF:* 5 mg/kg rapid IV bolus. *Perfusing supraventricular and ventricular arrhythmias:* Loading dose: 5 mg/kg IV/IO over 20–60 min (repeat, max 15 mg/kg/day)

Aspirin Uses: In the acute setting, administer to all patients with acute coronary syndrome (ACS) **Supplied:** Tabs 160, 325 mg **Dose:** 160–325 mg PO (chewing preferred ASAP after onset of ACS)

Atropine Sulfate Uses: First drug for symptomatic bradycardia (but not Mobitz II). Second drug (after epinephrine or vasopressin) for asystole or bradycardic PEA **Supplied:**

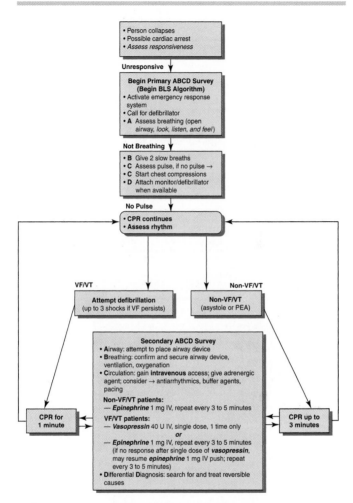

FIGURE 21–2 Comprehensive emergency cardiac care (ECC) algorithm. VF = ventricular fibrillation; VT = ventricular tachycardia; BLS = basic life support; PEA = pulseless electrical activity. (Reproduced, with permission, from *Circulation* 2000;**102** supplement 1, part 6.)

0.1 mg/mL in 10-mL syringe (total = 1 mg) **Dose:** *Adults. Asystole or PEA* 1 mg IV push. Repeat every 3–5 min (if asystole persists) to 0.03–0.04 mg/kg max. *Bradycardia:* 0.5–1.0 mg IV every 3–5 min as needed; max 3 mg or 0.04 mg/kg. *Endotracheal administration:* 2–3 mg in 10 mL NS. *Peds.* IV administration: 0.02 mg/kg. Min single dose: 0.1 mg, max: 0.5 mg. Max adolescent single dose: 1.0 mg. May double for second IV dose. Max child total dose: 1.0 mg. Max adolescent total dose: 2.0 mg. Endotracheal administration: 0.02 mg/kg (larger doses than IV may be required)

Beta Blockers: **Uses:** All patients with suspected MI; may reduce chance of VF and reduce damage. Second-line agents after adenosine, diltiazem, or

21

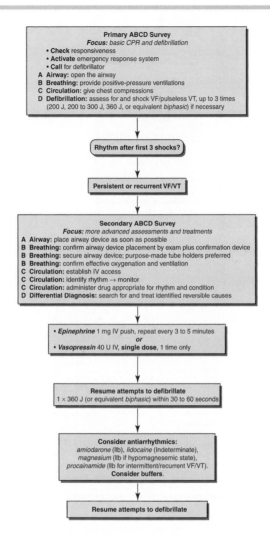

FIGURE 21–3 Ventricular fibrillation and pulseless ventricular tachycardia algorithm. VF = ventricular fibrillation; VT = ventricular tachycardia; BLS = basic life support (Reproduced, with permission, from *Circulation* 2000;**102** supplement 1, part 6.)

digoxin to slow ventricular response in supraventricular tachyarrhythmias. Antihypertensive for hemorrhagic and ischemic stroke. Do **not** administer along with calcium channel blockers due to risk of hypotension. Cardioselectivity increased in metoprolol, esmolol, and atenolol and are better choices in patients with asthma, COPD, and diabetes.

21

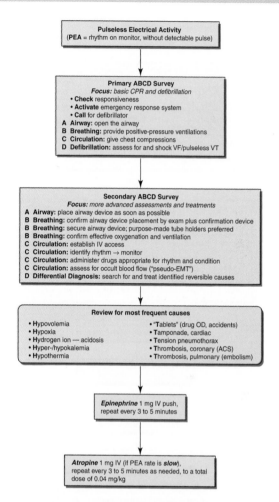

FIGURE 21–4 Pulseless electrical activity algorithm. VF = ventricular fibrillation; VT = ventricular tachycardia; EMT = emergency medical treatment; ACS = acute coronary syndrome; PEA = pulseless electrical activity. (Reproduced, with permission, from *Circulation* 2000;**102** supplement 1, part 6.)

- Metoprolol (Lopressor) **Supplied:** 1 mg/mL in 5-mL vial **Dose:** *Adults.* 5 mg slow IV q 5 min, total 15 mg
- Atenolol (Tenormin) **Supplied:** 0.5 mg/mL in 10-mL amp **Dose:** *Adults.* 5 mg slow IV (over 5 min). In 10 min, second dose 5 mg slow IV. In 10 min, if tolerated, start 50 mg PO, then 50 mg PO bid

21

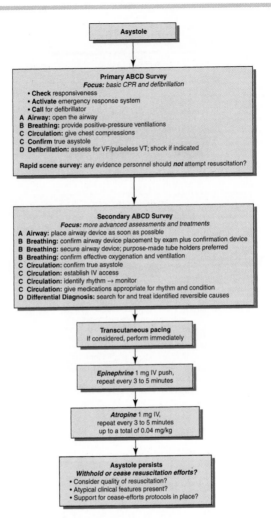

FIGURE 21-5 Asystole: the silent heart algorithm. VF = ventricular fibrillation; VT = ventricular tachycardia. (Reproduced with permission from *Circulation* 2000;**102** supplement 1, part 6)

- Propranolol (Inderal) **Supplied:** 1.0 mg/mL in 1 amp, 4 mg/mL in 5-mL amp **Dose:** *Adults.* 1 mg slow IV push, repeat every 5 mn, PRN to maximum of 5 mg min intervals, max 1 mg/min. Repeat after 2 min, PRN
- Esmolol (Brevibloc) **Supplied:** 10 mg/mL in 10-mL amp **Dose:** *Adults.* 0.5 mg/kg over 1 min, then 0.05 mg/kg/min. May increase infusion by 0.05 mg/kg every 4 min., up to 0.2 mg/kg.
- Labetalol **Supplied:** 5 mg/mL (Amps 20, 40, 60 mL) **Dose:** 20 mg IV push over 1–2 min. Repeat or double dose every 10 min (max: 300 mg); or initial bolus, then 2–8 mcg/min

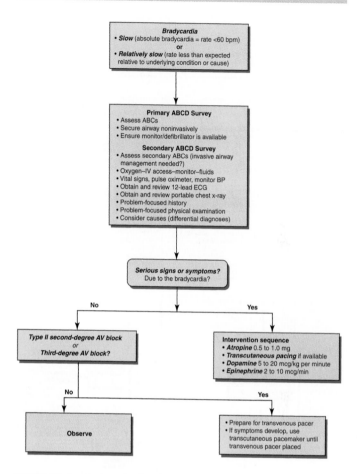

FIGURE 21–6 Bradycardia algorithm. BP = blood pressure; ECG = electrocardiogram; AV = atrioventricular. (Reproduced, with permission, from *Circulation* 2000; **102** supplement 1, part 6.)

Calcium Chloride **Uses:** Known/suspected hyperkalemia, hypocalcemia (eg, multiple transfusions), antidote for calcium channel blocker overdose, prophylactically before IV calcium channel blockers (prevent hypotension) **Supplied:** 100 mg/mL in 10-mL vial (total = 1 g; 10% soln) **Dose:** *Adults.* 2–4 mg/kg (usually 2 mL) IV before IV calcium blockers may repeat every 10 min. *Peds.* 20 mg/kg (0.2–0.25 mL/kg) slow push. Repeat PRN

Calcium Gluconate **Supplied:** 10% = 100 mg/10 mL = 9 mg/mL Ca **Dose:** *Peds.* 60–100 mg/kg (0.6–1.0 mL/kg) IV slow push. Repeat for documented conditions

Digibind Digoxin-specific antibody therapy **Uses:** Digoxin toxicity with uncontrolled life-threatening arrhythmias, shock, CHF; hyperkalemia > 5 mEq/L with serum dig levels above 10–15 ng/mL **Supplied:** 40-mg vial (each vial binds about 0.6 mg digoxin)

21

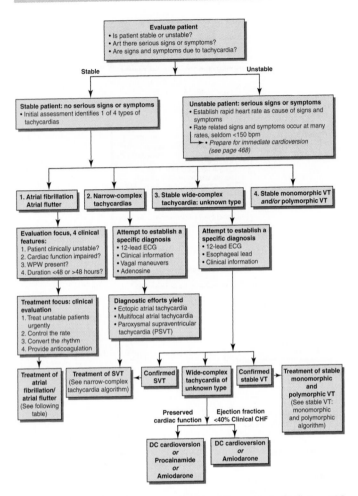

FIGURE 21–7 Tachycardia overview algorithm. VF = ventricular fibrillation; ECG = electrocardiogram; PSVT = paroxysmal supraventricular tachycardia; SVT = supraventricular tachycardia. (Reproduced, with permission, from *Circulation* 2000;**102** supplement 1, part 6.)

Dose: *Adults.* Chronic intoxication: 3–5 vials may be effective. *Acute overdose:* See Chapter 22, page 533; based on dose ingested (average dose is 10 vials (400 mg), but may require up to 20 vials (800 mg).

Digoxin   **Uses:** Slow ventricular response in AF or atrial flutter. Second-line for PSVT **Supplied:** 0.15 mg/mL or 0.1 mg/mL in 1- or 2-mL amp **Dose:** *Adults.* Loading 10–15 mcg/kg. Maintenance dose see Chapter 22, page 533.

Diltiazem (Cardizem)   **Uses:** Control ventricular rate in AF and atrial flutter. Use after adenosine to convert refractory PSVT in patients with narrow QRS complex and adequate BP. **Supplied:** 5 mg/mL in 5 or 10-mL vial (total = 25 or 50 mg) **Dose:** *Adults. Acute*

21

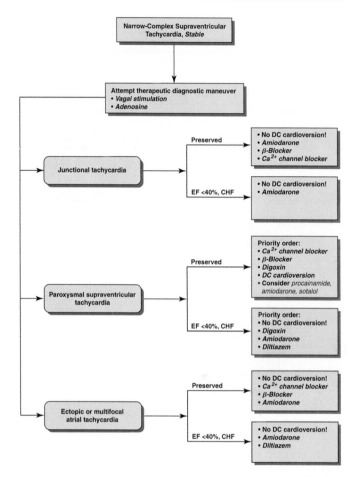

FIGURE 21–8 Narrow-complex SVT algorithm. EF = ejection fraction; CHF = congestive heart failure. (Reproduced, with permission, from *Circulation* 2000;**102** supplement 1, part 6.)

rate control: 15–20 mg (0.25 mg/kg) IV over 2 min. Repeat in 15 min at 20–25 mg (0.35 mg/kg) over 2 min. *Maintenance:* 5–15 mg/h, titrated to heart rate

Dobutamine (Dobutrex) **Uses:** Use alone in cardiac decompensation with BP 70–100 mm Hg and no signs of shock. May be added to dopamine in cardiogenic shock. **Supplied:** 12.5 mg/mL in 20-mL vial (total = 250 mg). IV inf: Dilute 250 mg (20 mL) in 250 mL NS or D_5W **Dose: *Adults.*** 2–20 mcg/kg/min; titrate to heart rate not > 10% of baseline. Hemodynamic monitoring recommended. *Peds.* Cont IV inf: Titrate to effect (initial dose 5–10 mcg/kg/min). Typical inf dose: 2–20 mcg/kg/min

Dopamine (Intropin) **Uses:** Hypotension (BP < 70–100 mm Hg) with signs of symptoms of shock. Second line for symptomatic bradycardia. **Supplied:** 40 mg/mL or 160 mg/mL. *IV inf:* Mix 400–800 mg in 250 mL NS or D_5W. **Dose: *Adults.*** Titrate to response. *Low:* 1–5 mcg/kg/min ("renal doses"). *Moderate:* 5–10 mcg/kg/min ("cardiac doses").

21

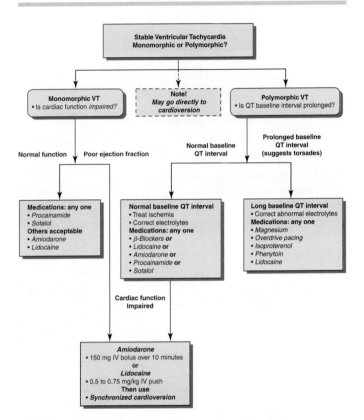

FIGURE 21–9 Stable SVT algorithm. VT = ventricular tachycardia. (Reproduced, with permission, from *Circulation* 2000;**102** supplement 1, part 6.)

High: 10–20 mcg/kg/min ("vasopressor doses"). **Peds.** Titrate to effect. Initial, 5–10 mcg/kg/min; typical: 2–20 mcg/kg/min
Note: If > 20 mcg/kg/min is required, consider use of alternative adrenergic agent (eg, epinephrine)

Epinephrine Uses: *Cardiac arrest:* VF, pulseless VT, asystole, PEA. *Symptomatic bradycardia:* After atropine and transcutaneous pacing. *Anaphylaxis, severe allergic reactions:* Combine with large fluid volumes, corticosteroids, antihistamines. **Supplied:** 1.0 mg/10 mL (1:10,000) in preloaded 10-mL syringe (total = 1 mg), 1 mg/mL in glass 1-mL amp (total = 1 mg) **Dose:** *Adults. Cardiac arrest:* IV dose: 1.0 mg IV push, repeat every 3–5 min; doses up to (0.2 mg/kg) if 1 mg dose fails (not AHA recommended). Inf: 30 mg epinephrine (30 mL of 1:1000 solution) to 250 mL NS or D_5W, run at 100 mL/h, titrate. Endotracheal: 2.0–2.5 mg in 20 mL NS. *Profound bradycardia/hypotension:* 2–10 mcg/min (1 mg of 1:1000 in 500 mL NS, infuse 1–5 mL/min). **Peds.** *Asystole, pulseless arrest:* First dose: 0.1 mg/kg IV (0.1 mL/kg of 1:10,000 "standard concentration"). Second and subsequent doses: 0.1 mg/kg IV (0.1 mL/kg of 1:1000 "High" concentration. Administer every 3–5 min during arrest; up to 0.2 mg/kg may be effective. Endotracheal: 0.1 mg/kg (0.1 mL/kg of 1:1000 ["high"] concentration) continue every 3–5 min of arrest until IV access is achieved; then begin with first IV dose. *Symptomatic bradycardia:* 0.01 mg/kg IV (0.1 mL/kg of 1:10,000 ["standard"] concentration). Endotracheal doses: 0.1 mg/kg (0.1 mL/kg

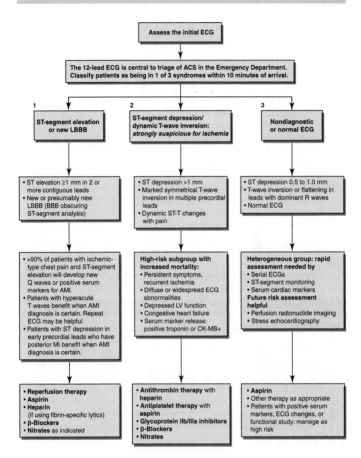

FIGURE 21–10 Acute coronary syndromes algorithm. ECG = electrocardiogram; LBBB = left bundle branch block; BBB = bundle branch block; AMI = acute myocardial infarction; MI = myocardial infarction; LV = left ventricle; CK-MB+ = positive for myocardial muscle creatine kinase isoenzyme. (Reproduced, with permission, from *Circulation* 2000;**102** supplement 1, part 6.)

of 1:1000 ["high"] concentration). Cont IV inf: Begin with rapid infusion; then titrate to response. Typical inf: 0.1–1.0 mcg/kg/min (Higher doses may be effective)

Flumazenil (Romazicon) Uses: Reverse iatrogenic benzodiazepine toxicity (do **not** use in benzodiazepine dependent pt, tricyclic overdose or in unknown poisoning) **Supplied:** 0.1 mg/mL in 5- and 10-mL vials **Dose:** *Adults.* 0.2 mg IV over 15 s then 0.3 mg IV over 30 s, if no response, give 0.5 mg IV given over 30 s, repeat once per min until response, or total of 3 mg.

Furosemide (Lasix) Uses: Acute pulmonary edema in BP > 90–100. Hypertensive emergencies or increased intracranial pressure **Supplied:** 10 mg/mL in 2-, 4-, and 10-mL amp or vials **Dose:** *Adults.* 0.5–1.0 mg/kg over 1–2 min. If no response, double the dose to 2.0 mg/kg over 1–2 min

Glucagon Uses: Reverse effects of calcium channel blocker or beta-blocker **Supplied:** 1- and 10-mg vials **Dose:** *Adults.* 1–5 mg over 2–5 min

21

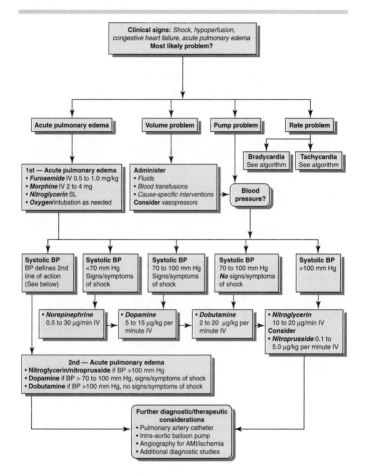

FIGURE 21–11 Acute pulmonary edema, hypotension, and shock. BP = blood pressure; AMI = acute myocardial infarction. (Reproduced, with permission, from *Circulation* 2000;**102** supplement 1, part 6.)

Glycoprotein IIb/IIIa Inhibitors: **Uses:** ACS undergoing percutaneous interventions (PCI), ACS without ST elevation. Do **not** use with history of active bleeding or surgery within 30 d or if platelets < 150,000/mm³. Note that optimum dosing and duration not established; check package insert.

- Abciximab (ReoPro) **Supplied:** 2 mg/mL in 5-mL vial **Dose:** ACS with planned PCI within 24 h: 0.25 mg/kg IV bolus up to 1 h before procedure, then 0.125 mcg/kg/IV; must use with heparin. Platelet recovery within 48 h; redosing may cause hypersensitivity reaction.
- Eptifibatide (Integrilin) **Supplied:** 0.75 and 2 mg/mL in 10-mL vial **Dose:** *ACS:* 180 mcg/kg IV bolus (max 22.6 mg) then 2 mcg/kg/min infusion, max 15 mg/hr *PCI:* 180 mcg/kg IV bolus then 0.5 mcg/kg/min infusion; repeat bolus in 10 min.

21

- Tirofiban (Aggrastat) **Supplied:** 250 mcg/mL in 50 mL or premixed 50 mcg/mL **Dose:** *ACS or PCI:* 0.4 mcg/kg/min IV for 30 min, then 0.1 mcg/kg/min infusion

Heparin (Unfractionated) **Uses:** Adjuvant therapy in AMI. Begin heparin with fibrinolytics. **Supplied:** 0.5–1.0 mL amp, vials, and prefilled syringes. Multidose vials 1, 2, 5 and 30 mL. Concentrations range from 1000 to 40,000 IU/mL. **Dose:** *Adults.* Bolus 80 IU/kg (max bolus: 4000 IU). Continue 18 IU/kg/h (max 1000 IU/h for patients > 70 kg) round to the nearest 50 IU. Adjust to maintain PTT 1.5–2.0 × control values for 48 h or until angiography.

Heparin (Low-Molecular-Weight) (Fragmin, Lovenox) **Uses:** ACS with non-Q wave or unstable angina **Supplied:** Dalteparin (Fragmin), Enoxaparin (Lovenox) **Dose:** 1 mg/kg bid SQ for 2–8 d with aspirin Doses differ for each drug. Dalteparin = 120 units/kg (max 10,000 units) q 12h

Ibutilide (Corvert) **Uses:** Supraventricular arrhythmias (AFiB, A flutter); short-acting **Supplied:** 1 mg/10 mL **Dose:** 1 mg IV over 10 min (if < 60 kg 0.01 mg/kg)

Isoproterenol (Isuprel) **Uses:** Torsades de pointes unresponsive to magnesium sulfate. Temporary control of bradycardia in heart transplant patients. Class IIb at low doses for symptomatic bradycardias **Supplied:** 0.1 mg/mL in 1-mL vial. IV inf: Mix 1 mg in 250 mL NS or D_5W **Dose:** *Adults.* 2–10 mcg/min. Titrate to effect.

Lidocaine **Uses:** VF/VT. Stable VT, **Supplied:** 20 mg/mL in preloaded 5-mL syringe, 10 mg/mL in 5-mL vial. Can be given via endotracheal tube. **Dose:** *Adults. Cardiac arrest from VF/VT:* Initial dose: 1.5 mg/kg IV. For stable VT 0.5–0.75 mg/kg every 5–10 min; max total dose, 3 mg/kg. Maintenance inf: 1–4 mg/min (30–50 mcg/min)

Magnesium Sulfate **Uses:** with torsades de pointes or suspected hypomagnesemic state, refractory VF, life-threatening ventricular arrhythmias due to digitalis toxicity, tricyclic overdose. **Supplied:** Amps of 2 and 10 mL of 50% $MgSO_4$ (total = 1 g and 5 g). 10 mL in preloaded syringe (total = 5 g/10 mL) **Dose:** *Adults.* 1–2 g, mixed in 50–100 mL of D_5W, over 5–60 min IV. Follow with 0.5–1.0 g/h IV for up to 24 h.

Mannitol **Uses:** Increased intracranial pressure in management of neurologic emergencies **Supplied:** 150-, 250-, and 1000-mL IV containers (strengths: 5%, 10%, 15%, 20%, and 25%). **Dose:** *Adults.* Administer 0.5–1.0 g/kg over 5–10 min. Additional doses of 0.25-2 g/kg can be given every 4–6 h as needed. Use in conjunction with oxygenation, ventilation and neurosurgical consultation.

Morphine Sulfate **Uses:** Chest pain and anxiety associated with AMI or cardiac ischemia, acute cardiogenic pulmonary edema (if blood pressure adequate) **Supplied:** 2–10 mg/mL in a 1-mL syringe **Dose:** *Adults.* 2–4 mg IV (over 1–5 min) every 5–30 min

Naloxone (Narcan) **Uses:** To reverse effects of narcotic toxicity, including respiratory depression, hypotension, and hypoperfusion **Dose:** *Adults.* 0.4–2.0 mg IV every 2 min; up to 10 mg over < 30 min. *Peds.* Bolus IV dose: For total reversal of narcotic effects (smaller doses may be used if total reversal not required), as follows: *Birth–5 y* (≤ 10 kg): 0.1 mg/kg. *> 5 y* (> 20 kg): 2.0 mg. May be necessary to repeat doses frequently. Cont inf: 0.04–0.16 mg/kg/h

Nitroglycerin **Uses:** Chest pain of suspected cardiac origin; unstable angina; complications of AMI, including CHF, left ventricular failure; HTN crisis or urgency with chest pain **Supplied:** *Parenteral:* Amps: 5 mg in 10 mL, 8 mg in 10 mL, 10 mg in 10 mL, vials: 25 mg in 5 mL, 50 mg in 10 mL, 100 mg in 10 mL. *SL tabs:* 0.3 and 0.4 mg. *Aerosol spray:* 0.4 mg/dose **Dose:** *Adults.* IV 5 mcg/min, increase by 5 mcg/min every 3–5 min PRN to 20 mcg/min. Route of choice for emergencies. Use IV sets provided by manufacturer. *SL route:* 0.3–0.4 mg, repeat every 5 min. Max 3 doses. *Aerosol spray:* Spray for 0.5–1.0 s at 5-min intervals. Max 3 doses.

Nitroprusside (Sodium Nitroprusside, Nipride) **Uses:** HTN crisis, reduce afterload in CHF **Supplied:** 50-mg amp, mix in 250 mL D_5W only (keep covered with opaque material) **Dose:** 0.10 mcg/kg/min, titrate up to 5.0 mcg/kg/min. Use infusion pump; hemodynamic monitoring for optimal safety

Norepinephrine **Uses:** Severe cardiogenic shock and significant hypotension. Last resort for ischemic heart disease and shock **Supplied:** 1 mg/mL in 4-mL amp. Mix 4 mg in

21

250 mL of D_5W or D_5NS **Dose:** *Adults.* 0.5–1.0 mcg/min titrated to 30 mcg/min. *Peds.* IV inf: Initial 0.1–2 mcg/kg/min to effect. Do **not** administer with alkaline solutions.

Procainamide (Pronestyl)   Uses: Recurrent VT **Supplied:** 100 mg/mL in 10-mL vial, 500 mg/mL in 2-mL vial **Dose:** *Adults. Recurrent VF/VT:* 30 mg/min IV (max total 17 mg/kg). In urgent situations up to 50 mg/min to a total dose of 17 mg/kg. *Other indications:* 30 mg/min IV until one of the following occurs: arrhythmia suppression, hypotension, QRS widens by more than 50%, total dose of 17 mg/kg is given. *Maintenance:* 1–4 mg/min

Sodium Bicarbonate   Uses: Known preexisting hyperkalemia (Class I—usually indicated). Known preexisting bicarbonate-responsive acidosis, TCA overdose, alkalinize urine in aspirin overdose (Class IIa—accepted, possibly controversial). Prolonged resuscitation with effective ventilation, on return of spontaneous circulation after long arrest interval (Class IIb—accepted, but may not help, probably not harmful). Hypoxic lactic acidosis (eg, cardiac arrest and CPR without intubation)(Class III—harmful) **Supplied:** 50-mL syringe (8.4% sodium bicarbonate provides 50 mEq/50 mL) **Dose:** *Adults.* IV inf: 1 mEq/kg IV bolus. Repeat half this dose every 10 min thereafter. If rapidly available, use ABG analysis to guide therapy. *Peds.* 1 mEq/kg. Dose may be calculated to correct ¼–½ of base deficit.

Thrombolytic Agents (Fibrinolytic Agents):   Uses: *AMI in adults:* ST-segment elevation of 1 mm or more in at least two contiguous leads in the setting of AMI.

- Alteplase, Recombinant   **Supplied:** Vials 20, 50, and 100 mg, reconstituted with sterile water to 1 mg/mL **Dose:** *Adults.* Recommended dose based on patient's weight, not to exceed 100 mg. *AMI:* Accelerated inf: Give 15 mg bolus. Then 0.75 mg/kg over next 30 min (not to exceed 50 mg). Then 0.50 mg/kg over next 60 min (not to exceed 35 mg). 3-h infusion: 60 mg in first hour (initial 6–10 mg as a bolus). Then 20 mg/h for 2 additional hours. *Acute ischemic stroke:* 0.9 mg/kg (max 90 mg) infused over 60 min. 10% of total dose as initial IV bolus over 1 min. Give the remaining 90% over the next 60 min.
- Streptokinase   **Supplied:** Reconstitute to 1 mg/mL **Dose:** *Adults.* 1.5 million IU in a 1-h inf. PE: 3 million U ng 24 hr
- Anistreplase APSAC   **Supplied:** Reconstitute 30 U in 50 mL water or D_5W. Use two peripheral IV lines, one exclusively for thrombolytic administration. **Dose:** *Adults.* 30 IU IV over 2–5 min
- Reteplase, recombinant (Retavase)   **Supplied:** 10-U vials reconstituted with sterile water to 1 U/mL **Dose:** *Adults.* 10 U IV bolus over 2 min. 30 min later, give second 10 U IV bolus over 2 min. NS flush before and after each bolus
- Tenecteplase, variant of alteplase (TNKase)   **Supplied:** 50-mg vial in packet with 10 mL sterile water for reconstitution **Dose:** *Adults.* A single bolus given IV push over 5 s based on the patient's weight. < 60 kg = 30 mg; > 60 to < 70 kg = 35 mg; > 70 to < 80 kg = 40 mg; > 80 to < 90 kg = 45 mg; > 90 kg = 50 mg

Verapamil (Calan, Isoptin)   Uses: Second line for PSVT with narrow QRS complex and adequate BP **Supplied:** 2.5 mg/mL in 2-, 4-, and 5-mL vials (totals = 5, 10, and 12.5 mg) **Dose:** *Adults.* 2.5–5.0 mg IV over 1–2 min. Repeat 5–10 mg, if needed, in 15–30 min (30 mg max). Alternative: 5-mg bolus every 15 min to total dose of 30 mg

21   **Electrical Defibrillation and Cardioversion**

Although the defibrillator is the basic piece of equipment for both defibrillation and cardioversion, they are two distinctly different procedures. New devices include shock advisory defibrillators (AED or automated external defibrillators). The energy level is the watt-second or joule.

Standard Defibrillation Procedure (conventional device)

1. This is the primary therapy for VF or pulseless VT. Asystole is not routinely shocked.
2. Use paste or pads on skin (see step 3 for location).
3. **Shout** "Charging defibrillator—stand clear," **synchronization switch off** (if **on,** the defibrillator may not fire). In *adults,* energy levels begin at 200 J. In *children,* use 2 J/kg advance to 6 J/kg max.
4. Place paddles as directed on the handles: one at the right upper sternum and one at the left anterior axillary line (apex).
5. Apply paddles with firm pressure (approximately 25 lb).
6. Shout "I am going to shock on three. Stand clear!" and make sure no one is touching the patient or bed *including yourself.*
7. Shout "Clear," and visually check for other team members.
8. Press both paddle buttons simultaneously to fire the unit, and observe for any change in the dysrhythmia.
9. Defibrillate up to three times with increasing joules (200, > 200–300, > 360). If fails to convert, continue full output (360 J) for all future shocks. If VT recurs, shock again at last energy level.
10. If a patient is **hypothermic** (Core temperature < 30°C) shock only three times as in step 8. Resume shocks only after temperature rises above 30°C.
11. If patient has automated implantable defibrillator and device is delivering shocks, wait 60 s for cycle to complete. If defibrillation attempted, place paddles several inches from the implanted pacer unit.

Automated External Defibrillator (AED)

1. Familiarize yourself with the features of the unit in advance of using it, if possible. These computerized devices "analyze" the rhythm and shock if appropriate and are appearing in public emergency boxes such as shopping malls and airports.
2. Place the pads on the patient (upper right sternum and cardiac apex). Press the "analyze" button.
3. If appropriate (VT or VF), the unit charges and the "shock" sign is given.
4. Announce "Shock is indicated.\Stand clear," and verify that no one is touching patient. Depress "shock" button to administer shock.
5. Repeat until arrhythmia is cleared ("no shock indicated" signal will flash). In general, shock in sets of three without interposing CPR. After three shocks, do 1 min of CPR.

Cardioversion: Used for VT with a pulse, atrial arrhythmias with rapid ventricular response (PAT, AF, or atrial flutter); an attempt to slow the heart or convert rhythm. Procedure is like that for defibrillation, **except:**

1. **Consider sedation if patient is conscious.** Agents can include diazepam, midazolam with or without a narcotic such as morphine, or fentanyl. Deep sedation is also useful if you are trained and credentialed. If not, anesthesia support is helpful if readily available.
2. Start with lower energy levels than for defibrillation. Start at 100 J and increase to 200, 300, and finally 360.

21

3. **Keep the synchronizer switch on** (prevents shocking during vulnerable part of QRS complex when shock may cause VF, so-called R-on-T phenomenon). Observe for the markers on the R waves indicating that the synch mode is engaged.
4. Place paddles, apply pressure, and verify area is cleared as for the defibrillation steps.
5. Most defibrillators default back to the unsynchronized mode to allow rapid shock in case of VF. Reset synch mode if multiple cardioversions needed.

Transcutaneous Pacing

Primarily for hemodynamically unstable bradycardia. External pacemakers can be set in the asynchronous (nondemand or fixed mode) or demand mode in the range of 30–180 bpm with current outputs from 0–200 mA.

1. Place electrode pads on chest as per unit's instructions.
2. Turn unit on and set pacer to 80 bpm initially.
3. Adjust current upward until capture is achieved (ie, wide QRS after each pacer spike on ECG for bradycardia.
4. For asystole (not routinely used) begin at full output. If capture occurs, decrease to threshold and increase by 2 mA.

OTHER COMMON EMERGENCIES

Anaphylaxis

Allergic Reaction with Systolic BP < 90 mm Hg or Airway Failure

Epinephrine   Drug of choice/cornerstone of therapy **Dose: *Adults.*** IV bolus: 100 mcg of 1:100,000 over 5–10 min.(mix 0.1 mL of 1:1,000 epi in 10 mL NS). IV inf: 1–4 mcg/min. ***Peds.*** IV inf: 0.1–0.3 mcg/kg/min, max 1.5 mcg/kg/min

Allergic Reaction with Systolic BP > 90 mm Hg

- Epinephrine   **Dose:** 1:1000 SQ. ***Adults.*** 0.3–0.5 mL SQ. ***Peds.*** 0.01 mL/kg, max 0.5 mL

Supplemental drugs for anaphylaxis include:

- Diphenhydramine   **Dose: *Adults.*** IV/IM/PO 50 mg. ***Peds.*** IV/IM/PO 1 mg/kg
- Methylprednisolone   Dose: 1–2 mg/kg IV
- Ranitidine (Zantac)   **Dose: *Adults.*** IV 50 mg over 5 min. ***Peds.*** IV 0.5 mg/kg over 5 min
- Albuterol   **Dose: *Adults.*** 2.5 mg nebulized. ***Peds.*** 1.25 mg nebulized

Asthmatic Attack: Mild

Albuterol (Nebulized)   Dose: *Adults.* 2.5–5.0 mg at 20 min for up to 3 doses in first h. *Peds.* 1.25–2.5 mg at 20 min for up to 3 doses/first hour. **Supplemental oxygen to keep sats > 90%**

Asthmatic Attack: Moderate to Severe

Ipratropium Bromide (nebulized)   Dose: *Adults.* 0.5 mg combined with first albuterol treatment. *Peds.* 250 mcg with first albuterol treatment. Give treatments continuously or every 20 min for first hour.

Methylprednisolone Dose: *Adults.* 60–125 mg IV. *Peds.* 2 mg/kg IV **Supplemental oxygen to keep sats > 90%**

Asthmatic Attack: Severe

Administer aerosolized beta-agonists with anticholinergic continuously, intubate and ventilate with 100% oxygen if impending or actual respiratory arrest, IV corticosteroid

Methylprednisolone Dose: *Adults.* 60–125 mg IV. *Peds.* 2 mg/kg IV

Anticholinergic Toxicity

Usually related to drug overdose. Patients present: "Hot as Hades, Blind as a Bat, Dry as a Bone, Red as a Beet, Mad as a Hatter."

Physostigmine (**controversial**—use probably only when seizures/coma/hypotension/agitation are refractory to conventional therapy) **Dose:** 0.5–2.0 mg IV

Note: Administer S-L-O-W-L-Y (may cause seizures if given rapidly). Have cardiac monitor attached and resuscitation equipment at the bedside.

Coma

1. Establish/secure airway(protect C-spine if trauma).
2. Assess for respiratory failure and shock (ACLS).
3. Supply oxygen, IV access, cardiac monitor, and pulse oximetry.
4. Administer 1 amp (50 mL) of D_{50} IV manually; some recommend checking a stat glucose first.
5. Administer 100 mg thiamine IV.
6. Give 0.4 mg naloxone (Narcan) IV (see following section on Narcotics Overdose).
7. Obtain fingerstick glucose, SMA, CBC, urinalysis, and ABG. Consider EKG, CT head. See Shock and Seizure.

Dental Emergencies

Not including facial fractures, there are generally two major categories of dental emergencies: toothaches with associated abscesses and avulsed (knocked-out) teeth. Most toothaches may be managed with antibiotics (usually penicillin-V 500 mg, q6h) and analgesics until proper dental attention can be obtained. Fluctuant abscesses may be drained if convenient. The exception to this rule is submandibular or infraorbital swelling. With submandibular infections, Ludwig's angina may develop, a life-threatening occurrence. These patients should be held for observation with special attention to maintaining the airway until a dental consult can be obtained. Infraorbital infections can lead to a cavernous sinus thrombosis if allowed to progress.

Avulsed teeth may or may not have an associated dentoalveolar fracture. The best treatment is to reposition the displaced tooth back in the socket within 30 min or as soon as possible. If the tooth root is dirty, wash it gently with sterile saline. Do not scrub or scrape the root. Get a dental consult to arrange to have the tooth splinted back in the socket.

21

Hypercalcemia

See Chapter 9, page 184

Hyperkalemia

See Chapter 9, page 181

Hypertensive Crisis

1. Treat only if signs of end organ damage.
2. MAP should not be reduced more than 20–25% over 30–60 min.

$$MAP = [\frac{1}{3}(SBP - DBP) + DBP]$$

- Labetalol **Dose:** 20 mg IV bolus then 2 mg/min IV to target BP or
- Sodium Nitroprusside **Dose:** 0.5 mcg /kg/min ↑ to max (10 mcg/kg) min

Hypoglycemia

1. Draw a STAT serum glucose. **Do not wait for result before treating if hypoglycemia is strongly suspected. A finger Dextro stick can usually be quickly checked.**
2. Give orange juice with sugar if the patient is awake and alert; if not, give 1 amp of D_{50} IV (**Peds.** 1 mL/kg).
3. If IV access is not possible, give glucagon 1 mg IM or SC.

Opioid Overdose

Naloxone (Narcan) **Dose:** *Adults.* 0.4–2.0 mg IV or IM, repeat as needed. (*Note:* If you suspect the patient is a narcotic addict give 0.4 mg instead and repeat as needed to avoid precipitating severe withdrawal. *Peds.* 0.01–0.02 mg/kg IV or IM, repeat as needed. Observe patient for at least 6 h after treatment. Manage airway by intubation if airway failure not immediately responsive to naloxone. See Coma (page 485)

Poisonings (common agents)

1. Support airway, respiration, and circulation, as needed.
2. Determine ingested substance; give specific antidote, if available. **Call Regional Poison Center for assistance (1-800-222-1222).** Some common poisons with their antidotes (Dosages for *adults,* unless otherwise specified) can be found in Table 21–1, page 487.
3. Prevent further absorption as described if conscious/unconscious level

Unconscious Patient
- Protect airway with an endotracheal tube.
- Consider lavage with an Ewald tube or 28 Fr or larger NG tube, if ingestion occurred < 1 h.
- Use 300 mL NS boluses at a time through the NG or Ewald tube for adults and 20 mL/kg in children.
- Consider activated charcoal with sorbitol unless an oral antidote is to be given.

Conscious Patient
- Consider activated charcoal 1 g/kg, contraindicated for iron, lithium, lead, alkali, acid. Also give 70% sorbitol solution (2 mL/kg body weight). Anyone given sorbitol should be monitored for hypokalemia and hypomagnesemia.
- Attempt to promote excretion through IV hydration.
- Alkalinization (0.5–1 mEq/kg/L in IV fluids) for salicylates, barbiturates, tricyclics

21

TABLE 21–1
Antidotes for Common Poisoning Emergencies

Acetaminophen	N-acetylcysteine, 140 mg/kg PO, then 70 mg/kg × 17
Anticholinesterases	Atropine 0.5–2 mg IV; may need up to 5 mg IV every 15 min if severe poisoning
Benzodiazepines	Flumazenil 0.2 mg IV (see page 479 and 545)
Beta-blockers	Glucagon 0.05 mg/kg IV bolus for BP <90, then infusion of 75–150 mg/kg/h
Carbon monoxide	High-flow oxygen
Calcium channel blockers	Calcium chloride 10–20 mL/kg of 1% solution then 20 mg/kg/h
Cyanide	Amyl nitrate pearls inhale every 2 min then sodium nitrite 10 mL 3% IV over 3 min (0.33 mL/kg of 3% solution in children) or sodium thiosulfate 50 mL of 25% solution over 10 min or 1.65 mL/kg in children
Cyclic antidepressants	NaHCO$_3$ 3 amps (50 mg/50 mL) in 1 L D5W at 2–3 mL/kg/h
Digoxin	Digoxin-specific Fab Number of vials = Serum digoxin level × $\dfrac{\text{Patient's weight (kg)}}{100}$
Ethylene glycol	Fomepizole 15 mg/kg slow infusion
Methanol	Fomepizole (see above) or Ethanol—Loading dose 1 g/kg of a 10% solution slowly IV, followed by an infusion of 130 mg/kg/h to keep serum level of 100–150 mg/dL.
Opiates	Naloxone see page 486

Seizures/Status Epilepticus

Status epilepticus refers to 30 min or more of continuous seizure activity or two or more seizures without recovery of consciousness in between.

Initial Supportive Care
- Maintain airway with C-spine precautions.
- Deliver oxygen by nasal cannula.
- Monitor ECG and blood pressure.
- Maintain normal temperature.

Pharmacologic Therapy (Table 21–2, page 488).
- Establish IV.
- Administer thiamine 100 mg IV.
- Administer 1 amp of D$_{50}$ IV in an adult (2 mL/kg D$_{25}$ in children) unless obviously hyperglycemic.

TABLE 21-2
Drugs for the Treatment of Status Epilepticus

Drug	Pediatric Dose (mg/kg)	Adult Dose	Maximum Rate (mg/min)
Diazepam (Valium)	0.10–0.20 IV	5–10 mg IV (up to 30 mg)	3–5
Fosphenytoin	N/A	20 mg/kg IV	150
Paraldehyde[a]	0.15–0.3 mL/kg PR	30 mL PR	NA
Phenytoin (Dilantin)[b]	15 IV	Same as for child	50
Phenobarbital[c]	10 IV or IM	120–140 mg IV	100

[a]When given rectally, mix 2:1 with cottonseed or olive oil.
[b]When given IV, use a maximum dose of 50 mg/min and monitor ECG and vital signs closely. Can cause severe hypotension and bradycardia. Mix with NS to prevent precipitation.
[c]Indicated when the patient is allergic to phenytoin, patients may require intubation.

- Administer IV lorazepam or diazepam initially (midazolam 0.2 mg/kg) can be given IM in children if no IV.
- If seizures persist, give fosphenytoin or phenytoin.
- If seizures persist, administer phenobarbital, paraldehyde.
- If still no response, obtain emergency neurosurgical and anesthesiology consultation.

COMMONLY USED MEDICATIONS

INTRODUCTION

The style of drug presentation used in this section includes key elements of commonly used medications that are essential information for both the student and practicing physician. Key medication elements include generic and selected brand names, common uses, mechanism of action, adult and pediatric dosages with key dosing modifiers (elderly, renal/hepatic disease), major cautions and contraindications (pregnancy, breast-feeding, and others), and available dosing formulations along with key notes and common side effects for the medication. A unique feature is the inclusion of common uses of medications rather than just the official labeled indications. These recommendations are based on the actual uses of the medication supported by publications and community standards of care. All common uses have been reviewed by our editorial board.

It is essential that students and residents in training learn more than the name and dose of the medications they prescribe. Certain common side effects and significant contraindications are associated with most prescription medications. Although a physician or other health care practitioner should ideally be completely familiar with the entire package insert of any medication being prescribed, such a requirement is unreasonable. References such as the *Physician's Desk Reference* and, in many cases, the drug manufacturer's Web site make package inserts readily available for many medications but may not provide key data for generic drugs and those available over the counter. The limitations of difficult-to-read package inserts were acknowledged by the Food and Drug Administration in early 2001, when it noted that physicians do not have time to read the many pages of small print in the typical package insert. In the future, package inserts will be redesigned to ensure that important drug interactions, contraindications, and common side effects are highlighted for easier practitioner reference. We have made this key prescribing information available to you now in this section. Information in this section is meant for use by health care professionals who order commonly prescribed medications.

MEDICATION KEY

Medications are listed by prescribing class, and the individual medications are then listed in alphabetical order by generic name. Some of the more commonly recognized trade names are listed for each medication (in parentheses after the generic name).

Controlled Substance Classification

Medications under the control of the U.S. Drug Enforcement Agency (Schedule I–V controlled substances) are indicated by the symbol [C]. Most medications are "uncontrolled" and do not require a DEA prescriber number on the prescription. The following is a general description for the schedules of DEA controlled substances:

Schedule (CI) I: All nonresearch use forbidden (eg, heroin, LSD, mescaline, etc).

Schedule (CII) II: High addictive potential; medical use accepted. No telephone call-in prescriptions; no refills. Some states require special prescription form (eg, cocaine, morphine, methadone).

Schedule (CIII) III: Low to moderate risk of physical dependence, high risk of psychologic dependence; prescription must be rewritten after 6 months or five refills (eg, acetaminophen plus codeine).

Schedule (CIV) IV: Limited potential for dependence; prescription rules same as for schedule III (eg, benzodiazepines, propoxyphene)

Schedule (CV) V: Very limited abuse potential; prescribing regulations often same as for uncontrolled medications; some states have additional restrictions.

FDA Fetal Risk Categories

Category A: Adequate studies in pregnant women have not demonstrated a risk to the fetus in the first trimester of pregnancy; there is no evidence of risk in the last two trimesters.

Category B: Animal studies have not demonstrated a risk to the fetus, but no adequate studies have been done in pregnant women.
or
Animal studies have shown an adverse effect, but adequate studies in pregnant women have not demonstrated a risk to the fetus during the first trimester of pregnancy and there is no evidence of risk in the last two trimesters.

Category C: Animal studies have shown an adverse effect on the fetus, but no adequate studies have been done in humans. The benefits from the use of the drug in pregnant women may be acceptable despite its potential risks.
or
No animal reproduction studies and no adequate studies in humans have been done.

Category D: There is evidence of human fetal risk, but the potential benefits from the use of the drug in pregnant women may be acceptable despite its potential risks.

Category X: Studies in animals or humans or adverse reaction reports, or both, have demonstrated fetal abnormalities. The risk of use in pregnant women clearly outweighs any possible benefit.

Category ?: No data available (not a formal FDA classification; included to provide complete data set).

Breast-Feeding

No formally recognized classification exists for drugs and breast-feeding. This shorthand was developed for the *Clinician's Pocket Drug Reference.*

+	Compatible with breast-feeding
M	Monitor patient or use with caution
±	Excreted, or likely excreted, with unknown effects or at unknown concentrations
?/–	Unknown excretion, but effects likely to be of concern
–	Contraindicated in breast-feeding
?	No data available

Generic Drug Name (Selected Common Brand Names [Controlled Substance])

WARNING: Summary of the "Black Box" precautions that are deemed necessary by the FDA. These are significant precautions and contraindications concerning the individual medication. **Uses:** This includes both FDA labeled indications and other "off label" uses of the medication. Because many medications are used to treat various conditions based on the medical literature and not listed in their package insert, we list common uses of the medication rather than the official "labeled indications" (FDA approved) based on input from our editorial board **Action:** How the drug works. This information is helpful in comparing classes of drugs and understanding side effects and contraindications **Dose:** *Adults.* Where no specific pediatric dose is given, the implication is that this drug is not commonly used or indicated in that age group. At the end of the dosing line, important dosing modifications may be noted (ie, take with food, avoid antacids, etc) **Caution/Contra:** [pregnancy/fetal risk categories, breast-feeding] Other common contraindications or cautions **Supplied:** Common dosing forms **Notes/SE:** Lists other key information about the drug as well as the more common or significant side effects.

CLASSIFICATION (GENERIC AND COMMON BRAND NAMES)

Allergy

Antihistamines

Cetirizine (Zyrtec)
Chlorpheniramine (Chlor-Trimeton)
Clemastine fumarate (Tavist)

Cyproheptadine (Periactin)
Desloratadine (Clarinex)
Diphenhydramine (Benadryl)
Fexofenadine (Allegra)

Hydroxyzine (Atarax, Vistaril)
Loratadine (Claritin)

Miscellaneous Antiallergenic Agents

Budesonide (Pulmicort)
Cromolyn (Cromolyn sodium)

Montelukast (Singulair)

Antidotes

Acetylcysteine (Mucomyst)
Amifostine (Ethyol)
Charcoal (Activated Charcoal, Actidose-Aqua, CharcoAid, Charcodote)

Dexrazoxane (Zinecard)
Digoxin Immune FAB (Digibind)
Flumazenil (Romazicon)
Ipecac Syrup (OTC Syrup)

Mesna (Mesnex)
Naloxone (Narcan)
Physostigmine (Antilirium, Isopto, Eserine)
Succimer (Chemet)

Antimicrobial Agents

Antibiotics

Aminoglycosides

Amikacin (Amikin)
Gentamicin (Garamycin)
Neomycin (Mycifradin)

Streptomycin (Streptomycin sulfate)
Tobramycin (Nebcin)

22

Carbapenems

Ertapenem (Invanz)
Imipenem-Cilastatin
  (Primaxin)

Meropenem (Merrem)

Cephalosporins, First Generation

Cefadroxil (Duricef)
Cefazolin (Ancef, Kefzol)

Cephalexin (Keflex, Keftab)
Cephalothin (Keflin)

Cephradine (Velosef)

Cephalosporins, Second Generation

Cefaclor (Ceclor)
Cefmetazole (Zefazone)
Cefonicid (Monocid)

Cefotetan (Cefotan)
Cefoxitin (Mefoxin)
Cefprozil (Cefzil)

Cefuroxime (Ceftin [oral],
  Zinacef [parenteral])
Loracarbef (Lorabid)

Cephalosporins, Third Generation

Cefdinir (Omnicef)
Cefditoren (Spectracef)
Cefixime (Suprax)
Cefoperazone (Cefobid)

Cefotaxime (Claforan)
Cefpodoxime (Vantin)
Ceftazidime (Fortaz, Ceptaz,
  Tazidime, Tazicef)

Ceftizoxime (Cefizox)
Ceftriaxone (Rocephin)

Cephalosporins, Fourth Generation

Cefepime (Maxipime)

Fluoroquinolones

Ciprofloxacin (Cipro)
Gatifloxacin (Tequin)
Levofloxacin (Levaquin)

Lomefloxacin (Maxaquin)
Moxifloxacin (Avelox)
Norfloxacin (Noroxin)

Ofloxacin (Floxin, Ocuflox
  Ophthalmic)
Sparfloxacin (Zagam)

Macrolides

Azithromycin (Zithromax)
Clarithromycin (Biaxin)
Dirithromycin (Dynabac)

Erythromycin (E-Mycin,
  Ilosone, Erythrocin)

Erythromycin and Sulfisoxazole (Eryzole, Pediazole)

Penicillins

Amoxicillin (Amoxil,
  Polymox)
Amoxicillin-Clavulanate
  (Augmentin)
Ampicillin (Amcill,
  Omnipen)
Ampicillin-Sulbactam
  (Unasyn)
Dicloxacillin (Dynapen,
  Dycill)

Mezlocillin (Mezlin)
Nafcillin (Nallpen)
Oxacillin (Bactocill,
  Prostaphlin)
Penicillin G Aqueous
  (potassium or sodium)
  (Pfizerpen, Pentids)
Penicillin G Benzathine
  (Bicillin)

Penicillin G Procaine
  (Wycillin)
Penicillin V (Pen-Vee K,
  Veetids)
Piperacillin (Pipracil)
Piperacillin-Tazobactam
  (Zosyn)
Ticarcillin (Ticar)
Ticarcillin-Clavulanate
  (Timentin)

Tetracyclines

Doxycycline (Vibramycin)
Tetracycline (Achromycin
  V, Sumycin)

Miscellaneous Antibacterial Agents

Aztreonam (Azactam)
Clindamycin (Cleocin,
  Cleocin-T)
Fosfomycin (Monurol)
Linezolid (Zyvox)

Metronidazole (Flagyl,
  MetroGel)
Quinupristin-Dalfopristin
  (Synercid)

Trimethoprim-Sulfamethox-
  azole [Co-trimoxazole]
  (Bactrim, Septra)
Vancomycin (Vancocin,
  Vancoled)

22

Antifungals

Amphotericin B (Fungizone)
Amphotericin B Cholesteryl (Amphotec)
Amphotericin B Lipid Complex (Abelcet)
Amphotericin B Liposomal (AmBisome)

Caspofungin (Cancidas)
Clotrimazole (Lotrimin, Mycelex)
Clotrimazole and Betamethasone (Lotrisone)
Econazole (Spectazole)
Fluconazole (Diflucan)
Itraconazole (Sporanox)

Ketoconazole (Nizoral)
Miconazole (Monistat)
Nystatin (Mycostatin)
Oxiconazole (Oxistat)
Terbinafine (Lamisil)
Triamcinolone and Nystatin (Mycolog-II)
Voriconazole (VFEND)

Antimycobacterials

Clofazimine (Lamprene)
Dapsone (Avlosulfon)
Ethambutol (Myambutol)

Isoniazid (INH)
Pyrazinamide)
Rifabutin (Mycobutin)

Rifampin (Rifadin)
Rifapentine (Priftin)
Streptomycin

Antiprotozoals

Nitazoxanide (Alinia)

Antiretrovirals

Abacavir (Ziagen)
Amprenavir (Agenerase)
Delavirdine (Rescriptor)
Didanosine [ddI] (Videx)
Efavirenz (Sustiva)
Indinavir (Crixivan)

Lamivudine (Epivir, Epivir-HBV)
Lopinavir/Ritonavir (Kaletra)
Nelfinavir (Viracept)
Nevirapine (Viramune)
Ritonavir (Norvir)
Saquinavir (Fortovase)

Stavudine (Zerit)
Tenofovir (Viread)
Zalcitabine (Hivid)
Zidovudine (Retrovir)
Zidovudine and Lamivudine (Combivir)

Antivirals

Acyclovir (Zovirax)
Adefovir (Hepsera)
Amantadine (Symmetrel)
Cidofovir (Vistide)
Famciclovir (Famvir)
Foscarnet (Foscavir)
Ganciclovir (Cytovene, Vitrasert)

Interferon Alfa-2b and Ribavirin Combination (Rebetron)
Oseltamivir (Tamiflu)
Palivizumab (Synagis)
Peg interferon alfa 2 a (Pegasys)
Penciclovir (Denavir)

Ribavirin (Virazole)
Rimantadine (Flumadine)
Valacyclovir (Valtrex)
Valganciclovir (Valcyte)
Zanamivir (Relenza)

Miscellaneous Antimicrobial Agents

Atovaquone (Mepron)
Atovaquone/Proguanil (Malarone)

Pentamidine (Pentam 300, NebuPent)

Trimetrexate (Neutrexin)

Antineoplastic Agents

Alkylating Agents

Altretamine (Hexalen)
Busulfan (Myleran)
Carboplatin (Paraplatin)

Cisplatin (Platinol AQ)
Procarbazine (Matulane)

Triethylenetriphosphamide (Thio-Tepa, TESPA, TSPA)

Nitrogen Mustards

Chlorambucil (Leukeran)
Cyclophosphamide (Cytoxan, Neosar)

Ifosfamide (Ifex, Holoxan)
Mechlorethamine (Mustargen)

Melphalan [l-PAM] (Alkeran)

Nitrosoureas

Carmustine [BCNU] (BiCNU)

Streptozocin (Zanosar)

22

Antibiotics

Bleomycin sulfate (Blenoxane)
Dactinomycin (Cosmegen)
Daunorubicin (Dauno-mycin, Cerubidine)
Doxorubicin (Adriamycin, Rubex)
Idarubicin (Idamycin)
Mitomycin (Mutamycin)
Pentostatin (Nipent)
Plicamycin (Mithracin)

Antimetabolites

Cytarabine [ARA-C] (Cytosar-U)
Cytarabine Liposomal (DepoCyt)
Floxuridine (FUDR)
Fludarabine (Fludara)
Fluorouracil [5-FU] (Adrucil)
Gemcitabine (Gemzar)
Mercaptopurine [6-MP] (Purinethol)
Methotrexate (Folex, Rheumatrex)
6-Thioguanine (Tabloid)

Hormones

Anastrozole (Arimidex)
Bicalutamide (Casodex)
Estramustine phosphate (Estracyt, Emcyt)
Fluoxymesterone (Halotestin)
Flutamide (Eulexin)
Fulvestrant (Faslodex)
Goserelin (Zoladex)
Leuprolide acetate (Lupron, Viadur)
Levamisole (Ergamisol)
Megestrol acetate (Megace)
Nilutamide (Nilandron)
Tamoxifen acetate (Nolvadex)
Triptorelin (Trelstar Depot, Trelstar LA)

Mitotic Inhibitors

Etoposide [VP-16] (VePesid)
Vinblastine (Velban, Velbe)
Vincristine (Oncovin, Vin-casar PFS)
Vinorelbine(Navelbine)

Miscellaneous

Aldesleukin [Interleukin-2, IL-2] (Proleukin)
Aminoglutethimide (Cytadren)
L-Asparaginase (Elspar, Oncaspar)
BCG (TheraCys, Tice BCG)
Cladribine (Leustatin)
Dacarbazine (DTIC)
Docetaxel (Taxotere)
Hydroxyurea (Hydrea, Droxia)
Imatinib mesylate (Gleevec)
Irinotecan (Camptosar)
Letrozole (Femara)
Mitotane (Lysodren)
Mitoxantrone (Novantrone)
Paclitaxel (Taxol)
Pentostatin (Nipent)
Rasburicase (Elitek)
Topotecan (Hycamtin)
Tretinoin [Retinoic acid] (Vesanoid)

Cardiovascular Agents

Aldosterone Antagonist

Eplerenone (Inspra)

Alpha₁-Adrenergic Blockers

Doxazosin (Cardura)
Prazosin (Minipress)
Terazosin (Hytrin)

Angiotensin-Converting Enzyme Inhibitors

Benazepril (Lotensin)
Captopril (Capoten)
Enalapril and Enalaprilat (Vasotec)
Fosinopril (Monopril)
Lisinopril (Prinivil, Zestril)
Moexipril (Univasc)
Perindopril (Aceon)
Quinapril (Accupril)
Ramipril (Altace)
Trandolapril (Mavik)

Angiotensin II Receptor Antagonists

Candesartan (Atacand)
Eprosartan (Teveten)
Irbesartan (Avapro)
Losartan (Cozaar)
Olmesartan (Benicar)
Telmisartan (Micardis)
Valsartan (Diovan)

22

Antiarrhythmic Agents

Adenosine (Adenocard)
Amiodarone (Cordarone, Pacerone)
Atropine
Digoxin (Lanoxin, Lanoxicaps)
Disopyramide (Norpace, NAPAmide)

Dofetilide (Tikosyn)
Esmolol (Brevibloc)
Flecainide (Tambocor)
Ibutilide (Corvert)
Lidocaine (Anestacon Topical, Xylocaine)
Methoxamine (Vasoxyl)
Mexiletine (Mexitil)

Moricizine (Ethmozine)
Procainamide (Pronestyl, Procan)
Propafenone (Rythmol)
Quinidine
Sotalol (Betapace, Betapace AF)
Tocainide (Tonocard)

Beta-Adrenergic Blockers

Acebutolol (Sectral)
Atenolol (Tenormin)
Atenolol and Chlorthalidone (Tenoretic)
Betaxolol (Kerlone)
Bisoprolol (Zebeta)

Carteolol (Cartrol, Ocupress Ophthalmic)
Carvedilol (Coreg)
Labetalol (Trandate, Normodyne)
Metoprolol (Lopressor, Toprol XL)

Nadolol (Corgard)
Penbutolol (Levatol)
Pindolol (Visken)
Propranolol (Inderal)
Timolol (Blocadren)

Calcium Channel Antagonists

Amlodipine (Norvasc)
Bepridil (Vascor)
Diltiazem (Cardizem, Dilacor, Tiazac)
Felodipine (Plendil)

Isradipine (DynaCirc)
Nicardipine (Cardene)
Nifedipine (Procardia, Procardia XL, Adalat, Adalat CC)

Nimodipine (Nimotop)
Nisoldipine (Sular)
Verapamil (Calan, Isoptin)

Centrally Acting Antihypertensive Agents

Clonidine (Catapres)

Methyldopa (Aldomet)

Diuretics

Acetazolamide (Diamox)
Amiloride (Midamor)
Bumetanide (Bumex)
Chlorothiazide (Diuril)
Chlorthalidone (Hygroton)
Furosemide (Lasix)
Hydrochlorothiazide (HydroDIURIL, Esidrix)

Hydrochlorothiazide and Amiloride (Moduretic)
Hydrochlorothiazide and Spironolactone (Aldactazide)
Hydrochlorothiazide and Triamterene (Dyazide, Maxzide)

Indapamide (Lozol)
Mannitol
Metolazone (Zaroxolyn)
Spironolactone (Aldactone)
Torsemide (Demadex)
Triamterene (Dyrenium)

Inotropic/Pressor Agents

Amrinone (Inocor)
Digoxin (Lanoxin, Lanoxicaps)
Dobutamine (Dobutrex)
Dopamine (Intropin)

Epinephrine (Adrenalin, Sus-Phrine)
Isoproterenol (Isuprel, Medihaler-Iso)
Methoxamine (Vasoxyl)

Milrinone (Primacor)
Nesiritide (Natrecor)
Norepinephrine (Levophed)
Phenylephrine (Neo-Synephrine)

Lipid-Lowering Agents

Atorvastatin (Lipitor)
Cholestyramine (Questran)
Colesevelam (Welchol)
Colestipol (Colestid)

Ezitimibe (Zetia)
Fenofibrate (Tricor)
Fluvastatin (Lescol)
Gemfibrozil (Lopid)

Lovastatin (Mevacor)
Niacin (Nicolar)
Pravastatin (Pravachol)
Simvastatin (Zocor)

Vasodilators

Alprostadil [Prostaglandin E_1] (Prostin VR)
Epoprostenol (Flolan)
Fenoldopam (Corlopam)
Hydralazine (Apresoline)
Isosorbide Dinitrate (Isordil, Sorbitrate)

Isosorbide Mononitrate (Ismo, Imdur)
Minoxidil (Loniten, Rogaine)
Nitroglycerin (Nitrostat, Nitrolingual, Nitro-Bid Ointment, Nitro-Bid IV, Nitrodisc, Transderm-Nitro)

Nitroprusside (Nipride, Nitropress)
Tolazoline (Priscoline)
Treprostinil sodium (Remodulin)

22

Central Nervous System Agents

Antianxiety Agents

Alprazolam (Xanax)
Buspirone (BuSpar)
Chlordiazepoxide (Librium)
Clorazepate (Tranxene)
Diazepam (Valium)

Doxepin (Sinequan, Adapin)
Hydroxyzine (Atarax, Vistaril)
Lorazepam (Ativan, others)

Meprobamate (Equanil, Miltown)
Oxazepam (Serax)

Anticonvulsants

Carbamazepine (Tegretol)
Clonazepam (Klonopin)
Diazepam (Valium)
Ethosuximide (Zarontin)
Fosphenytoin (Cerebyx)
Gabapentin (Neurontin)

Lamotrigine (Lamictal)
Levetiracetam (Keppra)
Lorazepam (Ativan, others)
Oxcarbazepine (Trileptal)
Pentobarbital (Nembutal)
Phenobarbital

Phenytoin (Dilantin)
Tiagabine (Gabitril)
Topiramate (Topamax)
Valproic acid (Depakene, Depakote)
Zonisamide (Zonegran)

Antidepressants

Amitriptyline (Elavil)
Bupropion (Wellbutrin, Zyban)
Citalopram (Celexa)
Desipramine (Norpramin)
Doxepin (Sinequan, Adapin)
Escitalopram (Lexapro)

Fluoxetine (Prozac, Sarafem)
Fluvoxamine (Luvox)
Imipramine (Tofranil)
Maprotiline (Ludiomil)
Mirtazapine (Remeron)
Nefazodone (Serzone)

Nortriptyline (Aventyl, Pamelor)
Paroxetine (Paxil)
Phenelzine (Nardil)
Sertraline (Zoloft)
Trazodone (Desyrel)
Trimipramine (Surmontil)
Venlafaxine (Effexor)

Antiparkinson Agents

Amantadine (Symmetrel)
Benztropine (Cogentin)
Bromocriptine (Parlodel)
Carbidopa/Levodopa (Sinemet)

Entacapone (Comtan)
Pergolide (Permax)
Pramipexole (Mirapex)
Procyclidine (Kemadrin)

Selegiline (Eldepryl)
Trihexyphenidyl (Artane)

Antipsychotics

Aripiprazole (Abilify)
Chlorpromazine (Thorazine)
Clozapine (Clozaril)
Fluphenazine (Prolixin, Permitil)
Haloperidol (Haldol)
Lithium carbonate (Eskalith)

Mesoridazine (Serentil)
Molindone (Moban)
Olanzapine (Zyprexa)
Perphenazine (Trilafon)
Prochlorperazine (Compazine)

Quetiapine (Seroquel)
Risperidone (Risperdal)
Thioridazine (Mellaril)
Thiothixene (Navane)
Trifluoperazine (Stelazine)
Ziprasidone (Geodon)

Sedative Hypnotics

Chloral hydrate
Diphenhydramine (Benadryl)
Estazolam (ProSom)
Flurazepam (Dalmane)
Hydroxyzine (Atarax, Vistaril)

Midazolam (Versed)
Pentobarbital (Nembutal)
Phenobarbital
Propofol (Diprivan)
Quazepam (Doral)
Secobarbital (Seconal)

Temazepam (Restoril)
Triazolam (Halcion)
Zaleplon (Sonata)
Zolpidem (Ambien)

Miscellaneous CNS Agents

Atomoxetine (Strattera)
Galantamine (Reminyl)

Nimodipine (Nimotop)
Rivastigmine (Exelon)

Sodium oxybate (Xyrem)
Tacrine (Cognex)

Dermatologic Agents

Acitretin (Soriatane)
Acyclovir (Zovirax)
Anthralin (Anthra-Derm)

Amphotericin B (Fungizone)
Bacitracin (Baci-IM)

Bacitracin, Topical (Baciguent)
Bacitracin and Polymyxin

B, Topical (Polysporin)
Bacitracin, Neomycin and Polymyxin B, Topical (Neosporin Ointment)
Bacitracin, Neomycin, Polymyxin B and Hydrocortisone, Topical (Cortisporin)
Bacitracin, Neomycin, Polymyxin B and Lidocaine, Topical (Clomycin)
Calcipotriene (Dovonex)
Capsaicin (Capsin, Zostrix)
Ciclopirox (Loprox)
Ciprofloxacin (Cipro)
Clindamycin, Topical (Cleocin-T)
Clotrimazole and Betamethasone (Lotrisone)
Dibucaine (Nupercainal)
Doxepin, Topical (Zonalon)
Econazole (Spectazole)
Erythromycin, Topical
Gentamicin, Topical
Haloprogin (Halotex)
Imiquimod (Aldara)
Isotretinoin [13-*cis* Retinoic acid] (Accutane)
Ketoconazole (Nizoral)
Lactic Acid and Ammonium Hydroxide (Lac-Hydrin)
Lindane (Kwell)
Metronidazole (MetroGel)
Miconazole (Monistat)
Minoxidil (Loniten, Rogaine)
Mupirocin (Bactroban)
Naftifine (Naftin)
Nystatin (Mycostatin, Nilstat)
Nystatin and Triamcinolone
Oxiconazole (Oxistat)
Penciclovir (Denavir)
Permethrin (Nix, Elimite)
Pimecrolimus (Elidel)
Pramoxine (Anusol Ointment, Proctofoam-NS)
Pramoxine and Hydrocortisone (Enzone, Proctofoam-HC)
Podophyllin (Podocon-25, Condylox Gel 0.5%, Condylox)
Tretinoin, Topical [Retinoic Acid] (Retin-A, Avita)
Selenium Sulfide (Exsel Shampoo, Selsun Blue Shampoo, Selsun Shampoo)
Silver Sulfadiazine (Silvadene)
Steroids, Topical (Table 5, page 612)
Tacrolimus (Prograf)
Tazarotene (Tazorac)
Terbinafine (Lamisil)
Tolnaftate (Tinactin)
Witch Hazel

Dietary Supplements

Calcium acetate (Calphron, Phos-Ex, PhosLo)
Calcium Glubionate (Neo-Calglucon [OTC])
Calcium Gluceptate
Calcium salts [calcium chloride and gluconate]
Cholecalciferol [Vitamin D_3] (Delta D)
Cyanocobalamin [Vitamin B_{12}]
Ferric gluconate Complex (Ferrlecit)
Ferrous gluconate (Fergon)
Ferrous sulfate
Folic acid
Iron Dextran (DexFerrum, InFeD)
Leucovorin (Wellcovorin)
Magnesium Oxide (Mag-Ox 400)
Magnesium sulfate
Phytonadione [Vitamin K] (Aqua-MEPHYTON)
Potassium Supplements (Kaon, Kaochlor, K-Lor, Slow-K, Micro-K, Klorvess)
Pyridoxine [Vitamin B_6]
Sodium bicarbonate [Bicarbonate]
Thiamine [Vitamin B_1]

Ear (Otic) Agents

Acetic acid and Aluminum acetate (Otic Domeboro)
Benzocaine and Antipyrine (Auralgan)
Ciprofloxacin and Hydrocortisone (Cipro HC Otic)
Neomycin, Colistin and Hydrocortisone (Cortisporin-TC Otic Drops)
Neomycin, Colistin, Hydrocortisone and Thonzonium (Cortisporin-TC Otic Suspension)
Neomycin, Polymyxin and Hydrocortisone (Cortisporin Ophthalmic and Otic)
Polymyxin B and Hydrocortisone(Otobiotic Otic)
Sulfacetamide and Prednisolone (Blephamide)
Triethanolamine (Cerumenex)

Endocrine System Agents

Antidiabetic Agents

Acarbose (Precose)
Chlorpropamide (Diabinese)
Glimepiride (Amaryl)
Glipizide (Glucotrol)
Glyburide (DiaBeta, Micronase)
Glyburide/Metformin (Glucovance)
Insulins (Table 6, page 616)
Metformin (Glucophage)
Miglitol (Glyset)
Nateglinide (Starlix)
Pioglitazone (Actos)
Repaglinide (Prandin)
Rosiglitazone (Avandia)
Tolazamide (Tolinase)
Tolbutamide (Orinase)

Hormone and Synthetic Substitutes

Calcitonin (Cibacalcin, Miacalcin)
Calcitriol (Rocaltrol)
Cortisone
Desmopressin (DDAVP, Stimate)

22

Dexamethasone (Decadron)
Fludrocortisone acetate (Florinef)
Glucagon
Hydrocortisone (Cortef, Solu-Cortef)
Methylprednisolone (Solu-Medrol)
Metyrapone (Metopirone)
Prednisolone (Delta-Cortef, others)
Prednisone (Deltasone, others)
Vasopressin (Pitressin)

Hypercalcemia Agents

Etidronate (Didronel)
Gallium nitrate (Ganite)
Pamidronate (Aredia)
Plicamycin (Mithracin)
Zoledronic acid (Zometa)

Obesity

Sibutramine (Meridia)

Osteoporosis Agents

Alendronate (Fosamax)
Raloxifene (Evista)
Risedronate (Actonel)
Teriparatide (Forteo)
Zoledronic acid (Zometa)

Thyroid/Antithyroid

Levothyroxine (Synthroid)
Liothyronine (Cytomel)
Methimazole (Tapazole)
Potassium iodide (SSKI)
Propylthiouracil [PTU]

Miscellaneous Endocrine Agents

Demeclocycline (Declomycin)
Diazoxide (Hyperstat, Proglycem)
Metyrosine (Demser)

Eye (Ophthalmic) Agents

Glaucoma Agents

Acetazolamide (Diamox)
Apraclonidine (Iopidine)
Betaxolol (Kerlone)
Brimonidine (Alphagan)
Brinzolamide (Azopt)
Carteolol (Cartrol, Ocupress Ophthalmic)
Dipivefrin (Propine)
Dorzolamide (Trusopt)
Dorzolamide and Timolol (Cosopt)
Echothiophate Iodine (Phospholine Ophthalmic)
Latanoprost (Xalatan)
Levobunolol (A-K Beta, Betagan)
Levocabastine (Livostin)
Lodoxamide (Alomide Ophthalmic)
Timolol (Blocadren)

Ophthalmic Antibiotics

Bacitracin (AK-Tracin Ophthalmic)
Bacitracin and Polymyxin B (AK-Poly-Bac Ophthalmic, Polysporin Ophthalmic)
Bacitracin, Neomycin and Polymyxin B (AK Spore Ophthalmic, Neosporin Ophthalmic)
Bacitracin, Neomycin, Polymyxin B and Hydrocortisone (AK Spore HC Ophthalmic, Cortisporin Ophthalmic)
Ciprofloxacin (Ciloxan)
Erythromycin (Ilotycin Ophthalmic)
Gentamicin (Garamycin, Genoptic, Gentacidin, Gentak)
Neomycin and Dexamethasone (AK-Neo-Dex Ophthalmic, NeoDecadron Ophthalmic)
Neomycin, Polymyxin-B and Dexamethasone (Maxitrol)
Neomycin, Polymyxin-B and Prednisolone (Poly-Pred Ophthalmic)
Ofloxacin (Ocuflox Ophthalmic)
Silver Nitrate (Dey-Drop)
Sulfacetamide (Bleph-10, Cetamide, Sodium Sulamyd)
Sulfacetamide and Prednisolone (Blephamide)
Tobramycin (AKTob, Tobrex)
Tobramycin and Dexamethasone (TobraDex)
Trifluridine (Viroptic)

Other Ophthalmic Agents

Artificial Tears (Tears Naturale)
Cromolyn (Opticrom)
Cyclopentolate (Cyclogyl)
Dexamethasone, Ophthalmic (AK-Dex Ophthalmic, Decadron Ophthalmic)
Emedastine (Emadine)
Ketorolac (Acular)
Ketotifen (Zaditor)
Lodoxamide (Alomide)

Naphazoline and Antazoline (Albalon-A Ophthalmic)

Naphazoline and Pheniramine (Naphcon A)

Olopatadine (Patanol)

Gastrointestinal Agents

Antacids

Alginic acid (Gaviscon)
Aluminum carbonate (Basaljel)
Aluminum hydroxide (Amphojel, AlternaGEL)
Aluminum hydroxide with Magnesium carbonate (Gaviscon)

Aluminum hydroxide with Magnesium hydroxide (Maalox)
Aluminum hydroxide with Magnesium hydroxide and Simethicone (Mylanta, Mylanta II, Maalox Plus)

Aluminum hydroxide with Magnesium Trisilicate (Gaviscon, Gaviscon-2)
Calcium carbonate (Tums, Alka-Mints)
Magaldrate (Riopan, Lowsium)
Simethicone (Mylicon)

Antidiarrheals

Bismuth Subsalicylate (Pepto-Bismol)
Diphenoxylate with Atropine (Lomotil)

Kaolin/Pectin (Kaodene, Kao-Spen, Kapectolin, Parepectolin)
Lactobacillus (Lactinex Granules)

Loperamide (Imodium)
Octreotide (Sandostatin, Sandostatin LAR)
Paregoric [Camphorated Tincture of Opium]

Antiemetics

Chlorpromazine (Thorazine)
Dimenhydrinate (Dramamine, others)
Dolasetron (Anzemet)
Dronabinol (Marinol)
Droperidol (Inapsine)

Granisetron (Kytril)
Meclizine (Antivert)
Metoclopramide (Reglan, Octamide)
Ondansetron (Zofran)
Prochlorperazine (Compazine)

Promethazine (Phenergan)
Scopolamine (Transderm-Scop)
Thiethylperazine (Torecan)
Trimethobenzamide (Tigan)

Antiulcer Agents

Cimetidine (Tagamet)
Esomeprazole (Nexium)
Famotidine (Pepcid)
Lansoprazole (Prevacid)

Nizatidine (Axid)
Omeprazole (Prilosec)
Pantoprazole (Protonix)
Rabeprazole (Aciphex)

Ranitidine (Zantac)
Sucralfate (Carafate)

Cathartics/Laxatives

Bisacodyl (Dulcolax)
Docusate calcium (Surfak)
Docusate potassium (Dialose)
Docusate sodium (Doss, Colace)
Glycerin Suppositories

Lactulose (Chronulac, Cephulac)
Magnesium citrate
Magnesium hydroxide (Milk of Magnesia)
Mineral Oil

Polyethylene Glycol-Electrolyte Solution (GoLYTELY, CoLyte)
Psyllium (Metamucil, Serutan, Effer-Syllium)
Sorbitol

Enzymes

Pancreatin (Creon)
Pancrelipase [Lipase, Protease, Amylase] (Pancrease, others)

Miscellaneous GI Agents

Alosetron (Lotronex)
Balsalazide (Colazal)
Dexpanthenol (Ilopan-Choline Oral, Ilopan)
Dibucaine (Nupercainal)
Dicyclomine (Bentyl)

Hydrocortisone, Rectal (Anusol-HC Suppository, Cortifoam Rectal, Proctocort)
Hyoscyamine (Anaspaz, Cystospaz, Levsin)

Hyoscyamine, Atropine, Scopolamine and Phenobarbital (Donnatal)
Infliximab (Remicade)
Mesalamine (Rowasa, Asacol, Pentasa)

22

Metoclopramide (Reglan, Clopra, Octamide)
Misoprostol (Cytotec)
Olsalazine (Dipentum)
Pramoxine (Anusol Ointment, Proctofoam-NS)
Pramoxine with Hydrocortisone (Enzone, Proctofoam-HC)
Propantheline (Pro-Banthine)
Sulfasalazine (Azulfidine)
Tegaserod maleate (Zelnorm)
Vasopressin (Pitressin)

Hematologic Agents

Anticoagulants

Ardeparin (Normiflo)
Argatroban (Acova)
Bivalirudin (Angiomax)
Dalteparin (Fragmin)
Enoxaparin (Lovenox)
Fondaparinux (Arixtra)
Heparin
Lepirudin (Refludan)
Protamine
Tinzaparin (Innohep)
Warfarin (Coumadin)

Antiplatelet Agents

Abciximab (ReoPro)
Aspirin (Bayer, St. Joseph)
Clopidogrel (Plavix)
Dipyridamole (Persantine)
Dipyridamole and Aspirin (Aggrenox)
Eptifibatide (Integrilin)
Reteplase (Retavase)
Ticlopidine (Ticlid)
Tirofiban (Aggrastat)

Antithrombotic Agents

Alteplase, Recombinant [TPA] (Activase)
Aminocaproic acid (Amicar)
Anistreplase (Eminase)
Aprotinin (Trasylol)
Dextran 40 (Rheomacrodex)
Reteplase (Retavase)
Streptokinase (Streptase, Kabikinase)
Tenecteplase (TNKase)
Urokinase (Abbokinase)

Hematopoietic Stimulants

Epoetin Alfa [Erythropoietin, EPO] (Epogen, Procrit)
Darbepoetin alfa (Aranesp)
Filgrastim [G-CSF] (Neupogen)
Oprelvekin (Neumega)
Pegfilgrastim (Neulasta)
Sargramostim [GM-CSF] (Prokine, Leukine)

Volume Expanders

Albumin (Albuminar, Buminate, Albutein)
Dextran 40 (Rheomacrodex)
Hetastarch (Hespan)
Plasma Protein Fraction (Plasmanate)

Miscellaneous Hematologic Agents

Antihemophilic Factor VIII (Monoclate)
Desmopressin (DDAVP, Stimate)
Pentoxifylline (Trental)

Immune System Agents

Immunomodulators

Anakinra (Kineret)
Etanercept (Enbrel)
Interferon Alfa (Roferon-A, Intron A)
Interferon Alfacon-1 (Infergen)
Interferon Beta-1b (Betaseron)
Interferon Gamma-1b (Actimmune)
Peg interferon alfa 2b (PEG-Intron)

Immunosuppressive Agents

Azathioprine (Imuran)
Basiliximab (Simulect)
Cyclosporine (Sandimmune, Neoral)
Daclizumab (Zenapax)
Lymphocyte Immune Globulin [Antithymocyte Globulin, ATG] (Atgam)
Muromonab-CD3 (Orthoclone OKT3)
Mycophenolate Mofetil (CellCept)
Sirolimus (Rapamune)
Steroids, Systemic (Table 4, page 612)
Tacrolimus (Prograf, Protopic)

Vaccines/Serums/Toxoids

CMV Immune Globulin [CMV-IG IV](CytoGam)

Diphtheria and Tetanus Toxoids

Diphtheria, Tetanus Toxoids, and Acellular Pertussis Adsorbed

Diphtheria, Tetanus Toxoids, and Acellular Pertussis Adsorbed, Hepatitis B (recombinant), and Inactivated Poliovirus Vaccine (IPV) Combined (Pediarix)

Haemophilus B Conjugate Vaccine (ActHIB, HibTITER, PedvaxHIB, Prohibit, Comvax)

Hepatitis A Vaccine (Havrix, Vaqta)

Hepatitis A (inactivated) and Hepatitis B Recombinant Vaccine (Twinrix)

Hepatitis B Immune Globulin (HyperHep, H-BIG)

Hepatitis B Vaccine (Engerix-B, Recombivax HB)

Immune Globulin, Intravenous (Gamimune N, Sandoglobulin, Gammar IV)

Influenza (Fluzone, FluShield, Fluvirin)

Meningococcal Polysaccharide Vaccine (Menomune)

Pneumococcal Vaccine, Polyvalent (Pneumovax-23)

Pneumococcal 7-Valent Conjugate (Prevnar)

Tetanus Immune Globulin

Tetanus Toxoid

Varicella Virus Vaccine (Varivax)

Musculoskeletal Agents

Antigout Agents

Allopurinol (Zyloprim, Lopurin, Alloprim)

Colchicine

Probenecid (Benemid)

Sulfinpyrazone (Anturane)

Muscle Relaxants

Baclofen (Lioresal)

Carisoprodol (Soma)

Chlorzoxazone (Paraflex, Parafon Forte DSC)

Cyclobenzaprine (Flexeril)

Dantrolene (Dantrium)

Diazepam (Valium)

Metaxalone (Skelaxin)

Methocarbamol (Robaxin)

Orphenadrine (Norflex)

Neuromuscular Blockers

Atracurium (Tracrium)

Mivacurium (Mivacron)

Pancuronium (Pavulon)

Pipecuronium (Arduan)

Succinylcholine (Anectine, Quelicin, Sucostrin)

Vecuronium (Norcuron)

Miscellaneous Musculoskeletal Agents

Edrophonium (Tensilon)

Leflunomide (Arava)

Methotrexate (Folex, Rheumatrex)

OB/GYN Agents

Contraceptives

Estradiol Cypionate and Medroxyprogesterone acetate (Lunelle)

Etonogestrel/Ethinyl Estradiol (NuvaRing)

Levonorgestrel Implants (Norplant)

Medroxyprogesterone (Provera, Depo-Provera)

Norgestrel (Ovrette)

Norelgestromin and Ethinyl Estradiol, Ortho Evra (Ortho)

Oral Contraceptives, Monophasic (Table 7, page 619)

Oral Contraceptives, Biphasic (Table 7, page 618)

Oral Contraceptives, Triphasic (Table 7, page 619)

Oral Contraceptives, Progestin Only (Table 7, page 619)

22

Emergency Contraceptives

Ethinyl Estradiol, Lev-
onorgestrel (Preven)

Levonorgestrel (Plan B)

Estrogen Supplementation Agents

Esterified Estrogens (Es-
tratab, Menest)
Esterified Estrogens with
Methyltestosterone
(Estratest)
Estradiol (Estrace)
Estradiol Transdermal
(Estraderm)
Estrogen, Conjugated
(Premarin)

Estrogen, Conjugated, Syn-
thetic (Cenestin)
Estrogen, Conjugated with
Medroxyprogesterone
(Prempro, Premphase)
Estrogen, Conjugated with
Methyl progesterone
(Premarin with Methyl
Progesterone)

Estrogen, Conjugated with
Methyltestosterone (Pre-
marin with Methyltestos-
terone)
Ethinyl Estradiol (Estinyl,
Feminone)

Vaginal Preparations

Amino-Cerv pH 5.5 Cream
Miconazole (Monistat)

Nystatin (Mycostatin,
Nilstat)

Terconazole (Terazol 7)
Tioconazole (Vagi stat)

Miscellaneous Ob/Gyn Agents

Dinoprostone (Cervidil
Vaginal Insert, Prepidil
Vaginal Gel)
Gonadorelin (Lutrepulse)
Leuprolide (Lupron)

Magnesium Sulfate
Medroxyprogesterone
(Provera, Depo-Provera)
Methylergonovine
(Methergine)

Mifepristone [RU486]
(Mifeprex)
Oxytocin (Pitocin)
Terbutaline (Brethine,
Bricanyl)

Pain Medications

Local Anesthetics

Benzocaine and Antipyrine
(Auralgan)
Bupivacaine (Marcaine)
Capsaicin (Capsin, Zostrix)

Cocaine
Dibucaine (Nupercainal)
Lidocaine (Anestacon Topi-
cal, Xylocaine)

Lidocaine/ELA-Max)
Lidocaine and Prilocaine
(EMLA)
Pramoxine

Migraine Headache Medications

Acetaminophen with Butal-
bital w/wo Caffeine
(Fioricet, Medigesic,
Repan, Sedapap-10 Two-
Dyne, Triapin, Axocet,
Phrenilin Forte)

Almotriptan (Axert)
Aspirin with Butalbital and
Caffeine (Fiorinal with
Codeine)
Naratriptan (Amerge)
Rizatriptan (Maxalt)

Serotonin 5-HT$_1$ Receptor
Agonists (See Table 11,
page 623)
Sumatriptan (Imitrex)
Zolmitriptan (Zomig)

Narcotics

Acetaminophen with
Codeine (Tylenol No. 1,
2, 3, 4)
Alfentanil Alfenta)
Aspirin with Codeine (Em-
pirin No. 2, 3, 4)
Buprenorphine (Buprenex)
Butorphanol (Stadol)
Codeine
Dezocine (Dalgan)
Fentanyl (Sublimaze)
Fentanyl Transdermal
(Duragesic)
Fentanyl Transmucosal
(Actiq, Fentanyl Oralet)

Hydrocodone and Acetamin-
ophen (Lorcet, Vicodin)
Hydrocodone and Aspirin
(Lortab ASA)
Hydrocodone and Ibuprofen
(Vicoprofen)
Hydromorphone (Dilaudid)
Levorphanol (Levo-
Dromoran)
Meperidine (Demerol)
Methadone (Dolophine)
Morphine (Roxanol, Du-
ramorph, MS Contin)
Nalbuphine (Nubain)

Oxycodone (OxyContin,
OxyIR, Roxicodone)
Oxycodone and Acetamin-
ophen (Percocet, Tylox)
Oxycodone and Aspirin (Per-
codan, Percodan-Demi)
Oxymorphone (Numorphan)
Pentazocine (Talwin)
Propoxyphene (Darvon)
Propoxyphene and Aceta-
minophen (Darvocet)
Propoxyphene and Aspirin
(Darvon Compound-65,
Darvon-N with Aspirin)
Sufentanil (Sufenta)

22

Nonnarcotic Agents

Acetaminophen [APAP] (Tylenol)

Aspirin (Bayer, St. Joseph)
Tramadol (Ultram)

Tramadol/Acetaminophen (Ultracet)

Nonsteroidal Antiinflammatory Agents

Celecoxib (Celebrex)
Diclofenac (Cataflam, Voltaren)
Diflunisal (Dolobid)
Etodolac (Lodine)
Fenoprofen (Nalfon)
Flurbiprofen (Ansaid)
Ibuprofen (Motrin, Rufen, Advil)

Indomethacin (Indocin)
Ketoprofen (Orudis, Oruvail)
Ketorolac (Toradol)
Meloxicam (Mobic)
Nabumetone (Relafen)
Naproxen (Aleve, Naprosyn, Anaprox)

Oxaprozin (Daypro)
Rofecoxib (Vioxx)
Piroxicam (Feldene)
Sulindac (Clinoril)
Tolmetin (Tolectin)
Valdecoxib (Bextra)

Miscellaneous Pain Medications

Amitriptyline (Elavil)

Imipramine (Tofranil)

Tramadol (Ultram)

Respiratory Agents

Antitussives, Decongestants and Expectorants

Acetylcysteine (Mucomyst)
Benzonatate (Tessalon Perles)
Codeine
Dextromethorphan (Mediquell, Benylin DM, PediaCare 1)
Guaifenesin (Robitussin)
Guaifenesin and Codeine (Robitussin AC, Brontex)

Guaifenesin and Dextromethorphan (Many OTC Brands)
Hydrocodone and Guaifenesin (Hycotuss Expectorant, others)
Hydrocodone and Homatropine (Hycodan)

Hydrocodone and Pseudoephedrine (Entuss-D, Histussin-D, others)
Hydrocodone, Chlorpheniramine, Phenylephrine, Acetaminophen and Caffeine (Hycomine)
Potassium Iodide
Pseudoephedrine (Sudafed, Novafed, Afrinol)

Bronchodilators

Albuterol (Proventil, Ventolin)
Albuterol and Ipratropium (Combivent)
Aminophylline
Bitolterol (Tornalate)
Ephedrine
Epinephrine (Adrenalin, Sus-Phrine)

Formoterol (Foradil Aerolizer)
Isoetharine (generic)
Isoproterenol (Isuprel)
Levalbuterol (Xopenex)
Metaproterenol (Alupent, Metaprel)
Pirbuterol (Maxair)
Salmeterol (Serevent)

Terbutaline (Brethine, Bricanyl)
Theophylline (Theolair, Somophyllin-CRT)

Respiratory Inhalants

Acetylcysteine (Mucomyst, Mucosil)
Beclomethasone (Beconase, Vancenase Nasal Inhaler)
Beractant (Survanta)
Budesonide (Pulmicort)
Calfactant (Infasurf)
Colfosceril Palmitate (Exosurf Neonatal)

Cromolyn sodium (Intal, Nasalcrom, Opticrom)
Dexamethasone, Nasal (Dexacort Phosphate Turbinaire)
Flunisolide (AeroBid, Nasalide)
Fluticasone, Oral, Nasal (Flonase, Flovent)

Fluticasone Propionate and Salmeterol Xinafoate (Advair Diskus)
Ipratropium (Atrovent)
Nedocromil (Tilade)
Triamcinolone (Aristocort, Kenalog)

Miscellaneous Respiratory Agents

Alpha$_1$-Protease Inhibitor (Prolastin)

Dornase Alfa (Pulmozyme)
Montelukast (Singulair)

Zafirlukast (Accolate)
Zileuton (Zyflo)

22

Urinary/Genitourinary Agents

Alprostadil (Caverject, Edex)
Alprostadil Urethral Suppository (Muse)
Ammonium Aluminum Sulfate [Alum]
Belladonna and Opium Suppositories (B & O Supprettes)
Bethanechol (Urecholine, others)
Dimethyl Sulfoxide [DMSO] (Rimso-50)

Flavoxate (Urispas)
Hyoscyamine (Anaspaz, Cystospaz, Levsin)
Methenamine (Hiprex, Urex)
Nalidixic acid (NegGram)
Neomycin-Polymyxin Bladder Irrigant [GU Irrigant]
Nitrofurantoin (Macrodantin, Furadantin, Macrobid)
Oxybutynin (Ditropan, Ditropan XL)

Pentosan polysulfate (Elmiron)
Phenazopyridine (Pyridium)
Potassium citrate (Urocit-K)
Potassium citrate and Citric acid (Polycitra-K)
Sildenafil (Viagra)
Sodium citrate (Bicitra)
Tolterodine (Detrol, Detrol LA)
Trimethoprim (Trimpex, Proloprim)

Benign Prostatic Hyperplasia Medications

Doxazosin (Cardura)
Dutasteride (Avodart)

Finasteride (Proscar, Propecia)

Tamsulosin (Flomax)
Terazosin (Hytrin)

Wound Care

Becaplermin (Regranex Gel)

Silver nitrate (Dey-Drop)

Miscellaneous Therapeutic Agents

Drotrecogin alfa (Xigris)
Megestrol Acetate (Megace)
Metaraminol (Aramine)
Naltrexone (ReVia)
Nicotine Gum (Nicorette, Nicorette DS)

Nicotine Nasal Spray (Nicotrol NS)
Nicotine Transdermal (Habitrol, Nicoderm, Nicotrol, ProStep)
Potassium iodide

Sodium Polystyrene sulfonate (Kayexalate)
Triethanolamine (Cerumenex)

GENERIC DRUG DATA

Abacavir (Ziagen) **WARNING:** Hypersensitivity manifested as fever, rash, fatigue, GI, and respiratory reported; stop drug immediately and do not rechallenge; lactic acidosis and hepatomegaly/steatosis reported **Uses:** HIV infection **Action:** Nucleoside reverse transcriptase inhibitor **Dose:** *Adults.* 300 mg PO bid. *Peds.* 8 mg/kg bid **Caution/Contra:** [C, −] CDC recommends HIV-infected mothers not breast-feed due to risk of infant HIV transmission **Supplied:** Tabs 300 mg; soln 20 mg/mL **Notes/SE:** Numerous drug interactions

Abciximab (ReoPro) **Uses:** Prevent acute ischemic complications in PTCA **Action:** Inhibits platelet aggregation (glycoprotein IIb/IIIa inhibitor) **Dose:** 0.25 mg/kg bolus 10–60 min prior to PTCA, then 0.125 mcg/kg/min (max = 10 mcg/min) cont inf for 12 h **Caution/Contra:** [C, ?/−] Contra if active or recent (w/n 6 wk) internal hemorrhage, CVA w/n 2 y or CVA with significant neurologic deficit, bleeding diathesis or administration of oral anticoagulants w/n 7 d (unless PT ≥ 2× control), thrombocytopenia (<100,000 cells/μL), recent trauma or major surgery (w/n 6 wk), CNS tumor, AVM, aneurysm, severe uncontrolled HTN, vasculitis, use of dextran prior to or during PTCA, hypersensitivity to murine proteins **Supplied:** Inj 2 mg/mL **Notes/SE:** Use with heparin; allergic reactions, bleeding, thrombocytopenia possible

Acarbose (Precose) **Uses:** Type 2 DM **Action:** α-Glucosidase inhibitor; delays digestion of carbohydrates, thus ↓ glucose levels **Dose:** 25–100 mg PO tid with 1st bite each meal; avoid if CrCl <25 mL/min **Caution/Contra:** [B, ?] Contra in IBD **Supplied:** Tabs 25, 50, 100 mg **Notes/SE:** May take with sulfonylureas; can affect digoxin levels; abdominal pain, diarrhea, flatulence, ↑ LFTs; check LFTs q3mon for 1st year of therapy

Acebutolol (Sectral) **Uses:** HTN **Action:** Competitively blocks β-adrenergic receptors, β_1, and ISA **Dose:** 200–800 mg/d, ↓ if CrCl <50 mL/min **Caution/Contra:** [B, D in 2nd and 3rd trimesters, +] Contra in 2nd- and 3rd-degree heart block; can exacerbate ischemic heart disease, do not DC abruptly **Supplied:** Caps 200, 400 mg **Notes/SE:** Fatigue, HA, dizziness, bradycardia

22

Acetaminophen [APAP, N-acetyl-p-aminophenol] (Tylenol) Uses: Mild pain, HA, and fever **Action:** Nonnarcotic analgesic; inhibits synthesis of prostaglandins in the CNS; inhibits hypothalamic heat-regulating center **Dose:** *Adults.* 650 mg PO or PR q4–6h or 1000 mg PO q6h; max 4 g/24 h. See quick dosing Table 1 (page 505). Administer q6h if CrCl 10–50 mL/min and q8h if CrCl <10 mL/min; avoid alcohol intake **Caution/Contra:** [B, +]. G6PD deficiency; alcoholic liver disease; hepatotoxicity reported in elderly and with alcohol use at doses >4 g/day **Supplied:** Tabs 160, 325, 500, 650 mg; chew tabs 80, 160 mg; liq 100 mg/mL, 120 mg/2.5 mL, 120 mg/5 mL, 160 mg/5 mL, 167 mg/5 mL, 325 mg/5 mL, 500 mg/5 mL; gtt 48 mg/mL, 60 mg/0.6 mL; supp 80, 120, 125, 300, 325, 650 mg **Notes/SE:** No antiinflammatory or platelet-inhibiting action; overdose causes hepatotoxicity, which is treated with *N*-acetylcysteine

Acetaminophen + Butalbital +/– Caffeine (Fioricet, Medigesic, Repan, Sedapap-10, Two-Dyne, Triapin, Axocet, Phrenilin Forte) [C-III] Uses: Mild pain; HA, especially associated with stress **Action:** Nonnarcotic analgesic with barbiturate **Dose:** 1–2 tabs or caps PO q4/6h PRN; ↓ in renal/hepatic impairment; 4 g/24 h APAP max; avoid alcohol intake **Caution/Contra:** [D, +] G6PD deficiency; alcoholic liver disease **Supplied:** Caps *Medigesic, Repan, Two-Dyne:* Butalbital 50 mg, caffeine 40 mg, + APAP 325 mg. Caps *Axocet, Phrenilin Forte:* Butalbital 50 mg + APAP 650 mg; *Triapin:* Butalbital 50 mg + APAP 325 mg. Tabs *Medigesic, Fioricet, Repan:* Butalbital 50 mg, caffeine 40 mg, + APAP 325 mg; *Phrenilin:* Butalbital 50 mg + APAP 325 mg; *Sedapap-10:* Butalbital 50 mg + APAP 650 mg **Notes/SE:** Butalbital habit-forming; drowsiness, dizziness, "hangover" effect

Acetaminophen + Codeine (Tylenol No. 1, No. 2, No. 3, No. 4) [C-III, C-V] Uses: No. 1, No. 2, and No. 3 for mild–moderate pain; No. 4 for moderate–severe pain **Action:** Combined effects of APAP and a narcotic analgesic **Dose:** *Adults.* 1–2 tabs q3–4h PRN (max dose APAP = 4 g/d). *Peds.* APAP 10–15 mg/kg/dose; codeine 0.5–1.0 mg/kg dose q4–6h (useful dosing guide: 3–6 y, 5 mL/dose; 7–12 y, 10 mL/dose); ↓ in renal/hepatic impairment; do not exceed 4 g/24 h of APAP in adults **Caution/Contra:** [C, +] G6PD deficiency; alcoholic liver disease **Supplied:** Tabs 300 mg of APAP + codeine; caps 325 mg of APAP + codeine; helix, susp (C-V) APAP 120 mg + codeine 12 mg/5 mL **Notes/SE:** Codeine in No. 1 = 7.5 mg, No. 2 = 15 mg, No. 3 = 30 mg, No. 4 = 60 mg; drowsiness, dizziness, N/V

Acetazolamide (Diamox) Uses: Diuresis, glaucoma, prevent high-altitude sickness, and refractory epilepsy **Action:** Carbonic anhydrase inhibitor; ↓ renal excretion of hydrogen and ↑ renal excretion of Na, K, bicarbonate, and water **Dose:** *Adults.* Diuretic: 250–375 mg IV or PO q24h. *Glaucoma:* 250–1000 mg PO q24h in ÷ doses. *Epilepsy:* 8–30 mg/kg/d PO in ÷ doses. *Altitude sickness:* 125–250 mg PO q8–12h or SR 500 mg PO q12–24h start 24 h before ascent. *Peds. Epilepsy:* 8–30 mg/kg/24 h PO in ÷ doses; max 1 g/d. *Diuretic:* 5 mg/kg/24 h PO or IV. *Alkalinization of urine:* 5 mg/kg/dose PO bid–tid. *Glaucoma:* 5–15 mg/kg/24 h PO in ÷ doses; max 1 g/d; adjust in renal impairment (avoid if CrCl <10 mL/min) **Caution/Contra:** [C, +] Renal/hepatic failure, sulfa hypersensitivity **Supplied:** Tabs 125, 250 mg; SR caps 500 mg; inj 500 mg/vial **Notes/SE:** Follow Na⁺ and K⁺; watch for metabolic acidosis; SR dosage forms not recommended for use in epilepsy; malaise, metallic taste, drowsiness, photosensitivity, hyperglycemia

Acetic Acid and Aluminum Acetate (Otic Domeboro) Uses: Otitis externa **Action:** Antiinfective **Dose:** 4–6 gtt in ear(s) q2–3h **Caution/Contra:** [C, ?] **Supplied:** Otic soln

Acetylcysteine (Mucomyst) Uses: Mucolytic agent as adjuvant Rx for chronic bronchopulmonary diseases and CF; antidote to APAP hepatotoxicity, best results used within 24 h **Action:** Splits disulfide linkages between mucoprotein molecular complexes; protects liver by restoring glutathione levels in APAP overdose **Dose:** *Adults & Peds. Neb:* 3–5 mL of 20% soln diluted with an equal vol of water or NS tid–qid. *Antidote:* PO or NG: 140 mg/kg loading dose, then 70 mg/kg q4h for 17 doses. Dilute 1:3 in carbonated beverage or orange juice **Caution/Contra:** [C, ?] **Supplied:** Soln 10%, 20% **Notes/SE:** Bronchospasm when used by inhalation in asthmatics; N/V, drowsiness; activated charcoal adsorbs acetylcysteine when given PO for acute APAP ingestion

Acitretin (Soriatane) Uses: Severe psoriasis and other keratinization disorders (lichen planus, etc) **Action:** Retinoid-like activity **Dose:** 25–50 mg/d PO, with main meal; can ↑ if no response by 4 wk to 75 mg/d **Caution/Contra:** [X, –] caution in renal/hepatic

22

impairment; caution in women of reproductive potential **Supplied:** Caps 10, 25 mg **Notes/SE:** Teratogenic, contra in PRG; follow LFTs; response often takes 2–3 mon; cheilitis, skin peeling, alopecia, pruritus, rash, arthralgia, GI upset, photosensitivity, thrombocytosis, hypertriglyceridemia

Acyclovir (Zovirax) **Uses:** Herpes simplex and herpes zoster viral infections **Action:** Interferes with viral DNA synthesis **Dose:** *Adults. Oral: Initial genital herpes:* 200 mg PO q4h while awake, total of 5 caps/d for 10 d or 400 mg PO tid for 7–10 d. *Chronic suppression:* 400 mg PO bid. *Intermittent Rx:* As for initial treatment, except treat for 5 d, or 800 mg PO bid, initiate at earliest prodrome. *Herpes zoster:* 800 mg PO 5×/d for 7–10 d. *IV:* 5–10 mg/kg/dose IV q8h. *Topical initial herpes genitalis:* Apply q3h (6×/d) for 7 d. *Peds.* 5–10 mg/kg/dose IV or PO q8h or 750 mg/m²/24 h ÷ q8h. *Chickenpox:* 20 mg/kg/dose PO qid; ↓ for CrCl <50 mL/min **Caution/Contra:** [C, +] **Supplied:** Caps 200 mg; tabs 400, 800 mg; susp 200 mg/5 mL; inj 500 mg/vial; oint 5% **Notes/SE:** PO better than topical for herpes genitalis; dizziness, lethargy, confusion, rash, inflammation at IV inj site

Adefovir (Hepsera) WARNING: Acute exacerbations of hepatitis may occur on discontinuation of therapy (monitor hepatic function); chronic administration may lead to nephrotoxicity especially in patients with underlying renal dysfunction (monitor renal function); HIV resistance may emerge; lactic acidosis and severe hepatomegaly with steatosis have been reported when used alone or in combination with other antiretrovirals **Uses:** Chronic active hepatitis B virus **Action:** Nucleotide analogue **Dose:** CrCl ≥ 50 mL/min: 10 mg PO qd; CrCl 20–49 mL/min: 10 mg PO q 48h; CrCl 10–19 mL/min: 10 mg PO q 72h; Hemodialysis: 10 mg PO q 7 days postdialysis; Adjust dose when CrCl < 50 mL/min **Caution/Contra:** [C, –]**Supplied:** Tabs 10 mg **Notes/SE:** asthenia, headache, abdominal pain, see Warning

Adenosine (Adenocard) **Uses:** PSVT, including associated with WPW **Action:** Class IV antiarrhythmic; slows AV node conduction **Dose:** *Adults.* 6 mg IV bolus; may repeat in 1–2 min; max 12 mg IV. *Peds.* 0.05 mg/kg IV bolus; may repeat q1–2min to 0.25 mg/kg max **Caution/Contra:** [C, ?] 2nd- or 3rd-degree AV block or SSS (w/o pacemaker); recent MI or cerebral hemorrhage **Supplied:** Inj 6 mg/2 mL **Notes/SE:** Doses >12 mg not recommended; can cause momentary asystole when administered; caffeine and theophylline antagonize effects of adenosine; facial flushing, HA, dyspnea, chest pressure, hypotension

Albumin (Albuminar, Buminate, Albutein) **Uses:** Plasma volume expansion for shock (burns, surgery, hemorrhage, or other trauma) **Action:** Maint of plasma colloid oncotic pressure **Dose:** *Adults.* Initially, 25 g IV; subsequent dose based on response. 250 g/48h max. *Peds.* 0.5–1.0 g/kg/dose; infuse at 0.05–0.1 g/min **Caution/Contra:** [C, ?] Severe anemia, cardiac failure; caution with cardiac, renal, or hepatic insufficiency due to added protein load and possible hypervolemia **Supplied:** Soln 5%, 25% **Notes/SE:** Contains 130–160 mEq Na⁺/L; chills, fever, CHF, tachycardia, hypotension, hypervolemia

Albuterol (Proventil, Ventolin) **Uses:** Bronchospasm in reversible obstructive airway disease; prevent exercise-induced bronchospasm **Action:** β-Adrenergic sympathomimetic bronchodilator; relaxes bronchial smooth muscle **Dose:** *Adults.* 2 inhal q4–6h PRN; 1 Rotacap inhaled q4–6h; 2–4 mg PO tid–qid; *Neb:* 1.25–5 mg (0.25–1 mL of 0.5% soln in 2–3 mL of NS tid–qid). *Peds.* 2 inhal q4–6h; 0.1–0.2 mg/kg/dose PO; max 2–4 mg PO tid; *Neb:* 0.05 mg/kg (max 2.5 mg) in 2–3 mL of NS tid–qid **Caution/Contra:** [C, +] **Supplied:** Tabs 2, 4 mg; ER tabs 4, 8 mg; syrup 2 mg/5 mL; 90 mcg/dose met-dose inhaler; Rotacaps 200 µg; soln for neb 0.083, 0.5% **Notes/SE:** Palpitations, tachycardia, nervousness, GI upset

Albuterol and Ipratropium (Combivent) **Uses:** COPD **Action:** Combination of β-adrenergic bronchodilator and quaternary anticholinergic compound **Dose:** 2 inhal qid **Caution/Contra:** [C, +] **Supplied:** Met-dose inhaler, 18 µg ipratropium/103 mcg albuterol/puff **Notes/SE:** Palpitations, tachycardia, nervousness, GI upset, dizziness, blurred vision

Aldesleukin [IL-2] (Proleukin) WARNING: Use restricted to patients with normal pulmonary and cardiac function **Uses:** RCC, melanoma **Action:** Acts via IL-2 receptor; numerous immunomodulatory effects **Dose:** 600,000 IU/kg q8h × 14 doses (FDA-approved dose/schedule for RCC). Multiple cont inf and alternate schedules (including "high dose" using 24 × 10⁶ IU/m² IV q8h on days 1–5 and 12–16) **Caution/Contra:** [C, ?/–] **Supplied:** Inj 1.1 mg/mL (22 × 10⁶ IU) **Notes/SE:** Flu-like syndrome (malaise, fever, chills), N/V/D, ↑ bilirubin; capillary leak syndrome with ↓ BP, pulmonary edema, fluid retention, and weight gain; renal toxicity and mild hematologic toxicity (anemia, thrombocytopenia, leukopenia) and secondary eosinophilia; cardiac toxicity (myocardial ischemia, atrial arrhythmias); neurologic toxicity (CNS depression, somnolence, rarely coma, delirium). Pruritic rashes, urticaria, and erythroderma common. Cont inf schedules less likely to cause severe hypotension and fluid retention

Alendronate (Fosamax) **Uses:** Rx and prevention of osteoporosis, Rx of steroid-induced osteoporosis and Paget's disease **Action:** ↓Normal and abnormal bone resorption **Dose:** *Osteoporosis: Rx:* 10 mg/d PO or 70 mg/wk. *Steroid-induced osteoporosis: Rx:* 5 mg/d PO. *Prevention:* 5 mg/d PO or 35 mg/wk. *Paget's disease:* 40 mg/d PO; **Caution/Contra:** [C, ?]. Not recommended if CrCl <35 mL/min; abnormalities of the esophagus, inability to sit or stand upright for 30 min, hypocalcemia; caution with NSAID use **Supplied:** Tabs 5, 10, 35, 40, 70 mg **Notes/SE:** Take 1st thing in AM with water (8 oz) at least 30 min before 1st food or beverage of the day. Do not lie down for 30 min after taking. Adequate Ca and vitamin D supplement necessary; GI disturbances, HA, pain

Alfentanil (Alfenta) [C-II] **Uses:** Adjunct in the maint of anesthesia; analgesia **Action:** Short-acting narcotic analgesic **Dose:** *Adults & Peds >12 y.* 3–75 mcg/kg IV inf; total dose depends on duration of procedure **Caution/Contra:** [C, +/–]. ↑ ICP, respiratory depression **Supplied:** Inj 500 mcg/mL **Notes/SE:** Bradycardia, ↓ BP, cardiac arrhythmias, peripheral vasodilation, ↑ ICP, drowsiness, respiratory depression

Alginic Acid + Aluminum Hydroxide and Magnesium Trisilicate (Gaviscon) **Uses:** Heartburn; pain from hiatal hernia **Action:** Forms protective layer blocking reflux of gastric acid **Dose:** 2–4 tabs or 15–30 mL PO qid followed by water; avoid in renal impairment or with Na-restricted diet **Caution/Contra:** [B, –] **Supplied:** Tabs, susp **Notes/SE:** Diarrhea, constipation

Allopurinol (Zyloprim, Lopurin, Aloprim) **Uses:** Gout, hyperuricemia of malignancy, and uric acid urolithiasis **Action:** Xanthine oxidase inhibitor; ↓ uric acid production **Dose:** *Adults.* PO: Initially, 100 mg/d; usual 300 mg/d; max 800 mg/d. *IV:* 200–400 mg/m^2/d (max 600 mg/24 h). *Peds.* Use only for treating hyperuricemia of malignancy in <10 y: 10 mg/kg/24 h PO or 200 mg/m^2/d IV ÷ q6–8h (max 600 mg/24 h); ↓ in renal impairment; take after meal with plenty of fluid **Caution/Contra:** [C, M] **Supplied:** Tabs 100, 300 mg; inj 500 mg/30 mL (Aloprim) **Notes/SE:** Aggravates acute gout; begin after acute attack resolves; administer pc. IV dose of 6 mg/mL final conc as single daily inf or ÷ 6, 8, or 12-h intervals; skin rash, N/V, renal impairment, angioedema

Almotriptan (Axert) See Table 11, page 623

Alpha$_1$-Protease Inhibitor (Prolastin) **Uses:** Panacinar emphysema **Action:** Replacement of human α_1-protease inhibitor **Dose:** 60 mg/kg IV once/wk **Caution/Contra:** [C, ?]. Selective IgA deficiencies with known antibodies to IgA **Supplied:** Inj 500 mg/20 mL, 1000 mg/40 mL **Notes/SE:** Fever, dizziness, flu-like symptoms, allergic reactions

Alosetron (Lotronex) **WARNING:** Serious GI side effects, some fatal, including ischemic colitis have been reported. May be prescribed only through participation in the prescribing program for Lotronex. **Uses:** Treatment of severe diarrhea-predominant IBS in women who have failed conventional therapy. **Action:** Selective 5-HT$_3$ receptor antagonist **Dose:** *Adults:* 1 mg PO qd × 4 wk; titrate to max of 1 mg bid; DC after 4 wk at max dose if IBS symptoms not controlled. **Caution/Contra:** [B, ?/–] Hx chronic or severe constipation, intestinal obstruction, strictures, toxic megacolon, GI perforation, adhesions, ischemic colitis, Crohn's disease, ulcerative colitis, diverticulitis, thrombophlebitis, or hypercoagulable state. **Supplied:** Tabs 1 mg **Notes/SE:** DC immediately if constipation or symptoms of ischemic colitis develop; constipation, abdominal pain, nausea.

Alprazolam (Xanax) [C-IV] **Uses:** Anxiety and panic disorders + anxiety with depression **Action:** Benzodiazepine; antianxiety agent **Dose:** *Anxiety:* Initially, 0.25–0.5 mg tid; ↑ to a max of 4 mg/d in ÷ doses. *Panic:* Initially, 0.5 mg tid; may gradually ↑ to desired response; ↓ dose in elderly, debilitated, and hepatic impairment **Caution/Contra:** [D, –] **Supplied:** Tabs 0.25, 0.5, 1.0, 2.0 mg **Notes/SE:** Avoid abrupt discontinuation after prolonged use; drowsiness, fatigue, irritability, memory impairment, sexual dysfunction

Alprostadil [Prostaglandin E$_1$] (Prostin VR) **Uses:** Any state in which blood flow must be maintained through the ductus arteriosus to sustain either pulmonary or sys-

22

temic circulation until surgery can be performed (eg, pulmonary atresia, pulmonary stenosis, tricuspid atresia, transposition, severe tetralogy of Fallot) **Action:** Vasodilator, platelet aggregation inhibitor; smooth muscle of the ductus arteriosus is especially sensitive **Dose:** 0.05 mcg/kg/min IV; ↓ dose to lowest that maintains response **Caution/Contra:** [X, –] **Supplied:** Injectable forms **Notes/SE:** Cutaneous vasodilation, seizure-like activity, jitteriness, temperature elevation, hypocalcemia, apnea, thrombocytopenia, hypotension; may cause apnea; have an intubation kit at bedside if patient is not intubated

Alprostadil, Intracavernosal (Caverject, Edex)
Uses: Erectile dysfunction **Action:** Relaxes smooth muscles, dilates cavernosal arteries, increases lacunar spaces and entrapment of blood by compressing venules against tunica albuginea **Dose:** 2.5–60 mcg intracavernosal; adjusted to individual needs **Caution/Contra:** [X, –]. Conditions predisposing to priapism; anatomic deformities of the penis; penile implants; men in whom sexual activity is inadvisable **Supplied:** *Caverject:* 6–10- or 6–20-mcg vials +/– diluent syringes. *Caverject Impulse: self-contained syringe (29 gauge) 10 and 20 mcg Edex:* 5-, 10-, 20-, 40-mcg vials + syringes **Notes/SE:** Penile pain common; titrate dose at physician's office. Counsel patients about possible priapism, penile fibrosis, and hematoma; pain with inj

Alprostadil, Urethral Suppository (Muse)
Uses: Erectile dysfunction **Action:** Alprostadil (PGE$_1$) absorbed through urethral mucosa; vasodilator and smooth muscle relaxant of corpus cavernosa **Dose:** 125–1000 mcg system 5–10 min prior to sexual activity **Caution/Contra:** [X, –] **Supplied:** 125, 250, 500, 1000 mcg with a transurethral delivery system **Notes/SE:** Hypotension, dizziness, syncope, penile pain, testicular pain, urethral burning/bleeding, and priapism. Dose titration under physician's supervision

Alteplase, Recombinant [TPA] (Activase)
Uses: AMI, PE, and acute ischemic stroke **Action:** Thrombolytic; initiates local fibrinolysis by binding to fibrin in the thrombus **Dose:** *AMI and PE:* 100 mg IV over 3 h (10 mg over 2 min, then 50 mg over 1 h, then 40 mg over 2 h); *stroke:* 0.9 mg/kg (max 90 mg) infused over 60 min **Caution/Contra:** [C, ?] Active internal bleeding; uncontrolled HTN (systolic BP ≥ 185 mm Hg/diastolic ≥ 110 mm Hg); recent (w/n 3 mon) CVA, GI bleed, trauma, surgery, prolonged external cardiac massage; intracranial neoplasm, suspected aortic dissection, AV malformation or aneurysm, bleeding diathesis, hemostatic defects, seizure at the time of stroke, suspicion of subarachnoid hemorrhage **Supplied:** Powder for inj 50, 100 mg **Notes/SE:** Bleeding, bruising (especially from venipuncture sites), hypotension; give heparin to prevent reocclusion; in AMI doses of >150 mg associated with intracranial bleeding

Altretamine (Hexalen)
Uses: Epithelial ovarian CA **Action:** Unknown; cytotoxic agent, possibly alkylating agent; inhibits nucleotide incorporation into DNA and RNA **Dose:** 260 mg/m^2/d in 4 ÷ doses for 14–21 d of a 28-d treatment cycle; dose ↑ to 150 mg/m^2/d for 14 d in multiagent regimens (refer to specific protocols) **Caution/Contra:** [D, ?/–]. Preexisting severe bone marrow depression or neurologic toxicity **Supplied:** Caps 50, 100 mg **Notes/SE:** N/V/D and cramps; neurologic toxicity (peripheral neuropathy, CNS depression); minimally myelosuppressive

Aluminum Carbonate (Basaljel)
Uses: Hyperacidity (peptic ulcer, GERD, etc); supplement to the Rx of hyperphosphatemia **Action:** Neutralizes gastric acid; binds phosphate **Dose:** *Adults.* 2 caps or tabs or 10 mL (in water) q2h PRN. *Peds.* 50–150 mg/kg/24 h PO ÷ q4–6h **Caution/Contra:** [C, ?] **Supplied:** Tabs, caps, susp **Notes/SE:** Constipation

Aluminum Hydroxide (Amphojel, AlternaGEL)
Uses: Hyperacidity (peptic ulcer, hiatal hernia, etc); supplement to Rx of hyperphosphatemia **Action:** Neutralizes gastric acid; binds phosphate **Dose:** *Adults.* 10–30 mL or 2 tabs PO q4–6h. *Peds.* 5–15 mL PO q4–6h or 50–150 mg/kg/24 h PO ÷ q4–6h (hyperphosphatemia) **Caution/Contra:** [C, ?] **Supplied:** Tabs 300, 600 mg; chew tabs 500 mg; susp 320, 600 mg/5 mL **Notes/SE:** Can use in renal failure; constipation

Aluminum Hydroxide + Magnesium Carbonate (Gaviscon)
Uses: Hyperacidity (peptic ulcer, hiatal hernia, etc) **Action:** Neutralizes gastric acid **Dose:** *Adults.* 15–30 PO pc and hs. *Peds.* 5–15 mL PO qid or PRN; avoid in renal impairment; may affect absorption of some drugs **Caution/Contra:** [C, ?] **Supplied:** Liq containing aluminum hydroxide 95 mg + magnesium carbonate 358 mg/15 mL **Notes/SE:** Doses qid are best given pc and hs; may cause ↑ Mg^{2+} (with renal insufficiency), constipation, diarrhea

Aluminum Hydroxide + Magnesium Hydroxide (Maalox) Uses: Hyperacidity (peptic ulcer, hiatal hernia, etc) Action: Neutralizes gastric acid Dose: *Adults.* 10–60 mL or 2–4 tabs PO qid or PRN. *Peds.* 5–15 mL PO qid or PRN Caution/Contra: [C, ?] Supplied: Tabs, susp Notes/SE: Doses qid best given pc and hs; may cause ↑ Mg^{2+} in renal insufficiency, constipation, diarrhea

Aluminum Hydroxide + Magnesium Hydroxide and Simethicone (Mylanta, Mylanta II, Maalox Plus) Uses: Hyperacidity with bloating Action: Neutralizes gastric acid Dose: *Adults.* 10–60 mL or 2–4 tabs PO qid or PRN. *Peds.* 5–15 mL PO qid or PRN; avoid in renal impairment; may affect absorption of some drugs Caution/Contra: [C, ?] Supplied: Tabs, susp Notes/SE: Hypermagnesemia in renal insufficiency, diarrhea, constipation; Mylanta II contains twice the aluminum and magnesium hydroxide of Mylanta

Aluminum Hydroxide + Magnesium Trisilicate (Gaviscon, Gaviscon-2) Uses: Hyperacidity Action: Neutralizes gastric acid Dose: Chew 2–4 tabs qid; avoid in renal impairment; concomitant administration may affect absorption of some drugs Caution/Contra: [C, ?] Supplied: *Gaviscon:* Aluminum hydroxide 80 mg and magnesium trisilicate 20 mg; *Gaviscon-2:* Aluminum hydroxide 160 mg and magnesium trisilicate 40 mg Notes/SE: Constipation, diarrhea

Amantadine (Symmetrel) Uses: Rx or prophylaxis for influenza A viral infections and parkinsonism Action: Prevents release of infectious viral nucleic acid into the host cell; releases dopamine from intact dopaminergic terminals Dose: *Adults. Influenza A:* 200 mg/d PO or 100 mg PO bid. *Parkinsonism:* 100 mg PO qd–bid. *Peds.* 1–9 y: 4.4–8.8 mg/kg/24 h to 150 mg/24 h max ÷ doses qd–bid. *10–12 y:* 100–200 mg/d in 1–2 ÷ doses; ↓ in renal impairment Caution/Contra: [C, M] Supplied: Caps 100 mg; tabs 100 mg; soln 50 mg/5 mL Notes/SE: Orthostatic hypotension, edema, insomnia, depression, irritability, hallucinations, dream abnormalities

Amifostine (Ethyol) Uses: Xerostomia prophylaxis during RT (head and neck, ovarian, or non-small-cell lung CA). Reduces renal toxicity associated with repeated administration of cisplatin Action: Prodrug, dephosphorylated by alkaline phosphatase to the pharmacologically active thiol metabolite Dose: 910 mg/m^2/d as a 15-min IV inf 30 min prior to chemotherapy Caution/Contra: [C, +/–] Supplied: 500 mg vials of lyophilized drug with 500 mg of mannitol, reconstituted in sterile NS Notes/SE: Transient hypotension in >60%, N/V, flushing with hot or cold chills, dizziness, hypocalcemia, somnolence, and sneezing. Does not reduce the effectiveness of cyclophosphamide plus cisplatin chemotherapy

Amikacin (Amikin) Uses: Serious infections caused by gram– bacteria and mycobacteria Action: Aminoglycoside antibiotic; inhibits protein synthesis Dose: *Adults & Peds.* 5–7.5 mg/kg/dose ÷ q8–24h based on renal function. *Neonates <1200 g, 0–4 wk:* 7.5 mg/kg/dose q12h–18h. *Postnatal age <7 d, 1200–2000 g:* 7.5 mg/kg/dose q12h. *>2000 g:* 10 mg/kg/dose q12h. *Postnatal age >7 d, 1200–2000 g:* 7 mg/kg/dose q8h. *>2000 g:* 7.5–10 mg/kg/dose q8h Caution/Contra: [C, +/–] Supplied: Inj 100, 500 mg/2 mL Notes/SE: May be effective against gram– bacteria resistant to gentamicin and tobramycin; monitor renal function carefully for dosage adjustments; monitor serum levels (Table 2, page 607); nephrotoxicity, ototoxicity, neurotoxicity, avoid use with potent diuretics

Amiloride (Midamor) Uses: HTN and CHF Action: K^+-sparing diuretic; interferes with K^+/Na^+ exchange in the distal tubules Dose: *Adults.* 5–10 mg/d PO. *Peds.* 0.625 mg/kg/d; ↓ in renal impairment Caution/Contra: [B, ?] Supplied: Tabs 5 mg Notes/SE: Hyperkalemia possible; monitor serum K^+ levels; HA, dizziness, dehydration, impotence

Aminocaproic Acid (Amicar) Uses: Excessive bleeding resulting from systemic hyperfibrinolysis and urinary fibrinolysis Action: Inhibits fibrinolysis via inhibition of TPA substances Dose: *Adults.* 5 g IV or PO (1st h) followed by 1–1.25 g/h IV or PO. *Peds.* 100 mg/kg IV (1st h) (max dose/d: 30 g), then 1 g/m^2/h; max 18 g/m^2/d; ↓ in renal failure Caution/Contra: [C, ?] DIC, hematuria of upper urinary tract Supplied: Tabs 500 mg; syrup 250 mg/mL; inj 250 mg/mL Notes/SE: Administer for 8 h or until bleeding is controlled; not for upper urinary tract bleeding; ↓ BP, bradycardia, dizziness, HA, fatigue, rash, GI disturbance, ↓ platelet function

22

Amino-Cerv pH 5.5 Cream **Uses:** Mild cervicitis, postpartum cervicitis/cervical tears, postcauterization, postcryosurgery, and postconization **Action:** Hydrating agent; removes excess keratin in hyperkeratotic conditions **Dose:** 1 Applicatorful intravaginally hs for 2–4 wk **Caution/Contra:** [C, ?] Use in viral skin infection **Supplied:** Vaginal cream **Notes/SE:** Also called carbamide or urea; contains 8.34% urea, 0.5% Na propionate, 0.83% methionine, 0.35% cystine, 0.83% inositol, and benzalkonium chloride; transient stinging, local irritation

Aminoglutethimide (Cytadren) **Uses:** Adrenocortical carcinoma, Cushing's syndrome, breast and prostate CA **Action:** Inhibits adrenal steroidogenesis and adrenal conversion of androgens to estrogens **Dose:** 750–1500 mg/d in ÷ doses plus hydrocortisone 20–40 mg/d; ↓ in renal insufficiency **Caution/Contra:** [D, ?] **Supplied:** Tabs 250 mg **Notes/SE:** Adrenal insufficiency ("medical adrenalectomy"), hypothyroidism, masculinization, hypotension, vomiting, rare hepatotoxicity, rash, myalgia, fever

Aminophylline **Uses:** Asthma and bronchospasm **Action:** Relaxes smooth muscle of the bronchi, pulmonary blood vessels; stimulates diaphragm **Dose:** *Adults. Acute asthma:* Load 6 mg/kg IV, then 0.4–0.9 mg/kg/h IV cont inf. *Chronic asthma:* 24 mg/kg/24 h PO or PR ÷ q6h. *Peds.* Load 6 mg/kg IV, then 1.0 mg/kg/h IV cont inf; ↓ in hepatic insufficiency and with certain drugs (macrolide and quinolone antibiotics, cimetidine, and propranolol) **Caution/Contra:** [C, +] Uncontrolled arrhythmias, hyperthyroidism, peptic ulcers, uncontrolled seizure disorder **Supplied:** Tabs 100, 200 mg; soln 105 mg/5 mL; supp 250, 500 mg; inj 25 mg/mL **Notes/SE:** Individualize dosage. N/V, irritability, tachycardia, ventricular arrhythmias, and seizures; follow serum levels carefully (as theophylline, Table 2, page 607); aminophylline is about 85% theophylline; erratic absorption with rectal doses

Amiodarone (Cordarone, Pacerone) **Uses:** Recurrent VF or hemodynamically unstable VT, AF **Action:** Class III antiarrhythmic **Dose:** *Adults. Loading dose:* 800–1600 mg/d PO for 1–3 wk. *Maint:* 600–800 mg/d PO for 1 mon, then 200–400 mg/d. *IV:* 15 mg/min for 10 min, then 1 mg/min for 6 h, then maint 0.5 mg/min cont inf. *Peds.* 10–15 mg/kg/24 h ÷ q12h PO for 7–10 d, then 5 mg/kg/24 h ÷ q12h or qd (infants/neonates require a higher loading dose); ↓ in severe liver insufficiency **Caution/Contra:** [D, –]. Sinus node dysfunction, 2nd- or 3rd-degree AV block, sinus bradycardia (w/o pacemaker) **Supplied:** Tabs 200 mg; inj 50 mg/mL **Notes/SE:** Half-life is 53 d; pulmonary fibrosis, exacerbation of arrhythmias, prolongs QT interval; CHF, arrhythmias, hypo-/hyperthyroidism, ↑ LFTs, liver failure, corneal microdeposits, optic neuropathy/neuritis, peripheral neuropathy, photosensitivity; IV conc of >0.2 mg/mL administered via a central catheter; alters digoxin levels, may require ↓ digoxin dose

Amitriptyline (Elavil) **Uses:** Depression, peripheral neuropathy, chronic pain, and tension HAs **Action:** TCA; inhibits reuptake of serotonin and norepinephrine by the presynaptic neurons **Dose:** *Adults.* Initially, 30–50 mg PO hs; may ↑ to 300 mg hs. *Peds.* Not recommended if <12 y unless for chronic pain; initially 0.1 mg/kg PO hs, advance over 2–3 wk to 0.5–2 mg/kg PO hs; caution in hepatic impairment; taper when discontinuing **Caution/Contra:** [D, +/–]. With MAOIs, during acute recovery following MI, narrow-angle glaucoma **Supplied:** Tabs 10, 25, 50, 75, 100, 150 mg; inj 10 mg/mL **Notes/SE:** Strong anticholinergic side effects; overdose may be fatal, may cause urine retention and sedation, ECG changes, photosensitivity

Amlodipine (Norvasc) **Uses:** HTN, chronic stable angina, and vasospastic angina **Action:** Ca channel blocker; relaxation of coronary vascular smooth muscle **Dose:** 2.5–10 mg/d PO **Caution/Contra:** [C, ?] **Supplied:** Tabs 2.5, 5, 10 mg **Notes/SE:** May be taken without regard to meals; peripheral edema, HA, palpitations, flushing

Ammonium Aluminum Sulfate (Alum) **Uses:** Hemorrhagic cystitis when bladder irrigation fails **Action:** Astringent **Dose:** 1–2% soln used with constant bladder irrigation with NS **Caution/Contra:** [+/–] **Supplied:** Powder for reconstitution **Notes/SE:** Safe to use without anesthesia and with vesicoureteral reflux. Encephalopathy possible; obtain aluminum levels, especially in renal insufficiency; can precipitate and occlude catheters

Amoxicillin (Amoxil, Polymox) **Uses:** Infections resulting from susceptible gram+ bacteria (streptococci) and gram– bacteria (*H. influenzae, E. coli, P. mirabilis*) **Action:** β-Lactam antibiotic; inhibits cell wall synthesis **Dose:** *Adults.* 250–500 mg PO tid or 500–875 mg bid. *Peds.* 25–100 mg/kg/24 h PO ÷ q8h. 200–400 mg PO bid (equivalent to

125–250 mg tid); ↓ in renal impairment **Caution/Contra:** [B, +] **Supplied:** Caps 250, 500 mg; chew tabs 125, 200, 250, 400 mg; susp 50 mg/mL, 125, 250 mg/5 mL; tabs 500, 875 mg **Notes/SE:** Cross-hypersensitivity with penicillin; diarrhea; skin rash common; many hospital strains of *E. coli* are resistant

Amoxicillin and Clavulanic Acid (Augmentin, Augmentin 600 ES, Augmentin XR) **Uses:** Infections caused by β-lactamase-producing *H. influenzae, S. aureus,* and *E. coli;* XR used for acute bacterial sinusitis and CAP **Action:** Combination of a β-lactam antibiotic and a β-lactamase inhibitor **Dose:** *Adults.* 250–500 mg PO q8h or 875 mg q12h; XR 2000 mg PO q12h. *Peds.* 20–40 mg/kg/d as amoxicillin PO ÷ q8h or 45 mg/kg/d ÷ q12h; ↓ in renal impairment; take with food **Caution/Contra:** [B, ?] **Supplied** (expressed as amoxicillin/clavulanic acid): Tabs 250/125, 500/125, 875/125 mg; chew tabs 125/31.25, 200/28.5, 250/62.5, 400/57 mg; susp 125/31.25, 250/62.5, 200/28.5, 400/57 mg/5 mL;600-ES 600/42.9 mg tab; XR tab 1000/62.5 mg **Notes/SE:** Do NOT substitute two 250-mg tabs for one 500-mg tab or an overdose of clavulanic acid will occur; abdominal discomfort, N/V/D, allergic reaction, vaginitis

Amphotericin B (Fungizone) **Uses:** Severe, systemic fungal infections; oral and cutaneous candidiasis **Action:** Binds ergosterol in the fungal membrane, altering membrane permeability **Dose:** *Adults & Peds.* 1 mg adults or 0.1 mg/kg to 1 mg in children, then 0.25–1.5 mg/kg/24 h IV over 2–6 h (range 25–50 mg/d or qod). Total dose varies with indication. *Oral:* 1 mL qid. *Topical:* Apply bid–qid for 1–4 wk depending on infection; ↓ in renal impairment **Caution/Contra:** [B, ?] **Supplied:** Powder for inj 50 mg/vial, oral susp 100 mg/mL, cream, lotion, oint 3% **Notes/SE:** Monitor renal function/LFTs; ↓ K+/↓ Mg^{2+} from renal wasting; anaphylaxis reported; pretreatment with APAP and antihistamines (Benadryl) helps minimize adverse effects with IV inf (eg, fever, chills, HA, nephrotoxicity, hypotension, anemia)

Amphotericin B Cholesteryl (Amphotec) **Uses:** Refractory invasive fungal infection in persons intolerant to conventional amphotericin B **Action:** Binds to sterols in the cell membrane, alters membrane permeability **Dose:** *Adults & Peds.* Test dose 1.6–8.3 mg, over 15–20 min, followed by a dose of 3–4 mg/kg/d; 1 mg/kg/h inf; ↓ in renal insufficiency **Caution/Contra:** [B, ?] **Supplied:** Powder for inj 50 mg, 100 mg/vial (final conc 0.6 mg/mL) **Notes/SE:** Anaphylaxis reported; do not use in-line filter; monitor LFT and electrolytes; fever, chills, HA, ↓ K+, ↓ Mg, nephrotoxicity,↓ BP anemia

Amphotericin B Lipid Complex (Abelcet) **Uses:** Refractory invasive fungal infection in persons intolerant to conventional amphotericin B **Action:** Binds to sterols in the cell membrane, alters membrane permeability **Dose:** 5 mg/kg/d IV as a single daily dose; 2.5 mg/kg/h inf **Supplied:** Inj 5 mg/mL **Caution/Contra:** [B, ?] **Notes/SE:** Anaphylaxis reported; filter soln with a 5-mm filter needle; do not mix in electrolyte-containing solns. If inf >2 h, manually mix bag; fever, chills, HA, ↓ K+, ↓ Mg, nephrotoxicity, hypotension, anemia

Amphotericin B Liposomal (AmBisome) **Uses:** Refractory invasive fungal infection in persons intolerant to conventional amphotericin B **Action:** Binds to sterols in the cell membrane, resulting in changes in membrane permeability **Dose:** *Adults & Peds.* 3–5 mg/kg/d, infused over 60–120 min; ↓ in renal insufficiency **Caution/Contra:** [B, ?] **Supplied:** Powder for inj 50 mg **Notes/SE:** Anaphylaxis reported; filter with no less than 1 μm filter; fever, chills, HA, ↓K+, ↓ Mg^{2+} nephrotoxicity, hypotension, anemia

Ampicillin (Amcill, Omnipen) **Uses:** Susceptible gram– (*Shigella, Salmonella, E. coli, H. influenzae,* and *P. mirabilis*) and gram+ (streptococci) bacteria **Action:** β-Lactam antibiotic; inhibits cell wall synthesis **Dose:** *Adults.* 500 mg–2 g IM or IV q6h or 250–500 mg PO q6h. *Peds. Neonates <7 d:* 50–100 mg/kg/24 h IV ÷ q8h. *Term Infants:* 75–150 mg/kg/24 h ÷ q6–8h IV or PO. *Children >1 mon:* 100–200 mg/kg/24 h ÷ q4–6h IM or IV; 50–100 mg/kg/24 h ÷ q6h PO up to 250 mg/dose. *Meningitis:* 200–400 mg/kg/24 h ÷ q4–6h IV; ↓ in renal impairment, take on an empty stomach **Caution/Contra:** [B, M] Cross-hypersensitivity with penicillin **Supplied:** Caps 250, 500 mg; susp 100 mg/mL (reconstituted as drops), 125 mg/5 mL, 250 mg/5 mL, 500 mg/5 mL; powder for inj 125 mg, 250 mg, 500 mg, 1 g, 2 g, 10 g/vial **Notes/SE:** Diarrhea, skin rash, allergic reaction; many hospital strains of *E. coli* now resistant

Ampicillin-Sulbactam (Unasyn) **Uses:** Infections caused by β-lactamase-producing strains of *S. aureus, Enterococcus, H. influenzae, P. mirabilis,* and *Bacteroides* spp **Ac-**

tion: Combination of a β-lactam antibiotic and a β-lactamase inhibitor **Dose:** *Adults.* 1.5–3.0 g IM or IV q6h. *Peds.* 100–200 mg ampicillin/kg/d (150–300 mg Unasyn) q6h; ↓ in renal impairment; take on an empty stomach **Caution/Contra:** [B, M] **Supplied:** Powder for inj 1.5, 3.0 g/vial **Notes/SE:** A 2:1 ratio of ampicillin: sulbactam; ↓ in renal failure; hypersensitivity reactions, rash, diarrhea, pain at inj site

Amprenavir (Agenerase)   WARNING: Oral soln contra in children <4 y due to potential toxicity from large vol of excipient polypropylene glycol in the formulation **Uses:** HIV infection **Action:** Protease inhibitor; prevents the maturation of the virion to mature viral particle **Dose:** *Adults.* 1200 mg bid. *Peds.* 20 mg/kg bid or 15 mg/kg tid up to 2400 mg/d **Caution/Contra:** [C, ?] CDC recommends HIV-infected mothers not breast-feed due to risk of transmission of HIV to infant; previous allergic reaction to sulfonamides **Supplied:** Caps 50, 150 mg; soln 15 mg/mL **Notes/SE:** Caps and soln contain vitamin E exceeding RDA intake amounts; avoid high-fat meals with administration; many drug interactions; life-threatening rash, hyperglycemia, hypertriglyceridemia, fat redistribution, N/V/D, depression

Amrinone [Inamrinone] (Inocor) **Uses:** Short-term Rx low cardiac output states and pulmonary HTN **Action:** Positive inotropic with vasodilator activity **Dose:** *Adults & Peds.* Initial IV bolus 0.75 mg/kg over 2–3 min, then maint dose 5–10 mcg/ kg/min; 10 mg/kg/d max; ↓ if ClCr <10 mL/min **Caution/Contra:** [C, ?] Hypersensitivity to sulfites **Supplied:** Inj 5 mg/mL **Notes/SE:** Incompatible with dextrose-containing solns; monitor for fluid, electrolyte, and renal changes

Anakinra (Kineret)   WARNING: Associated with ↑ incidence of serious infections; DC with serious infection **Uses:** Reduce signs and symptoms of moderately to severely active RA, failed 1 or more disease-modifying antirheumatic drugs **Action:** Human IL-1 receptor antagonist **Dose:** 100 mg SC qd **Caution/Contra:** [B, ?]. Contra hypersensitivity to *E. coli*-derived proteins, active infection, <18 y **Supplied:** 100 mg prefilled syringes **Notes/SE:** Neutropenia especially when used with TNF-blocking agents, inj site reactions, infections

Anastrozole (Arimidex) **Uses:** Breast CA: postmenopausal women with metastatic breast CA, adjuvant treatment of postmenopausal women with early hormone-receptor-positive breast CA. **Action:** Selective nonsteroidal aromatase inhibitor, ↓ circulating estradiol **Dose:** 1 mg/d **Caution/Contra:** [C, ?] **Supplied:** Tabs 1 mg **Notes/SE:** No detectable effect on adrenal corticosteroids or aldosterone; may ↑ cholesterol levels; diarrhea, hypertension, flushing, ↑ bone and tumor pain, HA, somnolence

Anistreplase (Eminase) **Uses:** AMI **Action:** Thrombolytic agent; activates the conversion of plasminogen to plasmin, promoting thrombolysis **Dose:** 30 U IV over 2–5 min **Caution/Contra:** [C, ?] Active internal bleeding, Hx CVA, recent (<2 mon) intracranial or intraspinal surgery or trauma, intracranial neoplasm, AV malformation, aneurysm, bleeding diathesis, severe uncontrolled HTN; may not be effective if readministered >5 d after the previous dose of anistreplase or streptokinase, or streptococcal infection because of the production of antistreptokinase antibody. **Supplied:** Vials containing 30 U **Notes/SE:** Bleeding, hypotension, hematoma

Anthralin (Anthra-Derm) **Uses:** Psoriasis **Action:** Keratolytic **Dose:** Apply qd **Caution/Contra:** [C, ?] Acutely inflamed psoriatic eruptions, use on face or genitalia **Supplied:** Cream, oint 0.1, 0.2, 0.25, 0.4, 0.5, 1% **Notes/SE:** Irritation; discoloration of hair, fingernails, skin

Antihemophilic Factor [Factor VIII] [AHF] (Monoclate) **Uses:** Classical hemophilia A **Action:** Provides factor VIII needed to convert prothrombin to thrombin **Dose:** *Adults & Peds.* 1 AHF unit/kg ↑ factor VIII level ≅2%. Units required = (kg) (desired factor VIII ↑ as % normal) × (0.5). Prophylax spontaneous hemorrhage = 5% normal. Hemostasis after trauma/surgery = 30% normal. Head injuries, major surgery, or bleeding = 80–100% normal. Determine patient's % of normal factor VIII before dosing **Caution/Contra:** [C, ?] **Supplied:** Check each vial for units contained **Notes/SE:** Not effective in controlling bleeding in von Willebrand's disease; rash, fever, HA, chills, N/V

Apraclonidine (Iopidine) **Uses:** Glaucoma **Action:** α_2-Adrenergic agonist **Dose:** 1–2 gtt of 0.5% tid **Caution/Contra:** [C, ?] **Supplied:** 0.5, 1.0% soln **Notes/SE:** Ocular irritation, lethargy, xerostomia

Aprotinin (Trasylol) Uses: Reduce/prevent blood loss in patients undergoing CABG **Action:** Protease inhibitor, antifibrinolytic **Dose:** 1-mL IV test dose to assess for allergic reaction. *High dose:* 2 million KIU load, 2 million KIU to prime pump, then 500,000 KIU/h until surgery ends. *Low dose:* 1 million KIU load, 1 million KIU to prime pump, then 250,000 KIU/h until surgery ends. 7 million KIU max total **Caution/Contra:** [B, ?] Thromboembolic disease requiring anticoagulants or blood factor administration **Supplied:** Inj 1.4 mg/mL (10,000 KIU/mL) **Notes/SE:** 1000/KIU = 0.14 mg of aprotinin. AF, MI, heart failure, dyspnea, postoperative renal dysfunction

Ardeparin (Normiflo) Uses: Prevent DVT/PE following knee replacement **Action:** LMW heparin **Dose:** 35–50 U/kg SC q12h. Begin day of surgery, continue up to 14 d; caution in ↓ renal function **Caution/Contra:** [C, ?] Active hemorrhage; hypersensitivity to pork products **Supplied:** Inj 5000, 10,000 IU/0.5 mL **Notes/SE:** Laboratory monitoring usually not necessary; bleeding, bruising, thrombocytopenia, pain at inj site, ↑ serum transaminases

Argatroban (Acova) Uses: Prophylaxis or Rx of thrombosis in HIT **Action:** Anticoagulant, direct thrombin inhibitor **Dose:** 2 mcg/kg/min IV; adjust until aPTT 1.5–3× baseline value not to exceed 100 s; 10 mcg/kg/min max; ↓ in hepatic impairment. **Caution/Contra:** [B, ?]. Avoid oral anticoagulants, ↑ risk of bleeding; avoid concomitant use of thrombolytics **Supplied:** Inj 100 mg/mL **Notes/SE:** AF, cardiac arrest, cerebrovascular disorder, hypotension, VT, N/V/D, sepsis, cough, renal toxicity, ↓ Hgb

Aripiprazole (Abilify) Uses: Atypical antipsychotic used in the treatment of schizophrenia **Action:** Dopamine and serotonin antagonist **Dose:** *Adults:* 10-15 mg PO qd; ↓ when used in combination with potent CYP3A4 or CYP2D6 inhibitors; ↑ when used in combination with inducer of CYP3A4 **Caution/Contra:** [C, –] **Supplied:** Tabs 10, 15, 20, 30 mg **Notes/SE:;** Neuroleptic malignant syndrome, tardive dyskinesia, orthostatic hypotension, cognitive and motor impairment

Artificial Tears (Tears Naturale) Uses: Dry eyes **Action:** Ocular lubricant **Dose:** 1–2 gtt tid–qid **Supplied:** OTC soln

ʟ-Asparaginase (Elspar, Oncaspar) Uses: ALL (in combination with other agents) **Action:** Protein synthesis inhibitor **Dose:** 500–20,000 IU/m²/d for 1–14 d (refer to specific protocols) **Caution/Contra:** [C, ?] Active or Hx pancreatitis **Supplied:** Inj 10,000 IU **Notes/SE:** Hypersensitivity reactions in 20–35% (spectrum of urticaria to anaphylaxis), test dose recommended; rare GI toxicity (mild nausea/anorexia, pancreatitis)

Aspirin (Bayer, St. Joseph) Uses: Mild pain, HA, fever, inflammation, prevention of emboli, and prevention of MI **Action:** Prostaglandin inhibitor **Dose:** *Adults. Pain, fever:* 325–650 mg q4–6h PO or PR. *RA:* 3–6 g/d PO in ÷ doses. *Platelet inhibitory action:* 81–325 mg PO qd. *Prevention of MI:* 81–325 mg PO qd. *Peds.* Caution: Use linked to Reye's syndrome; avoid use with viral illness in children. *Antipyretic:* 10–15 mg/kg/dose PO or PR q4h up to 80 mg/kg/24 h. *RA:* 60–100 mg/kg/24 h PO ÷ q4–6h (monitor serum levels to maintain between 15 and 30 mg/dL); avoid use with CrCl <10 mL/min and in severe liver disease; avoid or limit alcohol intake **Caution/Contra:** [C, M] Allergy to ASA **Supplied:** Tabs 325, 500 mg; chew tabs 81 mg; EC tabs 165, 325, 500, 650, 975 mg; SR tabs 650, 800 mg; effervescent tabs 325, 500 mg; supp 120, 200, 300, 600 mg **Notes/SE:** GI upset and erosion common adverse reactions; DC use 1 wk prior to surgery to avoid postoperative bleeding complications

Aspirin and Butalbital Compound (Fiorinal) [C-III] Uses: Tension HA, pain **Action:** Combination barbiturate and analgesic **Dose:** 1–2 PO q4h PRN, max 6 tabs/d; avoid use with CrCl <10 mL/min and in severe liver disease; avoid or limit alcohol intake **Caution/Contra:** [C (D if used for prolonged periods or high doses at term), ?] **Supplied:** Caps Fiorgen PF, Fiorinal. Tabs Fiorinal, Lanorinal: ASA 325 mg/butalbital 50 mg/caffeine 40 mg **Notes/SE:** Butalbital habit-forming; drowsiness, dizziness, GI upset, ulceration, bleeding

Aspirin + Butalbital, Caffeine, and Codeine (Fiorinal + Codeine) [C-III] Uses: Mild pain; HA, especially when associated with stress **Action:** Sedative analgesic, narcotic analgesic **Dose:** 1–2 tabs (caps) PO q4–6h PRN **Caution/Contra:** [D, ?] **Supplied:** Each cap or tab contains 325 mg ASA, 40 mg caffeine, 50 mg of butalbital, codeine **Notes/SE:** Drowsiness, dizziness, GI upset, ulceration, bleeding

22

Aspirin + Codeine (Empirin No. 2, No. 3, No. 4) [C-III]   **Uses:** Mild–moderate pain **Action:** Combined effects of ASA and codeine **Dose:** *Adults.* 1–2 tabs PO q4–6h PRN. *Peds.* ASA 10 mg/kg/dose; codeine 0.5–1.0 mg/kg/dose q4h **Caution/Contra:** [M] **Supplied:** Tabs 325 mg of ASA and codeine as in Notes **Notes/SE:** Codeine in No. 2 = 15 mg, No. 3 = 30 mg, No. 4 = 60 mg; drowsiness, dizziness, GI upset, ulceration, bleeding

Atenolol (Tenormin)   **Uses:** HTN, angina, MI **Action:** Competitively blocks β-adrenergic receptors, β_1 **Dose:** *HTN and angina:* 50–100 mg/d PO. *AMI:* 5 mg IV ×2 over 10 min, then 50 mg PO bid if tolerated; adjust in renal impairment **Caution/Contra:** [D, M] Contra bradycardia, pulmonary edema; caution in DM, bronchospasm; abrupt DC can exacerbate angina and occurrence of MI **Supplied:** Tabs 25, 50, 100 mg; inj 5 mg/10 mL **Notes/SE:** Bradycardia, hypotension, 2nd- or 3rd-degree AV block, dizziness, fatigue

Atenolol and Chlorthalidone (Tenoretic)   **Uses:** HTN **Action:** β-Adrenergic blockade with diuretic **Dose:** 50–100 mg/d PO; ↓ in renal impairment **Caution/Contra:** [D, M] Contra bradycardia, pulmonary edema; caution in DM, bronchospasm **Supplied:** *Tenoretic 50:* Atenolol 50 mg/chlorthalidone 25 mg; *Tenoretic 100:* Atenolol 100 mg/chlorthalidone 25 mg **Notes/SE:** Bradycardia, hypotension, 2nd- or 3rd-degree AV block, dizziness, fatigue, hypokalemia, photosensitivity

Atomoxetine (Strattera)   **Uses:** Treatment of ADHD **Action:** Selective norepinephrine reuptake inhibitor **Dose:** *Adults and children* >70 kg: 40 mg × 3 days, then ↑ to 80–100 mg ÷ qd–bid; Peds ≤ 70 kg: 0.5 mg/kg × 3 days, then ↑ to max of 1.2 mg/kg given qd or bid. **Caution/Contra:** [C, ? /–] Narrow-angle glaucoma, use with or within 2 wk of discontinuing an MAOI **Supplied:** Caps 10, 18, 25, 40, 60 mg **Notes/SE:** ↓ dose with hepatic insufficiency; ↓ dose when used in combination with inhibitors of CYP2D6; HTN, tachycardia, weight loss, sexual dysfunction

Atorvastatin (Lipitor)   **Uses:** ↑ cholesterol and triglycerides **Action:** HMG-CoA reductase inhibitor **Dose:** Initial dose 10 mg/d, may be ↑ to 80 mg/d **Caution/Contra:** [X, –]. Active liver disease, unexplained persistent elevation of serum transaminases **Supplied:** Tabs 10, 20, 40, 80 mg **Notes/SE:** May cause myopathy, monitor LFTs regularly; HA, arthralgia, myalgia, GI upset

Atovaquone (Mepron)   **Uses:** Rx and prevention mild to moderate PCP **Action:** Inhibits nucleic acid and ATP synthesis **Dose:** *Rx:* 750 mg PO bid for 21 d. *Prevention:* 1500 mg PO once/d; take with meals **Caution/Contra:** [C, ?] **Supplied:** Suspension 750 mg/5 mL **Notes/SE:** Fever, HA, anxiety, insomnia, rash, N/V

Atovaquone/Proguanil (Malarone)   **Uses:** Prevention or Rx uncomplicated *P. falciparum* malaria **Action:** Antimalarial **Dose:** *Adult: Prevention:* 1 tab PO 2 d before, during, and 7 d after leaving endemic region; *Treatment:* 4 tabs PO as single dose qd ×3 d. *Peds.* See insert **Caution/Contra:** [C, ?]. **Supplied:** Tab atovaquone 250 mg/proguanil 100 mg; Ped 62.5/25 mg **Notes/SE:** HA, fever, myalgia

Atracurium (Tracrium)   **Uses:** Adjunct to anesthesia to facilitate ET intubation **Action:** Nondepolarizing neuromuscular blocker **Dose:** *Adults & Peds.* 0.4–0.5 mg/kg IV bolus, then 0.08–0.1 mg/kg q20–45min PRN **Caution/Contra:** [C, ?] **Supplied:** Inj 10 mg/mL **Notes/SE:** Patient must be intubated and on controlled ventilation. Use adequate amounts of sedation and analgesia; flushing

Atropine   **Uses:** Preanesthetic; symptomatic bradycardia and asystole **Action:** Antimuscarinic agent; blocks acetylcholine at parasympathetic sites **Dose:** *Adults.* ECC: 0.5–1.0 mg IV q3–5min. *Preanesthetic:* 0.3–0.6 mg IM. *Peds.* ECC: 0.01—0.03 mg/kg IV q2–5min, max 1.0 mg, min dose 0.1 mg. *Preanesthetic:* 0.01 mg/kg/dose SC/IV (max 0.4 mg) **Caution/Contra:** [C, +] **Supplied:** Tabs 0.3, 0.4, 0.6 mg; inj 0.05, 0.1, 0.3, 0.4, 0.5, 0.8, 1 mg/mL; ophth 0.5, 1, 2% **Notes/SE:** Blurred vision, urinary retention, constipation, dried mucous membranes

Azathioprine (Imuran)   **Uses:** Adjunct for the prevention of rejection following organ transplantation; RA; SLE **Action:** Immunosuppressive agent; antagonizes purine metabolism **Dose:** *Adults & Peds.* 1–3 mg/kg/d IV or PO; reduce in renal failure **Caution/Contra:** [D, ?] **Supplied:** Tabs 50 mg; inj 100 mg/20 mL **Notes/SE:** GI intolerance, fever, chills, leukopenia, thrombocytopenia; chronic use may ↑ neoplasia; inj should be handled with cytotoxic precautions; interaction with allopurinol

Azithromycin (Zithromax) Uses: Community-acquired pneumonia, pharyngitis, otitis media, skin infections, nongonococcal urethritis, and PID; Rx and prevention of MAC in HIV **Action:** Macrolide antibiotic; inhibits protein synthesis **Dose: *Adults.*** *Oral: Respiratory tract infections:* 500 mg day 1, then 250 mg/d PO ×4 d. *Nongonococcal urethritis:* 1 g PO single dose. *Prevention of MAC:* 1200 mg PO once/wk. *IV:* 500 mg ×2 d, then 500 mg PO ×7–10 d. ***Peds.*** *Otitis media:* 10 mg/kg PO day 1, then 5 mg/kg/d days 2–5. *Pharyngitis:* 12 mg/kg/d PO ×5 d **Caution/Contra:** [B, +] **Supplied:** Tabs 250, 600 mg (Z-Pack 5-day regimen); susp 1-g single-dose packet; susp 100, 200 mg/5 mL; inj 500 mg **Notes/SE:** Take susp on an empty stomach; tabs may be taken w/wo food; GI upset

Aztreonam (Azactam) Uses: Aerobic gram– bacterial infections, including *P. aeruginosa* **Action:** Monobactam antibiotic; inhibits cell wall synthesis **Dose: *Adults.*** 1–2 g IV/IM q6–12h. ***Peds.*** *Premature infants:* 30 mg/kg/dose IV q12h. *Term infants, children:* 30 mg/kg/dose q6–8h; ↓ in renal impairment **Caution/Contra:** [B, +] **Supplied:** Inj 500 mg, 1 g, 2 g **Notes/SE:** No gram+ or anaerobic activity; may be given to penicillin-allergic patients; N/V/D, rash, pain at inj site

Bacitracin, Topical (Baciguent)
Bacitracin and Polymyxin B, Topical (Polysporin)
Bacitracin, Neomycin, and Polymyxin B, Topical (Neosporin Ointment)
Bacitracin, Neomycin, Polymyxin B, and Hydrocortisone, Topical (Cortisporin)

Bacitracin, Neomycin, Polymyxin B, and Lidocaine, Topical (Clomycin)
Uses: Prevention and Rx of minor cuts, scrapes, and burns **Action:** Topical antibiotic with added effects based on components (antiinflammatory and analgesic) **Dose:** Apply sparingly bid–qid **Caution/Contra:** [C, ?] **Supplied:** Bacitracin 500 U/g oint. Bacitracin 500 U/polymyxin B sulfate 10,000 U/g oint and powder. Bacitracin 400 U/neomycin 3.5 mg/polymyxin B 5000 U/g oint (for Neosporin Cream, see page 571). Bacitracin 400 U/neomycin 3.5 mg/polymyxin B/10,000 U/hydrocortisone 10 mg/g oint. Bacitracin 500 U/neomycin 3.5 g/ polymyxin B 5000 U/lidocaine 40 mg/g oint **Notes/SE:** Systemic and irrigation forms of bacitracin available but not generally used due to potential toxicity

Bacitracin, Ophthalmic (AK-Tracin Ophthalmic)
Bacitracin and Polymyxin B, Ophthalmic (AK-Poly-Bac Ophthalmic, Polysporin Ophthalmic)
Bacitracin, Neomycin, and Polymyxin B, Ophthalmic (AK Spore Ophthalmic, Neosporin Ophthalmic)

Bacitracin, Neomycin, Polymyxin B, and Hydrocortisone, Ophthalmic (AK Spore HC Ophthalmic, Cortisporin Ophthalmic) Uses: Blepharitis, conjunctivitis, prophylactic Rx of corneal abrasions **Action:** Topical antibiotic with added effects based on components (antiinflammatory) **Dose:** Apply q3–4h into conjunctival sac **Caution/Contra:** [C, ?] **Supplied:** See Topical equivalents, above

Baclofen (Lioresal) Uses: Spasticity secondary to severe chronic disorders, eg, MS or spinal cord lesions, trigeminal neuralgia **Action:** Centrally acting skeletal muscle relaxant; inhibits transmission of both monosynaptic and polysynaptic reflexes at the spinal cord **Dose: *Adults.*** Initially, 5 mg PO tid; ↑ q3d to max effect; max 80 mg/d. ***Peds.*** *2–7 y:* 10–15 mg/d ÷ q8h; titrate to effect or max of 40 mg/d. *>8 y:* Max of 60 mg/d. *IT:* Through implantable pump; ↓ in renal impairment; avoid abrupt withdrawal; take with food or milk **Caution/Contra:** [C, +] Use caution in epilepsy and neuropsychiatric disturbances; withdrawal may occur with abrupt DC **Supplied:** Tabs 10, 20 mg; IT inj 10 mg/20 mL, 10 mg/5 mL **Notes/SE:** Dizziness, drowsiness, insomnia, ataxia, weakness, hypotension

Balsalazide (Colazal) Uses: Mild–moderate ulcerative colitis **Action:** 5-Aminosalicylic acid derivative, antiinflammatory, ↓ leukotriene synthesis **Dose:** 2.25 g (3 caps) tid ×8–12 wk **Caution/Contra:** [B, ?] Contra in severe renal/hepatic failure **Supplied:** Caps 750 mg **Notes/SE:** Dizziness, HA, nausea, agranulocytosis, pancytopenia, renal impairment, allergic reactions

22

Basiliximab (Simulect) Uses: Prevention of acute organ transplant rejections **Action:** IL-2 receptor antagonists **Dose:** *Adults.* 20 mg IV 2 h prior to transplant, then 20 mg IV 4 d posttransplant. *Peds.* 12 mg/m^2 up to a max of 20 mg 2 h prior to transplant, then the same dose IV 4 d posttransplant **Caution/Contra:** [B, ?/–]. Known hypersensitivity to murine proteins **Supplied:** Inj 20 mg **Notes/SE:** Murine/human monoclonal antibody; edema, HTN, HA, dizziness, fever, pain, infection, GI effects, electrolyte disturbances

BCG [Bacillus Calmette-Guérin] (TheraCys, Tice BCG) Uses: Bladder carcinoma, TB prophylaxis **Action:** Immunomodulator **Dose:** Bladder CA, contents of 1 vial prepared and instilled in bladder for 2 h. Repeat once weekly for 6 wk; repeat 3 weekly doses 3, 6, 12, 18, and 24 mon after initial therapy **Caution/Contra:** [C, ?] <14 d after TURBT, Hx BCG sepsis, immunosuppression, steroid use **Supplied:** Inj 27 mg (3.4 + 3 × 10^8 CFU)/vial (TheraCys), 1–8 × 10^8 CFU/vial (Tice BCG) **Notes/SE:** *Intravesical:* Hematuria, urinary frequency, dysuria, bacterial UTI, rare BCG sepsis; routine U.S. adult BCG immunization not recommended; occasionally used in high-risk children who are PPD– and cannot take INH

Becaplermin (Regranex Gel) Uses: Adjunct to local wound care in diabetic foot ulcers **Action:** Recombinant PDGF, enhanced formation of granulation tissue **Dose:** Based on size of lesion; 1⅓ in. ribbon from 2-g tube, ⅔ in. ribbon from 7.5- or 15-mg tube/in.^{2} of ulcer; apply and cover with moist gauze; rinse after 12 h; do not reapply; repeat process 12 h later **Caution/Contra:** [C, ?] neoplasm or active infection at site **Supplied:** 0.01% gel in 2-, 7.5-, 15-g tubes **Notes/SE:** Use along with good wound care; wound must be vascularized; erythema, local pain

Beclomethasone (Beconase, Vancenase Nasal Inhaler) Uses: Allergic rhinitis refractory to conventional therapy with antihistamines and decongestants **Action:** Inhaled steroid **Dose:** *Adults.* 1 spray intranasally bid–qid; *aqueous inhal:* 1–2 sprays/nostril qd–bid. *Peds.* 6–12 y: 1 spray intranasally tid; **Caution/ Contra:** [C, ?] **Supplied:** Nasal met-dose inhaler **Notes/SE:** Nasal spray delivers 42 mcg/dose and 84 mcg/dose; local irritation, burning, epistaxis

Beclomethasone (Beclovent Inhaler, Vanceril Inhaler, QVAR) Uses: Chronic asthma **Action:** Inhaled corticosteroid **Dose:** *Adults.* 2–4 inhal tid–qid (max 20/d); Vanceril double strength: 2 inhal bid (max 10/d); QVAR: 1–4 inhal BID. *Peds.* 1–2 inhal tid–qid (max 10/d); Vanceril double strength: 2 inhal bid (max 5/d); QVAR: 1–4 inhal BID **Caution/Contra:** [C, ?] **Supplied:** Oral met-dose inhal; 42, 84 mcg/inhal; QVAR 40, 80 mcg/inhal **Notes/SE:** Rinse mouth/throat after use. Not effective for acute asthmatic attacks; HA, cough, hoarseness, oral candidiasis

Belladonna and Opium Suppositories (B & O Supprettes) [C-II] Uses: Bladder spasms; moderate/severe pain **Action:** Antispasmodic **Dose:** Insert 1 supp PR q6h PRN. 15A = 30 mg powdered opium/16.2 mg belladonna extract. 16A = 60 mg powdered opium/16.2 mg belladonna extract **Caution/Contra:** [C, ?] **Supplied:** Supp 15A, 16A **Notes/SE:** Anticholinergic side effects (sedation, urinary retention, and constipation)

Benazepril (Lotensin) Uses: HTN, DN, CHF **Action:** ACE inhibitor **Dose:** 10–40 mg/d PO **Caution/Contra:** [C (1st trimester), D (2nd and 3rd trimesters), +] **Supplied:** Tabs 5, 10, 20, 40 mg **Notes/SE:** Symptomatic hypotension with diuretics; dizziness, HA, hyperkalemia, nonproductive cough

Benzocaine and Antipyrine (Auralgan) Uses: Analgesia in severe otitis media **Action:** Anesthetic and local decongestant **Dose:** Fill the ear and insert a moist cotton plug; repeat 1–2 h PRN **Caution/Contra:** [C, ?] **Supplied:** Soln **Notes/SE:** Do not use with perforated eardrum; local irritation

Benzonatate (Tessalon Perles) Uses: Symptomatic relief of cough **Action:** Anesthetizes the stretch receptors in the respiratory passages **Dose:** *Adults & Peds >10 y.* 100 mg PO tid **Caution/Contra:** [C, ?] **Supplied:** Caps 100 mg **Notes/SE:** Do not chew or puncture the caps; sedation, dizziness, GI upset

Benztropine (Cogentin) Uses: Parkinsonism and drug-induced extrapyramidal disorders **Action:** Partially blocks striatal cholinergic receptors **Dose:** *Adults.* 0.5–6 mg PO, IM, or IV in ÷ doses/d. *Peds. >3 y.* 0.02–0.05 mg/kg/dose 1–2/d **Caution/Contra:** [C, ?] **Supplied:** Tabs 0.5, 1.0, 2.0 mg; inj 1 mg/mL **Notes/SE:** Anticholinergic side effects; physostigmine 1–2 mg SC/IV can reverse severe symptoms

Bepridil (Vascor) **Uses:** Chronic stable angina **Action:** Ca channel-blocking agent **Dose:** 200–400 mg/d PO **Caution/Contra:** [C, ?] QT interval prolongation, Hx ventricular arrhythmias, sick sinus syndrome, hypotension (DBP <90 mm Hg) **Supplied:** Tabs 200, 300, 400 mg **Notes/SE:** Dizziness, nausea, agranulocytosis, bradycardia, and serious ventricular arrhythmias, including torsades de pointes

Beractant (Survanta) **Uses:** Prevention and Rx of RDS in premature infants **Action:** Replacement of pulmonary surfactant **Dose:** 100 mg/kg administered via ET tube. May be repeated 3 more × q6h for a max of 4 doses/48 h **Caution/Contra:** [N/A, N/A] **Supplied:** Suspension 25 mg of phospholipid/mL **Notes/SE:** Administer via 4-quadrant method; transient bradycardia, oxygen desaturation, apnea

Betaxolol (Kerlone) **Uses:** HTN **Action:** Competitively blocks β-adrenergic receptors, $β_1$ **Caution/Contra:** [C (1st trimester), D (2nd or 3rd trimester), +/–]. Sinus bradycardia, AV conduction abnormalities, cardiac failure **Dose:** 10–20 mg/d **Supplied:** Tabs 10, 20 mg **Notes/SE:** Dizziness, HA, bradycardia, edema, CHF

Betaxolol, Ophthalmic (Betoptic) **Uses:** Glaucoma **Action:** Competitively blocks β-adrenergic receptors, $β_1$ **Dose:** 1 gt bid **Caution/Contra:** [C (1st trimester), D (2nd or 3rd trimester), ?/–] **Supplied:** Soln 0.5%; susp 0.25% **Notes/SE:** Local irritation, photophobia

Bethanechol (Urecholine, Duvoid, others) **Uses:** Neurogenic bladder atony with retention, acute postoperative and postpartum functional (nonobstructive) urinary retention **Action:** Stimulates cholinergic smooth muscle receptors in bladder and GI tract **Dose:** *Adults.* 10–50 mg PO tid–qid or 2.5–5 mg SC tid–qid and PRN. *Peds.* 0.6 mg/kg/24 h PO ÷ tid–qid or 0.15–2 mg/kg/d SC ÷ 3–4×; on empty stomach **Caution/Contra:** [C, ?/–]. Bladder outlet obstruction, PUD, epilepsy, hyperthyroidism, bradycardia, COPD, AV conduction defects, parkinsonism, hypotension, vasomotor instability **Supplied:** Tabs 5, 10, 25, 50 mg; inj 5 mg/mL **Notes/SE:** Do not administer IM or IV; abdominal cramps, diarrhea, salivation, hypotension

Bicalutamide (Casodex) **Uses:** Advanced prostate CA (in combination with GnRH agonists such as leuprolide or goserelin) **Action:** Nonsteroidal antiandrogen **Dose:** 50 mg/d **Caution/Contra:** [X, ?] **Supplied:** Caps 50 mg **Notes/SE:** Hot flashes, loss of libido, impotence, diarrhea, N/V, gynecomastia, and LFT ↑

Bicarbonate (See Sodium Bicarbonate, page 590)

Bisacodyl (Dulcolax) **Uses:** Constipation; preoperative bowel preparation **Action:** Stimulates peristalsis **Dose:** *Adults.* 5–15 mg PO or 10 mg PR PRN. *Peds.*<2 y: 5 mg PR PRN. >2 y: 5 mg PO or 10 mg PR PRN; do not chew tabs; do not give within 1 h of antacids or milk **Caution/Contra:** [B, ?] Acute abdomen or bowel obstruction **Supplied:** EC tabs 5 mg; supp 10 mg **Notes/SE:** Abdominal cramps, proctitis, and inflammation with suppositories

Bismuth Subsalicylate (Pepto-Bismol) **Uses:** N/V/D; combination for treatment of *H. pylori* infection **Action:** Antisecretory and antiinflammatory effects **Dose:** *Adults.* 2 tabs or 30 mL PO PRN (max 8 doses/24 h). *Peds.* 3–6 y: 1/3 tab or 5 mL PO PRN (max 8 doses/24 h). 6–9 y: 2/3 tab or 10 mL PO PRN (max 8 doses/24 h). 9–12 y: 1 tab or 15 mL PO PRN (max 8 doses/24 h); avoid in patients with renal failure **Caution/Contra:** [C, D (3rd trimester), –] Contra with influenza or chickenpox (↑ risk of Reye's syndrome) **Supplied:** Chew tabs 262 mg; liq 262, 524 mg/15 mL **Notes/SE:** May turn tongue and stools black

Bisoprolol (Zebeta) **Uses:** HTN **Action:** Competitively blocks $β_1$-adrenergic receptors, **Dose:** 5–10 mg/d (max dose 20 mg/d); ↓ in renal impairment **Caution/Contra:** [C (D 2nd and 3rd trimesters), +/–]. Sinus bradycardia, AV conduction abnormalities, cardiac failure **Supplied:** Tabs 5, 10 mg **Notes/SE:** Fatigue, lethargy, HA, bradycardia, edema, CHF; not dialyzed

Bitolterol (Tornalate) **Uses:** Prophylaxis and Rx of asthma and reversible bronchospasm **Action:** Sympathomimetic bronchodilator; stimulates $β_2$-adrenergic receptors in the lungs **Dose:** *Adults & Peds >12 y.* 2 inhal q8h **Caution/Contra:** [C, ?] **Supplied:** Aerosol 0.8% **Notes/SE:** Dizziness, nervousness, trembling, HTN, palpitations

Bivalirudin (Angiomax) **Uses:** Anticoagulant used with ASA in unstable angina undergoing PTCA **Action:** Anticoagulant, direct thrombin inhibitor **Dose:** 1 mg/kg IV bolus, then 2.5 mg/kg/h over 4 h; if needed, use 0.2 mg/kg/h for up to 20 h; give with aspirin 300–325 mg/day; start pre-PTCA **Caution/Contra:** [B, ?] Contra in major bleeding **Supplied:** Powder for inj **Notes/SE:** Bleeding, back pain, nausea, HA

Bleomycin Sulfate (Blenoxane) **Uses:** Testicular carcinomas; Hodgkin's and NHLs; cutaneous lymphomas; and squamous cell carcinomas of the head and neck, larynx, cervix, skin, penis; sclerosing agent for malignant pleural effusion **Action:** Induces breakage (scission) of single- and double-stranded DNA **Dose:** 10–20 mg (U)/m^2 1–2/wk (refer to specific protocols); ↓ in renal impairment **Supplied:** Inj 15 mg (15 U) **Caution/Contra:** [D, ?] Contra severe pulmonary disease **Notes/SE:** Hyperpigmentation (skin staining) and hypersensitivity (rash to anaphylaxis); test dose of 1 mg (U) recommended, especially in lymphoma patients; fever in 50%; lung toxicity (idiosyncratic and dose-related); pneumonitis may progress to fibrosis; lung toxicity likely when the total dose >400 mg (U); Raynaud's phenomenon, N/V

Brimonidine (Alphagan) **Uses:** Open-angle glaucoma **Action:** α_2-Adrenergic agonist **Dose:** 1 gtt in eye(s) tid; wait 15 min to insert contacts **Caution/Contra:** [B, ?] MAOI therapy **Supplied:** 0.2% soln **Notes/SE:** Local irritation, HA, fatigue

Brinzolamide (Azopt) **Uses:** Open-angle glaucoma **Action:** Carbonic anhydrase inhibitor **Dose:** 1 gtt in eye(s) tid **Caution/Contra:** [C, ?] **Supplied:** 1.0% susp **Notes/SE:** Blurred vision, dry eye, blepharitis, taste disturbance

Bromocriptine (Parlodel) **Uses:** Parkinson's syndrome, hyperprolactinemia, acromegaly **Action:** Direct-acting on the striatal dopamine receptors; ↓ prolactin secretion **Dose:** Initially, 1.25 mg PO bid; titrate to effect **Caution/Contra:** [C, ?] Severe ischemic heart disease or peripheral vascular disease **Supplied:** Tabs 2.5 mg; caps 5 mg **Notes/SE:** Hypotension, Raynaud's phenomenon, dizziness, nausea, hallucinations

Budesonide (Rhinocort, Pulmicort) **Uses:** Allergic and nonallergic rhinitis, asthma **Action:** Steroid **Dose:** *Intranasal:* 2 sprays/nostril bid or 4 sprays/nostril/d. *Aqueous:* 1 spray/nostril/d. *Oral inhaled:* 1–4 inhal bid. *Peds.* 1–2 inhal bid; rinse mouth after oral use **Caution/Contra:** [C, ?/–] **Supplied:** Met-dose Turbuhaler, nasal inhaler, and aqueous spray **Notes/SE:** HA, cough, hoarseness, *Candida* infection, epistaxis

Bumetanide (Bumex) **Uses:** Edema from CHF, hepatic cirrhosis, and renal disease **Action:** Loop diuretic; inhibits reabsorption of Na and chloride in the ascending loop of Henle and the distal renal tubule **Dose:** *Adults.* 0.5–2 mg/d PO; 0.5–1 mg IV q8–24h (max 10 mg/d). *Peds.* 0.015–0.1 mg/kg/d PO, IV, or IM ÷ q6–24h **Caution/Contra:** [D, ?] Anuria or increasing azotemia **Supplied:** Tabs 0.5, 1, 2 mg; inj 0.25 mg/mL **Notes/SE:** Monitor fluid and electrolyte status during treatment; hypokalemia, hyperuricemia, hypochloremia, hyponatremia, dizziness, ↑ serum creatinine, ototoxicity

Bupivacaine (Marcaine) **Uses:** Peripheral nerve block **Action:** Local anesthetic **Dose:** *Adults & Peds.* Dose-dependent on procedure (ie, tissue vascularity, depth of anesthesia, etc) (Table 3, page 611) **Caution/Contra:** [C, ?] **Supplied:** Inj 0.25, 0.5, 0.75% **Notes/SE:** Hypotension, bradycardia, dizziness, anxiety

Buprenorphine (Buprenex) [C-V] **Uses:** Moderate/severe pain **Action:** Opiate agonist–antagonist **Dose:** 0.3–0.6 mg IM or slow IV push q6h PRN **Caution/Contra:** [C, ?/–] **Supplied:** Inj 0.324 mg/mL (= 0.3 mg of buprenorphine) **Notes/SE:** May induce withdrawal syndrome in opioid-dependent patients; sedation, hypotension, respiratory depression

Bupropion (Wellbutrin, Wellbutrin SR, Zyban) **Uses:** Depression, adjunct to smoking cessation **Action:** Weak inhibitor of neuronal uptake of serotonin and norepinephrine; inhibits the neuronal reuptake of dopamine **Dose:** *Depression:* 100–450 mg/d ÷ bid–tid. *Smoking cessation:* 150 mg/d × 3 d, then 150 mg bid ×8–12 wk; ↓ in renal/hepatic impairment **Caution/Contra:** [B, ?/–]. Seizure disorder, prior diagnosis of anorexia nervosa or bulimia **Supplied:** Tabs 75, 100 mg; SR tabs 100, 150 mg **Notes/SE:** Associated with seizures; avoid use of alcohol and other CNS depressants; agitation, insomnia, HA, tachycardia

Buspirone (BuSpar) **Uses:** Short-term relief of anxiety **Action:** Antianxiety agent; selectively antagonizes CNS serotonin receptors **Dose:** 5–10 mg PO tid; ↑ to desired response; usual dose 20–30 mg/d; max 60 mg/d; ↓ in severe hepatic/renal insufficiency

22

Caution/Contra: [B, ?/–] **Supplied:** Tabs 5, 10, 15 mg **Notes/SE:** No abuse potential or physical or psychologic dependence; drowsiness, dizziness; HA, nausea

Busulfan (Myleran, Busulfex)
Uses: CML, preparative regimens for allogeneic and ABMT in high doses **Action:** Alkylating agent **Dose:** 4–12 mg/d for several wk; 16 mg/kg once or 4 mg/kg/d for 4 d in conjunction with another agent in transplant regimens. Refer to specific protocol **Caution/Contra:** [D, ?] **Supplied:** Tabs 2 mg, inj 60 mg/10 mL **Notes/SE:** Myelosuppression, pulmonary fibrosis, nausea (high-dose therapy), gynecomastia, adrenal insufficiency, and skin hyperpigmentation

Butorphanol (Stadol) [C-IV]
Uses: Moderate–severe pain and HAs **Action:** Opiate agonist–antagonist with central analgesic actions **Dose:** 1–4 mg IM or IV q3–4h PRN. *HAs:* 1 spray in 1 nostril, may repeat ×1 if pain not relieved in 60–90 min; ↓ in renal impairment **Caution/Contra:** [C (D if used in high doses or for prolonged periods at term), +] **Supplied:** Inj 1, 2 mg/mL; nasal spray 10 mg/ mL **Notes/SE:** Drowsiness, dizziness, nasal congestion; may induce withdrawal in opioid-dependent patients

Calcipotriene (Dovonex)
Uses: Plaque psoriasis **Action:** Keratolytic **Dose:** Apply bid **Caution/Contra:** [C, ?] **Supplied:** Cream; oint; soln 0.005% **Notes/SE:** Skin irritation, dermatitis

Calcitonin (Cibacalcin, Miacalcin)
Uses: Paget's disease of bone; hypercalcemia; osteogenesis imperfecta, postmenopausal osteoporosis **Action:** Polypeptide hormone **Dose:** Paget's salmon form: 100 U/d IM/SC initially, 50 U/d or 50–100 U q1–3d maint. Paget's human form: 0.5 mg/d initially; maint 0.5 mg 2–3¥/wk or 0.25 mg/d, max 0.5 mg bid. Hypercalcemia salmon calcitonin: 4 U/kg IM/SC q12h; ≠ to 8 U/kg q12h, max q6h. Osteoporosis salmon calcitonin: 100 U/d IM/SC; intranasal 200 U = 1 nasal spray/d **Caution/Contra:** [C, ?] **Supplied:** Spray, nasal 200 U/activation; inj, human (Cibacalcin) 0.5 mg/vial, salmon 200 U/mL (2 mL) **Notes/SE:** Human (Cibacalcin) and salmon forms; human only approved for Paget's bone disease; facial flushing, nausea, edema at inj site, nasal irritation, polyuria

Calcitriol (Rocaltrol)
Uses: ↓ Elevated PTH levels, hypocalcemia associated with dialysis **Action:** 1,25-Dihydroxycholecalciferol, a vitamin D analogue **Dose:** *Adults. Renal failure:* 0.25 mcg/d PO, ↑ 0.25 mcg/d q4–6wk PRN; 0.5 mcg 3×/wk IV, ↑ PRN. *Hyperparathyroidism:* 0.5–2 mcg/d. *Peds. Renal failure:* 15 ng/kg/d, ↑ PRN; typical maint 30–60 ng/kg/d. *Hyperparathyroidism:* <5 y, 0.25–0.75 mcg/d; >6 y, 0.5–2 mcg/d **Caution/Contra:** [C, ?] **Supplied:** Inj 1, 2 mcg/mL (in 1-mL vol); caps 0.25, 0.5 mcg **Notes/SE:** Monitor dosing to keep Ca⁺ wnl; hypercalcemia possible

Calcium Acetate (Calphron, Phos-Ex, PhosLo)
Uses: ESRD-associated hyperphosphatemia **Action:** Ca supplement to treat ESRD hyperphosphatemia without aluminum **Dose:** 2–4 tabs PO with meals **Caution/Contra:** [C, ?] **Supplied:** Caps Phos-Ex 500 mg (125 mg Ca); tabs Calphron and PhosLo 667 mg (169 mg Ca) **Notes/SE:** Can cause ↑ Ca²⁺, monitor Ca²⁺ levels; hypophosphatemia, constipation

Calcium Carbonate (Tums, Alka-Mints)
Uses: Hyperacidity associated with peptic ulcer disease, hiatal hernia, etc **Action:** Neutralizes gastric acid **Dose:** 500 mg–2 g PO PRN; ↓ in renal impairment **Caution/Contra:** [C, ?] **Supplied:** Chew tabs 350, 420, 500, 550, 750, 850 mg; susp **Notes/SE:** Hypercalcemia, hypophosphatemia, constipation

Calcium Glubionate (Neo-Calglucon) [OTC]
Uses: Rx and prevention of Ca deficiency **Action:** Oral Ca supplementation **Dose:** *Adults.* 6–18 g/d ÷ doses. *Peds.* 600–2000 mg/kg/d ÷ qid (9 g/d max); ↓ in renal impairment **Caution/Contra:** [C, ?] **Supplied:** OTC syrup 1.8 g/5 mL = Ca 115 mg/5 mL **Notes/ SE:** Hypercalcemia, hypophosphatemia, constipation

Calcium Salts (Chloride, Gluconate, Gluceptate)
Uses: Ca replacement, VF, Ca blocker toxicity, Mg²⁺ intoxication, tetany, hyperphosphatemia in ESRD **Action:** Ca supplementation/replacement **Dose:** *Adults. Replacement:* 1–2 g/d PO. *Cardiac emergencies:* CaCl 0.5–1.0 g IV q 10 min or Ca gluconate 1–2 g IV q 10 min. *Tetany:* 1 g CaCl over 10–30 min; repeat in 6 h PRN. *Peds. Replacement:* 200–500 mg/kg/24 h PO or IV ÷ qid. *Cardiac emergency:* 100 mg/ kg/dose IV of gluconate salt q 10 min. *Tetany:* 10 mg/kg CaCl over 5–10 min; repeat in 6 h or use inf (200 mg/kg/d max). *Adult & Peds. Hypocalcemia due to citrated blood inf:* 0.45 mEq Ca/100 mL citrated blood infused; ↓ in renal impairment **Caution/Contra:** [C, ?] **Supplied:** CaCl inj 10% = 100 mg/mL = Ca 27.2 mg/mL =

10-mL amp. Ca gluconate inj 10% = 100 mg/mL = Ca 9 mg/mL; tabs 500 mg = 45 mg Ca, 650 mg = 58.5 mg Ca, 975 mg = 87.75 mg Ca, 1 g = 90 mg Ca. Ca gluceptate inj 220 mg/mL = 18 mg/mL Ca **Notes/SE:** CaCl contains 270 mg (13.6 mEq) elemental Ca/g, and Ca gluconate contains 90 mg (4.5 mEq) Ca/g. RDA for Ca: *Adults* = 800 mg/d; *Peds* = <6 mon 360 mg/d, 6 mon–1 y 540 mg/d, 1–10 y 800 mg/d, 10–18 y 1200 mg/d; bradycardia, cardiac arrhythmias, hypercalcemia

Calfactant (Infasurf) **Uses:** Prevention and Rx of RSD in infants **Action:** Exogenous pulmonary surfactant **Dose:** 3 mL/kg instilled into lungs. Can retreat for a total of 3 doses given 12 h apart **Caution/Contra:** [NA/NA] **Supplied:** Intratracheal susp 35 mg/mL **Notes/SE:** Monitor for cyanosis, airway obstruction, bradycardia during administration

Candesartan (Atacand) **Uses:** HTN, DN, CHF **Action:** Angiotensin II receptor antagonists **Dose:** 2–32 mg/d (usual 16 mg/d) **Caution/Contra:** [X, –] Primary hyperaldosteronism; bilateral renal artery stenosis **Supplied:** Tabs 4, 8, 16, 32 mg **Notes/SE:** Dizziness, HA, flushing, angioedema

Capsaicin (Capsin, Zostrix, others) [OTC] **Uses:** Pain due to postherpetic neuralgia, chronic neuralgia, arthritis, diabetic neuropathy, postoperative pain, psoriasis, intractable pruritus **Action:** Topical analgesic **Dose:** Apply tid–qid **Caution/Contra:** [?, ?] **Supplied:** OTC creams; gel; lotions; roll-ons **Notes/SE:** Local irritation, neurotoxicity, cough

Captopril (Capoten, others) **Uses:** HTN, CHF, LVD, DN **Action:** ACE inhibitor **Dose:** *Adults. HTN:* Initially, 25 mg PO bid–tid; ↑ to maint q1–2wk by 25-mg increments/dose (max 450 mg/d) to effect. *CHF:* Initially, 6.25–12.5 mg PO tid; titrate PRN *LVD:* 50 mg PO tid. *DN:* 25 mg PO tid. *Peds.* Infants <2 mon: 0.05–0.5 mg/kg/dose PO q8–24h. *Children:* Initially, 0.3–0.5 mg/ kg/dose PO; ↑ to 6 mg/kg/d max; take 1 h before meals **Caution/Contra:** [C (1st trimester; D 2nd and 3rd trimesters), +] **Supplied:** Tabs 12.5, 25, 50, 100 mg; ? in renal impairment **Notes/SE:** Rash, proteinuria, cough, ↑ K+

Carbamazepine (Tegretol) WARNING: Aplastic anemia and agranulocytosis have been reported with carbamazepine **Uses:** Epilepsy, trigeminal neuralgia, alcohol withdrawal **Action:** Anticonvulsant **Dose:** *Adults.* Initially, 200 mg PO bid; ↑ by 200 mg/d; usual 800–1200 mg/d in ÷ doses. *Peds. <6 y:* 5 mg/kg/d, ↑ to 10–20 mg/kg/d ÷ in 2–4 doses. *6–12 y:* Initially, 100 mg PO bid or 10 mg/kg/24 h PO ÷ qd–bid; ↑ to a maint of 20–30 mg/kg/24 h ÷ tid–qid; ↓ in renal impairment; take with food **Caution/Contra:** [D, +] **Supplied:** Tabs 200 mg; chew tabs 100 mg; XR tabs 100, 200, 400 mg; susp 100 mg/5 mL **Notes/SE:** Monitor CBC and serum levels (Table 2, page 607); generic products not interchangeable; drowsiness, dizziness, blurred vision, N/V, rash, ↓ Na+, leukopenia, agranulocytosis

Carbidopa/Levodopa (Sinemet) **Uses:** Parkinson's disease **Action:** ↑ CNS levels of dopamine **Dose:** 25/100 mg bid–qid; ↑ as needed (max 200/2000 mg/d) **Caution/Contra:** [C, ?] Narrow-angle glaucoma, suspicious skin lesion (may activate melanoma) **Supplied:** Tabs (mg carbidopa/mg levodopa) 10/100, 25/100, 25/250; tabs SR (mg carbidopa/mg levodopa) 25/100, 50/200 **Notes/SE:** Psychiatric disturbances, orthostatic hypotension, dyskinesias, and cardiac arrhythmias

Carboplatin (Paraplatin) **Uses:** Ovarian, lung, head and neck, testicular, and brain CAs and allogeneic and ABMT in high doses **Action:** DNA cross-linker; forms DNA-platinum adducts **Dose:** 360 mg/m² (ovarian carcinoma); AUC dosing 4–7 mg/mL (using Culvert's formula: mg = AUC × [25 + calculated GFR]); adjusted based on pretreatment platelet count, CrCl, and BSA (Egorin's formula); up to 1500 mg/m² used in ABMT setting (refer to specific protocols) **Caution/Contra:** [D, ?] Severe bone marrow suppression, excessive bleeding **Supplied:** Inj 50, 150, 450 mg **Notes/SE:** Physiologic dosing based on either Culvert's or Egorin's formula allows ↑ doses with ↓ toxicity; myelosuppression, N/V/D, nephrotoxicity, hematuria, neurotoxicity, ↑ LFTs

Carisoprodol (Soma) **Uses:** Adjunct to sleep and physical therapy for the relief of painful musculoskeletal conditions **Action:** Centrally acting muscle relaxant **Dose:** 350 mg PO tid–qid **Caution/Contra:** [C, M] Caution in renal/hepatic impairment **Supplied:** Tabs 350 mg **Notes/SE:** Avoid alcohol and other CNS depressants; available in combination with ASA or codeine; drowsiness, dizziness

Carmustine [BCNU] (BiCNU) **Uses:** Primary brain tumors, melanoma, Hodgkin's and NHLs, multiple myeloma, and induction for allogeneic and ABMT in high doses **Action:** Alkylating agent; nitrosourea forms DNA cross-links; inhibitor of DNA synthesis

Dose: 75–100 mg/m^2/d for 2 d; 200 mg/m^2 in a single dose; 450–900 mg/m^2 in BMT (refer to specific protocols); ↓ in hepatic impairment **Caution/Contra:** [D, ?] Contra in myelosuppression **Supplied:** Inj 100 mg; wafer: 7.7 mg **Notes/SE:** Myelosuppression (especially leukocytes and platelets), phlebitis, facial flushing, hepatic and renal dysfunction, pulmonary fibrosis, and optic neuroretinitis. Hematologic toxicity may persist up to 4–6 wk after dose

Carteolol (Cartrol, Ocupress Ophthalmic) Uses: HTN, ↑ intraocular pressure **Action:** Competitively blocks β-adrenergic receptors, β$_1$, β$_2$, ISA **Dose:** PO 2.5–5 mg/d; ophth 1 gtt in eye(s) bid **Caution/Contra:** [C (1st trimester; D 2nd and 3rd trimesters), ?/–]. Bradycardia, AV conduction abnormalities, cardiac failure, asthma **Supplied:** Tabs 2.5, 5 mg; ophth soln 1% **Notes/SE:** Drowsiness, sexual dysfunction, edema, CHF; *ocular:* conjunctival hyperemia, anisocoria, keratitis, eye pain

Carvedilol (Coreg) Uses: HTN and CHF **Action:** Competitively blocks adrenergic receptors, β$_1$, β$_2$, α **Dose:** *HTN:* 6.25–12.5 mg bid. *CHF:* 3.125–25 mg bid; take with food to minimize hypotension **Caution/Contra:** [C (1st trimester; D 2nd and 3rd trimesters), ?/–]. Bradycardia, AV conduction abnormalities, uncompensated CHF, severe hepatic impairment, asthma **Supplied:** Tabs 3.125, 6.25, 12.5, 25 mg **Notes/SE:** Chest pain, dizziness, fatigue, hyperglycemia, bradycardia, edema, hypercholesterolemia; do not DC abruptly; increases digoxin levels

Caspofungin (Cancidas) Uses: Invasive aspergillosis refractory/intolerant to standard therapy **Action:** An echinocandin; inhibits fungal cell wall synthesis **Dose:** 70 mg IV load day 1, 50 mg/d IV; slow inf **Caution/Contra:** [C, ?/–] Do not use with cyclosporine. **Supplied:** IV inf **Notes:** Fever, N/V, thrombophlebitis at inj site, altered LFTs

Cefaclor (Ceclor) Uses: Infections caused by susceptible bacteria involving the upper and lower respiratory tract, skin, bone, urinary tract, abdomen, and gynecologic system **Action:** 2nd-gen. cephalosporin; inhibits cell wall synthesis **Dose:** *Adults.* 250–500 mg PO tid. *Peds.* 20–40 mg/kg/d PO ÷ tid; adjust in renal impairment **Caution/Contra:** [B, +] **Supplied:** Caps 250, 500 mg; ER tabs 375, 500 mg; susp 125, 187, 250, 375 mg/5 mL **Notes/SE:** More gram– activity than 1st-gen. cephalosporins; diarrhea, rash, eosinophilia, ↑ transaminases

Cefadroxil (Duricef, Ultracef) Uses: Infections caused by *Streptococcus, Staphylococcus, E. coli, Proteus,* and *Klebsiella* involving skin, bone, upper and lower respiratory tract, and urinary tract **Action:** 1st-gen. cephalosporin; inhibits cell wall synthesis **Dose:** *Adults.* 500–1000 mg PO bid–qd. *Peds.* 30 mg/kg/d ÷ bid; ↓ in renal impairment **Caution/Contra:** [B, +] **Supplied:** Caps 500 mg; tabs 1 g; susp 125, 250, 500 mg/5 mL **Notes/SE:** Diarrhea, rash, eosinophilia, ↑ transaminases

Cefazolin (Ancef, Kefzol) Uses: Infections caused by *Streptococcus, Staphylococcus, E. coli, Proteus,* and *Klebsiella* involving the skin, bone, upper and lower respiratory tract, and urinary tract **Action:** 1st-gen. cephalosporin; inhibits cell wall synthesis **Dose:** *Adults.* 1–2 g IV q8h. *Peds.* 50–100 mg/kg/d IV ÷ q8h; ↓ in renal impairment **Caution/Contra:** [B, +] **Supplied:** Inj **Notes/ SE:** Widely used for surgical prophylaxis; diarrhea, rash, eosinophilia, ↑ transaminases, pain at inj site

Cefdinir (Omnicef) Uses: Infections involving the respiratory tract, skin, bone, and urinary tract **Action:** 3rd-gen. cephalosporin; inhibits cell wall synthesis **Dose:** *Adults.* 300 mg PO bid or 600 mg/d PO. *Peds.* 7 mg/kg PO bid or 14 mg/kg/d PO; ↓ in renal impairment **Caution/Contra:** [B, +] **Supplied:** Caps 300 mg; susp 125 mg/5 mL **Notes/SE:** Crossreactions with penicillin, anaphylaxis, diarrhea, rare pseudomembranous colitis

Cefditoren (Spectracef) Uses: Acute exacerbations of chronic bronchitis, pharyngitis, tonsillitis; skin infections **Action:** 3rd-gen. cephalosporin **Dose:** *Adults & Peds >12 y.* Skin: 200 mg PO bid ×10 days. *Chronic bronchitis, pharyngitis, tonsillitis:* 400 mg PO bid ×10 days; avoid antacids within 2 h; ↓ dose in renal impairment **Caution/ Contra:** [B, ?] Contra cephalosporin/penicillin allergy, carnitine deficiency, milk sensitivities, or renal failure. **Supplied:** 200-mg tabs **Notes/SE:** HA, N/V/D, colitis, nephrotoxicity, hepatic dysfunction, Stevens-Johnson syndrome, toxic epidermal necrolysis, hypersensitivity reactions

Cefepime (Maxipime) Uses: UTI and pneumonia due to *S. pneumoniae, S. aureus, K. pneumoniae, E. coli, P. aeruginosa,* and *Enterobacter* spp **Action:** 4th-gen. cephalosporin; inhibits cell wall synthesis **Dose:** 1–2 g IV q12h; ↓ in renal impairment **Cau-**

22

tion/Contra: [B, +] **Supplied:** Inj 500 mg, 1, 2 g **Notes/SE:** Rash, pruritus, N/V/D, fever, HA, positive Coombs' test without hemolysis

Cefixime (Suprax)   **Uses:** Infections caused by susceptible bacteria involving the respiratory tract, skin, bone, and urinary tract **Action:** 3rd-gen. cephalosporin; inhibits cell wall synthesis **Dose:** *Adults.* 200–400 mg PO qd–bid. *Peds.* 8 mg/kg/d PO ÷ qd–bid; ↓ in renal impairment **Caution/Contra:** [B, +] **Supplied:** Tabs 200, 400 mg; susp 100 mg/5 mL **Notes/SE:** Use susp for otitis media; N/V/D, flatulence, and abdominal pain

Cefmetazole (Zefazone)   **Uses:** Infections involving the upper and lower respiratory tract, skin, bone, urinary tract, abdomen, and gynecologic system **Action:** 2nd-gen. cephalosporin; inhibits cell wall synthesis **Dose:** *Adults.* 1–2 mg IV q8h; ↓ in renal impairment **Caution/Contra:** [B, +] **Supplied:** Inj 1, 2 g **Notes/SE:** Has more gram– activity than 1st-gen. cephalosporins; has anaerobic activity; ↑ risk of bleeding; rash, diarrhea

Cefonicid (Monocid)   **Uses:** Susceptible bacterial infections (respiratory tract, skin, bone and joint, urinary tract, gynecologic, sepsis) **Action:** 2nd-gen. cephalosporin **Dose:** 1 g/24 h IM/IV; ↓ in renal impairment **Caution/Contra:** [B, +] **Supplied:** Powder for inj 500 mg, 1 g **Notes/SE:** Diarrhea, rash, eosinophilia, ↑ transaminases

Cefoperazone (Cefobid)   **Uses:** Susceptible bacterial infections (respiratory, skin, urinary tract, sepsis); as a 3rd-gen. cephalosporin, cefoperazone has activity against gram– organisms (eg, *E. coli, Klebsiella*); variable activity against *Streptococcus* and *Staphylococcus* spp; active against *P. aeruginosa* but less than ceftazidime **Action:** 3rd-gen. cephalosporin **Dose:** *Adults.* 2–4 g/d IM/IV ÷ q12h (12 g/d max). *Peds.* 100–150 mg/kg/d IM/IV ÷ bid–tid; ↓ in renal impairment **Caution/Contra:** [B, +] **Supplied:** Powder for inj 1, 2 g **Notes/SE:** Diarrhea, rash, eosinophilia, ↑ LFTs, hypoprothrombinemia, and bleeding (due to MTT side chain)

Cefotaxime (Claforan)   **Uses:** Infections involving the respiratory tract, skin, bone, urinary tract, meningitis, sepsis **Action:** 3rd-gen. cephalosporin; inhibits cell wall synthesis **Dose:** *Adults.* 1–2 g IV q4–12h. *Peds.* 100–200 mg/kg/d IV ÷ q6–8h; ↓ in renal impairment **Caution/Contra:** [B, +] **Supplied:** Powder for inj 500 mg, 1, 2 g **Notes/SE:** Diarrhea, rash, eosinophilia, ↑ transaminases

Cefotetan (Cefotan)   **Uses:** Infections involving the upper and lower respiratory tract, skin, bone, urinary tract, abdomen, and gynecologic system **Action:** 2nd-gen. cephalosporin; inhibits cell wall synthesis **Dose:** *Adults.* 1–2 g IV q12h. *Peds.* 40–80 mg/kg/d IV ÷ q12h; ↓ in renal impairment **Caution/Contra:** [B, +] **Supplied:** Powder for inj 1, 2 g **Notes/SE:** More gram– activity than 1st-gen. cephalosporins; has anaerobic activity; diarrhea, rash, eosinophilia, ↑ transaminases, hypoprothrombinemia, and bleeding (due to MTT side chain)

Cefoxitin (Mefoxin)   **Uses:** Infections involving the upper and lower respiratory tract, skin, bone, urinary tract, abdomen, and gynecologic system **Action:** 2nd-gen. cephalosporin; inhibits cell wall synthesis **Dose:** *Adults.* 1–2 mg IV q6h. *Peds.* 80–160 mg/kg/d ÷ q4–6h; ↓ in renal impairment **Caution/Contra:** [B, +] **Supplied:** Powder for inj 1, 2 g **Notes/SE:** More gram– activity than 1st-gen. cephalosporins; has anaerobic activity; diarrhea, rash, eosinophilia, ↑ transaminases

Cefpodoxime (Vantin)   **Uses:** Infections involving the respiratory tract, skin, and urinary tract **Action:** 3rd-gen. cephalosporin; inhibits cell wall synthesis **Dose:** *Adults.* 200–400 mg PO q12h. *Peds.* 10 mg/kg/d PO ÷ bid; ? in renal impairment, take with food **Caution/Contra:** [B, +] **Supplied:** Tabs 100, 200 mg; susp 50, 100 mg/5 mL **Notes/SE:** Drug interactions with agents that increase gastric pH; diarrhea, rash, eosinophilia, ↑ transaminases

Cefprozil (Cefzil)   **Uses:** Infections involving the upper and lower respiratory tract, skin, and urinary tract **Action:** 2nd-gen. cephalosporin; inhibits cell wall synthesis **Dose:** *Adults.* 250–500 mg PO qd–bid. *Peds.* 7.5–15 mg/kg/d PO ÷ bid; ↓ in renal impairment **Caution/Contra:** [B, +] **Supplied:** Tabs 250, 500 mg; susp 125, 250 mg/5 mL **Notes/SE:** More gram– activity than 1st-gen cephalosporins; use higher doses for otitis and pneumonia; diarrhea, rash, eosinophilia, ↑ transaminases

Ceftazidime (Fortaz, Ceptaz, Tazidime, Tazicef)   **Uses:** Infections involving the respiratory tract, skin, bone, urinary tract, meningitis, and septicemia **Action:** 3rd-gen

22

cephalosporin; inhibits cell wall synthesis **Dose:** *Adults.* 1–2 g IV q8h. *Peds.* 30–50 mg/kg/d IV ÷ q8h; ↓ in renal impairment **Caution/Contra:** [B, +] **Supplied:** Powder for inj 1, 2 g **Notes/SE:** Diarrhea, rash, eosinophilia, ↑ transaminases

Ceftibuten (Cedax) **Uses:** Infections involving the respiratory tract, skin, and urinary tract **Action:** 3rd-gen cephalosporin; inhibits cell wall synthesis **Dose:** *Adults.* 400 mg/d PO. *Peds.* 9 mg/kg/d PO; ↓ in renal impairment; take on an empty stomach **Caution/Contra:** [B, +] **Supplied:** Caps 400 mg; susp 90, 180 mg/5 mL **Notes/SE:** Little activity against *Streptococcus;* diarrhea, rash, eosinophilia, ↑ transaminases

Ceftizoxime (Cefizox) **Uses:** Infections involving the respiratory tract, skin, bone, urinary tract, meningitis, and septicemia **Action:** 3rd-gen cephalosporin; inhibits cell wall synthesis **Dose:** *Adults.* 1–2 g IV q8–12h. *Peds.* 150–200 mg/kg/d IV ÷ q6–8h; ÷ in renal impairment **Caution/Contra:** [B, +] **Supplied:** Inj 500 mg, 1, 2 g **Notes/SE:** Diarrhea, rash, eosinophilia, ↑ transaminases

Ceftriaxone (Rocephin) **Uses:** Respiratory tract, skin, bone, urinary tract infections, meningitis, and septicemia; pneumonia and GC **Action:** 3rd-gen cephalosporin; inhibits cell wall synthesis **Dose:** *Adults.* 1–2 g IV q12–24h. *Peds.* 50–100 mg/kg/d IV ÷ q12–24h; ↓ in renal impairment **Caution/Contra:** [B, +] **Supplied:** Powder for inj 250 mg, 1, 2 g **Notes/SE:** Diarrhea, rash, eosinophilia, ↑ transaminases

Cefuroxime (Ceftin [oral], Zinacef [parenteral]) **Uses:** Upper and lower respiratory tract, skin, bone, urinary tract, abdomen, and gynecologic infections **Action:** 2nd-gen. cephalosporin; inhibits cell wall synthesis **Dose:** *Adults.* 750 mg–1.5 g IV q8h or 250–500 mg PO bid. *Peds.* 100–150 mg/kg/d IV ÷ q8h or 20–30 mg/kg/d PO ÷ bid; adjust in renal impairment; take with food **Caution/Contra:** [B, +] **Supplied:** Tabs 125, 250, 500 mg; susp 125, 250 mg/5 mL; powder for inj 750 mg, 1.5, 7.5 g **Notes/SE:** ↑ Gram– activity over 1st-gen cephalosporins; IV crosses blood–brain barrier; diarrhea, rash, eosinophilia, ↑ LFTs

Celecoxib (Celebrex) **Uses:** Osteoarthritis and RA; acute pain, primary dysmenorrhea; preventive in familial adenomatous polyposis **Action:** NSAID, inhibits the COX-2 pathway **Dose:** 100–200 mg/d or bid; caution in renal impairment; ↓ with hepatic impairment **Caution/Contra:** [C, ?] Allergy to sulfonamides **Supplied:** Caps 100, 200 mg **Notes/SE:** GI upset, HTN, edema, renal failure, HA, no effect on platelets/bleeding time; can affect drugs metabolized by P-450 pathway

Cephalexin (Keflex, Keftab) **Uses:** Infections due to *Streptococcus, Staphylococcus, E. coli, Proteus,* and *Klebsiella* involving skin, bone, upper and lower respiratory tract, and urinary tract **Action:** 1st-gen. cephalosporin; inhibits cell wall synthesis **Dose:** *Adults.* 250–500 mg PO qid. *Peds.* 25–100 mg/kg/d PO ÷ qid; ↓ in renal impairment; take on an empty stomach **Caution/Contra:** [B, +] **Supplied:** Caps 250, 500 mg; tabs 250, 500, 1000 mg; susp 125, 250 mg/5 mL **Notes/SE:** Diarrhea, rash, eosinophilia, ↑ LFTs

Cephradine (Velosef) **Uses:** Various bacterial infections (includes group A β-hemolytic strep) **Action:** 1st-gen. cephalosporin; inhibits cell wall synthesis **Dose:** *Adults.* 2–4 g/d PO/IV ÷ qid (8 g/d max). *Peds.* *>9 mon:* 25–100 mg/kg/d ÷ bid–qid (4 g/d max); ↓ in renal impairment **Caution/Contra:** [B, +] **Supplied:** Caps: 250, 500 mg; powder for susp 125, 250 mg/5 mL, injectable **Notes/SE:** Diarrhea, rash, eosinophilia, ↑ LFTs

Cetirizine (Zyrtec) **Uses:** Allergic rhinitis and chronic urticaria **Action:** Nonsedating antihistamine **Dose:** *Adults & Children >6 y:* 5–10 mg/d. **Peds:** 6-11 mon 2.5 mg/d, 12–23 mon 2.5 mg qd–bid; ↓ in renal/hepatic impairment **Caution/Contra:** [B, ?/–] **Supplied:** Tabs 5, 10 mg; syrup 5 mg/5 mL **Notes/SE:** HA, drowsiness, xerostomia

Charcoal, Activated (Superchar, Actidose, Liqui-Char) **Uses:** Emergency treatment in poisoning by most drugs and chemicals **Action:** Adsorbent detoxicant **Dose:** Also give 70% sorbitol solution (2 mL/kg body weight) *Adults.* Acute intoxication: 30–100 g/dose. *GI dialysis:* 25–50 g q4–6h. *Peds.* Acute intoxication: 1–2 g/kg/dose. *GI dialysis:* 5–10 g/dose q4–8h **Caution/Contra:** [C, ?] Iron, lithium, lead, alkali, acid poisonings **Supplied:** Powder, liq **Notes/SE:** Some liq dosage forms in sorbitol base (a cathartic). If sorbitol used, monitor for hypokalemia and hypomagnesemia. Protect the airway in lethargic or comatose patients; vomiting, diarrhea, black stools

Chloral Hydrate [C-IV] **Uses:** Nocturnal and preoperative sedation **Action:** Sedative hypnotic **Dose:** *Adults.* Hypnotic: 500 mg–1 g PO or PR 30 min hs or before procedure.

22

Sedative: 250 mg PO or PR tid. **Peds.** Hypnotic: 20–40 mg/kg/24 h PO or PR 30 min hs or before procedure. *Sedative:* 25–50 mg/kg/d ↓ q6–8h; avoid use in CrCl <50 mL/min or severe hepatic impairment **Caution/Contra:** [C, +] **Supplied:** Caps 500 mg; syrup 250, 500 mg/5 mL; supp 324, 500, 648 mg **Notes/SE:** Mix syrup in water or fruit juice; drowsiness, ataxia, dizziness, nightmares, rash

Chlorambucil (Leukeran) Uses: CLL, Hodgkin's disease, Waldenström's macroglobulinemia **Action:** Alkylating agent **Dose:** 0.1–0.2 mg/kg/d for 3–6 wk or 0.4 mg/kg q2wk (refer to specific protocol) **Caution/Contra:** [D, ?] **Supplied:** Tabs 2 mg **Notes/SE:** Myelosuppression, CNS stimulation, N/V, drug fever, skin rash, chromosomal damage that can result in secondary leukemias, alveolar dysplasia, pulmonary fibrosis, hepatotoxicity

Chlordiazepoxide (Librium) [C-IV] Uses: Anxiety, tension, alcohol withdrawal, and preoperative apprehension **Action:** Benzodiazepine; antianxiety agent **Dose:** *Adults.* Mild anxiety: 5–10 mg PO tid–qid or PRN. *Severe anxiety:* 25–50 mg IM, IV, or PO q6–8h or PRN. *Alcohol withdrawal:* 50–100 mg IM or IV; repeat in 2–4 h if needed, up to 300 mg in 24 h; gradually taper the daily dosage. **Peds.** >6 y: 0.5 mg/kg/24 h PO or IM ÷ q6–8h; ↓ in renal impairment, elderly; avoid in hepatic impairment **Caution/Contra:** [D, ?] **Supplied:** Caps 5, 10, 25 mg; tabs 10, 25 mg; inj 100 mg **Notes/SE:** Erratic IM absorption; drowsiness, fatigue, memory impairment, xerostomia, weight gain

Chlorothiazide (Diuril) Uses: HTN, edema **Action:** Thiazide diuretic **Dose:** *Adults.* 500 mg–1 g PO or IV qd–bid. **Peds.** 20–30 mg/kg/24 h PO ÷ bid **Caution/Contra:** [D, +] Contra in cross-sensitivity to thiazides/sulfonamides, anuria **Supplied:** Tabs 250, 500 mg; susp 250 mg/5 mL; inj 500 mg/vial **Notes/SE:** Hypokalemia, hyponatremia, dizziness, hyperglycemia, hyperuricemia, hyperlipidemia, photosensitivity

Chlorpheniramine (Chlor-Trimeton, others) Uses: Allergic reactions **Action:** Antihistamine **Dose:** *Adults.* 4 mg PO q4–6h or 8–12 mg PO bid of SR. **Peds.** 0.35 mg/kg/24 h PO ÷ q4–6h or 0.2 mg/kg/24 h SR **Caution/Contra:** [C, ?/–] **Supplied:** Tabs 4 mg; chew tabs 2 mg; SR tabs 8, 12 mg; syrup 2 mg/5 mL; inj 10, 100 mg/mL **Notes/SE:** Anticholinergic SE and sedation common, orthostatic hypotension, QT changes, extrapyramidal reactions, photosensitivity

Chlorpromazine (Thorazine) Uses: Psychotic disorders, apprehension, intractable hiccups, N/V **Action:** Phenothiazine antipsychotic; antiemetic **Dose:** *Adults.* Psychosis: 10–25 mg PO or PR bid–tid (usual 30–800 mg/d in ÷ doses). *Children.* Psychosis & N/V: 0.5–1 mg/kg/dose PO q4–6h or IM/IV q6–8h. *Severe symptoms:* 25 mg IM; can repeat in 1 h; then 25–50 mg PO or PR tid. *Hiccups:* 25–50 mg PO bid–tid; avoid in severe hepatic impairment **Caution/Contra:** [C, ?/–] **Supplied:** Tabs 10, 25, 50, 100, 200 mg; SR caps 30, 75, 150 mg; syrup 10 mg/5 mL; conc 30, 100 mg/mL; supp 25, 100 mg; inj 25 mg/mL **Notes/SE:** Extrapyramidal SE and sedation; α-adrenergic blocking properties; prolongs QT interval

Chlorpropamide (Diabinese) Uses: Type 2 DM **Action:** Sulfonylurea; ↑ release of insulin from pancreas; ↑ insulin sensitivity at peripheral sites; ↓ hepatic glucose output **Dose:** 100–500 mg/d; avoid use in CrCl <50 mL/min; ↓ in hepatic impairment; take with food, avoid alcohol (disulfiram-like reaction) **Caution/ Contra:** [C, ?/–] **Supplied:** Tabs 100, 250 mg **Notes/SE:** HA, dizziness, rash, photosensitivity, hypoglycemia, SIADH

Chlorthalidone (Hygroton) Uses: HTN **Action:** Thiazide diuretic **Dose:** *Adults.* 50–100 mg/d PO qd. **Peds.** 2 mg/kg/dose PO 3×/wk or 1–2 mg/kg/d PO; ↓ in renal impairment **Caution/Contra:** [D, +] Anuria **Supplied:** Tabs 15, 25, 50, 100 mg **Notes/SE:** Hypokalemia, dizziness, photosensitivity, hyperglycemia, hyperuricemia, sexual dysfunction

Chlorzoxazone (Paraflex, Parafon Forte DSC) Uses: Adjunct to rest and physical therapy for the relief of discomfort associated with acute, painful musculoskeletal conditions **Action:** Centrally acting skeletal muscle relaxant **Dose:** *Adults.* 250–500 mg PO tid–qid. **Peds.** 20 mg/kg/d in 3–4 ÷ doses **Caution/Contra:** [C, ?] Contra in severe liver disease **Supplied:** Tabs 250, 500 mg; caps 250, 500 mg **Notes/SE:** Drowsiness, tachycardia, dizziness, hepatotoxicity, angioedema

Cholecalciferol [Vitamin D₃] (Delta D) Uses: Dietary supplement for treatment of vitamin D deficiency **Action:** Enhances intestinal Ca absorption **Dose:** 400–1000 IU/d PO **Caution/Contra:** [A (D doses above the RDA), +] Hypercalcemia **Supplied:** Tabs 400,

22

1000 IU **Notes/SE:** 1 mg of cholecalciferol = 40,000 IU of vitamin D activity; vitamin D toxicity (renal failure, HTN, psychosis)

Cholestyramine (Questran) Uses: Hypercholesterolemia; Rx pruritus associated with partial biliary obstruction **Action:** Binds intestinal bile acids to form insoluble complexes **Dose:** *Adults.* Individualize: 4 g/d–bid ($\uparrow$ to max 24 g/d and 6 doses/d). *Peds.* 240 mg/kg/d in 3 ÷ doses **Caution/Contra:** [C, ?] **Supplied:** 4 g of cholestyramine resin/9 g of powder; with aspartame: 4 g resin/5 g of powder **Notes/SE:** Mix 4 g of cholestyramine in 2–6 oz of noncarbonated beverage; take other meds 1–2 h before or 6 h after cholestyramine; constipation, abdominal pain, bloating, HA

Ciclopirox (Loprox) Uses: Tinea pedis, tinea cruris, tinea corporis, cutaneous candidiasis, tinea versicolor **Action:** Antifungal antibiotic **Dose:** *Adults & Peds >10 y.* Massage into affected area bid **Caution/Contra:** [B, ?] **Supplied:** Cream; gel; lotion 1% **Notes/SE:** Pruritus, local irritation

Cidofovir (Vistide) **WARNING:** Renal impairment is the major toxicity. Follow administration instructions Uses: CMV retinitis **Action:** Selective inhibition of viral DNA synthesis **Dose:** *Rx:* 5 mg/kg IV once/wk for 2 wk; administered with probenecid. *Maint:* 5 mg/kg IV once/2 wk; administered with probenecid. *Probenecid:* 2 g PO 3 h prior to cidofovir, and then 1 g PO at 2 h and 8 h after cidofovir; $\downarrow$ in renal impairment **Caution/Contra:** [C, –]. SCr >1.5 mg/dL or CrCl ≤55 mL/min or urine protein >100 mg/dL; other nephrotoxic drugs, hypersensitivity to probenecid or sulfa **Supplied:** Inj 75 mg/mL **Notes/SE:** Hydrate with NS prior to each inf; renal toxicity, follow renal function, chills, fever, HA, N/V/D, thrombocytopenia, neutropenia

Cimetidine (Tagamet) Uses: Duodenal ulcer; ulcer prophylaxis in hypersecretory states, eg, trauma, burns, surgery; and GERD **Action:** H_2 receptor antagonist **Dose:** *Adults.* *Active ulcer:* 2400 mg/d IV cont inf or 300 mg IV q6h; 400 mg PO bid or 800 mg hs. *Maint:* 400 mg PO hs. *GERD:* 800 mg PO bid; maint 800 mg PO hs. *Peds. Infants:* 10–20 mg/kg/24 h PO or IV ÷ q6–12h. *Children:* 20–40 mg/kg/24 h PO or IV ÷ q6h; $\uparrow$ dosing interval with renal insufficiency; $\downarrow$ dose in the elderly **Caution/Contra:** [B, +] Many drug interactions **Supplied:** Tabs 200, 300, 400, 800 mg; liq 300 mg/5 mL; inj 300 mg/2 mL **Notes/SE:** Dizziness, agitation, thrombocytopenia, gynecomastia

Ciprofloxacin (Cipro) Uses: Broad-spectrum activity against a variety of gram+ and gram– aerobic bacteria **Action:** Quinolone antibiotic; inhibits DNA gyrase **Dose:** *Adults.* 250–750 mg PO q12h or 200–400 mg IV q12h; $\downarrow$ in renal impairment; avoid antacids; reduce/restrict caffeine intake **Caution/Contra:** [C, ?/–]. Children <18 y **Supplied:** Tabs 100, 250, 500, 750 mg; susp 5 g/100 mL, 10 g/100 mL; inj 200, 400 mg **Notes/SE:** Little activity against streptococci; interactions with theophylline, caffeine, sucralfate, warfarin, antacids; restlessness, N/V/D, rash, ruptured tendons, $\uparrow$ LFTs

Ciprofloxacin, Ophthalmic (Ciloxan) Uses: Rx and prevention of ocular infections, eg, conjunctivitis, blepharitis, cornea; abrasions **Action:** Quinolone antibiotic; inhibits DNA gyrase **Dose:** 1–2 gtt in eye(s) q2h while awake for 2 d, then 1–2 gtt q4h while awake for 5 d **Caution/Contra:** [C, ?/–] **Supplied:** Soln 3.5 mg/mL **Notes/SE:** Local irritation

Ciprofloxacin, Otic (Cipro HC Otic) Uses: Otitis externa **Action:** Quinolone antibiotic; inhibits DNA gyrase **Dose:** *Adult & Peds >1 mon.* 1–2 gtt in ear(s) bid for 7 d **Caution/Contra:** [C, ?/?] Perforated tympanic membrane, viral infections of the external canal **Supplied:** Susp ciprofloxacin 0.2% and hydrocortisone 1% **Notes/SE:** HA, pruritus

Cisplatin (Platinol AQ) Uses: Testicular, small-cell and non-small-cell lung, bladder, ovarian, breast, head and neck, and penile CAs; osteosarcoma; pediatric brain tumors **Action:** DNA-binding; intrastrand cross-linking; formation of DNA adducts **Dose:** 20 mg/m^2/d for 5 d q3wk; 120 mg/m^2 q3–4wk; 100 mg/m^2 on days 1 and 8 q20d (refer to specific protocols); $\downarrow$ in renal impairment **Caution/Contra:** [D, –] Preexisting renal insufficiency, myelosuppression, hearing impairment **Supplied:** Inj 1 mg/mL **Notes/SE:** Allergic reactions, N/V, nephrotoxicity (exacerbated by concurrent administration of other nephrotoxic drugs and minimized by NS inf and mannitol diuresis), high-frequency hearing loss in 30%, peripheral "stocking glove"-type neuropathy, cardiotoxicity (ST-,T-wave changes), hypomagnesemia, mild myelosuppression, hepatotoxicity; renal impairment is dose-related and cumulative

Citalopram (Celexa) Uses: Depression **Action:** SSRI **Dose:** Initial 20 mg/d, may be $\uparrow$ to 40 mg/d **Caution/Contra:** [C, +/–] Contra if used with MAOI or within 14 d of MAOI

22

administration **Supplied:** Tabs 20, 40 mg **Notes/SE:** Somnolence, insomnia, anxiety, xerostomia, sexual dysfunction

Cladribine (Leustatin) **Uses:** HCL **Action:** Induces DNA strand breakage; interferes with DNA repair/synthesis **Dose:** 0.09 mg/kg/d cont IV inf for 7 d (refer to specific protocols) **Caution/Contra:** [D, ?/–] **Supplied:** Inj 1 mg/mL **Notes/SE:** Myelosuppression; T-lymphocyte suppression may be prolonged (26–34 wk); fever in 46% (possibly tumor lysis); infections (especially lung and IV sites); rash (50%)

Clarithromycin (Biaxin) **Uses:** Upper and lower respiratory tract infections, skin and skin structure infections, *H. pylori* infections, and infections caused by nontuberculosis (atypical) *Mycobacterium;* prevention of MAC infections in HIV-infected individuals. **Action:** Macrolide antibiotic; inhibits protein synthesis **Dose:** *Adults.* 250–500 mg PO bid or 1000 mg (2 × 500 mg ER tab)/d. *Mycobacterium:* 500–1000 mg PO bid. *Peds.* 7.5 mg/kg/dose PO bid; ↓ in renal/hepatic impairment **Caution/Contra:** [C, ?] **Supplied:** Tabs 250, 500 mg; susp 125, 250 mg/ 5 mL; 500 mg ER tab **Notes/SE:** Increases theophylline and carbamazepine levels; prolongs QT interval, multiple drug interactions; causes metallic taste, diarrhea, nausea, abdominal pain, HA

Clemastine Fumarate (Tavist) **Uses:** Allergic rhinitis **Action:** Antihistamine **Dose:** *Adults & Peds >12 y.* 1.34 mg bid–2.68 mg tid; max 8.04 mg/d.*<12 y:* 0.4 mg PO bid **Caution/Contra:** [C, M] Narrow-angle glaucoma **Supplied:** Tabs 1.34, 2.68 mg; syrup 0.67 mg/5 mL **Notes/SE:** Drowsiness

Clindamycin (Cleocin, Cleocin-T) **Uses:** Susceptible strains of streptococci, pneumococci, staphylococci, and gram+ and gram– anaerobes; no activity against gram– aerobes and bacterial vaginosis; topical for severe acne and vaginal infections **Action:** Bacteriostatic; interferes with protein synthesis **Dose:** *Adults.* 150–450 mg PO qid; 300–600 mg IV q6h or 900 mg IV q8h. *Vaginal:* 1 applicatorful hs for 7 d. *Topical:* Apply 1% gel, lotion, or soln bid. *Peds.* Neonates: 10–15 mg/kg/24 h ÷ q8–12h. *Children >1 mon:* 10–30 mg/kg/ 24 h ÷ q6–8h, to a max of 1.8 g/d oral or 4.8 g/d IV. *Topical:* Apply 1%, gel, lotion, or soln bid; adjust in severe hepatic impairment **Caution/Contra:** [B, +] **Supplied:** Caps 75, 150, 300 mg; susp 75 mg/5 mL; inj 300 mg/2 mL; vaginal cream 2% **Notes/SE:** Diarrhea may be pseudomembranous colitis caused by *C. difficile;* rash, ↑ LFTs

Clofazimine (Lamprene) **Uses:** Leprosy and combination therapy for MAC in AIDS **Action:** Bactericidal; inhibits DNA synthesis **Dose:** *Adults.* 100–300 mg PO qd. *Peds.* 1 mg/kg/d; take with meals **Caution/Contra:** [C, +/–] **Supplied:** Caps 50 mg **Notes/SE:** Pink to brownish-black discoloration of the skin and conjunctiva, dry skin, GI intolerance

Clonazepam (Klonopin) [C-IV] **Uses:** Lennox-Gastaut syndrome, akinetic and myoclonic seizures, absence seizures, panic attacks **Action:** Benzodiazepine; anticonvulsant **Dose:** *Adults.* 1.5 mg/d PO in 3 ÷ doses; ↑ by 0.5–1.0 mg/d q3d PRN up to 20 mg/d. *Peds.* 0.01–0.03 mg/kg/24 h PO ÷ tid; ↑ to 0.1–0.2 mg/kg/24 h–tid; avoid abrupt withdrawal **Caution/Contra:** [D, M] Severe hepatic impairment, narrow-angle glaucoma **Supplied:** Tabs 0.5, 1.0, 2.0 mg **Notes/ SE:** CNS side effects, including drowsiness, dizziness, ataxia, memory impairment

Clonidine, Oral (Catapres) **Uses:** HTN; opioid, alcohol, and tobacco withdrawal **Action:** Centrally acting α-adrenergic stimulant **Dose:** *Adults.* 0.10 mg PO bid adjust daily by 0.1- to 0.2-mg increments (max 2.4 mg/d). *Peds.* 5–10 mcg/ kg/d ÷ q8–12h (max 0.9 mg/d) **Caution/Contra:** [C, +/–] Avoid with β-blocker **Supplied:** Tabs 0.1, 0.2, 0.3 mg **Notes/SE:** More effective for HTN if combined with diuretics; rebound HTN with abrupt cessation of doses >0.2 mg bid; drowsiness, orthostatic hypotension, xerostomia, constipation; bradycardia

Clonidine, Transdermal (Catapres TTS) **Uses:** HTN **Action:** Centrally acting α-adrenergic stimulant **Dose:** Apply 1 patch q7–10d to hairless area (upper arm/torso); titrate to effect; ↓ in severe renal impairment, do not DC abruptly (rebound HTN) **Caution/Contra:** [C, +/–] Avoid with β-blocker **Supplied:** TTS-1, TTS-2, TTS-3 (delivers 0.1, 0.2, 0.3 mg, respectively, of clonidine/d for 1 wk) **Notes/SE:** Doses >2 TTS-3 usually not associated with ↑ efficacy; steady state in 3 d; drowsiness, orthostatic hypotension, xerostomia, constipation, bradycardia

Clopidogrel (Plavix) **Uses:** Reduction of atherosclerotic events **Action:** Inhibits platelet aggregation **Dose:** 75 mg/d **Caution/Contra:** [B, ?] Active bleeding **Supplied:** Tabs 75 mg **Notes/SE:** Prolongs bleeding time, use with caution in persons at risk of bleeding from trauma and other causes; GI intolerance, HA, dizziness, rash, thrombocytopenia, leukopenia; platelet aggregation returns to baseline ≅5 d after DC; platelet transfusion reverses effects acutely

Clorazepate (Tranxene) [C-IV]   **Uses:** Acute anxiety disorders, acute alcohol withdrawal symptoms, adjunctive therapy in partial seizures **Action:** Benzodiazepine; antianxiety agent **Dose:** *Adults.* 15–60 mg/d PO single or ÷ doses. *Elderly and debilitated patients:* Start at 7.5–15 mg/d in ÷ doses. *Alcohol withdrawal:* Day 1: Initially, 30 mg; then 30–60 mg in ÷ doses. Day 2: 45–90 mg in ÷ doses. Day 3: 22.5–45 mg in ÷ doses. Day 4: 15–30 mg in ÷ doses. *Peds.* 3.75–7.5 mg/dose bid to 60 mg/d max ÷ bid–tid; monitor patients with renal/hepatic impairment, avoid abrupt withdrawal **Caution/Contra:** [D, ?/–] **Supplied:** Tabs 3.75, 7.5, 11.25, 15, 22.5 mg **Notes/SE:** Monitor patients with renal/hepatic impairment (drug may accumulate); CNS depressant effects (drowsiness, dizziness, ataxia, memory impairment); hypotension

Clotrimazole (Lotrimin, Mycelex)   **Uses:** Candidiasis and tinea infections **Action:** Antifungal agent; alters cell wall permeability **Dose:** *Oral:* One troche dissolved in mouth 5 ×/d for 14 d. *Vaginal:* Cream 1 applicatorful hs for 7–14 d. Tabs 100 mg vaginally hs for 7 d or 200 mg (2 tabs) vaginally hs for 3 d or 500-mg tabs vaginally hs once. *Topical:* Apply bid for 10–14 d **Caution/Contra:** [B, (C if oral)/?] **Supplied:** 1% cream; soln; lotion; troche 10 mg; vaginal tabs 100, 500 mg; vaginal cream 1% **Notes/SE:** Oral prophylaxis common in immunosuppressed patients; *topical SE:* Local irritation; *oral:* N/V, ↑ LFTs

Clotrimazole and Betamethasone (Lotrisone)   **Uses:** Fungal skin infections **Action:** Imidazole antifungal and antiinflammatory **Dose:** Apply and massage into area bid for 2–4 wk **Caution/Contra:** [C, ?] Children, varicella infection **Supplied:** Cream 15, 45 g **Notes/SE:** Local irritation, rash

Clozapine (Clozaril)   WARNING: Myocarditis, agranulocytosis, seizures, and orthostatic hypotension have been associated with clozapine **Uses:** Refractory severe schizophrenia **Action:** Tricyclic "atypical" antipsychotic **Dose:** Initially, 25 mg qd–bid; ↑ to 300–450 mg/d over 2 wk. Maintain at the lowest dose possible; do not DC abruptly **Caution/Contra:** [B, +/–] WBC count = 3500 cells/mm³ before Rx or <3000 cells/mm³ during Rx **Supplied:** Tabs 25, 100 mg **Notes/SE:** CBC weekly for the 1st 6 mon, then every other wk; tachycardia, drowsiness, weight gain, constipation, urinary incontinence, rash, seizures

Cocaine [C-II]   **Uses:** Topical anesthetic for mucous membranes **Action:** Narcotic analgesic, local vasoconstrictor **Dose:** Apply lowest amount of topical soln that provides relief; 1 mg/kg max **Caution/Contra:** [C, ?] **Supplied:** Topical soln and viscous preparations 4, 10%; powder, soluble tabs (135 mg) for soln **Notes/SE:** CNS stimulation, nervousness, loss of taste/smell, chronic rhinitis

Codeine [C-II]   **Uses:** Mild–moderate pain; symptomatic relief of cough **Action:** Narcotic analgesic; depresses cough reflex **Dose:** *Adults.* Analgesic: 15–60 mg PO or IM qid PRN. *Antitussive:* 10–20 mg PO q4h PRN; max 120 mg/d. *Peds. Analgesic:* 0.5–1 mg/kg/dose PO or IM q4–6h PRN. *Antitussive:* 1–1.5 mg/ kg/24 h PO ÷ q4h; max 30 mg/24 h; ↓ in renal/hepatic impairment **Caution/Contra:** [C, (D if prolonged use or high doses at term), +] **Supplied:** Tabs 15, 30, 60 mg; soln 15 mg/5 mL; inj 30, 60 mg/mL **Notes/SE:** Usually combined with APAP for pain or with agents (eg, terpin hydrate as an antitussive); 120 mg IM = 10 mg IM morphine; drowsiness, constipation

Colchicine   **Uses:** Acute gout **Action:** Inhibits migration of leukocytes; reduces production of lactic acid by leukocytes **Dose:** *Initially:* 0.5–1.2 mg PO, then 0.5–0.6 mg q1–2h until relief or GI side effects develop (max 8 mg/d); do not repeat for 3 d. *IV:* 1–3 mg, then 0.5 mg q6h until relief (max 4 mg/d); do not repeat for 7 d. *Prophylaxis:* PO: 0.5–0.6 mg/d or 3–4 d/wk; ↓ renal impairment; caution in elderly **Caution/Contra:** [D, +] Serious renal, hepatic, cardiac, or GI disorder **Supplied:** Tabs 0.5, 0.6 mg; inj 1 mg/2 mL **Notes/SE:** Colchicine 1–2 mg IV within 24–48 h of an acute attack diagnostic/therapeutic in monoarticular arthritis; N/V/D, abdominal pain, bone marrow suppression, hepatotoxicity

Colesevelam (Welchol)   **Uses:** Reduction of LDL and total cholesterol **Action:** Bile acid sequestrant **Dose:** 3 tabs PO bid with meals **Caution/Contra:** [B, ?] Bowel obstruction **Supplied:** Tabs 625 mg **Notes/SE:** Constipation, dyspepsia, myalgia

Colestipol (Colestid)   **Uses:** Adjunct to ↓ serum cholesterol in primary hypercholesterolemia **Action:** Binds intestinal bile acids to form an insoluble complex **Dose:** Granules:

5–30 g/d ÷ into 2–4 doses; tabs: 2–16 g/d qd–bid **Caution/ Contra:** [C, ?] Avoid in patients with high triglycerides **Supplied:** Tabs 1 g; granules **Notes/SE:** Do NOT use dry powder; mix with beverages, soups, cereals, etc; constipation, abdominal pain, bloating, HA

Colfosceril Palmitate (Exosurf Neonatal) **Uses:** Prophylaxis and Rx for RSD in infants **Action:** Synthetic lung surfactant **Dose:** 5 mL/kg/dose through ET tube as soon after birth as possible and again at 12 and 24 h **Caution/ Contra:** [?, ?] **Supplied:** Suspension 108 mg **Notes/SE:** Monitor pulmonary compliance and oxygenation carefully; pulmonary hemorrhage possible in infants weighing <700 g at birth; mucous plugging

Cortisone See Steroids, Table 22–4, page 612 and Table 22–5 page 613

Cromolyn Sodium (Intal, Nasalcrom, Opticrom) **Uses:** Adjunct to the Rx of asthma; prevent exercise-induced asthma; allergic rhinitis; ophth allergic manifestations **Action:** Antiasthmatic; mast cell stabilizer **Dose:** *Adults & Children >12 y. Inhal:* 20 mg (as powder in caps) inhaled qid or met-dose inhal 2 puffs qid. *Oral:* 200 mg qid 15–20 min ac, up to 400 mg qid. *Nasal instillation:* Spray once in each nostril 2–6×/d. *Ophth:* 1–2 gtt in each eye 4–6×/d. *Peds. Inhal:* 2 puffs qid of met-dose inhal. *Oral: Infants <2 y:* 20 mg/kg/d in 4 ÷ doses. *2–12 y:* 100 mg qid ac **Caution/Contra:** [B, ?] **Supplied:** Oral conc 100 mg/ 5 mL; soln for neb 20 mg/2 mL; met-dose inhal; nasal soln 40 mg/mL; ophth soln 4% **Notes/SE:** No benefit in acute Rx; 2–4 wk for maximal effect in perennial allergic disorders; unpleasant taste, hoarseness, coughing

Cyanocobalamin [Vitamin B₁₂] **Uses:** Pernicious anemia and other vitamin B_{12} deficiency states **Action:** Dietary supplement of vitamin B_{12} **Dose:** *Adults.* 100 mcg IM or SC qd for 5–10 d, then 100 mcg IM 2×/wk for 1 mon, then 100 mcg IM monthly. *Peds.* 100 mcg/d IM or SC for 5–10 d, then 30–50 mcg IM q4wk **Caution/Contra:** [A (C if dose exceeds RDA), +] **Supplied:** Tabs 25, 50, 100, 250, 500, 1000 mcg; inj 30, 100, 1000 mcg/mL **Notes/SE:** Oral absorption erratic, altered by many drugs and not recommended; for use with hyperalimentation; itching, diarrhea

Cyclobenzaprine (Flexeril) **Uses:** Relief of muscle spasm **Action:** Centrally acting skeletal muscle relaxant; reduces tonic somatic motor activity **Dose:** 10 mg PO 2–4×/d (2–3 wk max) **Caution/Contra:** [B, ?] **Supplied:** Tabs 10 mg **Notes/SE:** Sedative and anticholinergic

Cyclopentolate (Cyclogyl) **Uses:** Diagnostic procedures requiring cycloplegia and mydriasis **Action:** Cycloplegic and mydriatic agent (can last up to 24 h) **Dose:** 1 gtt then another in 5 min **Caution/Contra:** [C, ?] Narrow-angle glaucoma **Supplied:** Soln, 0.5, 1, 2% **Notes/SE:** Blurred vision, ↑ sensitivity to light, tachycardia, restlessness

Cyclophosphamide (Cytoxan, Neosar) **Uses:** Hodgkin's and NHLs, multiple myeloma, small-cell lung, breast, and ovarian CAs, mycosis fungoides, neuroblastoma, retinoblastoma, acute leukemias, CA, and allogeneic and ABMT in high doses; severe rheumatologic disorders **Action:** Converted to acrolein and phosphoramide mustard, the active alkylating moieties **Dose:** 500–1500 mg/m² as a single dose at 2–4-wk intervals; 1.8 g/m² to 160 mg/kg (or ≅12 g/m² in a 75-kg individual) in the BMT setting (refer to specific protocols); ↓ in renal/hepatic impairment **Caution/Contra:** [D, ?] **Supplied:** Tabs 25, 50 mg; inj 100 mg **Notes/SE:** Myelosuppression (leukopenia and thrombocytopenia); hemorrhagic cystitis, SIADH, alopecia, anorexia; N/V; hepatotoxicity and rarely interstitial pneumonitis; irreversible testicular atrophy possible; cardiotoxicity rare; 2nd malignancies (bladder CA and acute leukemias); cumulative risk 3.5% at 8 y, 10.7% at 12 y. Hemorrhagic cystitis prophylaxis: continuous bladder irrigation and mesna uroprotection

Cyclosporine (Sandimmune, Neoral) **Uses:** Organ rejection in kidney, liver, heart, and BMT with steroids; RA; psoriasis **Action:** Immunosuppressant; reversible inhibition of immunocompetent lymphocytes **Dose:** *Adults & Peds. Oral:* 15 mg/kg/d 12 h pretransplant; after 2 wk, taper by 5 mg/wk to 5–10 mg/kg/d. *IV:* If NPO, give ½ oral dose IV; ↓ in renal/hepatic impairment **Caution/Contra:** [C, ?] **Supplied:** Caps 25, 50, 100 mg; oral soln 100 mg/mL; inj 50 mg/mL **Notes/SE:** May ↑ BUN and creatinine and mimic transplant rejection; administer in glass containers; many drug interactions; Neoral and Sandimmune not interchangeable; HTN; interaction with St. John's wort. See Table 2, page 607

Cyproheptadine (Periactin) **Uses:** Allergic reactions; itching **Action:** Phenothiazine antihistamine **Dose:** *Adults.* 4–20 mg PO ÷ q8h; max 0.5 mg/kg/d. *Peds. 2–6 y:* 2 mg bid–tid (max 12 mg/24 h). *7–14 y:* 4 mg bid–tid; ↓ in hepatic impairment **Caution/Contra:**

[B, ?] **Supplied:** Tabs 4 mg; syrup 2 mg/5 mL **Notes/SE:** Anticholinergic, drowsiness, may stimulate appetite

Cytarabine [ARA-C] (Cytosar-U)   **Uses:** Acute leukemias, CML, NHL; IT administration for leukemic meningitis or prophylaxis **Action:** Antimetabolite; interferes with DNA synthesis **Dose:** 100–150 mg/m²/d for 5–10 d (low dose); 3 g/m² q12h for 8–12 doses (high dose); 1 mg/kg 1–2×/wk (SC maint regimens); 5–70 mg/m² up to 3×/wk IT (refer to specific protocols); ↓ in renal/hepatic impairment **Caution/Contra:** [D, ?] **Supplied:** Inj 100, 500 mg, 1, 2 g **Notes/SE:** Myelosuppression, N/V/D, stomatitis, flu-like syndrome, rash on palms/soles, hepatic dysfunction; toxicity of high-dose regimens (conjunctivitis) ameliorated by corticosteroid ophth soln, cerebellar dysfunction, noncardiogenic pulmonary edema; neuropathy

Cytarabine Liposome (DepoCyt)   **Uses:** Lymphomatous meningitis **Action:** Antimetabolite; interferes with DNA synthesis **Dose:** 50 mg IT q14d for 5 doses, then 50 mg IT q28d for 4 doses; use dexamethasone prophylaxis **Caution/Contra:** [D, ?] **Supplied:** IT inj 50 mg/5 mL **Notes/SE:** Neck pain/rigidity, HA, confusion, somnolence, fever, back pain, N/V, edema, neutropenia, thrombocytopenia, anemia

Cytomegalovirus Immune Globulin [CMV-IG IV] (CytoGam)   **Uses:** Attenuation of primary CMV disease associated with transplantation **Action:** Exogenous IgG antibodies to CMV **Dose:** Administer for 16 wk posttransplant; see product information for dosing schedule **Caution/Contra:** [C, ?] **Supplied:** Inj 50–10 mg/mL **Notes/SE:** Flushing, N/V, muscle cramps, wheezing, HA, fever

Dacarbazine (DTIC)   **Uses:** Melanoma, Hodgkin's disease, sarcoma **Action:** Alkylating agent; antimetabolite activity as a purine precursor; inhibits synthesis of protein, RNA, and especially DNA **Dose:** 2–4.5 mg/kg/d for 10 consecutive d or 250 mg/m²/d for 5 d (refer to specific protocols); ↓ in renal impairment **Caution/Contra:** [C, ?] **Supplied:** Inj 100, 200, 500 mg **Notes/SE:** Myelosuppression, severe N/V, hepatotoxicity, flu-like syndrome, hypotension, photosensitivity, alopecia, facial flushing, facial paresthesias, urticaria, phlebitis at inj site

Daclizumab (Zenapax)   **Uses:** Prevent acute organ rejection **Action:** IL-2 receptor antagonist **Dose:** 1 mg/kg IV/dose; 1st dose pretransplant, then 4 doses 14 d apart posttransplant **Caution/Contra:** [C, ?] **Supplied:** Inj 5 mg/mL **Notes/SE:** Hyperglycemia, edema, HTN, hypotension, constipation, HA, dizziness, anxiety, nephrotoxicity, pulmonary edema, pain

Dactinomycin (Cosmegen)   **Uses:** Choriocarcinoma, Wilms' tumor, Kaposi's sarcoma, Ewing's sarcoma, rhabdomyosarcoma, testicular CA **Action:** DNA intercalating agent **Dose:** 0.5 mg/d for 5 d; 2 mg/wk for 3 consecutive wk; 15 mcg/kg or 0.45 mg/m²/d (max 0.5 mg) for 5 d q3–8wk in pediatric sarcoma (refer to specific protocols); ↓?in renal impairment **Caution/Contra:** [C, ?] **Supplied:** Inj 0.5 mg **Notes/SE:** Myelosuppression, immunosuppression, severe N/V, alopecia, acne, hyperpigmentation, radiation recall phenomenon, tissue damage with extravasation, hepatotoxicity

Dalteparin (Fragmin)   **Uses:** Unstable angina, non-Q-wave MI, prevention of ischemic complications due to clot formation in patients on concurrent ASA, prevention and Rx of DVT following surgery **Action:** LMW heparin **Dose:** *Angina/MI:* 120 IU/kg (max 10,000 IU) SC q12h with ASA. *DVT prophylaxis:* 2500–5000 IU SC 1–2 h preop, then qd for 5–10 d. *Systemic anticoagulation:* 200 IU/kg/d SC or 100 IU/kg bid SC **Caution/Contra:** [B, ?] Active hemorrhage, cerebrovascular disease, cerebral aneurysm, severe uncontrolled HTN **Supplied:** Inj 2500 IU (16 mg/0.2 mL), 5000 IU (32 mg/0.2 mL), 10,000 IU (64 mg/mL) **Notes/SE:** Predictable antithrombotic effects eliminate need for laboratory monitoring; bleeding, pain at inj site, thrombocytopenia

Dantrolene (Dantrium)   **Uses:** Clinical spasticity due to upper motor neuron disorders, eg, spinal cord injuries, strokes, CP, MS; Rx of malignant hyperthermia **Action:** Skeletal muscle relaxant **Dose:** *Adults.* Spasticity: Initially, 25 mg PO qd; ↑ to effect by 25 mg to a max dose of 100 mg PO qid PRN. *Peds.* Initially, 0.5 mg/ kg/dose bid; ↑ by 0.5 mg/kg to effect to a max dose of 3 mg/kg/dose qid PRN. *Adults & Peds.* Malignant hyperthermia: Treatment: Continuous rapid IV push beginning at 1 mg/kg until symptoms subside or 10 mg/kg is reached. *Postcrisis follow-up:* 4–8 mg/kg/d in 3–4 ÷ doses for 1–3 d to prevent recurrence **Caution/Contra:**[C, ?] Active hepatic disease **Supplied:** Caps 25, 50, 100 mg;

22

powder for inj 20 mg/vial **Notes/SE:** Monitor transaminases; drowsiness, dizziness, rash, muscle weakness, pleural effusion with pericarditis, diarrhea, blurred vision, hepatitis

Dapsone (Avlosulfon)   **Uses:** Rx and prevent PCP; toxoplasmosis prophylaxis; leprosy **Action:** Unknown; bactericidal **Dose:** *Adults.* Prophylaxis of PCP 50–100 mg/d PO; Rx of PCP 100 mg/d PO with TMP 5 mg/kg for 21 d. *Peds.* Prophylaxis of PCP 1–2 mg/kg/24 h PO qd; max 100 mg/d **Caution/Contra:** [C, +] Caution in G6PD deficiency **Supplied:** Tabs 25, 100 mg **Notes/SE:** Absorption ↑ by an acidic environment; with leprosy, combine with rifampin and other agents; hemolysis, methemoglobinemia, agranulocytosis, rash, cholestatic jaundice

Darbepoetin Alfa (Aranesp)   **Uses:** Anemia associated with CRF **Action:** Stimulates erythropoiesis, recombinant variant of erythropoietin **Dose:** 0.45 mcg/kg single IV or SC qwk; titrate dose, do not exceed target Hgb of 12 g/dL; see insert for converting from Epogen **Caution/Contra:** [C, ?] Contra uncontrolled hypertension, allergy to components **Supplied:** 25, 40, 60, 100 mcg/ mL, in polysorbate or albumin excipient **Notes/SE:** Longer ½-life than Epogen; follow weekly CBC until stable; may ↑ risk of cardiac events, chest pain, hypo-/hypertension, N/V/D, myalgia, arthralgia, dizziness, edema, fatigue, fever, ↑ risk infection

Daunorubicin (Daunomycin, Cerubidine)   WARNING: Cardiac function should be monitored due to potential risk for cardiac toxicity and CHF **Uses:** Acute leukemias **Action:** DNA intercalating agent; inhibits topoisomerase II; generates oxygen free radicals **Dose:** 45–60 mg/m²/d for 3 consecutive d; 25 mg/m²/wk (refer to specific protocols); ↓ in renal/hepatic impairment **Caution/Contra:** [D, ?] **Supplied:** Inj 20 mg **Notes/SE:** Myelosuppression, mucositis, N/V, alopecia, radiation recall phenomenon, hepatotoxicity (hyperbilirubinemia), tissue necrosis on extravascular extravasation, and cardiotoxicity (1–2% CHF risk with 550 mg/m² cumulative dose); prevent cardiotoxicity with dexrazoxane

Delavirdine (Rescriptor)   **Uses:** HIV infection **Action:** Nonnucleoside reverse transcriptase inhibitor **Dose:** 400 mg PO tid; avoid antacids **Caution/Contra:** [C, ?] CDC recommends HIV-infected mothers not breast-feed due to risk of HIV transmission to infant **Supplied:** Tabs 100 mg **Notes/SE:** Inhibits cytochrome P-450 enzymes. Numerous drug interactions; HA, fatigue, rash, ↑ serum transaminases, N/V/D

Demeclocycline (Declomycin)   **Uses:** SIADH **Action:** Antibiotic, antagonizes action of ADH on renal tubules **Dose:** 300–600 mg PO q12h on an empty stomach; ↓ in renal failure; avoid antacids **Caution/Contra:** [D, +] Avoid use in hepatic/renal dysfunction **Supplied:** Caps 150 mg; tabs 150, 300 mg **Notes/SE:** Diarrhea, abdominal cramps, photosensitivity, DI

Desipramine (Norpramin)   **Uses:** Endogenous depression, chronic pain, and peripheral neuropathy **Action:** TCA; increases synaptic conc of serotonin or norepinephrine in CNS **Dose:** 25–200 mg/d single or ÷ doses; usually a single hs dose (max 300 mg/d) **Caution/Contra:** [C, ?/–] Caution in cardiovascular disease, seizure disorder, hypothyroidism **Supplied:** Tabs 10, 25, 50, 75, 100, 150 mg; caps 25, 50 mg **Notes/SE:** Anticholinergic (blurred vision, urinary retention, xerostomia); prolongs QT interval, numerous drug interactions

Desloratadine (Clarinex)   **Uses:** Symptoms of seasonal and perennial allergic rhinitis; chronic idiopathic urticaria **Action:** The active metabolite of Claritin, H₁-antihistamine, blocks inflammatory mediators **Dose:** *Adults & Peds >12 y.* 5 mg PO qid; hepatic/renal impairment, 5 mg PO qod **Caution/Contra:** [C, ?/–] **Supplied:** Tabs 5 mg **Notes/SE:** Hypersensitivity reactions, anaphylaxis somnolence, HA, dizziness, fatigue, pharyngitis, xerostomia, nausea, dyspepsia, myalgia

Desmopressin (DDAVP, Stimate)   **Uses:** DI (intranasal and parenteral); bleeding due to uremia, hemophilia A, and type I von Willebrand's disease (parenteral), nocturnal enuresis **Action:** Synthetic analogue of vasopressin, a naturally occurring human ADH; ↑ factor VIII **Dose:** *DI: Intranasal: Adults.* 0.1–0.4 mL (10–40 mcg)/d in 1–4 ÷ doses. *Peds 3 mon–12 y.* 0.05–0.3 mL/d in 1 or 2 doses. *Parenteral: Adults.* 0.5–1 mL (2–4 mcg)/d in 2 ÷ doses. If converting from nasal to parenteral, use ½ nasal dose. *Oral: Adults.* 0.05 mg bid; ↑ to max of 1.2 mg. *Hemophilia A and von Willebrand's disease (type I): Adults & Peds >10 kg.* 0.3 mcg/kg in 50 mL NS, infuse over 15–30 min. *Peds <10 kg.* As above with dilution to 10 mL with NS. *Nocturnal enuresis: Peds >6 y.* 20 mcg intranasally hs. **Caution/Contra:** [B, M] **Supplied:** Tabs 0.1, 0.2 mg; inj 4 mcg/mL; nasal soln 0.1, 1.5 mg/mL **Notes/SE:** In very young and old patients, ↓ fluid intake to avoid water intoxication and hyponatremia; facial flushing, HA, dizziness, vulval pain, nasal congestion, pain at inj site, hyponatremia, water intoxication

Dexamethasone, Nasal (Dexacort Phosphate Turbinaire)
Uses: Chronic nasal inflammation or allergic rhinitis **Action:** Antiinflammatory corticosteroid **Dose:** *Adult and Peds >12 y.* 2 sprays/nostril bid–tid, max 12 sprays/d. *Peds 6–12 y.* 1–2 sprays/nostril, bid, max 8 sprays/d **Caution/Contra:** [C, ?] **Supplied:** Aerosol, 84 mcg/activation **Notes/SE:** Local irritation

Dexamethasone, Ophthalmic (AK-Dex Ophthalmic, Decadron Ophthalmic)
Uses: Inflammatory or allergic conjunctivitis **Action:** Antiinflammatory corticosteroid **Dose:** Instill 1–2 gtt tid–qid **Caution/Contra:** [C, ?/–] Contra in active untreated bacterial, viral, and fungal eye infections **Supplied:** Susp and soln 0.1%; oint 0.05% **Notes/SE:** Long-term use associated with cataract formation

Dexamethasone Systemic, Topical (Decadron)
See Steroids, Systemic, page 612, and and Topical, page 613

Dexpanthenol (Ilopan-Choline Oral, Ilopan)
Uses: Minimize paralytic ileus, Rx postop distention **Action:** Cholinergic agent **Dose:** *Adults.* Relief of gas: 2–3 tabs PO tid. *Prevent postop ileus:* 250–500 mg IM stat, repeat in 2 h, then q6h PRN. *Ileus:* 500 mg IM stat, repeat in 2 h, followed by doses q6h, if needed **Caution/Contra:** [C, ?] Hemophilia, mechanical obstruction **Supplied:** Inj; tabs 50 mg; cream **Notes/SE:** GI cramps

Dexrazoxane (Zinecard)
Uses: Prevent anthracycline-induced cardiomyopathy **Action:** Chelates heavy metals; binds intracellular iron and prevents anthracycline-induced free radicals **Dose:** 10:1 ratio dexrazoxane: doxorubicin 30 min prior to each dose **Caution/Contra:** [C, ?] **Supplied:** Inj 10 mg/mL **Notes/SE:** Myelosuppression (especially leukopenia), fever, infection, stomatitis, alopecia, N/V/D; mild ↑ transaminase, pain at inj site

Dextran 40 (Rheomacrodex)
Uses: Shock, prophylaxis of DVT and thromboembolism, adjunct in peripheral vascular surgery **Action:** Expands plasma volume; ↓ blood viscosity **Dose:** *Shock:* 10 mL/kg infused rapidly; 20 mL/kg max in the 1st 24 h; beyond 24 h 10 mL/kg max; DC after 5 d. *Prophylaxis of DVT and thromboembolism:* 10 mL/kg IV day of surgery, then 500 mL/d IV for 2–3 d, then 500 mL IV q2–3d based on risk for up to 2 wk **Caution/Contra:** [C, ?] **Supplied:** 10% dextran 40 in 0.9% NaCl or 5% dextrose **Notes/SE:** Hypersensitivity/anaphylactoid reaction (observe patient closely during 1st min of inf), arthralgia, cutaneous reactions, fever; monitor renal function and electrolytes

Dextromethorphan (Mediquell, Benylin DM, PediaCare 1, others)
Uses: Controlling nonproductive cough **Action:** Depresses the cough center in the medulla **Dose:** *Adults.* 10–30 mg PO q4h PRN. *Peds.* 7 mon–1 y: 2–4 mg q6–8h; *2–6 y:* 2.5–7.5 mg q4–8h (max 30 mg/24 h). *7–12 y:* 5–10 mg q4–8h (max 60 mg/24/h) **Caution/Contra:** [C,?/–] **Supplied:** Caps 30 mg; lozenges 2.5, 5, 7.5, 15 mg; syrup 15 mg/15 mL, 10 mg/5 mL; liq 10 mg/15 mL, 3.5, 7.5, 15 mg/5 mL; sustained-action liq 30 mg/5 mL **Notes/SE:** May be found in combination products with guaifenesin; GI disturbances

Dezocine (Dalgan)
Uses: Moderate–severe pain **Action:** Narcotic agonist–antagonist **Dose:** 5–20 mg IM or 2.5–10 mg IV q2–4h PRN;↓ in renal impairment **Caution/Contra:** [C, ?] Not recommended for patients <18 y **Supplied:** Inj 5, 10, 15 mg/mL **Notes/SE:** Withdrawal possible in patients dependent on narcotics

Diazepam (Valium) [C-IV]
Uses: Anxiety, alcohol withdrawal, muscle spasm, status epilepticus, panic disorders, amnesia, preoperative sedation **Action:** Benzodiazepine **Dose:** *Adults. Status epilepticus:* 5–10 mg q10–20min to 30 mg max in 8-h period. *Anxiety, muscle spasm:* 2–10 mg PO bid–qid or IM/IV q3–4h PRN. *Preop:* 5–10 mg PO or IM 20–30 min or IV just prior to procedure. *Alcohol withdrawal:* Initial 2–5 mg IV, then 5–10 mg q5–10min, 100 mg in 1 h max. May require up to 1000 mg in 24-h period for severe withdrawal. Titrate to agitation; avoid excessive sedation; may lead to aspiration or respiratory arrest. *Peds. Status epilepticus:* <5 y: 0.05–0.3 mg/kg/dose IV q15–30min up to a max of 5 mg. >5 y: Give up to max of 10 mg. *Sedation, muscle relaxation:* 0.04–0.3 mg/kg/dose q2–4h IM or IV to max of 0.6 mg/kg in 8 h, or 0.12–0.8 mg/kg/24 h PO ÷ tid–qid; ↓ in hepatic impairment; avoid abrupt withdrawal **Caution/Contra:** [D, ?/–] **Supplied:** Tabs 2, 5, 10 mg; soln 1,

22

5 mg/mL; inj 5 mg/mL; rectal gel 5 mg/mL **Notes/SE:** Do not exceed 5 mg/min IV in adults or 1–2 mg/min in Peds because respiratory arrest possible; IM absorption erratic; sedation, amnesia, bradycardia, hypotension, rash, decreased respiratory rate

Diazoxide (Hyperstat, Proglycem) **Uses:** Hypoglycemia due to hyperinsulinism (Proglycem); hypertensive crisis (Hyperstat) **Action:** Inhibits pancreatic insulin release; antihypertensive **Dose:** *Hypertensive crisis:* IV: 1–3 mg/kg (maximum: 150 mg in a single inj); repeat dose in 5–15 min until BP controlled; repeat every 4–24 h; monitor BP closely. *Adults & Peds.* 3–8 mg/kg/24 h PO ÷ q8–12h. *Neonates.* 8–15 mg/kg/24 h ÷ in 3 equal doses; maint 8–10 mg/kg/24 h PO in 2–3 equal doses **Caution/Contra:** [C, ?] Hypersensitivity to thiazides or other sulfonamide-containing products; HTN associated with aortic coarctation, arteriovenous shunt, or pheochromocytoma **Supplied:** Inj 15 mg/mL; caps 50 mg; oral susp 50 mg/mL **Notes/SE:** Hyperglycemia, hypotension, dizziness, Na and water retention, N/V, weakness

Dibucaine (Nupercainal) **Uses:** Hemorrhoids and minor skin conditions **Action:** Topical anesthetic **Dose:** Insert PR with applicator bid and after each bowel movement; apply sparingly to skin **Caution/Contra:** [C, ?] **Supplied:** 1% oint with rectal applicator; 0.5% cream **Notes/SE:** Local irritation, rash

Diclofenac (Cataflam, Voltaren) **Uses:** Arthritis and pain **Action:** NSAID **Dose:** 50–75 mg PO bid; take with food or milk **Caution/Contra:** [B (D 3rd trimester or near delivery), ?] Caution in CHF, HTN, renal/hepatic dysfunction, and Hx PUD. **Supplied:** Tabs 50 mg; tabs DR 25, 50, 75, 100 mg; XR tabs 100 mg; ophth soln 0.1% **Notes/SE:** Abdominal cramps, heartburn, GI ulceration, rash, interstitial nephritis

Dicloxacillin (Dynapen, Dycill) **Uses:** Infections due to susceptible strains of *S. aureus* and *Streptococcus* **Action:** Bactericidal; inhibits cell wall synthesis **Dose:** *Adults.* 250–500 mg qid. *Peds <40 kg.* 12.5–25 mg/kg/d ÷ qid; take on empty stomach **Caution/Contra:** [B, ?] **Supplied:** Caps 125, 250, 500 mg; soln 62.5 mg/5 mL **Notes/SE:** Diarrhea, nausea, abdominal pain

Dicyclomine (Bentyl) **Uses:** Functional irritable bowel syndromes **Action:** Smooth muscle relaxant **Dose:** *Adults.* 20 mg PO qid; ↑ to a max dose of 160 mg/d or 20 mg IM q6h. *Peds. Infants >6 mon:* 5 mg/dose tid–qid. *Children:* 10 mg/dose tid–qid **Caution/Contra:** [B, –] Infants >6 mon, narrow-angle glaucoma, MyG, severe UC, obstructive uropathy **Supplied:** Caps 10, 20 mg; tabs 20 mg; syrup 10 mg/5 mL; inj 10 mg/mL **Notes/SE:** Anticholinergic side effects may limit dose

Didanosine [ddI] (Videx) **WARNING:** Hypersensitivity manifested as fever, rash, fatigue, GI/respiratory symptoms reported; stop drug immediately and do not rechallenge; lactic acidosis and hepatomegaly/steatosis reported **Uses:** HIV infection in zidovudine-intolerant patients **Action:** Nucleoside antiretroviral agent **Dose:** *Adults.* >60 kg: 400 mg/d PO or 200 mg PO bid. *<60 kg:* 250 mg/d PO or 125 mg PO bid; adults should take 2 tabs/administration. *Peds.* Dose by following table; ↓ in renal impairment, thoroughly chew tablets, do not mix with fruit juice or other acidic beverages; reconstitute powder with water **Caution/Contra:** [B, –] CDC recommends HIV-infected mothers not breast-feed due to risk of transmission of HIV to their infant. **Supplied:** Chew tabs 25, 50, 100, 150, 200 mg; powder packets 100, 167, 250, 375 mg; powder for soln 2, 4 g **Notes/SE:** Pancreatitis, peripheral neuropathy, diarrhea, HA

BSA (m²)	Tablets (mg)	Powder (mg)
1.1–1.4	100 bid	125 bid
0.8–1	75 bid	94 bid
0.5–0.7	50 bid	62 bid
<0.4	25 bid	31 bid

Diflunisal (Dolobid) Uses: Mild–moderate pain; osteoarthritis **Action:** NSAID **Dose:** *Pain:* 500 mg PO bid. *Osteoarthritis:* 500–1500 mg PO in 2–3 ÷ doses; ↓ in renal impairment, take with food/milk **Caution/Contra:** [C (D 3rd trimester or near delivery), ?] Caution in CHF, HTN, renal/hepatic dysfunction, and Hx PUD. **Supplied:** Tabs 250, 500 mg **Notes/SE:** May prolong bleeding time; HA, abdominal cramps, heartburn, GI ulceration, rash, interstitial nephritis, fluid retention

Digoxin (Lanoxin, Lanoxicaps) Uses: CHF, AF and flutter, and PAT **Action:** Positive inotrope; ↑ AV node refractory period **Dose:** *Adults.* PO digitalization: 0.50–0.75 mg PO, then 0.25 mg PO q6–8h to total 1.0–1.5 mg. *IV or IM digitalization:* 0.25–0.5 mg IM or IV, then 0.25 mg q4–6h to total ≅1 mg. *Daily maint:* 0.125–0.5 mg/d PO, IM, or IV (average daily dose 0.125–0.25 mg). **Peds.** *Preterm infants: Digitalization:* 30 mcg/kg PO or 25 mcg/kg IV; give ½ of dose initially, then ¼ of dose at 8–12-h intervals for 2 doses. *Maint:* 5–7.5 mcg/kg/24 h PO or 4–6 mcg/ kg/24 h IV ÷ q12h. *Term infants: Digitalization:* 25–35 mcg/kg PO or 20–30 mcg/kg IV; give ½ the dose initially, then ⅓ of the dose at 8–12 h. *Maint:* 6–10 mcg/kg/24 h PO or 5–8 mcg/kg/24 h ÷ q12h. *1 mon–2 y: Digitalization:* 35–60 mcg/kg PO or 30–50 mcg/kg IV; give ½ the dose initially, then ⅓ of the dose at 8–12-h intervals for 2 doses. *Maint:* 10–15 mcg/kg/24 h PO or 7.5–15 mcg/kg/24 h IV ÷ q12h. *2–10 y: Digitalization:* 30–40 mcg/kg PO or 25 mcg/kg IV; give ½ dose initially, then ⅓ of the dose at 8–12-h intervals for 2 doses. *Maint:* 8–10 mcg/kg/24 h PO or 6–8 mcg/ kg/24 h IV ÷ q12h. *7–10 y:* Same as for adults; ↓ in renal impairment, follow serum levels **Caution/Contra:** [C, +] Contra AV block **Supplied:** Caps 0.05, 0.1, 0.2 mg; tabs 0.125, 0.25, 0.5 mg; elixir 0.05 mg/mL; inj 0.1, 0.25 mg/mL **Notes/SE:** See Drug Levels, Table 2, page 607. IM inj painful and erratic absorption; can cause heart block; ↓ K⁺ potentiates toxicity; N/V, HA, fatigue, visual disturbances (yellow-green halos around lights), cardiac arrhythmias, multiple drug interactions

Digoxin Immune Fab (Digibind) Uses: Life-threatening digoxin intoxication **Action:** Antigen-binding fragments bind and inactivate digoxin **Dose:** *Adults & Peds.* Based on serum level and patient's weight; see charts provided with the drug **Caution/Contra:** [C, ?] Hypersensitivity to sheep products **Supplied:** Inj 38 mg/vial **Notes/SE:** Each vial binds ≅ 0.6 mg of digoxin; in renal failure may require redosing in several days because of breakdown of the immune complex; worsening of cardiac output or CHF, hypokalemia, facial swelling, and redness

Diltiazem (Cardizem, Cardizem CD, Cardizem SR, Cartia XT, Dilacor XR, Diltia XT, Tiamate, Tiazac) Uses: Angina, prevention of reinfarction, HTN, AF or flutter, and PAT **Action:** Ca channel blocker **Dose:** *Oral:* Initially, 30 mg PO qid; ↑ to 180–360 mg/d in 3–4 ÷ doses PRN. *SR:* 60–120 mg PO bid; ↑ to 360 mg/d max. *CD:* 120–360 mg/d (max 480 mg/d). *IV:* 0.25 mg/kg IV bolus over 2 min; may repeat in 15 min at 0.35 mg/kg; may begin inf of 5–15 mg/h **Caution/Contra:** [C, +] Sick sinus syndrome, AV block, hypotension, AMI, pulmonary congestion **Supplied:** Cardizem CD: Caps 120, 180, 240, 300, 360 mg; Cardizem SR: caps 60, 90, 120 mg; Cardizem: Tabs 30, 60, 90, 120mg; Cartia XT: Caps 120, 180, 240, 300 mg; Dilacor XR: Caps 180, 240 mg; Diltia XT: Caps 120, 180, 240 mg; Tiazac: Caps 120, 180, 240, 300, 360, 420 mg; Tiamate (ER): Tabs 120, 180, 240 mg; inj: 5 mg/mL **Notes/SE:** Cardizem CD, Dilacor XR, and Tiazac not interchangeable; gingival hyperplasia, bradycardia, AV block, ECG abnormalities, peripheral edema, dizziness, HA

Dimenhydrinate (Dramamine, others) Uses: Prevention and Rx of nausea, vomiting, dizziness, or vertigo of motion sickness **Action:** Antiemetic **Dose:** *Adults.* 50–100 mg PO q4–6h, max 400 mg/d; 50 mg IM/IV PRN. *Peds.* 5 mg/kg/24 h PO or IV ÷ qid (max 300 mg/d) **Caution/Contra:** [B, ?] **Supplied:** Tabs 50 mg; chew tabs 50 mg; liq 12.5 mg/4 mL, 12.5 mg/5 mL, 15.62 mg/5 mL; inj 50 mg/mL **Notes/SE:** Anticholinergic side effects

Dimethyl Sulfoxide [DMSO] (Rimso-50) Uses: Interstitial cystitis **Action:** Unknown **Dose:** Intravesical, 50 mL, retain for 15 min; repeat q2wk until relief **Caution/Contra:** [C, ?] **Supplied:** 50% soln in 50 mL **Notes/SE:** Cystitis, eosinophilia, GI, and taste disturbance

Dinoprostone (Cervidil Vaginal Insert, Prepidil Vaginal Gel) Uses: Induce labor; terminate pregnancy (12–28 wk); evacuate uterus in missed abortion or fetal death; **Action:** prostaglandin, changes consistency, dilatation, and effacement of the cervix; induces uterine contraction. **Dose:** Gel 0.5 mg; if no cervical/uterine response, repeat 0.5 mg q 6 h (max 24 h dose 1.5 mg); vaginal insert: 1 insert (10 mg = 0.3 mg dinoprostone/h over

22

12-h); remove with onset of labor or 12 h after insertion; Vaginal supp: 20 mg repeated every 3-5 h; adjust PRN Suppository: 1 high in vagina, repeat at 3–5-h intervals until abortion, (240 mg max); **Supplied** gel, endocervical: 0.5 mg in 3 g syringes [each package contains a 10-mm and 20-mm shielded catheter] **Caution/Contra: [X, ?]** ruptured membranes, hypersensitivity to prostaglandins, placenta previa or unexplained vaginal bleeding during pregnancy, when oxytocic drugs contraindicated or if prolonged uterine contractions are inappropriate (Hx C-section or major uterine surgery, presence of cephalopelvic disproportion, etc) **Supplied** *Vaginal Gel:* 0.5 mg/3 g; *Vaginal supp:* 20 mg; *Vaginal insert, CR:* 0.3 mg/h **Notes:** N/V/D, dizziness, flushing, headache, fever

Diphenhydramine (Benadryl) **Uses:** Treat and prevent allergic reactions, motion sickness, potentiate narcotics, sedation, cough suppression, and treatment of extrapyramidal reactions **Action:** Antihistamine, antiemetic **Dose:** *Adults.* 25–50 mg PO, IV, or IM bid–tid. *Peds.* 5 mg/kg/24 h PO or IM ÷ q6h (max 300 mg/d); ↑ dosing interval in moderate/severe renal failure **Caution/Contra: [B, –]** **Supplied:** Tabs and caps 25, 50 mg; chew tabs 12.5 mg; elixir 12.5 mg/5 mL; syrup 12.5 mg/5 mL; liq 6.25 mg/5 mL, 12.5 mg/5 mL; inj 50 mg/mL **Notes/SE:** Anticholinergic side effects (xerostomia, urinary retention, sedation)

Diphenoxylate + Atropine (Lomotil) [C-V] **Uses:** Diarrhea **Action:** Constipating meperidine congener **Dose:** *Adults.* Initially, 5 mg PO tid–qid until under control, then 2.5–5.0 mg PO bid. *Peds >2 y:* 0.3–0.4 mg/kg/24 h (of diphenoxylate) bid–qid **Caution/Contra:** [C, +] Contra obstructive jaundice, diarrhea due to bacterial infection **Supplied:** Tabs 2.5 mg of diphenoxylate/0.025 mg of atropine; liq 2.5 mg diphenoxylate/0.025 mg atropine/5 mL **Notes/SE:** Drowsiness, dizziness, xerostomia, blurred vision, urinary retention, constipation

Diphtheria and Tetanus Toxoids [DT and Td] **Uses:** Vaccine against diphtheria, tetanus, when pertussis vaccination contraindicated **Actions:** Active immunization **Dose:** *Adults and Peds > 7* y: (Use Td) two 0.5-mL doses IM @ 4–6-wk intervals, reinforcing dose 6–12 mon later, booster every 10 y; *Peds* (use DT): 6 wk–1 y: three 0.5-mL doses IM @ 4-wk intervals, reinforcing dose @ 6–12 mon after 3rd inj; 1–6 y 2 0.5 mL doses IM @ 4 wk intervals, reinforcing dose @ 6–12 mon after 2nd dose (use adult formula [Td] if last dose after 7th birthday. **Contra/Caution:** [C, ?] Immunosuppressed, Hx allergy to any component of the vaccine, previous neurologic reaction to dose **Supplied:** Single-dose vials, varying concs of diphtheria and tetanus toxoids: 0.5-mL DT for peds ≤ 6 y; Td if >7 y and adults **Notes/SE:** DT contains higher conc of diphtheria toxoid than Td; dTaP preferred in children in U.S.; drowsiness, restlessness, fever, nodule redness, pain, and swelling at site

Diphtheria and Tetanus Toxoids and Acellular Pertussis Adsorbed [DTaP] (Tripedia, ACEL-IMUNE, Infanrix) **Uses:** Vaccine against diphtheria, tetanus, and pertussis **Actions:** Active immunization **Dose:** *Peds:* 0.5 mL IM 2, 4, 6, and 15–18 mon and 4–6 y; 5th dose not needed if 4th dose given on/after 4th birthday **Contra/Caution:** [C, ?] Immunosuppressed, HX allergy to any component of the vaccine, previous neurologic reaction to dose, Hx of seizures **Supplied:** Single-dose vials **Notes/SE:** Acellular pertussis is currently recommended over whole-cell pertussis vaccines due to lower incidence of side effects; local and febrile reactions, prolonged crying, rashes, hypotonic-hyporesponsive episodes, rare anaphylaxis and seizures

Diphtheria and Tetanus Toxoids and Acellular Pertussis Adsorbed, Hepatitis B (recombinant), and Inactivated Poliovirus Vaccine (IPV) Combined (Pediarix) **Uses:** Vaccine against diphtheria, tetanus, pertussis, HBV, polio(types 1, 2, 3) as a three-dose primary series in infants and children younger than age 7, born to HB$_s$Ag-negative mothers **Actions:** Active immunization **Dose:** Infants: 3 0.5-mL doses IM , at 6–8-wk intervals, start at 2 mon; child given 1 dose of hepatitis B vaccine, same; Child previously vaccinated with one or more doses of Infanrix or IPV, use to complete series **Contra/Caution:** [C, N/A] Contra if HB$_s$AG + mother, adults, children >7 y, immunosuppressed, in hypersensitivity to yeast, neomycin, or polymyxin B, Hx allergy to any component of the vaccine, encephalopathy, or progressive neurologic disorders; caution in bleeding disorders. **Supplied:** Single-dose vials: 0.5-mL **Notes:** drowsiness, restlessness, fever, fussiness. ↓ appetite; nodule redness, pain, and swelling at site

Dipivefrin (Propine) **Uses:** Open-angle glaucoma **Action:** α-Adrenergic agonist **Dose:** 1 gtt into eye q12h **Caution/Contra: [B, ?]** Contra closed-angle glaucoma **Supplied:** 0.1% soln **Notes/SE:** HA, local irritation, blurred vision, photophobia, HTN

Dipyridamole (Persantine) **Uses:** Prevent postoperative thromboembolic disorders, often in combination with ASA or warfarin (eg, CABG, vascular graft; with warfarin after artificial heart valve; chronic angina; with ASA to prevent coronary artery thrombosis); dipyridamole IV used in place of exercise stress test for CAD **Action:** Antiplatelet activity; coronary vasodilator **Dose:** *Adults.* 75–100 mg PO tid–qid; stress test 0.14 mg/kg/min (max 60 mg over 4 min). *Peds >12 y.* 3–6 mg/kg/d divided tid **Caution/Contra:** [B, ?/–] Caution with other drugs that affect coagulation **Supplied:** Tabs 25, 50, 75 mg; inj 5 mg/mL **Notes:** IV can worsen angina; HA, hypotension, nausea, abdominal distress, flushing rash, dyspnea

Dipyridamole and Aspirin (Aggrenox) **Uses:** Reduce rate of reinfarction after MI; prevent occlusion after CABG; ↓ risk of stroke **Action:** ↓ platelet aggregation (both agents) **Dose:** 1 cap PO bid **Caution/Contra:** [C, ?] Contra in ulcers, bleed diathesis **Supplied:** Dipyridamole (extended release) 200 mg/aspirin 25 mg **Notes/SE:** ASA component: allergic reactions, skin reactions, ulcers/GI bleed, bronchospasm; dipyridamole component: dizziness, HA, rash

Dirithromycin (Dynabac) **Uses:** Bronchitis, community-acquired pneumonia, and skin and skin structure infections **Action:** Macrolide antibiotic **Dose:** 500 mg/d PO; take with food **Caution/Contra:** [C, M] **Supplied:** Tabs 250 mg **Notes/SE:** Abdominal discomfort, HA, rash, hyperkalemia

Disopyramide (Norpace, NAPAmide) **Uses:** Suppression and prevention of VT **Action:** Class 1A antiarrhythmic **Dose:** *Adults.* 400–800 mg/d ÷ q6h for regular and q12h for SR. *Peds.* *<1 y:* 10–30 mg/kg/24 h PO (÷ qid). *1–4 y:* 10–20 mg/kg/24 h PO (÷ qid). *4–12 y:* 10–15 mg/kg/24 h PO (÷ qid). *12–18 y:* 6–15 mg/kg/24 h PO (÷ qid); ↓ in renal/hepatic impairment **Caution/Contra:** [C, +] AV block, cardiogenic shock **Supplied:** Caps 100, 150 mg; SR caps 100, 150 mg **Notes/SE:** See Drug Levels, Table 2, page 607. Anticholinergic side effects; negative inotropic properties may induce CHF

Dobutamine (Dobutrex) **Uses:** Short-term use in cardiac decompensation secondary to depressed contractility **Action:** Positive inotropic agent **Dose:** *Adults & Peds.* Cont IV inf of 2.5–15 mcg/kg/min; rarely, 40 mcg/kg/min may be required; titrate according to response **Caution/Contra:** [C, ?] **Supplied:** Inj 250 mg/20 mL **Notes/SE:** Monitor PWP and cardiac output if possible, check ECG for ↑ heart rate, ectopic activity, follow BP; chest pain, HTN, dyspnea

Docetaxel (Taxotere) **Uses:** Breast (anthracycline-resistant), ovarian, lung, and prostate CAs **Action:** Antimitotic agent; promotes microtubular aggregation; semisynthetic taxoid **Dose:** 100 mg/m² over 1 h IV q3wk. (refer to specific protocols) Start dexamethasone 8 mg bid prior to docetaxel and continue for 3–4 d; ↓ dose with ↑ bilirubin levels **Caution/Contra:** [D, –] **Supplied:** Inj 20, 40, 80 mg/mL **Notes/SE:** Myelosuppression, neuropathy, N/V; fluid retention syndrome; cumulative doses of 300–400 mg/m² w/o steroid prep and posttreatment and 600–800 mg/m² with steroid prep; hypersensitivity reactions possible, but rare with steroid prep

Docusate Calcium (Surfak)/Docusate Potassium (Dialose)/ Docusate Sodium (DOSS, Colace) **Uses:** Constipation; adjunct to painful anorectal conditions (hemorrhoids) **Action:** Stool softener **Dose:** *Adults.* 5 ÷ qd–qid; *3–6 y:* 20–60 mg/24 h ÷ qd–qid. *6–12 y:* 40–150 mg/24 h ÷ qd–qid **Caution/Contra:**[C, ?] **Supplied:** *Ca:* Caps 50, 240 mg. *K:* Caps 100, 240 mg. *Na:* Caps 50, 100 mg; syrup 50, 60 mg/15 mL; liq 150 mg/15 mL; soln 50 mg/mL **Notes/SE:** No significant side effects, rare abdominal cramping, diarrhea; no laxative action

Dolasetron (Anzemet) **Uses:** Prevent chemotherapy-associated N/V **Action:** 5-HT₃ receptor antagonist **Dose:** *Adults & Peds.* 1.8 mg/kg IV as single dose 30 min prior to chemotherapy. *Adults.* 100 mg PO as a single dose 1 h prior to chemotherapy. *Peds.* 1.8 mg/kg PO to max 100 mg as single dose **Caution/Contra:** [B, ?] **Supplied:** Tabs 50, 100 mg; inj 20 mg/mL **Notes/SE:** Prolongs QT interval, HTN, HA, abdominal pain, urinary retention, transient ↑ LFTs

Dofetilide (Tikosyn) **WARNING:** To minimize the risk of induced arrhythmia, patients initiated or reinitiated on Tikosyn should be placed for a minimum of 3 d in a facility that can provide calculations of CrCl, continuous ECG monitoring, and cardiac resuscitation **Uses:** Maintain NSR in AF/A flutter after conversion **Action:** Type III antiarrhythmic **Dose:** 125–500 mcg PO bid based on CrCl and QTc (See insert) **Caution/Contra:** [C, –] Contra in

22

prolonged QT interval, verapamil, cimetidine, trimethoprim, or ketoconazole **Supplied:** Caps 125, 250, 500 mcg **Notes/SE:** Ventricular arrhythmias, HA, chest pain, dizziness

Dopamine (Intropin) **Uses:** Short-term use in cardiac decompensation secondary to decreased contractility; increases organ perfusion (at low dose) **Action:** Positive inotropic agent with dose-related response. 2–10 mcg/kg/min β-effects (increases cardiac output and renal perfusion). 10–20 mcg/kg/min β-effects (peripheral vasoconstriction, pressor). >20 mcg/kg/min peripheral and renal vasoconstriction **Dose:** *Adults & Peds.* 5 mcg/kg/min by cont inf, ↑ increments of 5 mcg/kg/min to 50 mcg/kg/min max based on effect **Caution/Contra:** [C, ?] **Supplied:** Inj 40, 80, 160 mg/mL **Notes/SE:** Dosage >10 mcg/kg/min may ↓ renal perfusion; monitor urinary output; monitor ECG for ↑ in heart rate, BP, and ectopic activity; monitor PCWP and cardiac output if possible

Dornase Alfa (Pulmozyme) **Uses:** ↓ Frequency of respiratory infections in patients with CF **Action:** Enzyme that selectively cleaves DNA **Dose:** Inhal 2.5 mg/d **Caution/Contra:** [B, ?] **Supplied:** Soln for inhal 1 mg/mL **Notes/SE:** Use with recommended neb; pharyngitis, voice alteration, chest pain, rash

Dorzolamide (Trusopt) **Uses:** Glaucoma **Action:** Carbonic anhydrase inhibitor **Dose:** 1 gtt in eye(s) tid **Caution/Contra:** [C, ?] **Supplied:** 2% soln **Notes/SE:** Local irritation, bitter taste, superficial punctate keratitis, ocular allergic reaction

Dorzolamide and Timolol (Cosopt) **Uses:** Glaucoma MOA: Carbonic anhydrase inhibitor with β-adrenergic blocker **Dose:** 1 gtt in eye(s) bid **Caution/Contra:** [C, ?] **Supplied:** Soln dorzolamide 2% and timolol 0.5% **Notes/SE:** See Dorzolamide

Doxazosin (Cardura) **Uses:** HTN and symptomatic BPH **Action:** α_1-Adrenergic blocker; relaxes bladder neck smooth muscle **Dose:** *HTN:* Initially 1 mg/d PO; may be ↑ to 16 mg/d PO. *BPH:* Initially 1 mg/d PO, may be ↑ to 8 mg/d PO **Caution/Contra:** [B, ?] **Supplied:** Tabs 1, 2, 4, 8 mg **Notes/SE:** Doses >4 mg ↑ likelihood of orthostatic hypotension, dizziness, HA, drowsiness, sexual dysfunction

Doxepin (Sinequan, Adapin) **Uses:** Depression, anxiety, chronic pain **Action:** TCA; increases the synaptic CNS concs of serotonin or norepinephrine **Dose:** 25–150 mg/d PO, usually hs but can be in ÷ doses; ↓ hepatic impairment **Caution/Contra:** [C, ?/–] **Supplied:** Caps 10, 25, 50, 75, 100, 150 mg; oral conc 10 mg/mL **Notes/SE:** Anticholinergic side effects, hypotension, tachycardia, drowsiness, photosensitivity

Doxepin, Topical (Zonalon) **Uses:** Short-term Rx pruritus (atopic dermatitis or lichen simplex chronicus) **Action:** Antipruritic; H_1- and H_2-receptor antagonism **Dose:** Apply thin coating qid for max 8 d **Caution/Contra:** [C, ?/–] **Supplied:** 5% cream **Notes/SE:** Limited application area to avoid systemic toxicity (hypotension, tachycardia, drowsiness, photosensitivity)

Doxorubicin (Adriamycin, Rubex) **Uses:** Acute leukemias; Hodgkin's and NHLs; breast CA; soft tissue and osteosarcomas; Ewing's sarcoma; Wilms' tumor; neuroblastoma; bladder, ovarian, gastric, thyroid, and lung CAs **Action:** Intercalates DNA; inhibits DNA topoisomerases I and II **Dose:** 60–75 mg/m^2 q3wk; ↓ cardiotoxicity with weekly (20 mg/m^2/wk) or cont inf (60–90 mg/m^2 over 96 h); (refer to specific protocols) **Caution/Contra:** [D, ?] **Supplied:** Inj 10, 20, 50, 75, 200 mg **Notes/SE:** Myelosuppression; extravasation leads to tissue damage; venous streaking and phlebitis, N/V/D, mucositis, radiation recall phenomenon. Cardiomyopathy rare but dose related; limit of 550 mg/m^2 cumulative dose (400 mg/m^2 if prior mediastinal irradiation); dexrazoxane may limit cardiac toxicity

Doxycycline (Vibramycin) **Uses:** Broad-spectrum antibiotic, activity against *Rickettsia* spp, *Chlamydia,* and *M. pneumoniae* **Action:** Tetracycline; interferes with protein synthesis **Dose:** *Adults.* 100 mg PO q12h on 1st day, then 100 mg PO qd–bid or 100 mg IV q12h. *Peds >8y.* 5 mg/kg/24 h PO, to a max of 200 mg/d ÷ qd–bid **Supplied:** Tabs 50, 100 mg; caps 20, 50, 100 mg; syrup 50 mg/5 mL; susp 25 mg/5 mL; inj 100, 200 mg/vial **Caution/Contra:** [D, +] **Notes/SE:** Useful for chronic bronchitis; tetracycline of choice in renal impairment; diarrhea, GI disturbance, photosensitivity

Dronabinol (Marinol) [C-II] **Uses:** N/V; appetite stimulation **Action:** Antiemetic; inhibits the vomiting center in the medulla **Dose:** *Adults & Peds. Antiemetic:* 5–15 mg/m^2/dose q4–6h PRN. *Adults. Appetite:* 2.5 mg PO before lunch and dinner

Caution/Contra: [C, ?] **Supplied:** Caps 2.5, 5, 10 mg **Notes/SE:** Principal psychoactive substance present in marijuana; drowsiness, dizziness, anxiety, mood change, hallucinations, depersonalization, orthostatic hypotension, tachycardia

Droperidol (Inapsine) **Uses:** N/V; anesthetic premedication **Action:** Tranquilization, sedation, and antiemetic **Dose:** *Adults. Nausea:* 2.5–5 mg IV or IM q3–4h PRN. *Premed:* 2.5–10 mg IV, 30–60 min preop. *Peds. Premed:* 0.1–0.15 mg/kg/dose **Caution/Contra:** [C, ?] **Supplied:** Inj 2.5 mg/mL **Notes/SE:** Drowsiness, moderate hypotension, occasional tachycardia and extrapyramidal reactions, QT interval prolongation, arrhythmias

Drotrecogin Alfa (Xigris) **Uses:** Reduce mortality in adults with severe sepsis (associated with acute organ dysfunction) who have a high risk of death (eg, as determined by APACHE II) **Action:** Recombinant form of human activated protein C; exact mechanism unknown **Dose:** 24 mcg/kg/h for a total of 96 h **Caution/Contra:** [C, ?] Contra in active bleeding, recent stroke or CNS surgery, head trauma, epidural catheter, CNS lesion at risk for herniation **Supplied:** 5, 20 mg vials for reconstitution **Notes/SE:** Bleeding most common SE

Dutasteride (Avodart) **Uses:** Symptomatic BPH **Action:** 5α-reductase inhibitor **Dose:** 0.5 mg PO qd **Caution/Contra:** [X,–] Women and children, caution in hepatic impairment, pregnant women should avoid handling pills **Supplied:** Caps 0.5 mg **Notes/SE:** Do not donate blood until 6 mon after discontinuation of this drug; ↓ PSA levels, impotence, ↓ libido, gynecomastia

Echothiophate Iodine (Phospholine Ophthalmic) **Uses:** Glaucoma **Action:** Cholinesterase inhibitor **Dose:** 1 gtt eye(s) bid with one dose hs **Caution/Contra:** [C, ?] **Supplied:** Powder to reconstitute 1.5 mg/0.03%; 3 mg/0.06%; 6.25 mg/0.125%; 12.5 mg/0.25% **Notes/SE:** Local irritation, myopia, blurred vision, hypotension, bradycardia

Econazole (Spectazole) **Uses:** Most tinea, cutaneous *Candida,* and tinea versicolor infections **Action:** Topical antifungal **Dose:** Apply to areas bid (qd for tinea versicolor) for 2–4 wk **Caution/Contra:** [C, ?] **Supplied:** Topical cream 1% **Notes/SE:** Symptom/clinical improvement seen early in treatment, must carry out course of therapy to avoid recurrence; local irritation, pruritus, erythema

Edrophonium (Tensilon) **Uses:** Diagnosis of MyG; acute MyG crisis; curare antagonist **Action:** Anticholinesterase **Dose:** *Adults.* Test for MyG: 2 mg IV in 1 min; if tolerated, give 8 mg IV; positive test is a brief ↑ in strength. *Peds. Test for MyG:* Total dose of 0.2 mg/kg. Give 0.04 mg/kg as a test dose. If no reaction occurs, give the remainder of the dose in 1-mg increments to max of 10 mg; ↓ in renal impairment **Caution/Contra:** [C, ?] GI or GU obstruction; hypersensitivity to sulfite **Supplied:** Inj 10 mg/mL **Notes/SE:** Can cause severe cholinergic effects; keep atropine available

Efavirenz (Sustiva) **Uses:** HIV infections **Action:** Antiretroviral; nonnucleoside reverse transcriptase inhibitor **Dose:** *Adults.* 600 mg/d PO. *Peds.* Refer to product information; take hs, avoid high-fat meals **Caution/Contra:** [C, ?] CDC recommends HIV-infected mothers not breast-feed due to risk of transmission of HIV to infant. **Supplied:** Caps 50, 100, 200 mg **Notes/SE:** Somnolence, vivid dreams, dizziness, rash, N/V/D

Emedastine (Emadine) **Uses:** Allergic conjunctivitis **Action:** Antihistamine; selective H_1-antagonist **Dose:** 1 gtt in eye/s up to qid **Caution/Contra:** [B, ?] **Supplied:** 0.5% soln **Notes/SE:** Blurred vision, burning, corneal infiltrates and staining, dry eyes, foreign body sensation, hyperemia, keratitis, tearing, HA, pruritus, rhinitis, sinusitis, asthenia, bad taste, dermatitis, discomfort

Enalapril (Vasotec) **Uses:** HTN, CHF, DN, and asymptomatic LVD **Action:** ACE inhibitor **Dose:** *Adults.* 2.5–5 mg/d PO; ↑ by effect to 10–40 mg/d as 1–2 ÷ doses, or 1.25 mg IV q6h. *Peds.* 0.05–0.08 mg/kg/dose PO q12–24h; ↓ in renal impairment **Caution/Contra:** [C (1st trimester); D 2nd and 3rd trimesters), +] **Supplied:** Tabs 2.5, 5, 10, 20 mg; inj 1.25 mg/mL **Notes/SE:** Symptomatic hypotension with initial dose, especially with concomitant diuretics; DC diuretic for 2–3 d prior to initiation; monitor for ↑ in K; may cause a nonproductive cough, angioedema

Enoxaparin (Lovenox) **Uses:** Prevent and Rx of DVT; Rx PE; unstable angina and non-Q-wave MI **Action:** LMW heparin **Dose:** *Prevention:* 30 mg bid SC or 40 mg SC q24h.

22

DVT/PE: 1 mg/kg SC q12h or 1.5 mg/kg SC q24h. *Angina:* 1 mg/kg SC q12h; ↓ or avoid with severe renal impairment **Caution/Contra:** [B, ?] Active bleeding; not recommended for thromboprophylaxis in prosthetic heart valves **Supplied:** Inj 10 mg/0.1 mL (30-, 40-, 60-, 80-, 100-mg syringes) **Notes/SE:** Does not significantly affect bleeding time, platelet function, PT, or aPTT; bleeding, bruising, thrombocytopenia, pain at inj site, ↑ serum transaminases

Entacapone (Comtan) Uses: Parkinson's disease **Action:** Selective reversible COMT inhibitor **Dose:** 200 mg concurrently with each levodopa/carbidopa dose to a max of 8×/d **Caution/Contra:** [C, ?] Hepatic impairment **Supplied:** Tabs 200 mg **Notes/SE:** Dyskinesia, hyperkinesia, nausea, dizziness, hallucinations, orthostatic hypotension, brown-orange urine

Ephedrine Uses: Acute bronchospasm, nasal congestion, hypotension, narcolepsy, enuresis, and MyG **Action:** Sympathomimetic; stimulates both α- and β-receptors **Dose:** *Adults.* 25–50 mg IM or IV q10min to a max of 150 mg/d or 25–50 mg PO q3–4h PRN. *Peds.* 0.2–0.3 mg/kg/dose IM or IV q4–6h PRN **Caution/Contra:** [C, ?/–] **Supplied:** Inj 25, 50 mg/mL; caps 25, 50 mg; syrup 11, 20 mg/5 mL **Notes/SE:** CNS stimulation, nervousness, anxiety, trembling, HTN, tachycardia

Epinephrine (Adrenalin, Sus-Phrine Epi Pen) Uses: Cardiac arrest, anaphylactic reactions, acute asthma **Action:** β-Adrenergic agonist with some α-effects **Dose:** *Adults.* Emergency cardiac care: 0.5–1.0 mg (5–10 mL of 1:10,000) IV q5min to response. *Anaphylaxis:* 0.3–0.5 mL of 1:1000 dilution SC; may repeat q10–15min to a max of 1 mg/dose and 5 mg/d. *Asthma:* 0.3–0.5 mL of 1:1000 dilution SC, repeated at 20-min–4-h intervals or 1 inhal (met-dose) repeat in 1–2 min or susp 0.1–0.3 mL SC for extended effect. *Peds.* Emergency cardiac care: 0.1 mL/kg of 1:10,000 dilution IV q3–5min to response **Caution/Contra:** [C, ?] **Supplied:** Inj 1:1000, 1:2000, 1:10,000, 1:100,000; Epi Pen Auto inserter 0.15, 0.3 mg susp for inj 1:200; aerosol; soln for inhal **Notes/SE:** Sus-Phrine offers sustained action. In acute cardiac settings, can give via ET tube if no central line; tachycardia, HTN, CNS stimulation, nervousness, anxiety, trembling

Eplerenone (Inspra) Uses: HTN **Action:** Aldosterone antagonist **Dose:** *Adults:* 50 mg PO qd; max dose 50 mg PO bid;↓ dose to 25 mg/d PO if with weak inhibitors of CYP3A4 (eg, erythromycin, fluconazole, verapamil, saquinavir) **Caution/Contra:** [B, +/–] K⁺> 5.5 mEq/L, type 2 DM with microalbuminuria, SCr > 2.0 mg/dL in males or > 1.8 mg/dL in females, CrCl < 50 mL/min, use of K⁺ supplements or K⁺-sparing diuretics, use of strong inhibitors of CYP3A4 **Supplied:** Tabs 25 mg **Notes/SE:** Hyperkalemia, HA, dizziness, gynecomastia, hypercholesterolemia, hypertriglyceridemia

Epoetin Alfa [Erythropoietin, EPO] (Epogen, Procrit) Uses: Anemia associated with CRF, zidovudine treatment in HIV-infected patients, CA chemotherapy; reduction in transfusions associated with surgery **Action:** Erythropoietin supplementation **Dose:** *Adults & Peds.* 50–150 U/kg 3×/wk; adjust the dose q4–6wk as needed. *Surgery:* 300 U/kg/d for 10 d prior to surgery **Caution/Contra:** [C, +] Uncontrolled HTN **Supplied:** Inj 2000, 3000, 4000, 10,000, 20,000 U/mL **Notes/SE:** HTN, HA, tachycardia, N/V; refrigerate

Epoprostenol (Flolan) Uses: Pulmonary HTN **Action:** Dilates the pulmonary and systemic arterial vascular beds; inhibits platelet aggregation **Dose:** 4 ng/kg/min IV cont inf; adjustments based on response and package insert guidelines **Caution/Contra:** [B, ?] Chronic use in CHF **Supplied:** Inj 0.5, 1.5 mg **Notes/SE:** Flushing, tachycardia, CHF, fever, chills, nervousness, HA, N/V/D, jaw pain, flu-like symptoms

Eprosartan (Teveten) Uses: HTN, DN, CHF **Action:** Angiotensin II receptor antagonist **Dose:** 400–800 mg/d single dose or bid **Caution/Contra:** [C (1st trimester; D 2nd and 3rd trimesters), ?] **Supplied:** Tabs 400, 600 mg **Notes/SE:** Fatigue, depression, hypertriglyceridemia, URI, UTI

Eptifibatide (Integrilin) Uses: Acute coronary syndrome **Action:** Glycoprotein IIb/IIIa inhibitor **Dose:** 180-mcg/kg IV bolus, then 2-mcg/kg/min inf; ↓ adjust in renal impairment (SCr = 2 mg/dL and = 4 mg/dL: 135 mcg/kg bolus and 0.5 mcg/kg/min inf) **Caution/Contra:** [B, ?] Hx abnormal bleeding or stroke (within 30 d), any hemorrhagic stroke, severe HTN, major surgery (within 6 wk), platelet count <100,000 cells/mm³, renal dialysis **Supplied:** Inj 0.75, 2 mg/mL **Notes/SE:** Bleeding, hypotension, inj site reaction

Ertapenem (Invanz) Uses: Complicated intraabdominal, urinary, and skin infections, acute pelvic infections, community-acquired pneumonia Action: A carbapenem; β-lactam antibiotic, inhibits cell wall synthesis; active against gram –/+ anaerobes, but not *Pseudomonas*, penicillin-resistant pneumococci, MRSA, *Mycoplasma*, *Chlamydia* Dose: 1 g IM/IV once daily; reduce dose by 50% if CrCl <30 mL/min Caution/Contra: [C, ?/–] Contra in <18 y, caution in penicillin allergy Supplied: Inj 1 g/vial Notes/SE: N/V/D, inj site reactions, ↑ LFTs

Erythromycin (E-Mycin, Ilosone, Erythrocin) Uses: Infections caused by group A streptococci (*S. pyogenes*), α-hemolytic streptococci, and *N. gonorrhoeae* in penicillin-allergic patients; *S. pneumoniae*, *M. pneumoniae*, and *Legionella* infections Action: Bacteriostatic; interferes with protein synthesis Dose: *Adults.* 250–500 mg PO qid or 500 mg–1 g IV qid. *Peds.* 30–50 mg/kg/24 h PO or IV ÷ q6h, to a max of 2 g/d; take with food to minimize GI upset Caution/Contra: [B, +] Supplied: *Powder for inj as lactobionate and gluceptate salts:* 500 mg, 1 g. *Base:* Tabs 250, 333, 500 mg; caps 250 mg. *Estolate:* Tabs 500 mg; caps 250 mg; susp 125, 250 mg/5 mL. *Stearate:* Tabs 250, 500 mg. *Ethylsuccinate:* Chew tabs 200 mg; tabs 400 mg; susp 200, 400 mg/5 mL Notes/SE: Mild GI disturbances; cholestatic jaundice (estolate); erythromycin base not well absorbed from the GI tract; some forms better tolerated with respect to GI irritation; lactobionate salt contains benzyl alcohol (caution in neonates); part of the Condon bowel prep

Erythromycin and Benzoyl Peroxide (Benzamycin) Uses: Topical Rx of acne vulgaris Action: Macrolide antibiotic with keratolytic Dose: Apply bid (AM & PM) Caution/Contra: [C, ?] Supplied: Gel erythromycin 30 mg/benzoyl peroxide 50 mg/g Notes/SE: Local irritation

Erythromycin and Sulfisoxazole (Eryzole, Pediazole) Uses: Upper and lower respiratory tract; bacterial infections; otitis media in children due to *H. influenzae;* infections in penicillin-allergic patients Action: Macrolide antibiotic with sulfonamide Dose: Based on erythromycin content. *Adults.* 400 mg erythromycin/1200 mg sulfisoxazole PO q6h. *Peds >2 mon.* 40–50 mg/kg/d of erythromycin PO ÷ tid–qid; max 2 g erythromycin or 6 g sulfisoxazole/d or estimated dose of 1.25 mL/kg/d ÷ tid–qid; ↓?in renal impairment Caution/Contra: [C (D if given near term), +] Infants <2 mon Supplied: Susp erythromycin ethylsuccinate 200 mg/sulfisoxazole 600 mg/5 mL Notes/SE: GI disturbance

Erythromycin, Ophthalmic (Ilotycin Ophthalmic) Uses: Conjunctival infections Action: Macrolide antibiotic Dose: Apply q6h Caution/Contra: [B, +] Supplied: 0.5% oint Notes/SE: Local irritation

Erythromycin, Topical (Akne-Mycin Topical, Del-Mycin Topical, Emgel Topical, Staticin Topical) Uses: Acne Action: Macrolide antibiotic Dose: Wash and dry area, apply 2% product over area bid Caution/Contra: [B, +] Supplied: Soln 1.5, 2%; gel; impregnated pads and swabs 2% Notes/SE: Local irritation

Escitalopram (Lexapro) Uses: Depression Action: SSRI Dose: *Adults:* 10–20 mg PO qd; 10 mg PO qd in elderly & hepatic impairment Caution/Contra: [C, +/–] Use with or within 14 d of discontinuing an MAOI Supplied: Tabs 10, 20 mg; Soln 5 mg/5 mL Notes/SE: N/V, sweating, insomnia, dizziness, xerostomia, sexual dysfunction

Esmolol (Brevibloc) Uses: SVT and noncompensatory sinus tachycardia Action: β-Adrenergic blocking agent; class II antiarrhythmic Dose: *Adults & Peds.* Initiate treatment with 500 mcg/kg load over 1 min, then 50 mcg/kg/min for 4 min; if inadequate response, repeat the loading dose and follow with maint inf of 100 mcg/kg/min for 4 min; titrate by repeating loading, then incremental ↑ in the maint dose of 50 mcg/kg/min for 4 min until desired heart rate reached or BP decreases; average dose 100 mcg/kg/min Caution/Contra: [C (1st trimester; D 2nd or 3rd trimester), ?] Sinus bradycardia, heart block, uncompensated CHF, cardiogenic shock Supplied: Inj 10, 250 mg/mL Notes/SE: Monitor for hypotension; ↓ or discontinuing inf reverses hypotension in ≅30 min; bradycardia, diaphoresis, dizziness, pain on inj

Esomeprazole (Nexium) Uses: Short-term (4–8 wk) Rx confirmed erosive esophagitis/GERD; Rx of *H. pylori* infection in combination with antibiotics to reduce risk of duodenal ulcer Action: Proton pump inhibitor, ↓?acid production Dose: *GERD/erosive gastritis:* 20–40 mg/d PO 4–8 wk; repeat PRN ×4–8 wk; maint 20 mg/d PO; can open capsule and sprinkle on applesauce. *H. pylori infection:* 40 mg/d PO, plus clarithromycin 500 mg PO bid and amoxicillin 1000 mg/d for 10 d Caution/Contra: [B, ?/–] Supplied: Caps, 20, 40 mg Notes/SE: Related to omeprazole; HA, diarrhea, abdominal pain

22

Estazolam (ProSom) [C-IV]   **Uses:** Insomnia **Action:** Benzodiazepine **Dose:** 1–2 mg PO hs PRN; ↓ in hepatic impairment; avoid abrupt withdrawal **Caution/Contra:** [X, –] **Supplied:** Tabs 1, 2 mg **Notes/SE:** Somnolence, weakness, palpitations

Esterified Estrogens (Estratab, Menest)   **Uses:** Vasomotor symptoms, atrophic vaginitis, or kraurosis vulvae associated with menopause; osteoporosis, female hypogonadism **Action:** Estrogen supplementation **Dose:** *Menopause:* 0.3–1.25 mg/d, administered cyclically 3 wk on and 1 wk off. *Hypogonadism:* 2.5 mg PO qd–tid; not recommended in severe hepatic impairment **Caution/Contra:** [X, –] Genital bleeding of unknown cause, breast CA, estrogen-dependent tumors, thromboembolic disorders, thrombosis, thrombophlebitis, recent MI **Supplied:** Tabs 0.3, 0.625, 1.25, 2.5 mg **Notes/SE:** Nausea, bloating, breast enlargement/tenderness, edema, HA, hypertriglyceridemia, gallbladder disease

Esterified Estrogens + Methyltestosterone (Estratest)   **Uses:** Moderate/severe menopausal vasomotor symptoms; postpartum breast engorgement **Action:** Estrogen and androgen supplementation **Dose:** 1 tab/d for 3 wk, then 1 wk off **Caution/Contra:** [X, –] Genital bleeding of unknown cause, breast CA, estrogen-dependent tumors, thromboembolic disorders, thrombosis, thrombophlebitis, recent MI **Supplied:** Tabs (estrogen/methyltestosterone) 0.625 mg/ 1.25 mg, 1.25 mg/2.5 mg **Notes/SE:** Nausea, bloating, breast enlargement/tenderness, edema, HA, hypertriglyceridemia, gallbladder disease

Estradiol (Estrace)   **Uses:** Atrophic vaginitis, kraurosis vulvae vasomotor symptoms associated with menopause, osteoporosis **Action:** Estrogen supplementation **Dose:** *Oral:* 1–2 mg/d, adjust PRN to control symptoms. *Vaginal cream:* 2–4 g/d for 2 wk, then 1 g 1–3×/wk **Caution/Contra:** [X,–] Genital bleeding of unknown cause, breast CA, estrogen-dependent tumors, thromboembolic disorders, thrombosis, thrombophlebitis; recent MI; not recommended in severe hepatic impairment **Supplied:** Tabs 0.5, 1, 2 mg; vaginal cream **Notes/SE:** Nausea, bloating, breast enlargement/tenderness, edema, HA, hypertriglyceridemia, gallbladder disease

Estradiol Cypionate and Medroxyprogesterone Acetate (Lunelle) **WARNING:** Cigarette smoking ↑ risk of serious cardiovascular SE from contraceptives containing estrogen. This risk ↑ with age and with heavy smoking (> 15 cigarettes/day) and is quite marked in women > 35 y. Women who use Lunelle should be strongly advised not to smoke. **Uses:** contraceptive **Action:** estrogen and progestin **Dose:** 0.5 mL IM (deltoid, ant thigh, buttock) monthly, do not exceed 33 d **Caution/Contra:** [X, M] Contra pregnancy, heavy smokers >35 y, DVT, PE, cerebro/cardiovascular disease, estrogen-dependent neoplasm, undiagnosed abnormal uterine bleeding, hepatic tumors, cholestatic jaundice. Caution HTN, gallbladder disease, ↑ lipids, migraines, sudden HA, valvular heart disease with complications **Supplied:** Estradiol cypionate (5 mg), medroxyprogesterone acetate (25 mg) single-dose vial or prefilled syringe (0.5 mL) **Notes/SE:** Start within 5 d of menstruation; arterial thromboembolism, HTN, cerebral hemorrhage, MI, amenorrhea, acne, breast tenderness

Estradiol, Transdermal (Estraderm)   **Uses:** Severe menopausal vasomotor symptoms; female hypogonadism **Action:** Estrogen supplementation **Dose:** 0.1 mg/d patch 1–2×/wk depending on product; adjust PRN to control symptoms **Caution/Contra:** [X, –] (See Estradiol cypionate) **Supplied:** TD patches (delivers mg/24 h) 0.025, 0.0375, 0.05, 0.075, 0.1 **Notes/SE:** Nausea, bloating, breast enlargement/tenderness, edema, HA, hypertriglyceridemia, gallbladder disease

Estramustine Phosphate (Estracyt, Emcyt)   **Uses:** Advanced prostate CA **Action:** Antimicrotubule agent; weak estrogenic and antiandrogenic activity **Dose:** 14 mg/kg/d in 3–4 ÷ doses; preferable to take on empty stomach, do not take with milk or milk products **Caution/Contra:** [NA, not used in females] Active thrombophlebitis or thromboembolic disorders **Supplied:** Caps 140 mg **Notes/SE:** N/V, exacerbation of preexisting CHF, thrombophlebitis, MI, PE; gynecomastia in 20–100%

Estrogen, Conjugated (Premarin)   **WARNING:** Should not be used for the prevention of cardiovascular disease. The WHI reported ↑ risk of MI, stroke, breast CA, PE, and DVT when combined with methoxyprogesterone over 5 y of treatment; ↑ risk of endometrial CA **Uses:** Moderate–severe menopausal vasomotor symptoms; atrophic vaginitis; palliative therapy of advanced prostatic carcinoma; prevention and treatment of estrogen deficiency-induced osteoporosis **Action:** Hormonal replacement **Dose:** 0.3–1.25 mg/d PO cyclically; prostatic carcinoma requires 1.25–2.5 mg PO tid; **Caution/Contra:** [X, –] Not

22

recommended in severe hepatic impairment, genital bleeding of unknown cause, breast CA, estrogen-dependent tumors, thromboembolic disorders, thrombosis, thrombophlebitis, recent MI **Supplied:** Tabs 0.3, 0.625, 0.9, 1.25, 2.5 mg; inj 25 mg/mL **Notes/SE:** ↑ Risk of endometrial carcinoma, gallbladder disease, thromboembolism, HA, and possibly breast CA; generic products not equivalent

Estrogen, Conjugated-Synthetic (Cenestin) **Uses:** Treatment of moderate–severe vasomotor symptoms associated with menopause **Action:** Hormonal replacement **Dose:** 0.625–1.25 mg/d PO **Caution/Contra:** [X,–]; see estrogen, conjugated **Supplied:** Tabs 0.625, 0.9, 1.25 mg **Notes:** Do not use in PRG, associated with an ↑ risk of endometrial CA, gallbladder disease, thromboembolism, and possibly breast CA

Estrogen, Conjugated + Medroxyprogesterone (Prempro, Premphase) **WARNING:** Should not be used for the prevention of cardiovascular disease; the WHI study reported ↑ risk of MI, stroke, breast CA, PE, and DVT over 5 y of treatment **Uses:** Moderate–severe menopausal vasomotor symptoms; atrophic vaginitis; prevention of postmenopausal osteoporosis **Action:** Hormonal replacement **Dose:** Prempro 1 tab PO qd; Premphase 1 tab PO qd **Caution/Contra:** [X,–] Not recommended in severe hepatic impairment, genital bleeding of unknown cause, breast CA, estrogen-dependent tumors, thromboembolic disorders, thrombosis, thrombophlebitis **Supplied:** (expressed as estrogen/ medroxyprogesterone) *Prempro:* Tabs 0.625/2.5, 0.625/5 mg; *Premphase:* Tabs 0.625/0 (days 1–14) & 0.625/5 mg (days 15–28) **Notes/SE:** See Warning; gallbladder disease, thromboembolism, HA, breast tenderness

Estrogen, Conjugated + Methylprogesterone (Premarin + Methylprogesterone) **Uses:** Menopausal vasomotor symptoms; osteoporosis **Action:** Estrogen and androgen combination **Dose:** 1 tab/d; not recommended in severe hepatic impairment **Caution/Contra:** [X, –] Genital bleeding of unknown cause, breast CA, estrogen-dependent tumors, thromboembolic disorders, thrombosis, thrombophlebitis **Supplied:** Tabs containing 0.625 mg of estrogen, conjugated, and 2.5 or 5 mg of methylprogesterone **Notes/SE:** Nausea, bloating, breast enlargement/tenderness, edema, HA, hypertriglyceridemia, gallbladder disease

Estrogen, Conjugated + Methyltestosterone (Premarin + Methyltestosterone) **Uses:** Moderate–severe menopausal vasomotor symptoms; postpartum breast engorgement **Action:** Estrogen and androgen combination **Dose:** 1 tab/d for 3 wk, then 1 wk off **Caution/Contra:** [X, –] Not recommended in severe hepatic impairment, genital bleeding of unknown cause, breast CA, estrogen-dependent tumors, thromboembolic disorders, thrombosis, thrombophlebitis **Supplied:** Tabs (estrogen/methyltestosterone) 0.625 mg/5 mg, 1.25 mg/10 mg **Notes/SE:** Nausea, bloating, breast enlargement/tenderness, edema, HA, hypertriglyceridemia, gallbladder disease

Etanercept (Enbrel) **Uses:** Reduce signs and symptoms in cases of refractory RA **Action:** Binds TNF (disease-modifying antirheumatic drug) **Dose:** *Adults.* 25 mg SC 2× wk; *Peds 4–17 y.* 0.4 mg/kg SC 2× wk, max 25 mg **Caution/Contra:** [B, ?] Contra with active infection; caution in conditions that predispose to infection (ie, DM) **Supplied:** Inj 25 mg/vial **Notes/SE:** HA, rhinitis, inj site reaction

Ethambutol (Myambutol) **Uses:** Pulmonary TB and other mycobacterial infections **Action:** Inhibits cellular metabolism **Dose:** *Adults & Peds >12 y.* 15–25 mg/kg/d PO as a single dose **Caution/Contra:** [B, +] Optic neuritis; ↓ in renal impairment, take with food, avoid antacids **Supplied:** Tabs 100, 400 mg; **Notes/SE:** HA, hyperuricemia, acute gout, abdominal pain, ↑ LFTs, optic neuritis, GI upset

Ethinyl Estradiol (Estinyl, Feminone) **Uses:** Menopausal vasomotor symptoms; female hypogonadism **Action:** Estrogen supplement **Dose:** 0.02–1.5 mg/d ÷ qd–tid; **Caution/Contra:** [X, –] Not recommended in severe hepatic impairment; genital bleeding of unknown cause, breast CA, estrogen-dependent tumors, thromboembolic disorders, thrombosis, thrombophlebitis **Supplied:** Tabs 0.02, 0.05, 0.5 mg **Notes/SE:** Nausea, bloating, breast enlargement/tenderness, edema, HA, hypertriglyceridemia, gallbladder disease

Ethinyl Estradiol and Levonogestrel (Preven) **Uses:** Emergency contraceptive ("morning-after pill"); prevent pregnancy after contraceptive failure or unprotected intercourse **Actions:** estrogen and progestin; interferes with implantation **Dose:** 4 tabs, take 2 tab q12 h × 2 (within 72 h of intercourse) **Supplied:** Kit ethinyl estradiol (0.05), levonorgestrel (0.25) blister pack with 4 pills and urine pregnancy test **Contra/Caution** [X, M]

22

Known/suspected PRG, abnormal uterine bleeding **Notes:** Will not induce abortion; may increase risk of ectopic pregnancy; N/V, abdominal pain , fatigue HA, and menstrual changes

Ethinyl Estradiol and Norelgestromin, Ortho Evra (Ortho) **Uses:** Contraceptive patch **Action:** estrogen and progestin **Dose:** Applying patch to abdomen, buttocks, upper torso (not breasts) or upper outer arm at the beginning of the menstrual cycle; new patch is applied weekly for 3 wk; wk 4 is patch-free. **Caution/Contra:** [X, M] **Supplied:** 20-cm^2 patch (6 mg norelgestromin (active metabolite norgestimate) and 0.75 mg of ethinyl estradiol. **Notes/SE:** Less effective in women > 90 kg; breast discomfort, HA, application site reactions, nausea, menstrual cramps; thrombosis risks similar to OCP

Ethosuximide (Zarontin) **Uses:** Seizures **Action:** Anticonvulsant; increases the seizure threshold **Dose:** *Adults.* Initially, 500 mg PO ÷ bid; ↑ by 250 mg/d q4–7d PRN (max 1500 mg/d) *Peds.* 20–40 mg/kg/24 h PO ÷ bid to a max of 1500 mg/d; use with caution in renal/hepatic impairment **Caution/Contra:** [C, +] **Supplied:** Caps 250 mg; syrup 250 mg/5 mL **Notes/SE:** Blood dyscrasias, GI upset, drowsiness, dizziness, irritability

Etidronate Disodium (Didronel) **Uses:** Hypercalcemia of malignancy, Paget's disease, and hypertropic ossification **Action:** Inhibition of normal and abnormal bone resorption **Dose:** 5–20 mg/kg/d, may be given in ÷ doses (duration 3–6 mon); 7.5 mg/kg/d IV inf over 2 h **Caution/Contra:** [B oral (C parenteral), ?] SCr >5 mg/dL **Supplied:** Tabs 200, 400 mg; inj 50 mg/mL **Notes/SE:** GI intolerance ↓ by ÷ oral daily doses; hypophosphatemia, hypomagnesemia, bone pain, abnormal taste, fever, convulsions, nephrotoxicity

Etodolac (Lodine) **Uses:** Arthritis and pain **Action:** NSAID **Dose:** 200–400 mg PO bid–qid (max 1200 mg/d) **Caution/Contra:** [C (D 3rd trimester), ?] Caution in CHF, HTN, renal/hepatic impairment, Hx PUD **Supplied:** Tabs 400, 500 mg; ER tabs 400, 500, 600 mg; caps 200, 300 mg **Notes/SE:** GI disturbance, dizziness, HA, rash, edema, renal impairment, hepatitis

Etonogestrel/Ethinyl Estradiol (NuvaRing) **Uses:** Contraceptive **Action:** Estrogen and progestin combination **Dose: Adults: Rule out pregnancy first;** Insert ring vaginally for 3 wk, remove for 1 wk; insert new ring 7 d after last removed (even if still bleeding) at same time of day ring removed. First day of menses is day 1, insert prior to day 5 even if still bleeding. Use other contraception for first 7 d of starting therapy. See insert if converting from other forms of contraception; Following delivery or 2nd trimester abortion, insert ring 4 wk postpartum (if not breast-feeding) **Caution/Contra: [X, ?/–]** Contra PRG, heavy smokers >35 y, DVT, PE, cerebro/cardiovascular disease, estrogen-dependent neoplasm, undiagnosed abnormal genital bleeding, hepatic tumors, cholestatic jaundice. Caution HTN, gallbladder disease, ↑ lipids, migraines, sudden HA **Supplied:** intravaginal ring: ethinyl estradiol 0.015 mg/d and etonogestrel 0.12 mg/d **Note:** If ring accidentally removed, rinse with cool/lukewarm water (not hot) and reinserted ASAP; if not reinserted w/n 3 h, effectiveness decreased. Do not use with diaphragm.

Etoposide [VP-16] (VePesid, Toposar) **Uses:** Testicular CA, non-small-cell lung CAs, Hodgkin's and NHLs, pediatric ALL, and allogeneic/autologous BMT in high doses **Action:** Topoisomerase II inhibitor **Dose:** 50 mg/m^2/d IV for 3–5 d; 50 mg/m^2/d PO for 21 d (oral bioavailability = 50% of the IV form); 2–6 g/m^2 or 25–70 mg/kg used in BMT (refer to specific protocols); ↓ in renal/hepatic impairment **Caution/Contra:** [D, –] IT administration **Supplied:** Caps 50 mg; inj 20 mg/mL **Notes/SE:** Myelosuppression, N/V, and alopecia; hypotension if infused too rapidly; anaphylaxis or lesser hypersensitivity reactions (wheezing) rare; potential for secondary leukemias

Ezitimibe (Zetia) **Uses:** Primary hypercholesterolemia alone or in combination with an HMG-CoA reductase inhibitor **Action:** Inhibits intestinal absorption of cholesterol and phytosterols **Dose:** 10 mg/d PO **Caution/Contra:** [C, +/–] Hepatic impairment **Supplied:** Tabs 10 mg **Notes/SE:** Diarrhea, abdominal pain, ↑ transaminases when used in combination with an HMG-CoA reductase inhibitor

Famciclovir (Famvir) **Uses:** Acute herpes zoster (shingles) and genital herpes **Action:** Inhibits viral DNA synthesis **Dose:** *Zoster:* 500 mg PO q8h. *Simplex:* 125–250 mg PO bid; ↓ in renal impairment **Caution/Contra:** [B, –] **Supplied:** Tabs 125, 250, 500 mg **Notes/SE:** Fatigue, dizziness, HA, pruritus, nausea, diarrhea, paresthesia

22 **Famotidine (Pepcid)** **Uses:** Short-term Rx of active duodenal ulcer and benign gastric ulcer; maint Rx for duodenal ulcer, hypersecretory conditions, GERD, and heartburn **Ac-**

tion: H$_2$-antagonist; inhibits gastric acid secretion **Dose:** *Adults.* Ulcer: 20–40 mg PO hs or 20 mg IV q12h. *Hypersecretion:* 20–160 mg PO q6h. *GERD:* 20 mg PO bid; maint 20 mg PO hs. *Heartburn:* 10 mg PO PRN. *Peds.* 1–2 mg/kg/d; ↓ dose in severe renal insufficiency **Caution/Contra:** [B, M] **Supplied:** Tabs 10, 20, 40 mg; chew tabs 10 mg; susp 40 mg/5 mL; inj 10 mg/mL **Notes/SE:** Dizziness, HA, constipation, diarrhea, acne, thrombocytopenia, neutropenia, ↑ serum transaminases

Felodipine (Plendil) **Uses:** HTN and CHF **Action:** Ca channel blocker **Dose:** 5–20 mg PO qd; ↓ in hepatic impairment **Caution/Contra:** [C, ?] **Supplied:** Tabs 2.5, 5, 10 mg **Notes/SE:** Follow BP in elderly and in impaired hepatic function; do not use doses >10 mg in these patients; bioavailability ↑ when administered with grapefruit juice; peripheral edema, flushing, tachycardia, HA, gingival hyperplasia

Fenofibrate (Tricor) **Uses:** Hypertriglyceridemia **Action:** Inhibits triglyceride synthesis **Dose:** 54–160 mg/d ↓?in renal impairment, take with meals **Caution/Contra:** [C, ?] **Supplied:** Tabs 54–160 mg **Notes/SE:** Take with meals to ↑ bioavailability; monitor LFTs; GI disturbances, cholecystitis, rash, arthralgia, myalgia, dizziness

Fenoldopam (Corlopam) **Uses:** HTN emergency **Action:** Rapid vasodilator **Dose:** Initial dose 0.03–0.1 mg/kg/min IV cont inf, titrate to effect q15min with 0.05–0.1 mg/kg/min increments **Caution/Contra:** [B, ?] **Supplied:** Inj 10 mg/mL **Notes/SE:** Avoid concurrent use with b-blockers; hypotension, edema, facial flushing, N/V/D, atrial flutter/fibrillation, ≠ intraocular pressure, ≠ portal pressure in cirrhotic patients

Fenoprofen (Nalfon) **Uses:** Arthritis and pain **Action:** NSAID **Dose:** 200–600 mg q4–8h, to 3200 mg/d max; take with food **Caution/Contra:** [B (D 3rd trimester), +/–] Caution in patients with CHF, HTN, renal/hepatic impairment, Hx PUD **Supplied:** Caps 200, 300 mg; tabs 600 mg **Notes/SE:** GI disturbance, dizziness, HA, rash, edema, renal impairment, hepatitis

Fentanyl (Sublimaze) [C-II] **Uses:** Short-acting analgesic used in conjunction with anesthesia **Action:** Narcotic **Dose:** *Adults & Peds.* 0.025–0.15 mg/kg IV/IM titrated to effect; ↓ in renal impairment **Caution/Contra:** [B, +] ↑ ICP, respiratory depression, severe renal/hepatic impairment **Supplied:** Inj 0.05 mg/mL **Notes/SE:** 0.1 mg of fentanyl = 10 mg of morphine IM; sedation, hypotension, bradycardia, constipation, nausea, respiratory depression, rash, miosis

Fentanyl, Transdermal (Duragesic) [C-II] **Uses:** Chronic pain **Action:** Narcotic **Dose:** Apply patch to upper torso q72h. Dose calculated from narcotic requirements in previous 24 h; ↓ in renal impairment **Caution/Contra:** [B, +] ↑ ICP, respiratory depression, severe renal/hepatic impairment **Supplied:** TD patches deliver 25, 50, 75, 100 mcg/h **Notes/SE:** 0.1 mg of fentanyl = 10 mg of morphine IM; sedation, ↓ BP, bradycardia, constipation, nausea, respiratory depression, rash, miosis

Fentanyl, Transmucosal System (Actiq, Fentanyl Oralet) [C-II] **Uses:** Induction of anesthesia; breakthrough CA pain **Action:** Narcotic **Dose:** *Adults & Peds.* Anesthesia: 5–15 mcg/kg. *Pain:* 200 mcg consumed over 15 min, titrate to effect; ↓ in renal impairment **Caution/Contra:** [B, +] ↑ ICP, respiratory depression, severe renal/hepatic impairment **Supplied:** Lozenges 100, 200, 300, 400 mcg; lozenges on stick 200, 400, 600, 800, 1200, 1600 mcg **Notes/SE:** Sedation, ↓ BP, bradycardia, constipation, nausea, respiratory depression, rash, miosis

Ferrous Gluconate (Fergon) **Uses:** Iron deficiency anemia and iron supplementation **Action:** Dietary supplementation **Dose:** *Adults.* 100–200 mg Fe/d in ÷ doses; take on empty stomach (may take with meals if GI upset occurs); avoid antacids **Caution/Contra:** [A, ?] Hemochromatosis, hemolytic anemia **Supplied:** Tabs 240 (27 mg Fe), 325 mg (36 mg Fe) **Notes/SE:** 12% Fe; GI upset, constipation, dark stools, discoloration of urine

Ferrous Gluconate Complex (Ferrlecit) **Uses:** Iron deficiency anemia or supplement to erythropoietin therapy **Action:** Supplemental iron **Dose:** Test dose: 2 mL (25 mg Fe) infused over 1 h. If no reaction, 125 mg (10 mL) IV over 1 h until favorable hematocrit achieved. Usual cumulative dose 1 g Fe administered over 8 sessions **Caution/Contra:** [B, ?] **Supplied:** Inj 12.5 mg/mL Fe **Notes/SE:** Dosage expressed as mg Fe; may be infused during dialysis; hypotension, serious hypersensitivity reactions, GI disturbance, inj site reaction

22

Ferrous Sulfate **Uses:** Iron deficiency anemia and iron Fe supplementation **Action:** Dietary supplementation **Dose:** *Adults.* 100–200 mg Fe in ÷ doses. *Peds.* 1–4 mg/kg/24 h ÷ qd–bid; take on empty stomach (take with meals if GI upset occurs); avoid antacids **Caution/Contra:** [A, ?] Hemochromatosis, hemolytic anemia **Supplied:** Tabs 187 (60 mg Fe), 200 (65 mg Fe), 324 (65 mg Fe), 325 mg (65 mg Fe); SR caplets and tabs 160 mg (50 mg Fe); gtt 75 mg/0.6 mL (15 mg Fe/0.6 mL); elixir 220 mg/5 mL (44 mg Fe/5 mL); syrup 90 mg/5 mL (18 mg Fe/5 mL) **Notes/SE:** Vitamin C taken with ferrous sulfate ↑ absorption of Fe; GI upset, constipation, dark stools, discolored urine

Fexofenadine (Allegra) **Uses:** Allergic rhinitis **Action:** Antihistamine **Dose:** *Adults & Peds >12 y.* 60 mg bid or 180 mg/d; adjust in renal impairment **Caution/Contra:** [C, ?] **Supplied:** Caps 60 mg, tabs 180 mg; also in combination with pseudoephedrine (60 mg fexofenadine/120 mg pseudoephedrine) **Notes/SE:** Drowsiness (uncommon)

Filgrastim [G-CSF] (Neupogen) **Uses:** Decrease incidence of infection in febrile neutropenic patients; Rx chronic neutropenia **Action:** Recombinant G-CSF **Dose:** *Adults & Peds.* 5 mcg/kg/d SC or IV single daily dose; DC therapy when ANC >10,000 **Caution/Contra:** [C, ?] **Supplied:** Inj 300 mcg/mL **Notes/SE:** Fever, alopecia, N/V/D, splenomegaly, bone pain, HA, rash

Finasteride (Proscar, Propecia) **Uses:** BPH and androgenetic alopecia **Action:** Inhibits 5α-reductase **Dose:** *BPH:* Proscar 5 mg/d PO. *Alopecia:* Propecia 1 mg/d PO **Caution/Contra:** [X, –] Caution in hepatic impairment; pregnant women should avoid handling pills **Supplied:** Tabs 1 (Propecia), 5 (Proscar) mg **Notes/SE:** ↓ PSA levels; reestablish PSA baseline at 6 mon; 3–6 mon for effect on urinary symptoms; to maintain new hair must continue therapy; ↓ libido, impotence (rare)

Flavoxate (Urispas) **Uses:** Symptomatic relief of dysuria, urgency, nocturia, suprapubic pain, urinary frequency, and incontinence **Action:** Antispasmodic **Dose:** 100–200 mg PO tid–qid **Caution/Contra:** [B, ?] Pyloric or duodenal obstruction, GI hemorrhage, GI obstruction, ileus, achalasia, BPH **Supplied:** Tabs 100 mg **Notes/SE:** Drowsiness, blurred vision, xerostomia

Flecainide (Tambocor) **Uses:** Prevent AF/flutter and PSVT, Rx life-threatening ventricular arrhythmias **Action:** Class 1C antiarrhythmic **Dose:** *Adults.* 100 mg PO q12h; ↑ in increments of 50 mg q12h q4d to a max of 400 mg/d. *Peds.* 3–6 mg/kg/d in 3 ÷ doses; ↓ in renal impairment, monitor closely in hepatic impairment **Caution/Contra:** [C, +] 2nd- or 3rd-degree AV block, bifascicular or trifascicular block, cardiogenic shock **Supplied:** Tabs 50, 100, 150 mg **Notes/SE:** May cause new/worsened arrhythmias; initiate Rx in hospital; may dose q8h if the patient is intolerant or condition is uncontrolled at 12-h intervals; drug interactions with propranolol, digoxin, verapamil, and disopyramide; dizziness, visual disturbances, dyspnea, palpitations, edema, tachycardia, CHF, HA, fatigue, rash, nausea

Floxuridine (FUDR) **Uses:** Colon, pancreatic, liver CAs; adenocarcinoma of the GI tract metastatic to the liver **Action:** Inhibitor of thymidylate synthase; interferes with DNA synthesis (S-phase specific) **Dose:** 0.1–0.6 mg/kg/d for 1–6 wk **Caution/Contra:** [D, –] **Supplied:** Inj 500 mg **Notes/SE:** Myelosuppression, anorexia, abdominal cramps, N/V/D, mucositis, alopecia, skin rash, and hyperpigmentation; rare neurotoxicity (blurred vision, depression, nystagmus, vertigo, and lethargy); intraarterial catheter-related problems (ischemia, thrombosis, bleeding, and infection)

Fluconazole (Diflucan) **Uses:** Oropharyngeal and esophageal candidiasis; cryptococcal meningitis; *Candida* infections of the lungs, peritoneum, and urinary tract; prevention of candidiasis in BMT patients on chemotherapy and radiation; candidal vaginitis **Action:** Antifungal; inhibits fungal cytochrome P-450 sterol demethylation **Dose:** *Adults.* 100–400 mg/d PO or IV. *Vaginitis:* 150 mg PO as a single dose. *Peds.* 3–6 mg/kg/d PO or IV; ↓ in renal impairment **Caution/Contra:** [C, –] **Supplied:** Tabs 50, 100, 150, 200 mg; susp 10, 40 mg/mL; inj 2 mg/mL **Notes/SE:** PO use produces the same blood levels as IV, PO preferred when possible; HA, rash, GI upset, hypokalemia, ↑ LFTs

Fludarabine Phosphate (Flamp, Fludara) **Uses:** CLL, low-grade lymphoma, mycosis fungoides **Action:** Inhibits ribonucleotide reductase; blocks DNA polymerase-induced DNA repair **Dose:** 18–30 mg/m²/d for 5 d, as a 30-min inf (refer to specific protocols) **Caution/Contra:** [D, –] **Supplied:** Inj 50 mg **Notes/SE:** Myelosuppression, N/V/D, and LFT elevations; edema, CHF, fever, chills, fatigue, dyspnea, nonproductive cough, pneumonitis; severe CNS toxicity rare in leukemia

22

Fludrocortisone Acetate (Florinef) Uses: Partial treatment for adrenocortical insufficiency **Action:** Mineralocorticoid replacement **Dose:** *Adults.* 0.05–0.2 mg/d PO. *Peds.* 0.05–0.1 mg/d PO **Caution/Contra:** [C, ?] **Supplied:** Tabs 0.1 mg **Notes/SE:** For adrenal insufficiency, must use with glucocorticoid supplement; dosage changes based on plasma renin activity; HTN, edema, CHF, HA, dizziness, convulsions, acne, rash, bruising, hyperglycemia, cataracts

Flumazenil (Romazicon) Uses: Reversal of the sedative effects of benzodiazepines (diazepam, etc) **Action:** Benzodiazepine receptor antagonist **Dose:** *Adults.* 0.2 mg IV over 15 s; repeat dose if desired level of consciousness not obtained, to 1 mg max. *Peds.* 0.01 mg/kg to max of 0.2 mg IV over 15 s. Repeat doses 0.005 mg/kg at 1-min intervals; ↓ in hepatic impairment **Caution/Contra:** [C, ?] **Supplied:** Inj 0.1 mg/mL **Notes/SE:** Does not reverse narcotic symptoms; N/V, palpitations, HA, anxiety, nervousness, hot flashes, tremor, blurred vision, dyspnea, hyperventilation, withdrawal syndrome

Flunisolide (AeroBid, Nasalide) Uses: Control of bronchial asthma in patients requiring chronic steroid therapy; relief of seasonal/perennial allergic rhinitis **Action:** Topical steroid **Dose:** *Adults.* 2–4 inhal bid. *Nasal:* 2 sprays/nostril bid. *Peds >6 y.* 2 inhal bid. *Nasal:* 1–2 sprays/nostril bid **Caution/Contra:** [C, ?] **Supplied:** Met-dose aerosol 250 mg; nasal spray 0.025% **Notes/SE:** Not for acute asthma attack; tachycardia, bitter taste, local effects, oral candidiasis

Fluorouracil [5-FU] (Adrucil) Uses: Colorectal, bladder, gastric, pancreatic, anal, head, neck, and breast CAs **Action:** Inhibitor of thymidylate synthetase (interferes with DNA synthesis, S-phase specific) **Dose:** 370–1000 mg/m^2/d for 1–5 d IV push to 24-h cont inf; protracted venous inf of 200–300 mg/m^2/d (See specific protocol) **Caution/Contra:** [D, ?] Bilirubin >5 mg/dL **Supplied:** Inj 50 mg/mL **Notes/SE:** Stomatitis, esophagopharyngitis, N/V/D, anorexia; myelosuppression (leukocytopenia, thrombocytopenia, and anemia); rash, dry skin, and photosensitivity frequent; tingling in hands/feet followed by pain (palmar–plantar erythrodysesthesia); phlebitis and discoloration at inj sites

Fluorouracil [5-FU], Topical [5-FU] (Efudex) Uses: Basal cell carcinoma of the skin, actinic and solar keratosis **Action:** Inhibitor of thymidylate synthetase (interferes with DNA synthesis, S-phase specific) **Dose:** Apply 5% cream bid for 4–6 wk **Caution/Contra:** [D, ?] **Supplied:** Cream 1, 5%; soln 1, 2, 5% **Notes/SE:** Rash, dry skin, photosensitivity

Fluoxetine (Prozac, Sarafem) Uses: Depression, OCD, bulimia, PMDD (Sarafem) **Action:** SSRI **Dose:** Initially, 20 mg/d PO; ↑ to a max of 80 mg/ 24 h; ÷ doses of 20 mg/d. Weekly regimen 90 mg/wk after 1–2 wk of standard dose. *Bulimia:* 60 mg/d in AM. *PMDD:* 20 mg/d or 20 mg intermittently starting 14 d prior to menses, repeat with each cycle; ↓ in hepatic failure **Caution/Contra:** [B, ?/–] Serious reactions with MAOI and thioridazine; wait 5 wk after DC before starting MAOI **Supplied:** *Prozac:* Caps 10, 20, 40 mg; scored tabs 10 mg; SR cap 90 mg; soln 20 mg/5 mL. *Sarafem:* 10, 20 mg caps **Notes/SE:** Nausea, nervousness, weight loss, HA, insomnia

Fluoxymesterone (Halotestin) Uses: Androgen-responsive metastatic breast CA **Action:** Inhibition of secretion of LH and FSH by feedback inhibition **Dose:** 10–40 mg/d **Caution/Contra:** [X, ?/–] Serious cardiac, liver, or kidney disease **Supplied:** Tabs 2, 5, 10 mg **Notes/SE:** Virilization, amenorrhea and menstrual irregularities, hirsutism, alopecia and acne, nausea, and cholestasis. *Hematologic toxicity symptoms:* Suppression of clotting factors II, V, VII, and X and polycythemia; ↑ libido, HA, and anxiety

Fluphenazine (Prolixin, Permitil) Uses: Psychotic disorders **Action:** Phenothiazine antipsychotic; blocks postsynaptic mesolimbic dopaminergic receptors in the brain **Dose:** 0.5–10 mg/d in ÷ doses PO q6–8h; average maint 5.0 mg/d or 1.25 mg IM initially, then 2.5–10 mg/d in ÷ doses q6–8h PRN; ↓ dose in elderly **Caution/Contra:** [C, ?/–] Narrow-angle glaucoma **Supplied:** Tabs 1, 2.5, 5, 10 mg; conc 5 mg/mL; elixir 2.5 mg/5 mL; inj 2.5 mg/mL; depot inj 25 mg/mL **Notes/SE:** Monitor LFT; may cause drowsiness; do not administer conc with caffeine, tannic acid, or pectin-containing products; extrapyramidal effects

Flurazepam (Dalmane) [C-IV] Uses: Insomnia **Action:** Benzodiazepine **Dose:** *Adults & Peds >15 y.* 15–30 mg PO hs PRN; ↓ in elderly **Caution/ Contra:** [X, ?/–] Respiratory depression, narrow-angle glaucoma **Supplied:** Caps 15, 30 mg **Notes/SE:** Hangover due to accumulation of metabolites, apnea

22

Flurbiprofen (Ansaid) Uses: Arthritis Action: NSAID Dose: 50–100 mg bid–qid to a max of 300 mg/d Caution/Contra: [B (D in 3rd trimester), +] Supplied: Tabs 50, 100 mg Notes/SE: Dizziness, GI upset, peptic ulcer disease

Flutamide (Eulexin) WARNING: Liver failure and death have been reported. Measure LFT before, monthly, and periodically after; DC immediately if ALT 2× uln or jaundice develops Uses: Advanced prostate CA (in combination with GnRH agonists, eg, leuprolide or goserelin); with radiation and GnRH for localized prostate CA Action: Nonsteroidal antiandrogen Dose: 250 mg PO tid (750 mg total) Caution/Contra: [D, ?] Severe hepatic impairment Supplied: Caps 125 mg Notes/SE: Hot flashes, loss of libido, impotence, diarrhea, N/V, gynecomastia; follow LFTs

Fluticasone, Nasal (Flonase) Uses: Seasonal allergic rhinitis Action: Topical steroid Dose: *Adults & Adolescents* Nasal: 1–2 sprays/nostril/d. *Peds 4–11 y.* Nasal: 1–2 sprays/nostril/d Caution/Contra: [C, M] Supplied: Nasal spray 50 mcg/actuation Notes/SE: HA, dysphonia, oral candidiasis

Fluticasone, Oral (Flovent, Flovent Rotadisk) Uses: Chronic Rx of asthma Action: Topical steroid Dose: *Adults & Adolescents.* 2–4 puffs bid. *Peds 4–11 y.* 50 mcg bid Caution/Contra: [C, M] Supplied: Multidose inhaler 44, 110, 220 mcg/activation; Rotadisk dry powder 50, 100, 250 mcg/activation; risk of thrush Notes/SE: Counsel patients carefully on use of device; HA, dysphonia, oral candidiasis

Fluticasone Propionate and Salmeterol Xinafoate (Advair Diskus) Uses: Maint therapy for asthma Action: corticosteroid and long-acting bronchodilator Dose: *Adults & Peds >12 y.* Caution/Contra: [C, M] Not for acute attack or in conversion from oral steroids Supplied: Met-dose inhal powder (fluticasone in mcg/salmeterol in mcg)100/50, 250/50, 500/50 Notes/SE: Not for acute asthma attack, combination of Flovent and Serevent; URI, pharyngitis, HA

Fluvastatin (Lescol) Uses: Adjunct to diet in the treatment of ↑ total cholesterol Action: HMG-CoA reductase inhibitor Dose: 20–40 mg PO hs, may be ↑ to 80 mg/d; ↓ dose with hepatic impairment Caution/Contra: [X, –]. Myopathy Supplied: Caps 20, 40 mg Notes/SE: Avoid concurrent use with gemfibrozil.

Fluvoxamine (Luvox) Uses: OCD Action: SSRI Dose: Initial 50 mg as single hs dose, may be ↑ to 300 mg/d in ÷ doses Caution/Contra: [C, ?/–] Numerous drug interactions (MAOIs) Supplied: Tabs 25, 50, 100 mg Notes/SE: ÷ Doses of >100 mg; HA, GI upset, somnolence, insomnia

Folic Acid Uses: Megaloblastic anemia; recommended for all women of childbearing age Action: Dietary supplementation Dose: *Adults. Supplement:* 0.4 mg/d PO. *PRG:* 0.8 mg/d PO. *Folate deficiency:* 1.0 mg PO qd–tid. *Peds. Supplement:* 0.04–0.4 mg/24 h PO, IM, IV, or SC. *Folate deficiency:* 0.5–1.0 mg/24 h PO, IM, IV, or SC Caution/Contra: [A, +] Supplied: Tabs 0.1, 0.4, 0.8, 1.0 mg; inj 5 mg/mL Notes/SE: ↓ Incidence of fetal neural tube defects by 50%; no effect on normocytic anemias; well tolerated

Fondaparinux (Arixtra) WARNING: When epidural/spinal anesthesia or spinal puncture is used, patients anticoagulated or scheduled to be anticoagulated with LMW heparins, heparinoids, or fondaparinux for prevention of thromboembolic complications are at risk for epidural or spinal hematoma, which can result in long-term or permanent paralysis Uses: Prevent DVT in hip fracture or replacement or knee replacement surgery Action: Synthetic and specific inhibitor of activated factor X; a LMW heparin Dose: 2.5 mg/d SC, up to 5–9 d; start at least 6 h postop Caution/Contra: [B, ?] Contra in weight <50 kg and CrCl <30 mL/min, active major bleeding, bacterial endocarditis, thrombocytopenia associated with antiplatelet antibody Supplied: Prefilled syringes 2.5 mg Notes/SE: Thrombocytopenia, DC if platelets <100,000 mm³; anemia, fever, nausea, constipation, reversible ↑ LFTs

Formoterol (Foradil Aerolizer) Uses: Long term in the maint treatment of asthma and prevention of bronchospasm with reversible obstructive airways disease Action: Long-acting β_2-adrenergic receptor agonist, bronchodilator Dose: *Adults & Peds >5 y.* Inhal of one 12-mcg capsule q12h using the aerosolizer inhaler, 24 mcg/d max; patient must not exhale into device; prevent exercise-induced bronchospasm. *Adults & Peds > 12 y.* One inhal 12-mcg cap 15 min before exercise Caution/Contra: [C, ?]. Do not start with significantly worsening or acutely deteriorating asthma, which may be life-threatening Supplied: 12-mcg blister pack for use in aerosolizer **Notes/SE:** Paradoxical bronchospasm, can be life-threatening; URI, pharyngitis, back pain

Foscarnet (Foscavir) **Uses:** CMV; acyclovir-resistant herpes infections **Action:** Inhibits viral DNA polymerase and reverse transcriptase **Dose:** *Induction:* 60 mg/kg IV q8h for 14–21 d. *Maint:* 90–120 mg/kg/d IV (Mon–Fri) **Caution/Contra:** [C, –] Significant renal impairment **Supplied:** Inj 24 mg/mL **Notes/SE:** Adjust in ↓ renal function; nephrotoxic; monitor ionized Ca closely (causes electrolyte abnormalities); administer through central line

Fosfomycin (Monurol) **Uses:** Uncomplicated UTI **Action:** Inhibits bacterial cell wall synthesis **Dose:** 3 g PO dissolved in 90–120 mL of water as single dose; ↓ in renal impairment **Caution/Contra:** [B, ?] **Supplied:** Granule packets 3 g **Notes/SE:** May take 2–3 d for symptoms to improve; HA, GI upset

Fosinopril (Monopril) **Uses:** HTN, CHF, DN **Action:** ACE inhibitor **Dose:** Initially 10 mg/d PO; may be ↑ to a max of 80 mg/d PO ÷ qd–bid; ↓ dose in elderly **Caution/Contra:** [D, +] Renal impairment **Supplied:** Tabs 10, 20, 40 mg **Notes/SE:** Nonproductive cough, dizziness, angioedema, hyperkalemia

Fosphenytoin (Cerebyx) **Uses:** Status epilepticus **Action:** Inhibits seizure spread in motor cortex **Dose:** Dosed as phenytoin equivalents (PEs), loading 15–20 mg PE/kg, maint 4–6 mg PE/kg/d; dosage adjustment/plasma monitoring necessary in hepatic impairment **Caution/Contra:** [D, +] Rash development during treatment **Supplied:** Inj **Notes/SE:** Requires 15 min to convert fosphenytoin to phenytoin; administer at <150 mg PE/min to prevent hypotension; administer with BP monitoring; hypotension, dizziness, ataxia, pruritus, nystagmus

Frovatriptan (Frova) See Table 11, page 613

Fulvestrant (Faslodex) **Uses:** Hormone receptor-positive metastatic breast CA in postmenopausal women with disease progression following antiestrogen therapy **Action:** Estrogen receptor antagonist **Dose:** 250 mg monthly, either a single 5-mL inj or two concurrent 2.5-mL IM injs into buttocks **Caution/Contra:** [X, ?/–] **Supplied:** Prefilled syringes 50 mg/mL; single 5 mL, dual 2.5 mL **Notes/SE:** N/V/D, constipation, abdominal pain, HA, back pain, hot flushes, pharyngitis, inj site reactions

Furosemide (Lasix) **Uses:** CHF, HTN, edema, ascites **Action:** Loop diuretic; inhibits Na and Cl reabsorption in ascending loop of Henle and distal tubule **Dose:** *Adults.* 20–80 mg PO or IV qd–bid. *Peds.* 1 mg/kg/dose IV q6–12h; 2 mg/kg/dose PO q12–24h; **Caution/Contra:** [C, +] Caution in hepatic disease, anuria **Supplied:** Tabs 20, 40, 80 mg; soln 10 mg/ mL, 40 mg/5 mL; inj 10 mg/mL **Notes/SE:** Monitor for hypokalemia; high doses of the IV form may cause ototoxicity; hypotension, hyperglycemia

Gabapentin (Neurontin) **Uses:** Adjunctive therapy in the treatment of partial seizures; chronic pain syndromes **Action:** Anticonvulsant **Dose:** 900–1800 mg/d PO in 3 ÷ doses; dosage adjustment in renal impairment **Caution/Contra:** [C, ?] **Supplied:** Caps 100, 300, 400 mg **Notes/SE:** Not necessary to monitor serum gabapentin levels; somnolence, dizziness, ataxia, fatigue

Galantamine (Reminyl) **Uses:** Alzheimer's disease **Action:** Acetylcholinesterase inhibitor **Dose:** 4 mg PO bid, ↑ to 8 mg bid after at least 4 wk; may ↑ to 12 mg in 4 wk **Caution/Contra:** [B, ?]. Do not use in severe renal or hepatic impairment; caution with urinary outflow obstruction, Parkinson's disease, severe asthma or COPD, severe heart disease or hypotension **Supplied:** Tabs 4, 8, 12 mg **Notes/SE:** GI disturbances, weight loss, sleep disturbances, dizziness, HA

Gallium Nitrate (Ganite) **Uses:** Hypercalcemia of malignancy; bladder CA **Action:** Inhibits resorption of Ca^{2+} from the bones **Dose:** *CA:* 350 mg/m^2 cont inf for 5 d to 700 mg/m^2 rapid IV inf q2wk in antineoplastic settings **Caution/Contra:** [C, ?] **Supplied:** Inj 25 mg/mL **Notes/SE:** Can cause renal insufficiency; hypocalcemia, hypophosphatemia, and decreased bicarbonate; <1% of patients developed acute optic neuritis; for bladder CA, use in combination with vinblastine and ifosfamide

Ganciclovir (Cytovene, Vitrasert) **Uses:** Rx and prevention of CMV retinitis and prevention of CMV disease in transplant recipients **Action:** Inhibits viral DNA synthesis **Dose:** *Adults & Peds.* IV: 5 mg/kg IV q12h for 14–21 d, then maint of 5 mg/kg/d IV for

7 d/wk or 6 mg/kg/d IV for 5 d/wk. *Ocular implant:* One implant q5–8mo. **Adults.** PO: Following induction, 1000 mg PO tid. *Prevention:* 1000 mg PO tid; take caps with food; ↓ dose in renal impairment **Caution/Contra:** [C, –] Neutropenia, thrombocytopenia **Supplied:** Caps 250, 500 mg; inj 500 mg; ocular implant 4.5 mg **Notes/SE:** Not a cure for CMV; inj should be handled with cytotoxic cautions; implant confers no systemic benefit; granulocytopenia/thrombocytopenia are major toxicities; fever, rash, GI upset

Gatifloxacin (Tequin) **Uses:** Acute exacerbation of chronic bronchitis, sinusitis, community-acquired pneumonia, UTI **Action:** Quinolone antibiotic, inhibits DNA-gyrase **Dose:** 400 mg/d PO or IV; avoid use with antacids; ↓ dose in renal impairment **Caution/Contra:** [C, M] Do not use in children <18 y or in pregnant or lactating women. **Supplied:** Tabs 200, 400 mg; inj **Notes/SE:** Reliable activity against *S. pneumoniae;* prolonged QT interval, HA, nausea, diarrhea; tendon rupture, photosensitivity

Gemcitabine (Gemzar) **Uses:** Pancreatic CA, gastric CA, and lung CA **Action:** Antimetabolite; inhibits ribonucleotide reductase; produces false nucleotide base-inhibiting DNA synthesis **Dose:** 1000 mg/m^2 as a 1-h IV inf/wk for 3–4 wk or 6–8 wk; dose modifications based on hematologic function **Caution/Contra:** [D, ?/–] **Supplied:** Inj 20 mg/mL **Notes/SE:** Myelosuppression, N/V/D, drug fever, and skin rash

Gemfibrozil (Lopid) **Uses:** Hypertriglyceridemia and reduction of CHD risk **Action:** Lipid-regulating agent **Dose:** 1200 mg/d PO in 2 ÷ doses 30 min ac AM and PM **Caution/Contra:** [C, ?] Avoid concurrent use with the HMG-CoA reductase inhibitors; renal/hepatic impairment, gallbladder disease **Supplied:** Tabs 600 mg; caps 300 mg **Notes/SE:** Monitor LFTs and serum lipids; cholelithiasis may occur secondary to treatment; may enhance the effect of warfarin; GI upset

Gentamicin (Garamycin, G-Myticin, others) **Uses:** Serious infections caused by *Pseudomonas, Proteus, E. coli, Klebsiella, Enterobacter,* and *Serratia* and initial treatment of gram– sepsis **Action:** Bactericidal; inhibits protein synthesis **Dose:** *Adults.* 3–5 mg/kg/24 h IV ÷ q8–24h. *Peds.* Infants <7 d <1200 g: 2.5 mg/kg/dose q18–24h. *Infants >1200 g:* 2.5 mg/kg/dose q12–18h. *Infants >7 d:* 2.5 mg/kg/dose IV q8–12h. *Children:* 2.5 mg/kg/d IV q8h; ↓?dose with renal insufficiency **Caution/Contra:** [C, +/–] Monitor CrCl and serum conc for dosage adjustments (Table 2, page 607). **Supplied:** Inj 10, 40 mg/mL, IT preservative-free 2 mg/mL **Notes/SE:** Nephrotoxic and ototoxic, ataxia; daily dosing becoming popular; follow Cr

Gentamicin, Ophthalmic (Garamycin, Genoptic, Gentacidin, Gentak, others) **Uses:** Conjunctival infections **Action:** Bactericidal; inhibits protein synthesis **Dose:** Oint apply bid or tid; soln: 1–2 gtt q2–4h, up to 2 gtt/h for severe infections **Caution/Contra:** [C, ?] **Supplied:** Soln and oint 0.3% **Notes/SE:** Local irritation

Gentamicin, Topical (Garamycin, G-Myticin) **Uses:** Skin infections caused by susceptible organisms **Action:** Bactericidal; inhibits protein synthesis **Dose:** *Adults & Peds >1 y.* Apply tid–qid **Caution/Contra:** [C, ?] **Supplied:** Cream; oint; soln 0.3% **Notes/SE:** Irritation

Gentamicin and Prednisolone, Ophthalmic (Pred-G Ophthalmic) **Uses:** Steroid-responsive ocular and conjunctival infections sensitive to gentamicin (eg, *Staphylococcus, E. coli, H. influenzae, Neisseria, Pseudomonas, Proteus,* and *Serratia* spp) **Action:** Bactericidal; inhibits protein synthesis plus antiinflammatory **Dose:** Oint apply bid or tid; Soln: 1–2 gtt q2–4h, up to 2 gtt/h for severe infections **Caution/Contra:** [C, ?] **Supplied:** *Oint, ophth:* Prednisolone acetate 0.6% and gentamicin sulfate 0.3% (3.5 g). *Susp, ophth:* Prednisolone acetate 1% and gentamicin sulfate 0.3% (2 mL, 5 mL, 10 mL). *Soln and oint:* 0.3% **Notes/SE:** Local irritation

Glimepiride (Amaryl) **Uses:** Type 2 DM **Action:** Sulfonylurea; stimulates pancreatic insulin release; ↑ peripheral insulin sensitivity; ↓ hepatic glucose output and production **Dose:** 1–4 mg/d, up to max of 8 mg **Caution/Contra:** [C, –] **Supplied:** Tabs 1, 2, 4 mg **Notes/SE:** HA, hypoglycemia

Glipizide (Glucotrol XL) **Uses:** Type 2 DM **Action:** Sulfonylurea; stimulates pancreatic insulin release; ↑ peripheral insulin sensitivity; ↓ hepatic glucose output and production; ↓ intestinal absorption of glucose **Dose:** 5–15 mg qd–bid **Caution/Contra:** [C, ?/–] Contra in type 1 DM, sensitivity to sulfonamides; caution in severe liver disease **Supplied:** Tabs 5, 10 mg; ER tabs 5, 10 mg **Notes/SE:** Counsel patient about diabetes management;

22

wait several days before adjusting dose; monitor glucose; HA, anorexia, N/V/D, constipation, fullness, rash, urticaria, photosensitivity

Glucagon Uses: Severe hypoglycemic reactions in DM with sufficient liver glycogen stores or β-blocker and Ca channel blocker overdose **Action:** Accelerates liver gluconeogenesis **Dose:** *Adults.* 0.5–1.0 mg SC, IM, or IV; repeat after 20 min PRN. β*-Blocker overdose:* 3–10 mg IV; repeat in 10 min PRN; may be given as cont inf. *Peds. Neonates:* 0.3 mg/kg/dose SC, IM, or IV q4h PRN. *Children:* 0.025–0.1 mg/kg/dose SC, IM, or IV; repeat after 20 min PRN **Caution/Contra:** [B, M] **Supplied:** Inj 1 mg **Notes/SE:** Administration of glucose IV necessary; ineffective in states of starvation, adrenal insufficiency, or chronic hypoglycemia; hypotension

Glyburide (DiaBeta, Micronase, Glynase) Uses: Type 2 DM **Action:** Sulfonylurea; stimulates pancreatic insulin release; ↑ peripheral insulin sensitivity; ↓ hepatic glucose output and production; ↓ intestinal absorption of glucose **Dose:** *Nonmicronized:* 1.25–10 mg qd–bid. *Micronized:* 1.5–6 mg qd–bid **Caution/Contra:** [C, ?] Not recommended in renal impairment **Supplied:** Tabs 1.25, 2.5, 5 mg; micronized tabs 1.5, 3, 4.5, 6 mg **Notes/SE:** HA, hypoglycemia

Glyburide/Metformin (Glucovance) Uses: Type 2 DM **Action:** Sulfonylurea; stimulates pancreatic insulin release; ↑ peripheral insulin sensitivity; ↓ hepatic glucose output and production; ↓ intestinal absorption of glucose **Dose:** 1st line (naive patients), 1.25/250 mg PO qd–bid; 2nd line, 2.5/500 mg or 5/500 mg bid, take with meals, ↑ dose gradually **Caution/Contra:** [C, –] Do not use if SCr >1.3 in females or >1.4 in males; contra in hypoxemic conditions (CHF, sepsis); avoid alcohol; hold dose prior to and 48 h after ionic contrast media **Supplied:** Tabs 1.25/250 mg, 2.5/500 mg, 5/500 mg **Notes/SE:** HA, hypoglycemia, lactic acidosis, anorexia, N/V, rash

Glycerin Suppository [OTC] Uses: Constipation **Action:** Hyperosmolar laxative **Dose:** *Adults.* 1 adult supp PR PRN. *Peds.* 1 infant supp PR qd–bid PRN **Caution/ Contra:** [C, ?] **Supplied:** Supp (adult, infant); liq 4 mL/applicatorful **Notes/SE:** Can cause diarrhea

Gonadorelin (Lutrepulse) Uses: Primary hypothalamic amenorrhea **Action:** Stimulates the pituitary to release the gonadotropins LH and FSH **Dose:** 5–20 mcg IV q90min for 21 d using a reservoir and pump **Caution/Contra:** [B, M] **Supplied:** Inj 0.8 mg, 3.2 mg **Notes/SE:** Risk of multiple PRG; inj site pain

Goserelin (Zoladex) Uses: Advanced prostate CA and with radiation for localized prostate CA; endometriosis **Action:** LHRH agonist, inhibits LH, resulting in ↓ testosterone **Dose:** 3.6 mg SC (implant) q28d or 10.8 mg SC q3mo; usually into lower abdominal wall **Caution/Contra:** [X, –] **Supplied:** Subcutaneous implant 3.6, 10.8 mg **Notes/SE:** Hot flashes, ↓ libido, gynecomastia, and transient exacerbation of CA-related bone pain ("flare reaction" 7–10 d after 1st dose)

Granisetron (Kytril) Uses: Prevention of N/V **Action:** Serotonin receptor antagonist **Dose:** *Adults & Peds.* 10 mg/kg IV 30 min prior to initiation of chemotherapy; 0.1–1 mg before end of operative case. *Adults.* 1 mg PO 1 h prior to chemotherapy, then 12 h later **Caution/Contra:** [B, +/–] **Supplied:** Tabs 1 mg; inj 1 mg/mL **Notes/SE:** HA

Guaifenesin (Robitussin, others) Uses: Symptomatic relief of dry, nonproductive cough **Action:** Expectorant **Dose:** *Adults.* 200–400 mg (10–20 mL) PO q4h. *Peds.* <2 y: 12 mg/kg/d in 6 ÷ doses. *2–5 y:* 50–100 mg (2.5–5 mL) PO q4h. *6–11 y:* 100–200 mg (5–10 mL) PO q4h **Caution/Contra:** [C, ?] **Supplied:** Tabs 100, 200, 1200 mg; SR tabs 600 mg; caps 200 mg; SR caps 300 mg; liq 100, 200 mg/5 mL **Notes/SE:** GI upset

Guaifenesin and Codeine (Robitussin AC, Brontex, others) [C-V] Uses: Symptomatic relief of dry, nonproductive cough **Action:** Antitussive with expectorant **Dose:** *Adults.* 10 mL or 1 tab PO q6–8h. *Peds. 2–6 y:* 1–1.5 kg/kg codeine/d ÷ dose q4–6h; *6–12 y:* 5 mL q4h; *>12 y:* 10 mL q4h, max 60 mL/24 h **Caution/Contra:** [C, +] **Supplied:** Brontex tab contains 10 mg codeine; Brontex liq 2.5 mg codeine/5 mL; others 10 mg codeine/5 mL **Notes/SE:** Somnolence

Guaifenesin and Dextromethorphan (many OTC brands) Uses: Cough due to upper respiratory tract irritation **Action:** Antitussive with expectorant **Dose:** *Adults & Peds >12 y.* 10 mL PO q6h. *Peds. 2–6 y:* 2.5 mL q6–8h, 10 mL/d max. *6–12 y:* 5 mL q6–8h, 20 mL max/d **Caution/Contra:** [C, +] **Supplied:** Many OTC formulations **Notes/SE:** Somnolence

Haemophilus B Conjugate Vaccine (ActHIB, HibTITER, PedvaxHIB, Prohibit, others) Uses: Routine immunization of children against *H. influenzae* type B diseases **Action:** Active immunization against *Haemophilus* B **Dose:** *Peds.* 0.5 mL (25 mg) IM in deltoid or vastus lateralis **Caution/Contra:** [C, +] Febrile illness, immunosuppression **Supplied:** Inj 7.5, 10, 15, 25 mcg/0.5 mL **Notes/SE:** Booster not required; observe for anaphylaxis

Haloperidol (Haldol) Uses: Psychotic disorders, agitation, Tourette's disorders, and hyperactivity in children **Action:** Antipsychotic, neuroleptic **Dose:** *Adults. Moderate symptoms:* 0.5–2.0 mg PO bid–tid. *Severe symptoms/agitation:* 3–5 mg PO bid–tid or 1–5 mg IM q4h PRN (max 100 mg/d). *Peds. 3–6 y:* 0.01–0.03 mg/kg/24 h PO qd. *6–12 y:* Initially, 0.5–1.5 mg/24 h PO; ↑ by 0.5 mg/24 h to maint of 2–4 mg/24 h (0.05–0.1 mg/kg/24 h) or 1–3 mg/dose IM q4–8h to a max of 0.1 mg/kg/24 h; Tourette's may require up to 15 mg/24 h PO; ↓ dose in elderly **Caution/Contra:** [C, ?] Narrow-angle glaucoma **Supplied:** Tabs 0.5, 1, 2, 5, 10, 20 mg; conc liq 2 mg/mL; inj 5 mg/mL; decanoate inj 50, 100 mg/mL **Notes/SE:** Extrapyramidal symptoms, hypotension, anxiety, dystonias

Haloprogin (Halotex) Uses: Topical Rx of tinea pedis, tinea cruris, tinea corporis, tinea manus **Action:** Topical antifungal **Dose:** *Adults.* Apply bid for up to 2 wk; intertriginous may require up to 4 wk **Caution/Contra:** [B, ?] **Supplied:** 1% Cream; soln **Notes/SE:** Local irritation

Heparin Uses: Rx and prevention of DVT and PE, unstable angina, AF with emboli formation, and acute arterial occlusion **Action:** Acts with antithrombin III to inactivate thrombin and inhibit thromboplastin formation **Dose:** *Adults. Prophylaxis:* 3000–5000 U SC q8–12h. *Thrombosis Rx:* Loading dose of 50–75 U/kg IV, then 10–20 U/kg IV qh (adjust based on PTT). *Peds. Infants:* Loading dose 50 U/kg IV bolus, then 20 U/kg/h IV by cont inf. *Children:* Loading dose 50 U/kg IV, then 15–25 U/kg cont inf or 100 U/kg/dose q4h IV intermittent bolus **Caution/Contra:** [B, +] Uncontrolled bleeding **Supplied:** Inj 10, 100, 1000, 2000, 2500, 5000, 7500, 10,000, 20,000, 40,000 U/mL **Notes/SE:** Follow PTT, thrombin time, or activated clotting time to assess effectiveness; little effect on the PT; therapeutic PTT is 2–3 for most conditions; thrombocytopenia (HIT); follow platelet counts

Hepatitis A Vaccine (Havrix, Vaqta) Uses: Prevent hepatitis A in high-risk individuals (eg, travelers, certain professions, or high-risk behaviors) **Action:** Provides active immunity **Dose:** (Expressed as ELISA units [EL.U]) *Havrix: Adults.* 1440 EL.U. single IM dose. *Peds >2 y.* 720 EL.U. single IM dose. *Vaqta: Adults.* 50 U single IM dose. *Peds.* 25 U single IM dose **Caution/Contra:** [C, +] **Supplied:** Inj 720 EL.U./0.5 mL, 1440 EL.U./1 mL.; 50 U/mL **Notes/SE:** Booster recommended 6–12 mon after primary vaccination. Fever, fatigue, pain at inj site, HA

Hepatitis A (inactivated) and Hepatitis B Recombinant Vaccine (Twinrix) Uses: Active immunization against hepatitis A/B **Action:** Provides active immunity **Dose:** 1 mL IM at 0, 1, and 6 mon **Caution/Contra:** [C, +] **Supplied:** Single-dose vials, syringes **Notes/SE:** Booster recommended 6–12 mon after primary vaccination; fever, fatigue, pain at inj site, HA

Hepatitis B Immune Globulin (HyperHep, H-BIG) Uses: Exposure to HBs Ag-positive materials, eg, blood, plasma, or serum (accidental needle-stick, mucous membrane contact, or oral ingestion) **Action:** Passive immunization **Dose:** *Adults & Peds.* 0.06 mL/kg IM to a max of 5 mL; within 24 h of needle-stick or percutaneous exposure; within 14 d of sexual contact; repeat 1 and 6 mon after exposure **Caution/Contra:** [C, ?] Thimerosal allergy **Supplied:** Inj **Notes/SE:** Administered in gluteal or deltoid muscle; if exposure continues, patient should also receive the hepatitis B vaccine; pain at inj site, dizziness

Hepatitis B Vaccine (Engerix-B, Recombivax HB) Uses: Prevention of hepatitis B **Action:** Active immunization **Dose:** *Adults.* 3 IM doses of 1 mL each, the 1st 2 doses given 1 mon apart, the 3rd 6 mon after the 1st. *Peds.* 0.5 mL IM given on the same schedule as for adults **Caution/Contra:** [C, +] Yeast hypersensitivity **Supplied:** *Engerix-B:* Inj 20 mcg/mL; peds inj 10 mcg/0.5 mL. *Recombivax HB:* Inj 10 and 40 mcg/mL; peds inj 5 mcg/0.5 mL **Notes/SE:** Administer IM injs for adults and older peds in the deltoid; in other peds, administer in the anterolateral thigh; may cause fever, inj site soreness; derived from recombinant DNA technology

Hetastarch (Hespan) Uses: Plasma volume expansion as an adjunct in the treatment of shock and leukapheresis **Action:** Synthetic colloid with actions similar to those of albumin **Dose:** 500–1000 mL (do not exceed 1500 mL/d) IV at a rate not to exceed 20 mL/kg/h. *Leukapheresis:* 250–700 mL; ↓ dose in renal failure **Caution/Contra:** [C, +] Severe bleeding disorders, severe CHF, or renal failure with oliguria or anuria **Supplied:** Inj 6 g/100 mL **Notes/SE:** Not a substitute for blood or plasma; bleeding side effect (prolongs PT, PTT, bleed time, etc)

Hydralazine (Apresoline, others) Uses: Moderate–severe HTN; CHF (with Isordil) **Action:** Peripheral vasodilator **Dose:** *Adults.* Begin at 10 mg PO qid, then ↑ to 25 mg qid to max of 300 mg/d. *Peds.* 0.75–3 mg/kg/24 h PO ÷ q12–6h; ↓ in renal impairment; check CBC and ANA before starting **Caution/Contra:** [C, +] Caution with impaired hepatic function and CAD **Supplied:** Tabs 10, 25, 50, 100 mg; inj 20 mg/mL **Notes/SE:** Compensatory sinus tachycardia eliminated with use of a β-blocker; chronically high doses cause SLE-like syndrome; SVT following IM administration, peripheral neuropathy

Hydrochlorothiazide (HydroDIURIL, Esidrix, others) Uses: Edema, HTN **Action:** Thiazide diuretic; inhibits Na^+ reabsorption in the distal tubule **Dose:** *Adults.* 25–100 mg/d PO in single or ÷ doses. *Peds.* *<6 mon:* 2–3 mg/ kg/d in 2 ÷ doses. *>6 mon:* 2 mg/kg/d in 2 ÷ doses **Caution/Contra:** [D, +] Contra in anuria; sulfonamide allergy **Supplied:** Tabs 25, 50, 100 mg; caps 12.5 mg; oral soln 50 mg/5 mL **Notes/SE:** Hypokalemia frequent; hyperglycemia, hyperuricemia, hyponatremia

Hydrochlorothiazide and Amiloride (Moduretic) Uses: HTN **Action:** Combined effects of a thiazide diuretic and a K^+-sparing diuretic **Dose:** 1–2 tabs/d PO **Caution/Contra:** [D, ?] Do not give to diabetics or patients with renal failure, sulfonamide allergy. **Supplied:** Tabs (amiloride/hydrochlorothiazide) 5 mg/50 mg **Notes/SE:** Hypotension, photosensitivity, hyper-/hypokalemia

Hydrochlorothiazide and Spironolactone (Aldactazide) Uses: Edema, HTN **Action:** Combined effects of a thiazide diuretic and a K^+-sparing diuretic **Caution/Contra:** [D, +] Sulfonamide allergy **Dose:** 25–200 mg each component/d in ÷ doses **Supplied:** Tabs (hydrochlorothiazide/spironolactone) 25 mg/25 mg, 50 mg/50 mg **Notes/SE:** Photosensitivity, hypotension, hyper-/hypokalemia

Hydrochlorothiazide and Triamterene (Dyazide, Maxzide) Uses: Edema and HTN **Action:** Combined effects of a thiazide diuretic and a K^+-sparing diuretic **Dose:** *Dyazide:* 1–2 caps PO qd–bid. *Maxzide:* 1 tab/d PO **Caution/Contra:** [D, +/–] Sulfonamide allergy **Supplied:** (triamterene/HCTZ) 37.5 mg/25 mg, 50 mg/25 mg, 75 mg/50 mg **Notes/SE:** HCTZ component in Maxzide more bioavailable than in Dyazide; can cause hyperkalemia as well as hypokalemia; follow serum K^+ levels; hypotension, photosensitivity

Hydrocodone and Acetaminophen (Lorcet, Vicodin, others) [C-III] Uses: Moderate–severe pain; hydrocodone has antitussive properties **Action:** Narcotic analgesic with nonnarcotic analgesic **Dose:** 1–2 caps or tabs PO q4–6h PRN **Caution/Contra:** [C, M] **Supplied:** Many different combinations; specify hydrocodone/APAP dose. Caps 5/500; tabs 2.5/500, 5/400, 5/500, 7.5/400, 10/400, 7.5/500, 7.5/650, 7.5/750, 10/325, 10/400, 10/500, 10/650; elixir and soln (fruit punch flavor) 2.5 mg hydrocodone/167 mg APAP/5 mL **Notes/SE:** GI upset, sedation, fatigue

Hydrocodone and Aspirin (Lortab ASA, others) [C-III] Uses: Moderate–severe pain **Action:** Narcotic analgesic with NSAID **Dose:** 1–2 PO q4–6h PRN **Caution/Contra:** [C, M] **Supplied:** 5 mg hydrocodone/500 mg ASA/tab **Notes/SE:** GI upset, sedation, fatigue

Hydrocodone and Guaifenesin (Hycotuss Expectorant, others) [C-III] Uses: Nonproductive cough associated with respiratory infection **Action:** Expectorant plus cough suppressant **Dose:** *Adults & Peds >12 y.* 5 mL q4h, pc and hs. *Peds. < 2 y:* 0.3 mg/kg/d ÷ qid. *2–12 y:* 2.5 mL q4h pc and hs **Caution/Contra:** [C, M] **Supplied:** Hydrocodone 5 mg/guaifenesin 100 mg/5 mL **Notes/SE:** GI upset, sedation, fatigue

Hydrocodone and Homatropine (Hycodan, others) [C-III] Uses: Relief of cough **Action:** Combination antitussive **Dose:** Dose based on hydrocodone. *Adults.* 5–10 mg q4–6h. *Peds.* 0.6 mg/kg/d ÷ tid–qid **Caution/Contra:** [C, M] Narrow-angle glaucoma **Supplied:** Syrup 5 mg hydrocodone/5 mL; tabs 5 mg hydrocodone **Notes/SE:** Sedation, fatigue, GI upset

22

Hydrocodone and Ibuprofen (Vicoprofen) [C-III] Uses: Moderate–severe pain (<10 d) Action: Narcotic with NSAID Dose: 1–2 tabs q4–6h PRN Caution/Contra: [C, M] Caution in renal insufficiency Supplied: Tabs 7.5 mg hydrocodone/200 mg ibuprofen Notes/SE: Sedation, fatigue, GI upset

Hydrocodone and Pseudoephedrine (Entuss-D, Histussin-D, others) [C-III] Uses: Cough and nasal congestion Action: Narcotic cough suppressant with decongestant Dose: 5 mL qid, PRN Caution/Contra: [C, M] MAOIs Supplied: *Entuss-D:* 5 mg hydrocodone/30 mg pseudoephedrine/5 mL. *Histussin-D:* 5 mg hydrocodone/60 mg pseudoephedrine/5 mL Notes/SE: ↑ blood pressure, GI upset, sedation, fatigue

Hydrocodone, Chlorpheniramine, Phenylephrine, Acetaminophen, and Caffeine (Hycomine Compound) [C-III] Uses: Cough and symptoms of URI Action: Narcotic cough suppressant with decongestants and analgesic Dose: 1 tab PO q4h PRN Caution/Contra: [C, M] Narrow-angle glaucoma Supplied: Hydrocodone 5 mg/chlorpheniramine 2 mg/phenylephrine 10 mg/APAP 250 mg/caffeine 30 mg/tab Notes/SE: ↑ BP, GI upset, sedation, fatigue

Hydrocortisone, Topical and Systemic (Cortef, Solu-Cortef) See Steroids, Tables 4 and 5, Pages 612 and 613 Caution/Contra: [B, –] Notes/SE: Systemic forms: ↑ appetite, insomnia, hyperglycemia, bruising

Hydrocortisone, Rectal (Anusol-HC Suppository, Cortifoam Rectal, Proctocort, others) Uses: Painful anorectal conditions; radiation proctitis; management of ulcerative colitis Action: Antiinflammatory steroid Dose: *Adults. Ulcerative colitis:* 10–100 mg rectally qd–bid 2–3 wk, 1–2×/d for 2–3 wk Caution/Contra: [B, ?/–] Supplied: *Hydrocortisone acetate:* Rectal aerosol 90 mg/applicator; supp 25 mg. *Hydrocortisone base:* Rectal 1%; rectal susp 100 mg/60 mL Notes/SE: Minimal systemic effect

Hydromorphone (Dilaudid) [C-II] Uses: Moderate–severe pain Action: Narcotic analgesic Dose: 1–4 mg PO, IM, IV, or PR q4–6h PRN; 3 mg PR q6–8h PRN; ↓ with hepatic failure Caution/Contra: [B (D if prolonged use or high doses near term), ?] Supplied: Tabs 1, 2, 3, 4, 8 mg; liq 5 mg/mL; inj 1, 2, 4, 10 mg/mL; supp 3 mg Notes/SE: 1.5 mg IM = 10 mg of morphine IM; sedation, dizziness, GI upset

Hydroxyurea (Hydrea, Droxia) Uses: CML, head and neck, ovarian and colon CA, melanoma, acute leukemia, sickle cell anemia, polycythemia vera, HIV Action: Probable inhibitor of the ribonucleotide reductase system Dose: 50–75 mg/kg for WBC counts of >100,000 cells/mL; 20–30 mg/kg in refractory CML. *HIV:* 1000–1500 mg/d in single or ÷ doses; ↓ in renal insufficiency Caution/Contra: [D, –] Severe anemia Supplied: Caps 200, 300, 400, 500 mg Notes/SE: Myelosuppression (primarily leukopenia), N/V, rashes, facial erythema, radiation recall reactions, and renal dysfunction

Hydroxyzine (Atarax, Vistaril) Uses: Anxiety, tension, sedation, itching Action: Antihistamine, anxiety Dose: *Adults. Anxiety or sedation:* 50–100 mg PO or IM qid or PRN (max 600 mg/d). *Itching:* 25–50 mg PO or IM tid–qid. *Peds.* 0.5–1.0 mg/kg/24 h PO or IM q6h; ↓ in hepatic failure Caution/Contra: [C, +/–] Supplied: Tabs 10, 25, 50, 100 mg; caps 25, 50, 100 mg; syrup 10 mg/5 mL; susp 25 mg/5 mL; inj 25, 50 mg/mL Notes/SE: Useful in potentiating effects of narcotics; not for IV use; drowsiness and anticholinergic effects

Hyoscyamine (Anaspaz, Cystospaz, Levsin, others) Uses: Spasm associated with GI and bladder disorders Action: Anticholinergic Dose: *Adults.* 0.125–0.25 mg (1–2 tabs) SL 3–4×/d, pc and hs; 1 SR caps q12h Caution/Contra: [C, +] Contra in obstructive uropathy, GI obstruction; narrow-angle glaucoma Supplied: (Cystospaz-M, Levsinex): cap timed release 0.375 mg; elixir (alcohol), soln 0.125 mg/5 mL; inj 0.5 mg/mL; tab 0.125 mg; tab (Cystospaz) 0.15 mg; ER tab (Levbid): 0.375 mg; SL (Levsin SL) 0.125 mg Notes/SE: Dry skin, xerostomia, constipation, anticholinergic SE

Hyoscyamine, Atropine, Scopolamine, and Phenobarbital (Donnatal, Barbidonna, others) Uses: Irritable bowel, spastic colitis, peptic ulcer, spastic bladder Dose: 0.125–0.25 mg (1–2 tabs) 3–4×/d, 1 cap q12h (SR), 5–10 mL elixir 3–4×/d or q8h Caution/Contra: [D, M] Narrow-angle glaucoma Supplied: Many combinations/manufacturers available. *Cap* (Donnatal, others): Hyoscyamine 0.1037 mg/atropine 0.0194 mg/scopolamine 0.0065 mg/phenobarbital 16.2 mg. *Tabs* (Donnatal, others): Hyoscyamine 0.1037 mg/atropine 0.0194 mg/scopolamine 0.0065 mg/phenobarbital 16.2 mg. *Long acting*

(Donnatal): Hyoscyamine 0.311 mg/atropine 0.0582 mg/scopolamine 0.0195 mg/phenobarbital 48.6 mg. *Elixirs* (Donnatal, others): Hyoscyamine 0.1037 mg/atropine 0.0194 mg/scopolamine 0.0065 mg/phenobarbital 16.2 mg/5 mL **Notes/ SE:** Sedation, xerostomia, constipation

Ibuprofen (Motrin, Rufen, Advil, others) Uses: Arthritis and pain **Action:** NSAID **Dose:** *Adults.* 200–800 mg PO bid–qid. *Peds.* 30–40 mg/kg/d in 3–4 ÷ doses; best taken with food, caution when combined with other NSAIDs **Caution/Contra:** [B, +] Avoid in severe hepatic impairment; hypersensitivity to NSAIDs, UGI bleed, or ulcers **Supplied:** Tabs 100, 200, 400, 600, 800 mg; chew tabs 50, 100 mg; caps 200 mg; susp 100 mg/2.5 mL, 100 mg/5 mL, 40 mg/mL (200 mg is OTC preparation) **Notes/SE:** Dizziness, peptic ulcer, platelet inhibition, worsening of renal insufficiency; increases in lithium levels

Ibutilide (Convert) Uses: Rapid conversion of AF or flutter **Action:** Class III antiarrhythmic agent **Dose:** 0.01 mg/kg (max 1 mg) IV inf over 1 min; may be repeated once **Caution/Contra:** [C, –] Do not administer class I or III antiarrhythmics concurrently or within 4 h of ibutilide inf. **Supplied:** Inj 0.1 mg/mL **Notes/SE:** Arrhythmias, HA

Idarubicin (Idamycin) Uses: AML (in combination with cytarabine), CML in blast crisis, and ALL **Action:** DNA intercalating agent; inhibits DNA topoisomerases I and II **Dose:** 10–12 mg/m^2/d for 3–4 d; ↓ in renal/hepatic dysfunction **Caution/Contra:** [D, –] **Supplied:** Inj 1 mg/mL (5-, 10-, 20-mg vials) **Notes/SE:** Myelosuppression, cardiotoxicity, N/V, mucositis, alopecia, and irritation at sites of IV administration; rare changes in renal/hepatic function

Ifosfamide (Ifex, Holoxan) Uses: Lung and testicular CA, soft tissue sarcoma, NHL **Action:** Alkylating agent **Dose:** 1.2 g/m^2/d for 5 d by bolus or cont inf; 2.4 g/m^2/d for 3 d; with mesna uroprotection; ↓ in renal, hepatic (consider) **Caution/Contra:** [D, M] **Supplied:** Inj 1, 3 g **Notes/SE:** Hemorrhagic cystitis, nephrotoxicity, N/V, mild–moderate leukopenia, lethargy and confusion, alopecia, and hepatic enzyme elevations; dosage adjustment in renal impairment

Imatinib (Gleevec) Uses: Treatment of CML, gastrointestinal stromal tumors (GIST) **Action:** Inhibits Bcl-Abl tyrosine kinase (signal transduction) **Dose:** *Chronic phase CML:* 400–600 mg/d PO. *Accelerated/blast crisis:* 600–800 mg/d PO. *GIST:* 400-600/d mg **Caution/Contra:** [D, ?/–] Metabolized by CYP3A4 **Supplied:** Caps 100 mg **Notes/SE:** GI upset, fluid retention, muscle cramps, musculoskeletal pain, arthralgia, rash, HA; neutropenia and thrombocytopenia, follow CBCs; LFTs at baseline and monthly; caution with warfarin, cyclosporine, azole antifungals, erythromycin, phenytoin, rifampin, carbamazepine

Imipenem-Cilastatin (Primaxin) Uses: Serious infections caused by a wide variety of susceptible bacteria; inactive against *S. aureus*, group A and B streptococci, etc **Action:** Bactericidal; interferes with cell wall synthesis **Dose:** *Adults.* 250–500 mg (imipenem) IV q6h. *Peds.* 60–100 mg/kg/24 h IV ÷ q6h; ↓ in renal disease if calculated CrCl is <70 mL/min **Caution/Contra:** [C, +/–] **Supplied:** Inj (imipenem/cilastatin) 250 mg/250 mg, 500 mg/500 mg **Notes/SE:** Seizures may occur if drug accumulates; GI upset, thrombocytopenia

Imipramine (Tofranil) Uses: Depression, enuresis, panic attack, and chronic pain **Action:** TCA; ↑ synaptic conc of serotonin or norepinephrine in the CNS **Dose:** *Adults. Hospitalized:* Start at 100 mg/24 h PO in ÷ doses; can ↑ over several wk to 250–300 mg/24 h. *Outpatient:* Maint of 50–150 mg PO hs, not to exceed 200 mg/24 h. *Peds. Antidepressant:* 1.5–5.0 mg/kg/24 h ÷ 1–4×/d. *Enuresis:>6 y:* 10–25 mg PO hs; ↑ by 10–25 mg at 1–2 wk intervals; treat for 2–3 mon, then taper **Caution/Contra:** [D, ?/–] Do not use with MAOIs, narrow-angle glaucoma **Supplied:** Tabs 10, 25, 50 mg; caps 75, 100, 125, 150 mg **Notes/SE:** Less sedation than with amitriptyline; cardiovascular symptoms, dizziness, xerostomia, discolored urine

Imiquimod Cream, 5% (Aldara) Uses: External genital warts **Action:** Unknown; may induce cytokines **Dose:** Applied 3×/wk; leave on skin for 6–10 h, continue therapy for a max of 16 wk **Caution/Contra:** [B, ?] **Supplied:** Single-dose packets (250 mg of the cream) **Notes/SE:** Local skin reactions common

Immune Globulin, Intravenous (Gamimune N, Sandoglobulin, Gammar IV) Uses: IgG antibody deficiency disease states, (eg, congenital agammaglobuline-

22

mia, CVH, and BMT) also ITP **Action:** IgG supplementation **Dose:** *Adults & Peds. Immunodeficiency:* 100–200 mg/kg/mon IV at a rate of 0.01–0.04 mL/kg/min to a max of 400 mg/kg/dose. *ITP:* 400 mg/kg/dose IV qd for ↓5 d. *BMT:* 500 mg/kg/wk; ↓ renal insufficiency **Caution/Contra:** [C, ?] **Supplied:** Inj **Notes/SE:** Adverse effects associated mostly with rate of inf; GI upset

Indapamide (Lozol) **Uses:** HTN and CHF **Action:** Thiazide diuretic; enhances Na⁺, Cl⁻, and water excretion in the proximal segment of the distal tubule **Dose:** 1.25–5 mg/d PO **Caution/Contra:** [D, ?] Thiazide/sulfonamide allergy **Supplied:** Tabs 1.25, 2.5 mg **Notes/SE:** Doses >5 mg do not have additional effects on lowering BP; hypotension, dizziness, photosensitivity

Indinavir (Crixivan) **Uses:** HIV infection **Action:** Protease inhibitor; inhibits maturation of immature noninfectious virions to mature infectious virus **Dose:** 800 mg PO q8h; use in combination with other antiretroviral agents; take on an empty stomach; ↓ in hepatic impairment **Caution/Contra:** [C, ?] Numerous drug interactions **Supplied:** Caps 200, 400 mg **Notes/SE:** Nephrolithiasis; drink six 8-oz glasses of water/d; dyslipidemia, lipodystrophy, GI effects

Indomethacin (Indocin) **Uses:** Arthritis; closure of the ductus arteriosus; tocolysis **Action:** Inhibits prostaglandin synthesis **Dose:** *Adults.* 25–50 mg PO bid–tid, to a max of 200 mg/d. *Tocolysis:* 50–100 10 PR, then 25 mg PO/PR q4–6h ×48 h. *Infants:* 0.2–0.25 mg/kg/dose IV; may be repeated in 12–24 h for up to 3 doses; take with food **Caution/Contra:** [B, +] ASA/NSAID sensitivity, peptic ulcer disease **Supplied:** Inj 1 mg/vial; caps 25, 50 mg; SR caps 75 mg; supp 50 mg; susp 25 mg/5 mL **Notes/SE:** Monitor renal function; GI bleeding or upset, dizziness, edema

Infliximab (Remicade) **Uses:** Moderate to severe Crohn's disease; RA (in combination with methotrexate) **Action:** IgG1κ neutralizes biologic activity of TNFα **Dose:** *Crohn's disease:* 5 mg/kg IV inf, may follow with subsequent doses given at 2 and 6 wk after initial inf. *RA:* 3 mg/kg IV inf at 0, 2, 6 wk, followed by q8wk **Caution/Contra:** [C, ?/–] Murine hypersensitivity, active infection **Supplied:** Inj **Notes/SE:** May cause hypersensitivity reaction, made up of human constant and murine variable regions; patients are predisposed to infection (especially TB); HA, fatigue, GI upset, inf reactions

Influenza Vaccine (Fluzone, FluShield, Fluvirin) **Uses:** Prevent influenza; all adults >65 y, children 6–23 mon, pregnant women (who will be in their 2nd or 3rd trimester during flu season, residents of nursing homes, patients with chronic diseases, health care workers and household contacts of high-risk patients, children < 9 y receiving vaccine for the first time **Actions:** Active immunization **Dose:** *Adults.* 0.5 mL/dose IM 0.5-mL IM *Peds:* ≥ 3 y 0.5-mL dose; 6–35 mon 0.25 mL IM; 6 to < 9 y who receive for the 1st time: 2 doses at least 4 wk apart, the 2nd dose before December if possible. **Caution, Contra:** [C, +] Egg or thimerosal allergy, active infection at site, Egg protein sensitivity **Supplied:** Based on specific manufacturer, 0.25 and 0.5 mL prefilled syringes **Notes:** Optimal dosing in the U.S. is Oct–Nov, protection begins 1–2 wk after and lasts up to 6 mon; Each y, specific vaccines manufactured based on predictions of the strains to be active in flu season (Dec–Spring in U.S.) Whole or split virus usually given to adults; give children <13 y split virus or purified surface antigen form to ↓ febrile reactions; soreness at the inj site, adverse fever, myalgia malaise, Guillain-Barré syndrome (controversial)

Insulin **Uses:** Type 1 or type 2 DM refractory to diet change or oral hypoglycemic agents; management of acute life-threatening hyperkalemia **Action:** Insulin supplementation **Dose:** Based on serum glucose levels; usually SC but can be given IV (only regular)/IM; typical start dose for type 1 0.5–1 U/kg/d; type 2 0.3–0.4 U/kg/d; renal failure may ↓ insulin needs **Caution/Contra:** [B, +] **Supplied:** Table 6 (page 616) **Notes/SE:** Highly purified insulins ↑ free insulin; monitor patients closely for several wk when changing doses/agents

Interferon Alfa (Roferon-A, Intron A) **Uses:** Hairy cell leukemia, Kaposi's sarcoma, multiple myeloma, CML, renal cell carcinoma, bladder CA, melanoma, and chronic hepatitis C **Action:** Direct antiproliferative action against tumor cells; modulation of the host immune response **Dose:** Dictated by treatment protocol. *Alfa-2a (Roferon-A):* 3 million IU/d for 16–24 wk SC or IM. *Alfa-2b (Intron A):* 2 million IU/m² IM or SC 3×/wk for 2–6 mon; intravesical 50–100 million IU in 50 mL/wk NS ×6 **Caution/Contra:** [C, +/–] Benzyl alcohol sensitivity **Supplied:** Injectable forms **Notes/SE:** May cause flu-like symptoms; fatigue common; anorexia occurs in 20–30% of patients; neurotoxicity may occur at high doses; neutralizing antibodies in up to 40% of patients receiving prolonged systemic therapy

Interferon Alfa-2b and Ribavirin Combination (Rebetron) **Uses:** Chronic hepatitis C in patients with compensated liver disease who have relapsed following α-interferon therapy **Action:** Combination antiviral agents **Dose:** 3 MU Intron A SC 3x/wk with 1000–1200 mg of Rebetron PO ÷ bid dose for 24 wk. *Patients <75 kg:* 1000 mg of Rebetron/d **Caution/Contra:** [X, ?] **Supplied:** *Patients <75 kg:* Combination packs: 6 vials Intron A (3 MU/0.5 mL) with 6 syringes and alcohol swabs, 70 Rebetron caps; one 18 million-IU multidose vial of Intron A inj (22.8 MU/3.8 mL; 3 MU/0.5 mL) and 6 syringes and swabs, 70 Rebetron caps; one 18 million-IU Intron A inj multidose pen (22.5 million IU/1.5 mL; 3 million IU/0.2 mL) and 6 disposable needles and swabs, 70 Rebetron caps. *Patients <75 kg:* Identical except 84 Rebetron caps/pack **Notes/SE:** Instruct patients in self-administration of SC Intron A; flu-like syndrome, HA, anemia

Interferon Alfacon-1 (Infergen) **Uses:** Management of chronic hepatitis C **Action:** Biologic response modifier **Dose:** 9 mcg SC 3x/wk **Caution/Contra:** [C, M] **Supplied:** Inj 9, 15 mcg **Notes/SE:** Allow at least 48 h between inj; flu-like syndrome, depression, blood dyscrasias

Interferon β-1b (Betaseron) **Uses:** Management of MS **Action:** Biologic response modifier **Dose:** 0.25 mg SC qod **Caution/Contra:** [C, ?] **Supplied:** Powder for inj 0.3 mg **Notes/SE:** Flu-like syndrome, depression, blood dyscrasias

Interferon γ-1b (Actimmune) **Uses:** ↓ Incidence of serious infections in chronic granulomatous disease (CGD), osteopetrosis **Action:** Biologic response modifier **Dose:** CGD: 50 mcg/m² SC (1.5 MU/m²) BSA >0.5 m²; if BSA <0.5 m², give 1.5 mcg/kg/dose; given 3x/wk **Caution/Contra:** [C, ?] **Supplied:** Inj 100 mcg (3 MU) **Notes/SE:** Flu-like syndrome, depression, blood dyscrasias

Ipecac Syrup **Uses:** Drug overdose and certain cases of poisoning **Action:** Irritation of the GI mucosa; stimulation of the chemoreceptor trigger zone **Dose:** *Adults.* 15–30 mL PO, followed by 200–300 mL of water; if no emesis occurs in 20 min, may repeat once. *Peds. 6–12 mon:* 5–10 mL PO, followed by 10–20 mL/kg of water; if no emesis in 20 min, repeat once. *1–12 y:* 15 mL PO followed by 10–20 mL/kg of water; if no emesis in 20 min, repeat once **Caution/Contra:** [C, ?] Do not use for ingestion of petroleum distillates or strong acid, base, or other corrosive or caustic agents; not for use in comatose or unconscious patients **Supplied:** Syrup 15, 30 mL **Notes/SE:** Caution in CNS depressant overdose; lethargy, cardiotoxicity, protracted vomiting

Ipratropium (Atrovent) **Uses:** Bronchospasm with COPD, bronchitis, emphysema, and rhinorrhea **Action:** Synthetic anticholinergic agent similar to atropine **Dose:** *Adults & Peds >12 y.* 2–4 puffs qid. *Nasal:* 2 sprays/nostril bid–tid **Caution/Contra:** [B, +] **Supplied:** Met-dose inhaler 18 mcg/dose; soln for inhal 0.02%; nasal spray 0.03%, 0.06% **Notes/SE:** Not for acute bronchospasm; nervousness, dizziness, HA, cough

Irbesartan (Avapro) **Uses:** HTN, DN, CHF **Action:** Angiotensin II receptor antagonist **Dose:** 150 mg/d PO, may be ↑ to 300 mg/d **Caution/Contra:** [C (in 1st trimester; D in 2nd and 3rd), ?/–] **Supplied:** Tabs 75, 150, 300 mg **Notes/SE:** Fatigue, hypotension

Irinotecan (Camptosar) **Uses:** Colorectal and lung CA **Action:** Topoisomerase I inhibitor; interferes with DNA synthesis **Dose:** 125–250 mg/m² weekly to qowk; ↓ hepatic dysfunction, as tolerated per toxicities **Caution/Contra:** [D, –] **Supplied:** Inj 20 mg/mL **Notes/SE:** Myelosuppression, N/V/D, abdominal cramping, alopecia. Diarrhea dose limiting in many studies; Rx acute diarrhea with atropine; Rx subacute diarrhea with loperamide. Diarrhea correlated to levels of metabolite SN-38

Iron Dextran (Dexferrum, INFeD) **Uses:** Iron deficiency when oral supplementation not possible **Action:** Parenteral iron supplementation **Dose:** Estimate iron deficiency, given IM/IV. A 0.5-mL test dose (0.25 mL in infants) prior to starting iron dextran. Total replacement dose (mL) = 0.0476 × weight (kg) × [desired hemoglobin (g/dL) – measured hemoglobin (g/dL)] + 1 mL/5 kg weight (max 14 mL). *Adults >50 kg. Max daily dose:* 100 mg Fe. *Peds. Max daily dose:* *<5 kg:* 25 mg Fe. *5–10 kg:* 50 mg Fe. *10–50 kg:* 100 mg Fe **Caution/Contra:** [C, M] **Supplied:** Inj 50 mg (Fe)/mL **Notes/SE:** Use test dose because

22

anaphylaxis possible; give deep IM using "Z-track" technique, IV route preferred; anaphylaxis, flushing, dizziness, inj site and inf reactions, metallic taste

Isoetharine (generic) **Uses:** Bronchial asthma and reversible bronchospasm **Action:** Sympathomimetic bronchodilator **Dose:** *Adults.* 0.25–1 mL diluted 1:3 with NS q4–6h. *Peds.* 0.01 mL/kg; min dose 0.1 mL; max dose 0.5 mL; dilute with NS q4–6h **Caution/Contra:** [C, ?] **Supplied:** Soln for inhal; aerosol **Notes/SE:** Tachycardia, HTN, dizziness, trembling

Isoniazid (INH) **Uses:** Rx and prophylaxis of *Mycobacterium* spp infections **Action:** Bactericidal; interferes with mycolic acid synthesis (disrupts cell wall) **Dose:** *Adults.* Active TB: 5 mg/kg/24 h PO or IM (usually 300 mg/d). *Prophylaxis:* 300 mg/d PO for 6–12 mon *Peds.* Active TB: 10–20 mg/kg/24 h PO or IM to a max of 300 mg/d. *Prophylaxis:* 10 mg/kg/24 h PO; ↓ in hepatic impairment **Caution/Contra:** [C, +] Acute liver disease, dialysis **Supplied:** Tabs 50, 100, 300 mg; syrup 50 mg/5 mL; inj 100 mg/mL **Notes/SE:** Given with 2–3 other drugs for active TB, based on INH resistance patterns where TB acquired; IM route rarely used. To prevent peripheral neuropathy, give pyridoxine 50–100 mg/d. Can cause severe hepatitis, peripheral neuropathy, GI upset, anorexia, nausea

Isoproterenol (Isuprel) **Uses:** Shock, cardiac arrest, and AV nodal block; antiasthmatic **Action:** β_1- and β_2-receptor stimulant **Dose:** *Adults.* Shock: 1–4 mg/min IV inf; titrate to effect. *AV nodal block:* 20–60 mg IV push; may repeat q3–5min; maint 1–5 mg/min IV inf. *Inhalation:* 1–2 inhal 4–6×/d. *Peds.* Inhal: 1–2 inhal 4–6×/d **Caution/Contra:** [C, ?] Tachycardia; pulse >130 may induce ventricular arrhythmias. **Supplied:** Met-inhaler; soln for neb 0.5%, 1%; inj 0.02 mg/mL, 0.2 mg/mL **Notes/SE:** Insomnia, arrhythmias, GI upset, trembling, dizziness

Isosorbide Dinitrate (Isordil, Sorbitrate) **Uses:** Rx and prevention of angina, CHF (with hydralazine) **Action:** Relaxation of vascular smooth muscle **Dose:** *Acute angina:* 5–10 mg PO (chew tabs) q2–3h or 2.5–10 mg SL PRN q5–10min; >3 doses should not be given in a 15–30-min period. *Angina prophylaxis:* 5–60 mg PO tid; do not give nitrates on a chronic q6h or qid basis >7–10 d because tolerance may develop **Caution/Contra:** [C, ?] Contra severe anemia, closed-angle glaucoma, orthostatic hypotension, cerebral hemorrhage, head trauma (can ↑ ICP) **Supplied:** Tabs 5, 10, 20, 30, 40 mg; SR tabs 40 mg; SL tabs 2.5, 5, 10 mg; chew tabs 5, 10 mg; SR caps 40 mg **Notes/SE:** HAs, ↓ BP, flushing, tachycardia, dizziness; higher oral dose usually needed to achieve same results as SL forms

Isosorbide Mononitrate (ISMO, Imdur) **Uses:** Prevention of angina pectoris **Action:** Relaxes vascular smooth muscle **Dose:** 20 mg PO bid, the 2 doses 7 h apart or ER (Imdur) 30–120 mg/d PO **Caution/Contra:** [C, ?] Contra in head trauma or cerebral hemorrhage (can ↑ ICP) **Supplied:** Tabs 10, 20 mg; ER 30, 60, 120 mg **Notes/SE:** HAs, dizziness, hypotension

Isotretinoin [13-*cis* Retinoic Acid] (Accutane) **WARNING:** Must not be used by pregnant females; patient must be capable of complying with mandatory contraceptive measures; Accutane must be prescribed under SMART (system to manage Accutane-related teratogenicity) **Uses:** Refractory severe acne **Action:** Retinoic acid derivative **Dose:** 0.5–2 mg/kg/d PO ÷ bid; ↓ in hepatic disease **Caution/Contra:** [X, –] Retinoid sensitivity **Supplied:** Caps 10, 20, 40 mg **Notes/SE:** Isolated reports of depression, psychosis, suicidal thoughts; dermatologic sensitivity, xerostomia, photosensitivity; SMART risk management programs requires 2 negative PRG tests before therapy and use 2 forms of contraception 1 mon before, during, and 1 mon after therapy; informed consent recommended

Isradipine (DynaCirc) **Uses:** HTN w/wo diuretics **Action:** Ca^{2+} channel blocker **Dose:** 2.5–10 mg PO bid **Caution/Contra:** [C, ?] Heart block, CHF **Supplied:** Caps 2.5, 5 mg; tabs CR 5, 10 mg **Notes/SE:** HA, edema, flushing, fatigue, dizziness, palpitations

Itraconazole (Sporanox) **WARNING:** Potential for negative inotropic effects on the heart; if signs or symptoms of CHF occur during administration, continued use should be assessed **Uses:** Systemic fungal infections (*Aspergillosis, Blastomycosis, Histoplasmosis, Candidiasis*) **Action:** Inhibits synthesis of ergosterol **Dose:** 200 mg PO or IV qd–bid with meals or cola/grapefruit juice **Caution/Contra:** [C, ?] Contra if CrCl <30 mL/min, Hx of CHF or ventricular dysfunction, or concurrently with H_2-antagonist, omeprazole, antacids; numerous other interactions **Supplied:** Caps 100 mg; soln 10 mg/mL; inj 10 mg/mL **Notes/SE:** Often used in patients who cannot take amphotericin B; nausea, rash, hepatitis

22

Kaolin-Pectin (Kaodene, Kao-Spen, Kapectolin, Parepectolin) Uses: Diarrhea **Action:** Absorbent demulcent **Dose:** *Adults.* 60–120 mL PO after each loose stool or q3–4h PRN. *Peds. 3–6 y:* 15–30 mL/dose PO PRN. *6–12 y:* 30–60 mL/dose PO PRN **Caution/Contra:** [C, +] **Supplied:** Multiple OTC forms; also available with opium (Parepectolin) **Notes/SE:** Constipation, dehydration

Ketoconazole (Nizoral, Nizoral AD Shampoo [OTC]) Uses: Systemic fungal infections; topical cream for localized fungal infections due to dermatophytes and yeast; shampoo for dandruff, short term in prostate CA when rapid reduction of testosterone needed (ie, cord compression) **Action:** Inhibits fungal cell wall synthesis **Dose:** *Adults. Oral:* 200 mg PO qd; $\uparrow$ to 400 mg/d PO for serious infections; prostate CA 400 mg PO tid (short term). *Topical:* Apply to the affected area qd (cream or shampoo). *Peds >2 y.* 5–10 mg/kg/24 h PO ÷ q12–24h; drug interaction with any agent increasing gastric pH will prevent absorption of ketoconazole; $\downarrow$ in hepatic disease **Caution/Contra:** [C, +/–] Contra in CNS fungal infections (poor CNS penetration); may enhance oral anticoagulants; may react with alcohol to produce a disulfiram-like reaction; numerous other drug interactions **Supplied:** Tabs 200 mg; topical cream 2%; shampoo 2% **Notes/SE:** Monitor LFTs with systemic use; can cause nausea; oral form multiple drug interactions

Ketoprofen (Orudis, Oruvail) Uses: Arthritis and pain **Action:** NSAID; inhibits prostaglandin synthesis **Dose:** 25–75 mg PO tid–qid to a max of 300 mg/d; take with food **Caution/Contra:** [B, D 3rd trimester, ?] NSAID/ASA sensitivity **Supplied:** Tabs 12.5 mg; caps 25, 50, 75 mg; caps, SR 100, 150, 200 mg **Notes/SE:** GI upset, peptic ulcers, dizziness, edema, rash

Ketorolac (Toradol) WARNING: Indicated for short term (up to 5 d) of moderately severe acute pain that requires analgesia at opioid level Uses: Pain **Action:** NSAID; inhibits prostaglandin synthesis **Dose:** 15–30 mg IV/IM q6h or 10 mg PO qid; max IV/IM 120 mg/d, max PO 40 mg/d; do not use for longer than 5 days; $\downarrow$ for age and renal dysfunction **Caution/Contra:** [B, D 3rd trimester, –] Contra peptic ulcer disease, NSAID sensitivity, advanced renal disease, CNS bleeding, anticipated major surgery, labor and delivery, nursing mothers **Supplied:** Tabs 10 mg; inj 15 mg/mL, 30 mg/mL **Notes/SE:** Bleeding, peptic ulcer disease, renal failure, edema, dizziness, hypersensitivity; PO used only as continuation of IM/IV therapy

Ketorolac Ophthalmic (Acular) Uses: Relief of ocular itching caused by seasonal allergic conjunctivitis **Action:** NSAID **Dose:** 1 gtt qid **Caution/Contra:** [C, +] **Supplied:** Soln 0.5% **Notes/SE:** Local irritation

Ketotifen (Zaditor) Uses: Allergic conjunctivitis **Action:** H_1-receptor antagonist and mast cell stabilizer **Dose:** *Adults & Peds.* 1 gtt in affected eye(s) q8–12h **Caution/Contra:** [C, ?/–] **Supplied:** Solution 0.025%/5 mL **Notes/SE:** Local irritation, HA, rhinitis

Labetalol (Trandate, Normodyne) Uses: HTN and hypertensive emergencies **Action:** α- and β-Adrenergic blocking agent **Dose:** *Adults. HTN:* Initially, 100 mg PO bid, then 200–400 mg PO bid. *Hypertensive emergency:* 20–80 mg IV bolus, then 2 mg/min IV inf, titrated to effect. *Peds. Oral:* 3–20 mg/ kg/d in ÷ doses. *Hypertensive emergency:* 0.4–1.5 mg/kg/h IV cont inf **Caution/ Contra:** [C (D in 2nd or 3rd trimester), +] Cardiogenic shock, uncompensated CHF, heart block **Supplied:** Tabs 100, 200, 300 mg; inj 5 mg/mL **Notes/SE:** Dizziness, nausea, $\downarrow$ BP, fatigue, cardiovascular effects

Lactic Acid and Ammonium Hydroxide [Ammonium Lactate] (Lac-Hydrin) Uses: Severe xerosis and ichthyosis **Action:** Emollient moisturizer **Dose:** Apply bid **Caution/Contra:** [C, ?] **Supplied:** Lactic acid 12% with ammonium hydroxide **Notes/SE:** Local irritation

Lactobacillus (Lactinex Granules) Uses: Control of diarrhea, especially after antibiotic therapy **Action:** Replaces normal intestinal flora **Dose:** *Adults & Peds >3 y.* 1 packet, 2 caps, or 4 tabs with meals or liq tid–qid **Caution/Contra:** [A, +] Contra in milk/lactose allergy **Supplied:** Tabs; caps; EC caps; powder in packets **Notes/SE:** Flatulence

Lactulose (Chronulac, Cephulac) Uses: Hepatic encephalopathy; laxative **Action:** Acidifies the colon, allowing ammonia to diffuse into the colon **Dose:** *Adults. Acute hepatic encephalopathy:* 30–45 mL PO q1h until soft stools, then tid–qid. *Chronic laxative therapy:*

30–45 mL PO tid–qid; adjust q1–2d to produce 2–3 soft stools/d. *Rectally:* 200 g in 700 mL of water PR. **Peds.** *Infants:* 2.5–10 mL/ 24 h ÷ tid–qid. *Children:* 40–90 mL/24 h ÷ tid–qid **Caution/Contra:** [B, ?] Galactosemia **Supplied:** Syrup 10 g/15 mL **Notes/SE:** Severe diarrhea, flatulence

Lamivudine (Epivir, Epivir-HBV) WARNING: Lactic acidosis and severe hepatomegaly with steatosis reported with nucleoside analogs **Uses:** HIV infection and chronic hepatitis B **Action:** Inhibits HIV reverse transcriptase, resulting in viral DNA chain termination **Dose:** *HIV: Adults & Peds >12 y.* 150 mg PO bid. *Peds <12 y.* 4 mg/kg bid. *HBV:* 100 mg/d. *Peds 2–17 y:* 3 mg/kg/d PO, 100 mg max; ↓ in renal impairment **Caution/Contra:** [C, ?] **Supplied:** Tabs 100, 150 mg (HBV); soln 5 mg/mL, 10 mg/mL **Notes/SE:** HA, pancreatitis, anemia, GI upset

Lamotrigine (Lamictal) WARNING: Serious rashes requiring hospitalization and DC of treatment reported with Lamictal use; this rash occurs more frequently in children than adults **Uses:** Partial seizures **Action:** Phenyltriazine antiepileptic **Dose:** *Adults.* Initial 50 mg/d PO, then 50 mg PO bid for 2 wk, then maint 300–500 mg/d in 2 ÷ doses. *Peds.* 0.15 mg/kg in 1–2 ÷ doses for wk 1 and 2, then 0.3 mg/kg for wk 3 and 4, then maint 1 mg/kg/d in 1–2 ÷ doses **Caution/Contra:** [C, –] **Supplied:** Tabs 25, 100, 150, 200 mg; chew tabs 5, 25 mg **Notes/SE:** May cause rash and photosensitivity; value of therapeutic monitoring not established; interacts with other antiepileptics; HA, GI upset, dizziness, ataxia, rash (potentially life-threatening in children > adults)

Lansoprazole (Prevacid) **Uses:** Duodenal ulcers, prevent and Rx NSAID gastric ulcers, *H. pylori* infection, erosive esophagitis, and hypersecretory conditions **Action:** Proton pump inhibitor **Dose:** 15–30 mg/d PO; NSAID ulcer prevention 15 mg/d PO up to 12 wk, NSAID ulcers 30 mg/d PO, ×8 wk; ↓ in severe hepatic impairment **Caution/Contra:** [B, ?/–] **Supplied:** Caps 15, 30 mg **Notes/SE:** HA, fatigue

Latanoprost (Xalatan) **Uses:** Refractory glaucoma **Action:** Prostaglandin **Dose:** 1 gtt eye(s) hs **Caution/Contra:** [C, ?] **Supplied:** 0.005% Soln **Notes/SE:** May darken light irides; blurred vision, ocular stinging, and itching

Leflunomide (Arava) WARNING: PRG must be excluded prior to start of treatment **Uses:** Active RA **Action:** Inhibits pyrimidine synthesis **Dose:** Initial 100 mg/d for 3 d, then 10–20 mg/d **Caution/Contra:** [X, –] **Supplied:** Tabs 10, 20, 100 mg **Notes/SE:** Monitor LFTs during initial therapy; diarrhea, infection, HTN, alopecia, rash, nausea, joint pain, hepatitis

Lepirudin (Refludan) **Uses:** Heparin-induced thrombocytopenia **Action:** Direct inhibitor of thrombin **Dose:** Bolus 0.4 mg/kg IV, then 0.15 mg/kg inf; ↓ dose and inf rate if CrCl <60 mL/min **Caution/Contra:** [B, ?/–] Caution in patients who have suffered hemorrhagic event **Supplied:** Inj 50 mg **Notes/SE:** Adjust dose based on aPTT ratio, maintain aPTT ratio of 1.5–2.0; bleeding, anemia, hematoma

Letrozole (Femara) **Uses:** Advanced breast CA **Action:** Nonsteroidal inhibitor of the aromatase enzyme system **Dose:** 2.5 mg/d **Caution/Contra:** [D, ?] **Supplied:** Tabs 2.5 mg **Notes/SE:** Requires periodic CBC, thyroid function, electrolyte, LFT, and renal monitoring; anemia, nausea, hot flashes, arthralgia

Leucovorin (Wellcovorin) **Uses:** Overdose of folic acid antagonist; augmentation of 5-FU **Action:** Reduced folate source; circumvents action of folate reductase inhibitors (ie, MTX) **Dose:** *Adults & Peds.* *MTX rescue:* 10 mg/m²/dose IV or PO q6h for 72 h until MTX level <10⁻⁸. *5-FU:* 200 mg/m²/d IV 1–5 d during daily 5-FU treatment or 500 mg/m²/wk with weekly 5-FU therapy. *Adjunct to antimicrobials:* 5–15 mg/d PO **Caution/Contra:** [C, ?/–] Pernicious anemia; should not be administered intrathecally/intraventricularly **Supplied:** Tabs 5, 15, 25 mg; inj **Notes/SE:** Many dosing schedules for leucovorin rescue following MTX therapy; allergic reaction

Leuprolide (Lupron, Lupron DEPOT, Lupron Depot-Ped, Viadur, Eligard) **Uses:** Advanced prostate CA (CAP), endometriosis, uterine fibroids, and CPP **Action:** LHRH agonist; paradoxically inhibits release of gonadotropin, resulting in decreased pituitary gonadotropins (ie, ↓ LH); in men ↓ testosterone **Dose:** *Adults.* *CAP:* 7.5 mg IM q28d or 22.5 mg IM q3mon or 30 mg IM q4mon. Viadur implant (CAP only); insert in inner upper arm using local anesthesia, replace q12mon. *Endometriosis (depot only):* 3.75 mg IM qmon ×6. *Fibroids:* 3.75 mg IM qmon ×3. *Peds.* *CPP:* 50 mcg/kg/d as a daily SC inj; ↑ by 10 mcg/kg/d until total down-regulation achieved. *Depot: <25 kg:* 7.5 mg IM q4wk.

>*25–37.5 kg:* 11.25 mg IM q4wk. >*37.5 kg:* 15 mg IM q4wk **Caution/Contra:** [X, ?] Contra in undiagnosed vaginal bleeding **Supplied:** Inj 5 mg/mL; Lupron depot 3.75 (1 mon for fibroids, endometriosis), Lupron depot for CAP: 7.5 (1 mon), 22.5 (3 mon), 30 mg (4 mon); Eligard depot for CAP: 7.5 mg (1 mon); Viadur 12-mon SC implant; Lupron-PED 7.5, 11.25, 15 mg **Notes/SE:** Hot flashes, gynecomastia, N/V, constipation, anorexia, dizziness, HA, insomnia, paresthesias, peripheral edema, and bone pain (transient "flare reaction" at 7–14 d after the 1st dose due to LH and testosterone surge before suppression)

Levalbuterol (Xopenex) **Uses:** Rx and prevention of bronchospasm **Action:** Sympathomimetic bronchodilator **Dose:** 0.63 mg neb q6–8h **Caution/Contra:** [C, +] **Supplied:** Soln for inhal 0.63, 1.25 mg/3 mL **Notes/SE:** Therapeutically active *R*-isomer of albuterol; tachycardia, nervousness, trembling

Levamisole (Ergamisol) **Uses:** Adjuvant therapy of Dukes C colon CA (in combination with 5-FU) **Action:** Poorly understood immunostimulatory effects **Dose:** 50 mg PO q8h for 3 d q14d during 5-FU therapy; ↓ in hepatic dysfunction **Caution/Contra:** [C, ?/–] **Supplied:** Tabs 50 mg **Notes/SE:** N/V/D, abdominal pain, taste disturbance, anorexia, hyperbilirubinemia, disulfiram-like reaction on alcohol ingestion, minimal bone marrow depression, fatigue, fever, conjunctivitis

Levetiracetam (Keppra) **Uses:** Partial onset seizures **Action:** Unknown **Dose:** 500 mg PO bid, may ↑ to max 3000 mg/d; ↓ in renal insufficiency **Caution/Contra:** [C, ?/–] **Supplied:** Tabs 250, 500, 750 mg **Notes/SE:** May cause dizziness and somnolence; may impair coordination

Levobunolol (A-K Beta, Betagan) **Uses:** Glaucoma **Action:** β-Adrenergic blocker **Dose:** 1–2 gtt/d 0.5% or 1–2 gtt 0.25% bid **Caution/Contra:** [C, ?] **Supplied:** Soln 0.25, 0.5% **Notes/SE:** Ocular stinging or burning; possible systemic effects if absorbed

Levocabastine (Livostin) **Uses:** Allergic seasonal conjunctivitis **Action:** Antihistamine **Dose:** 1 gtt in eye(s) qid up to 4 wk **Caution/Contra:** [C, +/–] **Supplied:** 0.05% gtt **Notes/SE:** Ocular discomfort

Levofloxacin (Levaquin, Quixin Ophthalmic) **Uses:** Lower respiratory tract infections, sinusitis, UTI; topical for bacterial conjunctivitis **Action:** Quinolone antibiotic, inhibits DNA gyrase **Dose:** 250–500 mg/d PO or IV; ophth 1–2 gtt in eye(s) q2h while awake for 2 d, then q4h while awake for 5 d; ↓ in renal insufficiency **Caution/Contra:** [C, –] **Supplied:** Tabs 250, 500 mg; premixed bags 250, 500 mg; ophth 0.5% soln **Notes/SE:** Reliable activity against *S. pneumoniae;* interactions with cation-containing products; dizziness, rash, GI upset, photosensitivity

Levonorgestrel (Plan B) **Uses:** Emergency contraceptive ("morning-after pill"); can prevent pregnancy if taken < 72 h after unprotected sex (contraceptive fails or if no contraception used) **Actions:** progestin **Dose:** 1 pill q12h × 2 **Supplied:** tablets, 0.75 mg, 2 blister pack **Contra/Caution:** [X, M]Contra known suspected PRG, abnormal uterine bleeding **Notes:** Will not induce abortion; may increase risk of ectopic pregnancy; N/V, abdominal pain, fatigue HA, menstrual changes.

Levonorgestrel Implant (Norplant) **Uses:** Contraceptive **Dose:** Implant 6 caps in the midforearm **Caution/Contra:** [X, +/–] Hepatic disease, thromboembolism, breast CA **Supplied:** Kits containing 6 implantable caps, each containing 36 mg **Notes/SE:** Prevents pregnancy for up to 5 y; may be removed if PRG desired; uterine bleeding, HA, acne, nausea

Levorphanol (Levo-Dromoran) [C-II] **Uses:** Moderate–severe pain **Action:** Narcotic analgesic **Dose:** 2 mg PO or SC PRN q6–8h; ↓ in hepatic failure **Caution/Contra:** [B, ?] **Supplied:** Tabs 2 mg; inj 2 mg/mL **Notes/SE:** Tachycardia, hypotension, drowsiness, GI upset, constipation, respiratory depression

Levothyroxine (Synthroid, others) **Uses:** Hypothyroidism **Action:** Supplementation of L-thyroxine **Dose:** *Adults.* Initially, 25–50 mcg/d PO or IV; ↑ by 25–50 μg/d every mon; usual dose 100–200 μg/d. *Peds. 0–1 y:* 8–10 mcg/kg/24 h PO or IV. *1–5 y:* 4–6 mcg/kg/24 h PO or IV. *>5 y:* 3–4 mcg/kg/24 h PO or IV; titrate dosage based on clinical response and thyroid function tests; dosage can ↑ more rapidly in young to middle-aged patients. **Caution/Contra:** [A, +] Contra recent MI, uncorrected renal insufficiency **Supplied:** Tabs 25, 50, 75, 88, 100, 112, 125, 150, 175, 200, 300 mcg; inj 200, 500 mcg **Notes/SE:** Insomnia, weight loss, alopecia, arrhythmia

Lidocaine (Anestacon Topical, Xylocaine, others) **Uses:** Local anesthetic; treatment of cardiac arrhythmias **Action:** Anesthetic; class IB antiarrhythmic **Dose:** *Adults. Antiarrhythmic, ET:* 5 mg/kg; follow with 0.5 mg/kg in 10 min if effective. *IV load:* 1 mg/kg/dose bolus over 2–3 min; repeat in 5–10 min up to 200–300 mg/h; cont inf of 20–50 mcg/kg/min or 1–4 mg/min. *Peds. Antiarrhythmic, ET, loading dose:* 1 mg/kg; repeat in 10–15 min max total dose of 5 mg/kg, then IV inf 20–50 mcg/kg/min. *Topical:* Apply max 3 mg/kg/dose. *Local inj anesthetic:* Max 4.5 mg/kg (Table 3, page 611) **Caution/Contra:** [C, +] Do not use lidocaine with epinephrine on the digits, ears, or nose because vasoconstriction may cause necrosis; heart block **Supplied:** *Inj local:* 0.5, 1, 1.5, 2, 4, 10, 20%. *Inj IV:* 1% (10 mg/mL, 2% 20 mg/mL); admixture 4, 10, 20%. *IV inf:* 0.2%, 0.4%; cream 2%; gel 2, 2.5%; oint 2.5, 5%; liq 2.5%; soln 2, 4%; viscous 2% **Notes/SE:** 2nd line to amiodarone in emergency cardiac care; dilute ET dose 1–2 mL with NS; epinephrine may be added for local anesthesia to ↑ effect and ↓ bleeding; for IV forms, ↓ with liver disease or CHF; dizziness, paresthesias, and convulsions associated with toxicity; Table 2 (page 607) for drug levels

Lidocaine (ELA-Max) **Uses:** Topical anesthetic; adjunct to phlebotomy or invasive dermal procedures **Action:** Topical anesthetic **Dose:** Apply a ¼-in. thick layer to intact skin at least 30 min before procedure; do not apply over area larger than 100 cm^2 in children **Caution/Contra:** [C, +]. Not for ophth use; methemoglobinemia **Supplied:** Cream 4% **Notes/SE:** Longer contact time gives greater effect; burning, stinging, methemoglobinemia

Lidocaine/Prilocaine (EMLA) **Uses:** Topical anesthetic; adjunct to phlebotomy or dermal procedures **Action:** Topical anesthetic **Dose:** *Adults. EMLA cream and anesthetic disc (1 g/10 cm^2):* Apply thick layer 2–2.5 g to intact skin and cover with an occlusive dressing (eg, Tegaderm) for at least 1 h. *Anesthetic disc:* 1 g/10 cm^2 for at least 1 h. *Peds. Max dose:* =3 mon or <5 kg: 1 g/10 cm^2 for 1 h. *3–12 mon and >5 kg:* 2 g/20 cm^2 for 4 h. *1–6 y and >10 kg:* 10 g/100 cm^2 for 4 h. *7–12 y and >20 kg:* 20 g/200 cm^2 for 4 h **Caution/Contra:** [B, +] Contra on mucous membranes, broken skin, ophth use; methemoglobinemia **Supplied:** Cream 2.5% lidocaine/2.5% prilocaine; anesthetic disc (1 g) **Notes/SE:** Longer contact time gives greater effect; burning, stinging, methemoglobinemia

Lindane (Kwell) **Uses:** Head lice, crab lice, scabies **Action:** Ectoparasiticide and ovicide **Dose:** *Adults & Peds. Cream or lotion:* Apply thin layer after bathing, leave on for 8–12 h (6–8 h children, 6 h infants), pour on laundry. *Shampoo:* Apply 30 mL, develop a lather with warm water for 4 min, comb out nits; repeat in 7 d if necessary **Caution/Contra:** [B, +/–] Premature infants, open wounds **Supplied:** Lotion 1%; shampoo 1% **Notes/SE:** Caution with overuse; may be absorbed into blood; arrhythmias, seizures, local irritation, GI upset

Linezolid (Zyvox) **Uses:** Infections caused by gram+ bacteria, including vancomycin-resistant and methicillin-resistant strains **Action:** Unique action, binds ribosomal bacterial RNA; bactericidal for strep, bacteriostatic for enterococci and Staph **Dose:** 400–600 mg IV or PO q12h **Caution/Contra:** [C, ?/–] Avoid foods containing tyramine; avoid cough and cold products containing pseudoephedrine; myelosuppression **Supplied:** Inj 2 mg/mL; tabs 400, 600 mg; susp 100 mg/5 mL **Notes/SE:** Reversible MAOI; follow weekly CBC; HTN, HA, insomnia, GI upset

Liothyronine (Cytomel) **Uses:** Hypothyroidism **Action:** T$_3$ replacement **Dose:** *Adults.* Initial dose of 25 mcg/24 h, then titrate q1–2wk according to clinical response and TFT to maint of 25–100 mcg/d PO. *Myxedema coma:* 25–50 mcg IV. *Peds.* Initial dose of 5 mcg/ 24 h, then titrate by 5-mcg/24 h increments at 1–2 wk intervals; maint 25–75 mcg/24 h PO qd; ↓ dose in elderly **Caution/Contra:** [A, +] Contra recent MI **Supplied:** Tabs 5, 25, 50 mcg; inj 10 mcg/mL **Notes/SE:** Monitor TFT; alopecia, arrhythmias, chest pain

Lisinopril (Prinivil, Zestril) **Uses:** HTN, CHF, prevent DN and AMI **Action:** ACE inhibitor **Dose:** 5–40 mg/24 h PO qd–bid. *AMI:* 5 mg within 24 h of MI, followed by 5 mg after 24 h, 10 mg after 48 h, then 10 mg/d; ↓ in renal insufficiency **Caution/Contra:** [D, –] **Supplied:** Tabs 2.5, 5, 10, 20, 30, 40 mg **Notes/SE:** Dizziness, HA, cough, hypotension, angioedema, hyperkalemia; to prevent DN, start when urinary microalbuminemia begins

Lithium Carbonate (Eskalith, others) **Uses:** Manic episodes of bipolar illness; maint therapy in recurrent disease **Action:** Effects shift toward intraneuronal metabolism of catecholamines **Dose:** *Adults. Acute mania:* 600 mg PO tid or 900 mg SR bid. *Maint:*

300 mg PO tid–qid. *Peds 6–12 y.* 15–60 mg/kg/d in 3–4 ÷ doses; dosage must be titrated; follow serum levels; ↓ in renal insufficiency, elderly **Caution/Contra:** [D, –] Severe renal impairment or cardiovascular disease **Supplied:** Caps 150, 300, 600 mg; tabs 300 mg; SR tabs 300, 450 mg; syrup 300 mg/5 mL **Notes/SE:** Table 2 (page 607) for drug levels. Polyuria, polydipsia, nephrogenic DI, tremor; Na retention or diuretic use may potentiate toxicity, arrhythmias, dizziness

Lodoxamide (Alomide) **Uses:** Seasonal allergic conjunctivitis **Action:** Stabilizes mast cells **Dose:** *Adults & Peds >2 y.* 1–2 gtt in eye(s) qid up to 3 mon **Caution/Contra:** [B, ?] **Supplied:** Soln 0.1% **Notes/SE:** Ocular burning, stinging, HA

Lomefloxacin (Maxaquin) **Uses:** UTI and lower respiratory tract infections caused by gram– bacteria; prophylaxis in transurethral procedures **Action:** Quinolone antibiotic; inhibits DNA gyrase **Dose:** 400 mg/d PO; ↓ in renal insufficiency **Caution/Contra:** [C, –] **Supplied:** Tabs 400 mg **Notes/SE:** Photosensitivity, seizures, HA, dizziness

Loperamide (Imodium) **Uses:** Diarrhea **Action:** Slows intestinal motility **Dose:** *Adults.* Initially 4 mg PO, then 2 mg after each loose stool, up to 16 mg/d. *Peds.* 0.4–0.8 mg/kg/24 h PO q6–12h until diarrhea resolves or for 7 d max **Caution/Contra:** [B, +] Do not use in acute diarrhea caused by *Salmonella, Shigella,* or *C. difficile.* **Supplied:** Caps 2 mg; tabs 2 mg; liq 1 mg/5 mL, 1 mg/mL **Notes/SE:** Constipation, sedation, dizziness

Lopinavir/Ritonavir (Kaletra) **Uses:** HIV infection **Action:** Protease inhibitor **Dose:** *Adults.* 3 caps or 5 mL PO bid with food. *Peds. 7–15 kg:* 12/3 mg/kg PO bid. *15–40 kg:* 10/2.5 mg/kg PO bid. *>40 kg:* adult dose. **Caution/Contra:** [C, ?/–] Numerous drug interactions **Supplied:** Caps 133.3 mg/33.3 mg (lopinavir/ritonavir), solution 400 mg/100 mg/5 mL **Notes/SE:** Soln contains alcohol, avoid disulfiram and metronidazole; GI upset, asthenia, ↑ cholesterol and triglycerides, pancreatitis; protease metabolic syndrome

Loracarbef (Lorabid) **Uses:** Upper and lower respiratory tract, skin, bone, urinary tract, abdomen, and gynecologic system bacterial infections **Action:** 2nd-gen. cephalosporin; inhibits cell wall synthesis **Dose:** *Adults.* 200–400 mg PO bid. *Peds.* 7.5–15 mg/kg/d PO ÷ bid; take on empty stomach; ↓ in severe renal insufficiency **Caution/Contra:** [B, +] **Supplied:** Caps 200, 400 mg; susp 125, 250 mg/5 mL **Notes/SE:** More gram– activity than 1st-gen. cephalosporins; causes diarrhea

Loratadine (Claritin) **Uses:** Allergic rhinitis, chronic idiopathic urticaria **Action:** Nonsedating antihistamine **Dose:** *Adults.* 10 mg/d PO; *Peds. 2–5 y:* 5 mg PO qd; *>6 y:* adult dose; should be taken on an empty stomach; ↓ in hepatic insufficiency **Caution/Contra:** [B, +/–] **Supplied:** Tabs 10 mg; rapid disintegration; Reditabs 10 mg; syrup 1 mg/mL **Notes/SE:** HA, somnolence, xerostomia

Lorazepam (Ativan, others) [C-IV] **Uses:** Anxiety and anxiety with depression; preop sedation; control of status epilepticus; alcohol withdrawal; antiemetic **Action:** Benzodiazepine; antianxiety agent **Dose:** *Adults. Anxiety:* 1–10 mg/d PO in 2–3 ÷ doses. *Preop sedation:* 0.05 mg/kg to 4 mg max IM 2 h before surgery. *Insomnia:* 2–4 mg PO hs. *Status epilepticus:* 4 mg/dose IV PRN q10–15 min; usual total dose 8 mg. *Antiemetic:* 0.5–2 mg IV or PO q4–6h PRN. *Peds. Status epilepticus:* 0.05 mg/kg/dose IV repeated at 1–20-min intervals × 2 PRN. *Antiemetic, 2–15 y:* 0.05 mg/kg (to 2 mg/dose) prechemotherapy; ↓ in elderly; do not administer IV >2 mg/min or 0.05 mg/kg/min **Caution/Contra:** [D, ?/–] Contra in severe pain, severe hypotension, narrow-angle glaucoma **Supplied:** Tabs 0.5, 1, 2 mg; soln, oral conc 2 mg/mL; inj 2, 4 mg/mL **Notes/SE:** May take up to 10 min to see effect when given IV; sedation, ataxia, tachycardia, constipation, respiratory depression

Losartan (Cozaar) **Uses:** HTN, CHF, DN **Action:** Angiotensin II antagonist **Dose:** 25–50 mg PO qd–bid; ↓ dose in elderly or hepatic impairment **Caution/Contra:** [C (1st trimester), D (2nd and 3rd trimesters), ?/–] **Supplied:** Tabs 25, 50, 100 mg **Notes/SE:** Symptomatic hypotension may occur in patients on diuretics; GI upset, angioedema

Lovastatin (Mevacor, Altocor) **Uses:** Hypercholesterolemia; slows progression of atherosclerosis **Action:** HMG-CoA reductase inhibitor **Dose:** 20 mg/d PO with PM meal; may ↑ at 4-wk intervals to a max of 80 mg/d taken with meals; avoid grapefruit juice **Caution/Contra:** [X, –] Avoid concurrent use with gemfibrozil if possible; active liver disease **Supplied:** Tabs 10, 20, 40 mg **Notes/SE:** Patient must maintain standard cholesterol-lowering diet throughout treatment; monitor LFT q12wk × 1 y, then q6mo; HA and GI intolerance

22

common; patient should promptly report any unexplained muscle pain, tenderness, or weakness (myopathy)

Lymphocyte Immune Globulin [Antithymocyte Globulin, ATG] (Atgam)
Uses: Allograft rejection in transplant patients; aplastic anemia if not candidates for BMT **Action:** ↓ Number of circulating, thymus-dependent lymphocytes **Dose:** *Adults.* Prevent rejection: 15 mg/kg/day IV ×14 d, then qod ×7; initial within 24 h before/after transplant. Treat rejection: Same except use 10–15 mg/kg/day **Caution/Contra:** [C, ?] Acute viral illness, Hx reaction to other equine γ-globulin preparation **Supplied:** Inj 50 mg/mL **Notes/SE:** Test dose 0.1 mL of a 1:1000 dilution in NS; DC with severe thrombocytopenia or leukopenia; rash, fever, chills, HA, ↑ K⁺

Magaldrate (Riopan, Lowsium) **Uses:** Hyperacidity associated with peptic ulcer, gastritis, and hiatal hernia **Action:** Low-Na antacid **Dose:** 5–10 mL PO between meals and hs **Caution/Contra:** [B, ?] Do not use in renal insufficiency due to Mg content. **Supplied:** Susp **Notes/SE:** <0.3 mg Na/tab or tsp; GI upset

Magnesium Citrate **Uses:** Vigorous bowel preparation; constipation **Action:** Cathartic laxative **Dose:** *Adults.* 120–240 mL PO PRN. *Peds.* 0.5 mL/kg/dose, to a max of 200 mL PO; take with a beverage **Caution/Contra:** [B, +] Renal insufficiency or intestinal obstruction **Supplied:** Effervescent soln **Notes/SE:** Abdominal cramps, gas

Magnesium Hydroxide (Milk of Magnesia) **Uses:** Constipation **Action:** NS laxative **Dose:** *Adults.* 15–30 mL PO PRN. *Peds.* 0.5 mL/kg/dose PO PRN **Caution/Contra:** [B, +] Renal insufficiency or intestinal obstruction **Supplied:** Tabs 311 mg, liq 400, 800 mg/5 mL **Notes/SE:** Diarrhea, abdominal cramps

Magnesium Oxide (Mag-Ox 400, others) **Uses:** Replacement for low plasma levels **Action:** Mg supplementation **Dose:** 400–800 mg/d ÷ qd–qid with full glass of water **Caution/Contra:** [B, +] Renal insufficiency **Supplied:** Caps 140 mg; tabs 400 mg **Notes/SE:** Diarrhea, nausea

Magnesium Sulfate **Uses:** Replacement for low Mg levels; refractory hypokalemia and hypocalcemia; preeclampsia and premature labor **Action:** Mg supplement **Dose:** *Adults. Supplement:* 1–2 g IM or IV; repeat PRN. *Preeclampsia/premature labor:* 4 g load then 1–4 g/h IV inf. *Peds.* 25–50 mg/kg/dose IM or IV q4–6h for 3–4 doses; repeat if ↓ Mg persists; ↓ dose with low urine output or renal insufficiency **Caution/Contra:** [B, +] Heart block, renal failure **Supplied:** Inj 100, 125, 250, 500 mg/mL; oral soln 500 mg/mL; granules 40 mEq/5 g **Notes/SE:** CNS depression, diarrhea, flushing, heart block

Mannitol **Uses:** Cerebral edema, oliguria, anuria, myoglobinuria **Action:** Osmotic diuretic **Dose:** *Adults. Diuresis:* 0.2 g/kg/dose IV over 3–5 min; if no diuresis within 2 h, DC. *Peds. Diuresis:* 0.75 g/kg/dose IV over 3–5 min; if no diuresis within 2 h, DC. *Adults & Peds. Cerebral edema:* 0.25 g/kg/dose IV push, repeated at 5-min intervals PRN; ↑ incrementally to 1 g/kg/dose PRN for ↑ ICP; caution with CHF or volume overload **Caution/Contra:** [C, ?] Anuria, dehydration, PE **Supplied:** Inj 5, 10, 15, 20, 25% **Notes/SE:** Initial volume increase may exacerbate CHF; monitor for volume depletion

Maprotiline (Ludiomil) **Uses:** Depressive neurosis, bipolar illness, major depressive disorder, anxiety with depression **Action:** Tetracyclic antidepressant **Dose:** 75–150 mg/d hs to a max of 300 mg/d; patients > 60 y, give only 50–75 mg/d **Caution/Contra:** [B, +/–] Contra with MAOIs or seizure Hx **Supplied:** Tabs 25, 50, 75 mg **Notes/SE:** Anticholinergic side effects, arrhythmias

Mechlorethamine (Mustargen) WARNING: Highly toxic agent, handle with care
Uses: Hodgkin's and NHL, cutaneous T-cell lymphoma (mycosis fungoides), lung CA, CLL, CML, and malignant pleural effusions **Action:** Alkylating agent (bifunctional) **Dose:** 0.4 mg/kg single dose or 0.1 mg/kg/d for 4 d; 6 mg/m² 1–2 ×/mon; highly volatile; must be administered within 30–60 min of preparation **Caution/Contra:** [D, ?] **Supplied:** Inj 10 mg **Notes/SE:** *Toxicity symptoms:* Myelosuppression, thrombosis, or thrombophlebitis at inj site; tissue damage with extravasation (Na thiosulfate may be used topically to treat); N/V, skin rash, amenorrhea, and sterility. High rates of sterility (especially in men) and secondary leukemia in patients treated for Hodgkin's disease

Meclizine (Antivert) **Uses:** Motion sickness; vertigo associated with diseases of the vestibular system **Action:** Antiemetic, anticholinergic, and antihistaminic properties **Dose:**

Adults & Peds >12 y. 25 mg PO tid–qid PRN **Caution/Contra:** [B, ?] **Supplied:** Tabs 12.5, 25, 50 mg; chew tabs 25 mg; caps 25, 30 mg **Notes/SE:** Drowsiness, xerostomia, and blurred vision common

Medroxyprogesterone (Provera, Depo-Provera) **Uses:** Contraception; secondary amenorrhea, and AUB caused by hormonal imbalance; endometrial CA **Action:** Progestin supplement **Dose:** *Contraception:* 150 mg IM q3mon or 450 mg IM q6mon. *Secondary amenorrhea:* 5–10 mg/d PO for 5–10 d. *AUB:* 5–10 mg/d PO for 5–10 d beginning on the 16th or 21st d of menstrual cycle. *Endometrial CA:* 400–1000 mg/wk IM; ↓ in hepatic insufficiency **Caution/Contra:** [X, +] Contra with Hx past thromboembolic disorders or with hepatic disease **Supplied:** Tabs 2.5, 5, 10 mg; depot inj 100, 150, 400 mg/mL **Notes/SE:** Perform breast exam and Pap smear before therapy; breakthrough bleeding, spotting, altered menstrual flow, anorexia, edema, thromboembolic complications, depression, weight gain

Megestrol Acetate (Megace) **Uses:** Breast and endometrial CAs; appetite stimulant in CA and HIV-related cachexia **Action:** Hormone; progesterone analogue **Dose:** *CA:* 40–320 mg/d PO in ÷ doses. *Appetite:* 800 mg/d PO **Caution/Contra:** [X, –] Thromboembolism **Supplied:** Tabs 20, 40 mg; soln 40 mg/mL **Notes/SE:** May induce DVT; do not DC therapy abruptly; edema, menstrual bleeding; photosensitivity, insomnia, rash, myelosuppression

Meloxicam (Mobic) **Uses:** Osteoarthritis **Action:** NSAID with ↑ COX-II activity **Dose:** 7.5–15 mg/d PO; ↓ in renal insufficiency; take with food **Caution/Contra:** [C, ?/–] Peptic ulcer, NSAID, or ASA sensitivity **Supplied:** Tabs 7.5 mg **Notes/SE:** HA, dizziness, GI upset, GI bleeding, edema

Melphalan [L-PAM] (Alkeran) WARNING: Severe bone marrow depression, leukemogenic, and mutagenic **Uses:** Multiple myeloma, breast, testicular, and ovarian CAs, melanoma; allogenic and ABMT in high doses **Action:** Alkylating agent (bifunctional) **Dose:** (Per protocol) 9 mg/m^2 or 0.25 mg/kg/d for 4–7 d, repeated at 4–6-wk intervals, or 1-mg/kg single dose once q4–6wk; 0.15 mg/kg/d for 5 d q6wk. *High dose for high-risk multiple myeloma:* Single dose 140–240 mg/m^2 IV; ↓ in renal insufficiency. *ABMT:* 140–240 mg/m^2 IV; ↓ in renal insufficiency, take on empty stomach **Caution/Contra:** [D, ?] **Supplied:** Tabs 2 mg; inj 50 mg **Notes/SE:** Myelosuppression (leukopenia and thrombocytopenia), secondary leukemia, alopecia, dermatitis, stomatitis, and pulmonary fibrosis; very rare hypersensitivity reactions

Meningococcal Polysaccharide Vaccine (Menomune) **Uses:** Immunize against *N. meningitidis* (meningococcus); recommended in certain complement deficiencies, asplenia, lab workers with exposure, recommended for college students by some professional groups **Action:** Live bacterial vaccine, active immunization **Dose:** *Adults & Peds >2 y.* 0.5 mL SC; do not inject intradermally or IV; epinephrine (1:1000) must be available for anaphylactic/allergic reactions **Caution/Contra:** [C, ?/–]. Contra in thimerosal sensitivity **Supplied:** Inj **Notes/SE:** Active against meningococcal serotypes groups A, C, Y, and W-135 but not group B; local inj site reactions, HA

Meperidine (Demerol) [C–II] **Uses:** Moderate to severe pain **Action:** Narcotic analgesic **Dose:** *Adults.* 50–150 mg PO or IM q3–4h PRN. *Peds.* 1–1.5 mg/kg/dose PO or IM q3–4h PRN, up to 100 mg/dose; ↓ dose in elderly and renal impairment **Caution/Contra:** [B, +] Do not use in renal failure; MAOIs **Supplied:** Tabs 50, 100 mg; syrup 50 mg/mL; inj 10, 25, 50, 75, 100 mg/mL **Notes/SE:** 75 mg IM = 10 mg of morphine IM; respiratory depression, seizures, sedation, constipation, analgesic effects potentiated with use of Vistaril

Meprobamate (Equanil, Miltown) [C–IV] **Uses:** Short-term relief of anxiety **Action:** Mild tranquilizer; antianxiety **Dose:** *Adults.* 400 mg PO tid–qid up to 2400 mg/d; SR 400–800 mg PO bid. *Peds. 6–12 y.* 100–200 mg bid–tid; SR 200 mg bid; ↓ in renal insufficiency **Caution/Contra:** [D, +/–] Narrow-angle glaucoma, porphyria **Supplied:** Tabs 200, 400, 600 mg; SR caps 200, 400 mg **Notes/SE:** May cause drowsiness, syncope, tachycardia, edema

Mercaptopurine [6-MP] (Purinethol) **Uses:** Acute leukemias, 2nd-line Rx of CML and NHL, maint therapy of ALL in children, and immunosuppressant therapy for autoimmune diseases (Crohn's disease) **Action:** Antimetabolite; mimics hypoxanthine **Dose:** 80–100 mg/m^2/d or 2.5–5 mg/kg/d; maint 1.5–2.5 mg/kg/d; concurrent allopurinol therapy requires a 67–75% dose reduction of 6-MP because of interference with metabolism by xanthine oxidase; ↓ in renal, hepatic insufficiency; empty stomach; adequate hydration **Cau-**

tion/Contra: [D, ?] Severe hepatic disease **Supplied:** Tabs 50 mg **Notes/SE:** Mild hematologic toxicity; uncommon GI toxicity, except mucositis, stomatitis, and diarrhea; rash, fever, eosinophilia, jaundice, and hepatitis

Meropenem (Merrem) **Uses:** Serious infections caused by a wide variety of bacteria; bacterial meningitis **Action:** Carbapenem; inhibits cell wall synthesis, a β-lactam **Dose:** *Adults.* 1 g IV q8h; *Peds.* 20–40 mg/kg IV q 8h; ↓ in renal insufficiency; beware of possible anaphylaxis **Caution/Contra:** [B, ?] β-Lactam sensitivity **Supplied:** Inj **Notes/SE:** Less seizure potential than imipenem; diarrhea, thrombocytopenia

Mesalamine (Rowasa, Asacol, Pentasa) **Uses:** Mild–moderate distal ulcerative colitis, proctosigmoiditis, or proctitis **Action:** Unknown; may topically inhibit prostaglandins **Dose:** Retention enema qd hs or insert 1 supp bid. *Oral:* 800–1000 mg PO 3–4×/d **Caution/Contra:** [B, M] Sulfite or salicylate sensitivity **Supplied:** Tabs 400 mg; caps 250 mg; supp 500 mg; rectal susp 4 g/60 mL **Notes/SE:** HA, malaise, abdominal pain, flatulence, rash, pancreatitis, pericarditis

Mesna (Mesnex) **Uses:** ↓ Incidence of ifosfamide- and cyclophosphamide-induced hemorrhagic cystitis **Action:** Antidote **Dose:** 20% of the ifosfamide dose (+/–) or cyclophosphamide dose IV 15 min prior to and 4 and 8 h after chemotherapy **Caution/Contra:** [B; ?/–] Thiol sensitivity **Supplied:** Inj 100 mg/mL **Notes/SE:** Hypotension, allergic reactions, HA, GI upset, taste perversion

Mesoridazine (Serentil) **WARNING:** Can prolong QT interval in a dose-related fashion; torsades de points reported **Uses:** Schizophrenia, acute and chronic alcoholism, chronic brain syndrome **Action:** Phenothiazine antipsychotic **Dose:** Initially, 25–50 mg PO or IV tid; ↑ to 300–400 mg/d max **Caution/Contra:** [C, ?/–] Phenothiazine sensitivity **Supplied:** Tabs 10, 25, 50, 100 mg; oral conc 25 mg/mL; inj 25 mg/mL **Notes/SE:** Low incidence of extrapyramidal side effects; hypotension, xerostomia, constipation, skin discoloration, tachycardia, lowered seizure threshold, blood dyscrasias, pigmentary retinopathy at high doses

Metaproterenol (Alupent, Metaprel) **Uses:** Asthma and reversible bronchospasm **Action:** Sympathomimetic bronchodilator **Dose:** *Adults.* *Inhal:* 1–3 inhal q3–4h, 12 inhal max/24 h; allow at least 2 min between inhal. *Oral:* 20 mg q6–8h. *Peds.* *Inhal:* 0.5 mg/kg/dose, 15 mg/dose max inhaled q4–6h by neb or 1–2 puffs q4–6h. *Oral:* 0.3–0.5 mg/kg/dose q6–8h **Caution/Contra:** [C, ?/–] Tachycardia or other arrhythmia **Supplied:** Aerosol 75, 150 mg; soln for inhal 0.4, 0.6, 5%; tabs 10, 20 mg; syrup 10 mg/5 mL **Notes/SE:** Fewer β₁ effects than isoproterenol and longer acting; nervousness, tremor, tachycardia, HTN

Metaraminol (Aramine) **Uses:** Prevention and Rx of hypotension due to spinal anesthesia **Action:** α-Adrenergic agent **Dose:** *Adults.* *Prevention:* 2–10 mg IM q10–15min PRN. *Rx:* 0.5–5 mg IV bolus followed by IV inf of 1–4 mg/kg/min titrated to effect. *Peds.* *Prevention:* 0.1 mg/kg/dose IM PRN. *Rx:* 0.01-mg/kg IV bolus followed by IV inf of 5 mg/kg/min titrated to effect **Caution/Contra:** [D, ?] **Supplied:** Injectable forms **Notes/SE:** Allow 10 min for max effect; use other shock management techniques, eg, fluid resuscitation, as needed; may cause cardiac arrhythmias, skin blanching, flushing

Metaxalone (Skelaxin) **Uses:** Relief of painful musculoskeletal conditions **Action:** Centrally acting skeletal muscle relaxant **Dose:** 800 mg PO 3–4×/d **Caution/Contra:** [X, ?/–] Do not use in hepatic/renal impairment; caution in anemia **Supplied:** Tabs 400 mg **Notes/SE:** N/V, HA, drowsiness, hepatitis

Metformin (Glucophage, Glucophage XR) **WARNING:** Associated with lactic acidosis **Uses:** Type 2 DM **Action:** decreases hepatic glucose production; ↓ intestinal absorption of glucose; improves insulin sensitivity **Dose:** Initial dose 500 mg PO bid; may ↑ 2500 mg/d max; administer with AM and PM meals; can convert total daily dose to qd dose of XR formulation **Caution/Contra:** [B, +/–] Do not use if SCr >1.4 in females or >1.5 in males; contra in hypoxemic conditions, including acute CHF/sepsis; avoid alcohol; hold dose before and 48 h after ionic contrast **Supplied:** Tabs 500, 850, 1000 mg; XR Tabs 500 mg **Notes/SE:** Anorexia, N/V, rash

Methadone (Dolophine) [C-II] **Uses:** Severe pain; detoxification and maint of narcotic addiction **Action:** Narcotic analgesic **Dose:** *Adults.* 2.5–10 mg IM q3–8h or 5–15 mg

PO q8h; titrate as needed. *Peds.* 0.7 mg/kg/24 h PO or IM ÷ q8h; ↑ slowly to avoid respiratory depression; ↓ in renal disease **Caution/Contra:** [B, + (with doses = 20 mg/24 h)] Severe liver disease **Supplied:** Tabs 5, 10, 40 mg; oral soln 5, 10 mg/5 mL; oral conc 10 mg/mL; inj 10 mg/mL **Notes/SE:** Equianalgesic with parenteral morphine; longer half-life; respiratory depression, sedation, constipation, urinary retention

Methenamine (Hiprex, Urex, others)
Uses: Suppression or elimination of bacteriuria associated with chronic/recurrent UTI **Dose:** *Adults. Hippurate:* 1 g bid. *Mandelate:* 1 g qid pc and hs. *Peds. 6–12 y. Hippurate:* 25–50 mg/kg/d ÷ bid. *Mandelate:* 50–75 mg/kg/d ÷ qid; take with food and ascorbic acid; adequate hydration **Caution/Contra:** [C, +] Contra in patients with renal insufficiency, severe hepatic disease, and severe dehydration; allergy to sulfonamides **Supplied:** *Methenamine hippurate (Hiprex, Urex):* 1-g tabs. *Methenamine mandelate:* 500 mg/1 g EC tabs **Notes/SE:** Rash, GI upset, dysuria, ↑ LFTs

Methimazole (Tapazole)
Uses: Hyperthyroidism and prep for thyroid surgery or radiation **Action:** Blocks the formation of T_3 and T_4 **Dose:** *Adults. Initial:* 15–60 mg/d PO ÷ tid. *Maint:* 5–15 mg PO qd. *Peds. Initial:* 0.4–0.7 mg/kg/24 h PO ÷ tid. *Maint:* $\frac{1}{3}$–$\frac{2}{3}$ of the initial dose PO qd; take with food **Caution/Contra:** [D] Avoid in nursing mothers **Supplied:** Tabs 5, 10 mg **Notes/SE:** Follow clinically and with TFT; GI upset, dizziness, blood dyscrasias

Methocarbamol (Robaxin)
Uses: Relief of discomfort associated with painful musculoskeletal conditions **Action:** Centrally acting skeletal muscle relaxant **Dose:** *Adults.* 1.5 g PO qid for 2–3 d, then 1-g PO qid maint therapy; IV form rarely indicated. *Peds.* 15 mg/kg/dose may repeat PRN (recommended for tetanus only) **Caution/Contra:** [C, +] Contra with myasthenia gravis, renal impairment; caution in seizure disorders **Supplied:** Tabs 500, 750 mg; inj 100 mg/mL **Notes/SE:** Can discolor urine; drowsiness, GI upset

Methotrexate (Folex, Rheumatrex)
Uses: ALL and AML (including leukemic meningitis), trophoblastic tumors (chorioepithelioma, choriocarcinoma, chorioadenoma destruens, hydatidiform mole), breast CA, Burkitt's lymphoma, mycosis fungoides, osteosarcoma, head and neck CA, Hodgkin's and NHL, lung CA; psoriasis; and RA **Action:** Inhibits dihydrofolate reductase-mediated gen. of tetrahydrofolate **Dose:** *CA, "conventional dose":* 15–30 mg PO or IV 1–2×/wk q1–3 wk. *"Intermediate dose":* 50–240 mg or 0.5–1 g/m^2 IV once q4d to 3 wk. *"High dose":* 1–12 g/m^2 IV once q1–3wk; 12 mg/m^2 (max 15 mg) IT, weekly until the CSF cell count returns to normal. *RA:* 7.5 mg/wk PO as a single dose or 2.5 mg q12h PO for 3 doses/wk; "high dose" RX requires leucovorin rescue to limit hematologic and mucosal toxicity; ↓ in renal/hepatic impairment **Caution/Contra:** [D, –] Severe renal/hepatic impairment **Supplied:** Tabs 2.5 mg; inj 2.5, 25 mg/mL; preservative-free inj 25 mg/mL **Notes/SE:** Myelosuppression, N/V/D, anorexia, mucositis, hepatotoxicity (transient and reversible; may progress to atrophy, necrosis, fibrosis, cirrhosis), rashes, dizziness, malaise, blurred vision, renal failure, pneumonitis, and, rarely, pulmonary fibrosis. Chemical arachnoiditis and HA with IT delivery; monitor blood counts and MTX levels

Methoxamine (Vasoxyl)
Uses: Support, restoration, or maint of BP during anesthesia; for termination of some episodes of PSVT **Action:** α-Adrenergic **Dose:** *Adults. Anesthesia:* 10–15 mg IM; if emergency, 3–5 mg slow IV push. *PSVT:* 10 mg by slow IV push. *Peds.* 0.25 mg/kg/dose IM or 0.08 mg/kg/dose slow IV push **Caution/Contra:** [C, ?] **Supplied:** Injectable forms **Notes/SE:** IM dose requires 15 min to act; use 5–10 mg phentolamine locally in case of extravasation; MAOIs and TCAs potentiate methoxamine effect

Methyldopa (Aldomet)
Uses: Essential HTN **Action:** Centrally acting antihypertensive **Dose:** *Adults.* 250–500 mg PO bid–tid (max 2–3 g/d) or 250 mg–1 g IV q6–8h. *Peds.* 10 mg/kg/24 h PO in 2–3 ÷ doses (max 40 mg/kg/24 h ÷ q6–12h) or 5–10 mg/kg/dose IV q6–8h to total dose of 20–40 mg/kg/24 h; ↓ dose in renal insufficiency and in elderly **Caution/Contra:** [B (oral), C (IV), +] Contra in liver disease; MAOIs **Supplied:** Tabs 125, 250, 500 mg; oral susp 50 mg/mL; inj 50 mg/mL **Notes/SE:** Can discolor urine; initial transient sedation or drowsiness frequent; edema, hemolytic anemia; hepatic disorders

Methylergonovine (Methergine)
Uses: Prevention and Rx postpartum hemorrhage caused by uterine atony **Action:** Ergotamine derivative **Dose:** 0.2 mg IM after delivery of placenta, may repeat at 2–4 h intervals or 0.2–0.4 mg PO q6–12h for 2–7 d **Caution/Contra:** [C, ?] HTN **Supplied:** Injectable forms; tabs 0.2 mg **Notes/SE:** IV doses should be given over a period of >1 min with frequent BP monitoring; HTN, N/V

Methylprednisolone (Solu-Medrol)   See Steroids, page 591, Table 4, page 612

Metoclopramide (Reglan, Clopra, Octamide)   Uses: Relief of diabetic gastroparesis, symptomatic GERD; chemotherapy-induced N/V; stimulate gut in prolonged postop ileus **Action:** Stimulates motility of the upper GI tract; blocks dopamine in the chemoreceptor trigger zone **Dose:** *Adults. Diabetic gastroparesis:* 10 mg PO 30 min ac and hs for 2–8 wk PRN, or same dose given IV for 10 d, then switch to PO. *Reflux:* 10–15 mg PO 30 min ac and hs. *Antiemetic:* 1–3 mg/kg/dose IV 30 min before chemotherapy, then q2h for 2 doses, then q3h for 3 doses. *Peds. Reflux:* 0.1 mg/kg/dose PO qid. *Antiemetic:* 1–2 mg/kg/dose IV as for adults **Caution/Contra:** [B, –] Seizure disorders **Supplied:** Tabs 5, 10 mg; syrup 5 mg/5 mL; soln 10 mg/mL; inj 5 mg/mL **Notes/SE:** Dystonic reactions common with high doses, treat with IV diphenhydramine; used to facilitate small-bowel intubation and radiologic evaluation of the upper GI tract; restlessness, drowsiness, diarrhea

Metolazone (Mykrox, Zaroxolyn)   Uses: Mild/moderate essential HTN and edema of renal disease or cardiac failure **Action:** Thiazide-like diuretic; inhibits Na reabsorption in the distal tubules **Dose:** *Adults. HTN:* 2.5–5 mg/d PO. *Edema:* 5–20 mg/d PO. *Peds.* 0.2–0.4 mg/kg/d PO ÷ q12h–qd **Caution/Contra:** [D, +] Thiazide or sulfonamide sensitivity **Supplied:** Tabs Mykrox (rapid acting) 0.5 mg, Zaroxolyn 2.5, 5, 10 mg **Notes/SE:** Monitor fluid and electrolyte status during treatment; dizziness, hypotension, tachycardia, chest pain, photosensitivity; Mykrox and Zaroxolyn not bioequivalent

Metoprolol (Lopressor, Toprol XL)   WARNING: Do not acutely stop therapy as marked worsening of angina can result **Uses:** HTN, angina, AMI, and CHF **Action:** Competitively blocks β-adrenergic receptors, β$_1$. **Dose:** *Angina:* 50–100 mg PO bid. *HTN:* 100–450 mg/d PO. *AMI:* 5 mg IV ×3 doses, then 50 mg PO q6h ×48 h, then 100 mg PO bid; *CHF:* 12–25 mg/d PO ×2 wk, increase at 2-wk intervals to 200 mg/max, use low dose in patients with greatest severity; ↓ in hepatic failure **Caution/Contra:** [C, +] Uncompensated CHF, bradycardia, heart block **Supplied:** Tabs 50, 100 mg; ER tabs 50, 100, 200 mg; inj 1 mg/mL **Notes/SE:** Drowsiness, insomnia, erectile dysfunction, bradycardia, bronchospasm

Metronidazole (Flagyl, MetroGel)   Uses: Amebiasis, trichomoniasis, *C. difficile*, *H. pylori*, anaerobic infections, and bacterial vaginosis **Action:** Interferes with DNA synthesis **Dose:** *Adults. Anaerobic infections:* 500 mg IV q6–8h. *Amebic dysentery:* 750 mg/d PO for 5–10 d. *Trichomoniasis:* 250 mg PO tid for 7 d or 2 g PO ×1. *C. difficile infection:* 500 mg PO or IV q8h for 7–10 d (PO preferred; IV only if patient NPO). *Vaginosis:* 1 applicatorful intravaginally bid or 500 mg PO bid for 7 d. *Acne rosacea/skin:* Apply bid. *Peds. Anaerobic infections:* 15 mg/kg/24 h PO or IV ÷ q6h. *Amebic dysentery:* 35–50 mg/kg/24 h PO in 3 ÷ doses for 5–10 d;?↓ in hepatic failure **Caution/Contra:** [B, M] Avoid alcohol **Supplied:** Tabs 250, 500 mg; ER tabs 750 mg; caps 375 mg; topical lotion and gel 0.75%; gel, vaginal 0.75% (5 g/applicator 37.5 mg in 70-g tube) **Notes/SE:** For *Trichomonas* infections, Rx patient's partner; no aerobic bacteria activity; used in combination in serious mixed infections; may cause disulfiram-like reaction; dizziness, HA, GI upset, anorexia, urine discoloration

Metyrosine (Demser)   Uses: Pheochromocytoma; short-term preop and long term when surgery contraindicated **Action:** Tyrosine hydroxylase inhibitor **Dose:** *Adults & Peds >12 y.* 250 mg PO qid, ↑ by 250–500 mg/d up to 4 g/d. *Maint dose:* 2–3 g/d ÷ qid **Caution/Contra:** [C, ?] **Supplied:** 250-mg caps **Notes/SE:** Hydrate well to prevent crystallization; Administer at least 5–7 d preop; drowsiness, extrapyramidal symptoms, diarrhea

Mexiletine (Mexitil)   Uses: Suppression of symptomatic ventricular arrhythmias; diabetic neuropathy **Action:** Class IB antiarrhythmic **Dose:** Administer with food or antacids; 200–300 mg PO q8h; 1200 mg/d max; drug interactions with hepatic enzyme inducers and suppressors requiring dosage changes **Caution/Contra:** [C, +] Contra in cardiogenic shock or 2nd/3rd-degree AV block w/o pacemaker; may worsen severe arrhythmias **Supplied:** Caps 150, 200, 250 mg **Notes/ SE:** Monitor LFTs; lightheadedness, dizziness, anxiety, incoordination, GI upset, ataxia, hepatic damage, blood dyscrasias

Mezlocillin (Mezlin)   Uses: Infections caused by susceptible gram– bacteria (including *Klebsiella, Proteus, E. coli, Enterobacter, P. aeruginosa,* and *Serratia*) involving the skin, bone, respiratory tract, urinary tract, abdomen, and septicemia **Action:** Bactericidal; inhibits cell wall synthesis **Dose:** *Adults.* 3 g IV q4–6h. *Peds.* 200–300 mg/kg/d ÷ q4–6h; ↓ in renal/hepatic insufficiency **Caution/ Contra:** [B, M] Penicillin sensitivity **Supplied:** Inj

22

Notes/SE: Often used in combination with aminoglycoside; GI upset, agranulocytosis, thrombocytopenia

Miconazole (Monistat, others) **Uses:** Various tinea forms; cutaneous candidiasis; vulvovaginal candidiasis; tinea versicolor; occasionally used for severe systemic fungal infections **Action:** Fungicidal; alters permeability of the fungal cell membrane **Dose:** *Adults.* Apply to area bid for 2–4 wk. *Intravaginally:* 1 applicatorful or supp hs for 7 d; 200–1200 mg/d IV, ÷ tid **Caution/Contra:** [C, ?] Azole sensitivity **Supplied:** Topical cream 2%; lotion 2%; powder 2%; spray 2%; vaginal supp 100, 200 mg; vaginal cream 2%; inj **Notes/SE:** Antagonistic to amphotericin B in vivo; may potentiate warfarin

Midazolam (Versed) [C-IV] **Uses:** Preoperative sedation, conscious sedation for short procedures, induction of general anesthesia **Action:** Short-acting benzodiazepine **Dose:** *Adults.* 1–5 mg IV or IM; titrate to effect. *Peds. Preop:* 0.25–1 mg/kg, 20 mg max PO. *Conscious sedation:* 0.08 mg/kg IM ×1. *General anesthesia:* 0.15 mg/kg IV, then 0.05 mg/kg/dose q2min for 1–3 doses PRN to induce anesthesia; ↓ in elderly, with use of narcotics or CNS depressants **Caution/Contra:** [D, +/–] Narrow-angle glaucoma; use of amprenavir, nelfinavir, ritonavir **Supplied:** Inj 1, 5 mg/mL; syrup 2 mg/mL **Notes/SE:** Monitor for respiratory depression; hypotension in conscious sedation, nausea

Mifepristone [RU 486] (Mifeprex) WARNING: Patient counseling and information required **Uses:** Termination of intrauterine pregnancies of <49 d **Action:** Antiprogestin; ↑ prostaglandins, resulting in uterine contraction **Dose:** Administered with 3 office visits: day 1, three 200-mg tabs PO; day 3 if no abortion, two 200-mg misoprostol PO; on or about day 14, verify termination of PRG **Caution/Contra:** [X, –] Must be administered under physician's supervision **Supplied:** Tabs 200 mg **Notes/SE:** Abdominal pain and 1–2 wk of uterine bleeding

Miglitol (Glyset) **Uses:** Type 2 DM **Action:** α-Glucosidase inhibitor; delays digestion of ingested carbohydrates **Dose:** Initial 25 mg PO tid with 1st bite of each meal; maint 50–100 mg tid with meals **Caution/Contra:** [B, –] Obstructive or inflammatory GI disorders; avoid if SCr >2 **Supplied:** Tabs 25, 50, 100 mg **Notes/SE:** Used alone or in combination with sulfonylureas; flatulence, diarrhea, abdominal pain

Milrinone (Primacor) **Uses:** CHF **Action:** Positive inotrope and vasodilator; little chronotropic activity **Dose:** 50 mcg/kg, then 0.375–0.75 mcg/kg/min inf; ↓ dose in renal impairment **Caution/Contra:** [C, ?] **Supplied:** Inj 1 mcg/mL **Notes/ SE:** Carefully monitor fluid and electrolyte status; arrhythmias, hypotension, HA

Mineral Oil **Uses:** Constipation **Action:** Emollient laxative **Dose:** *Adults.* 5–45 mL PO PRN. *Peds >6 y.* 5–20 mL PO bid **Caution/Contra:** [C, ?] N/V, difficulty swallowing, bedridden patients **Supplied:** Liq **Notes/SE:** Lipid pneumonia, anal incontinence, impaired vitamin absorption

Minoxidil (Loniten, Rogaine) **Uses:** Severe HTN; male and female pattern baldness **Action:** Peripheral vasodilator; stimulates vertex hair growth **Dose:** *Adults. Oral:* 2.5–10 mg PO bid–qid. *Topical:* Apply bid to affected area. *Peds.* 0.2–1 mg/kg/24 h ÷ PO q12–24h; ↓ oral dose in elderly **Caution/Contra:** [C, +] **Supplied:** Tabs 2.5, 5, 10 mg; topical soln (Rogaine) 2% **Notes/SE:** Pericardial effusion and volume overload may occur with oral use; hypertrichosis after chronic use; edema, ECG changes, weight gain

Mirtazapine (Remeron) **Uses:** Depression **Action:** Tetracyclic antidepressant **Dose:** 15 mg PO hs, up to 45 mg/d hs **Caution/Contra:** [C, ?] Contra with MAOIs within 14 d **Supplied:** Tabs 15, 30, 45 mg **Notes/SE:** Do not ↑ dose at intervals of less than 1–2 wk; somnolence, ↑ cholesterol, constipation, xerostomia, weight gain, agranulocytosis

Misoprostol (Cytotec) **Uses:** Prevention of NSAID-induced gastric ulcers; induction of labor, incomplete and therapeutic abortion **Action:** Prostaglandin with both antisecretory and mucosal protective properties **Dose:** ulcer prevention: 200 mcg PO qid with meals; in females, start on 2nd or 3rd of next normal menstrual period; 25–50 mcg 4 induction of labor (Term): 400 mcg 94 induction of labor (2nd trimester), 600 mcg **Caution/Contra:** [X, –] **Supplied:** Tabs 100, 200 mcg **Notes/SE:** Can cause miscarriage with potentially dangerous bleeding; HA, GI SE common (diarrhea, abdominal pain, constipation)

Mitomycin (Mutamycin) **Uses:** Stomach, breast, pancreas, colon CAs; squamous cell carcinoma of the anus; non-small-cell lung, head, and neck, cervical, and breast CAs;

bladder CA (intravesically) **Action:** Alkylating agent; may also generate oxygen free radicals, induces DNA strand breaks **Dose:** 20 mg/m^2 q6–8wk or 10 mg/m^2 in combination with other myelosuppressive drugs; bladder CA 20–40 mg in 40 mL NS via a urethral catheter once/wk for 8 wk, followed by monthly treatments for 1 y; ↓ dose in renal/hepatic impairment **Caution/Contra:** [D, –] Thrombocytopenia, leukopenia, serum creatinine (> 0.7 mg/dL **Supplied:** Inj **Notes/SE:** Myelosuppression (may persist up to 3–8 wk after dose and may be cumulative minimized by a lifetime dose <50–60 mg/m^2), N/V, anorexia, stomatitis, and renal toxicity; microangiopathic hemolytic anemia (similar to hemolytic-uremic syndrome) with progressive renal failure; venoocclusive disease of the liver, interstitial pneumonia, alopecia (rare); extravasation reactions can be severe

Mitotane (Lysodren) **Uses:** Palliative treatment of inoperable adrenocortical carcinoma **Action:** Unclear; induces mitochondrial injury in adrenocortical cells **Dose:** 8–10 g/d in 3–4 ÷ doses (begin at 2 g/d with glucocorticoid replacement); ↓ in hepatic insufficiency; adequate hydration necessary **Caution/Contra:** [C, ?] **Supplied:** Tabs 500 mg **Notes/SE:** Anorexia, N/V/D; acute adrenal insufficiency may be precipitated by physical stresses (shock, trauma, infection), Rx with steroids; allergic reactions (rare), visual disturbances, hemorrhagic cystitis, albuminuria, hematuria, HTN or hypotension, minor aches, fever

Mitoxantrone (Novantrone) **Uses:** AML (with cytarabine), ALL, CML, breast and prostate CA, NHL, MS **Action:** DNA-intercalating agent; inhibitor of DNA topoisomerase II **Dose:** 12 mg/m^2/d for 3 d (ALL induction), 12–14 mg/m^2 q3wk (advanced solid tumors); cumulative dose should not exceed 160 mg/m^2 with prior mediastinal radiation therapy or 120 mg/m^2 with prior anthracycline therapy; MS: 12 mg/m^2 over 5–15 min q3mon up to cumulative 140 mg/m^2; ↓ dose in hepatic failure, leukopenia, thrombocytopenia; maintain hydration **Caution/Contra:** [D, –] **Supplied:** Inj 20, 25, 30 mg **Notes/SE:** Myelosuppression, N/V, stomatitis, alopecia (infrequent), cardiotoxicity

Mivacurium (Mivacron) **Uses:** Adjunct to general anesthesia or mechanical ventilation **Action:** Nondepolarizing neuromuscular blocker **Dose:** *Adults.* 0.15 mg/kg/dose IV; repeat PRN at 15-min intervals. *Peds.* 0.2 mg/kg/dose IV; repeat PRN at 10-min intervals; ↓ dose in renal/hepatic impairment **Caution/Contra:** [C, ?] **Supplied:** Inj 0.5, 2 mg/mL **Notes/SE:** Flushing, hypotension, bronchospasm

Moexipril (Univasc) **Uses:** HTN, post-MI, DN **Action:** ACE inhibitor **Dose:** 7.5–30 mg in 1–2 ÷ doses 1 h ac **Caution/Contra:** [C (1st trimester), D (2nd and 3rd trimesters), ?] ACE inhibitor sensitivity **Supplied:** Tabs 7.5, 15 mg; ↓ dose in renal impairment **Notes/SE:** Hypotension, edema, angioedema, HA, dizziness, cough

Molindone (Moban) **Uses:** Psychotic disorders **Action:** Piperazine phenothiazine **Dose:** *Adults.* 50–75 mg/d, ↑ to 225 mg/d if necessary. *Peds. 3–5 y:* 1–2.5 mg/d in 4 ÷ doses. *5–12 y:* 0.5–1.0 mg/kg/d in 4 ÷ doses **Caution/Contra:** [C, ?] Narrow-angle glaucoma **Supplied:** Tabs 5, 10, 25, 50, 100 mg; conc 20 mg/mL **Notes/SE:** Hypotension, tachycardia, arrhythmias, extrapyramidal symptoms, seizures, constipation, xerostomia

Montelukast (Singulair) **Uses:** Prophylaxis and Rx of chronic asthma, seasonal allergic rhinitis **Action:** Leukotriene receptor antagonist **Dose:** *Asthma: Adults >15 y.* 10 mg/d PO taken in PM. *Peds. 2–5 y:* 4 mg/d PO taken in PM. *6–14 y:* 5 mg/d PO in PM; *Rhinitis:* Adult: 10 mg/d; *Peds:* 2–5 y 4 mg/d, 6–14 5 mg/d **Caution/Contra:** [B, M] **Supplied:** Tabs 10 mg; chew tabs 4, 5 mg **Notes/SE:** Not for acute asthma attacks; HA, dizziness, fatigue, rash, GI upset, Churg-Strauss syndrome

Moricizine (Ethmozine) WARNING: Proarrhythmic effects **Uses:** Ventricular arrhythmias **Action:** Class I antiarrhythmic **Dose:** 200–300 mg PO tid; ↓ dose in renal/hepatic insufficiency **Caution/Contra:** [B, +/–] AV block w/o pacemaker; cardiogenic shock **Supplied:** Tabs 200, 250, 300 mg **Notes/SE:** Dizziness, arrhythmias, CHF, HA, fatigue, GI upset, BP changes

Morphine (Avinza ER, Duramorph, MS Contin, Kadian SR, Oramorph SR, Roxanol) [C-II] **Uses:** Relief of severe pain **Action:** Narcotic analgesic **Dose:** *Adults. Oral:* 10–30 mg q4h PRN; SR tabs 30–60 mg q8–12h. *IV/IM:* 2.5–15 mg q2–6h. *Peds.* 0.1–0.2 mg/kg/dose IM/IV q2–4h PRN to a max of 15 mg/dose **Caution/Contra:** [B (D if prolonged use or high doses at term), +/–] Respiratory depression **Supplied:** Immediate release tabs 10, 14, 20 mg; MS Contin CR tabs 15, 30, 60, 100, 200 mg; Oramorph SR

CR tabs 15, 30, 60, 100 mg; Kadian SR caps 20, 30 50, 60, 100 mg; Avinza ER caps 30, 60, 90, 120 mg; soln 10, 20, 100 mg; supp 5, 10, 20 mg; inj 2, 4, 5, 8, 10, 15 mg/mL; Duramorph preservative-free inj 0.5, 1 mg/mL **Notes/SE:** May require scheduled dosing to relieve severe chronic pain; MS Contin commonly used SR form (do not crush); narcotic SE (respiratory depression, sedation, constipation, N/V, pruritus)

Moxifloxacin (Avelox) **Uses:** Acute sinusitis, acute bronchitis, and community-acquired pneumonia **Action:** Quinolone; inhibits DNA gyrase **Dose:** 400 mg/d once **Caution/Contra:** [C, ?/–] Quinolone sensitivity; interactions with Mg^{2+}-, Ca^{2+}-, Al^{2+}-, and Fe^{2+}-containing products and class IA and III antiarrhythmic agents **Supplied:** Tabs 400 mg **Notes/SE:** Active against gram– bacteria and *S. pneumoniae;* dizziness, nausea, QT prolongation, seizures, photosensitivity, tendon rupture: take 4 h before or 8 h after antacids

Mupirocin (Bactroban) **Uses:** Impetigo; eradication of MRSA in nasal carriers **Action:** Inhibits bacterial protein synthesis **Dose:** *Topical:* Apply small amount to affected area. *Nasal:* Apply bid in nostrils **Caution/Contra:** [B, ?] Do not use concurrently with other nasal products **Supplied:** Oint 2%; cream 2% **Notes/SE:** Local irritation, rash

Muromonab-CD3 (Orthoclone OKT3) **WARNING:** Can cause anaphylaxis; monitor fluid status **Uses:** Acute rejection following organ transplantation **Action:** Blocks T-cell function **Dose:** *Adults.* 5 mg/d IV for 10–14 d. *Peds.* 0.1 mg/kg/d for 10–14 d **Caution/Contra:** [C, ?/–] Murine sensitivity, fluid overload **Supplied:** Inj 5 mg/5 mL **Notes/SE:** Murine antibody; fever and chills after the 1st dose; monitor for anaphylaxis or pulmonary edema

Mycophenolate Mofetil (CellCept) **WARNING:** ↑ risk of infections, possible development of lymphoma **Uses:** Prevent organ rejection after transplant **Action:** Inhibits immunologically mediated inflammatory responses **Dose:** 1 g PO bid; used with steroids and cyclosporine; ↓ in renal insufficiency or neutropenia; take on empty stomach **Caution/Contra:** [C, ?/–] **Supplied:** Caps 250, 500 mg; inj 500 mg **Notes/SE:** Pain, fever, HA, infection, HTN, diarrhea, anemia, leukopenia, edema

Nabumetone (Relafen) **Uses:** Arthritis and pain **Action:** NSAID; inhibits prostaglandin synthesis **Dose:** 1000–2000 mg/d ÷ qd–bid with food **Caution/Contra:** [C (D 3rd trimester), +] Peptic ulcer, NSAID sensitivity **Supplied:** Tabs 500, 750 mg **Notes/SE:** Dizziness, rash, GI upset, edema, peptic ulcer

Nadolol (Corgard) **Uses:** HTN and angina **Action:** Competitively blocks β-adrenergic receptors, β_1, β_2 **Dose:** 40–80 mg/d; ↑ to 240 mg/d (angina) or 320 mg/d (HTN) may be needed; ↓ dose in renal insufficiency and elderly **Caution/Contra:** [C (1st trimester); D if 2nd or 3rd trimester), +] Uncompensated CHF, shock, heart block, asthma **Supplied:** Tabs 20, 40, 80, 120, 160 mg **Notes/ SE:** Nightmares, paresthesias, hypotension, bradycardia, fatigue

Nafcillin (Nallpen) **Uses:** Infections caused by susceptible strains of *Staphylococcus* and *Streptococcus* **Action:** Bactericidal; inhibits cell wall synthesis **Dose:** *Adults.* 1–2 g IV q4–6h. *Peds.* 50–200 mg/kg/d ÷ q4–6h **Caution/Contra:** [B, ?] Penicillin allergy **Supplied:** Inj **Notes/SE:** No adjustments for renal function; interstitial nephritis, diarrhea, fever, nausea

Naftifine (Naftin) **Uses:** Tinea cruris and tinea corporis **Action:** Antifungal antibiotic **Dose:** Apply bid **Caution/Contra:** [B, ?] **Supplied:** 1% cream; gel **Notes/SE:** Local irritation

Nalbuphine (Nubain) **Uses:** Moderate–severe pain; preop and obstetric analgesia **Action:** Narcotic agonist–antagonist; inhibits ascending pain pathways **Dose:** *Adults.* 10–20 mg IM or IV q4–6h PRN; max of 160 mg/d; single max dose, 20 mg. *Peds.* 0.2 mg/kg IV or IM to a max dose of 20 mg; ↓ in hepatic insufficiency **Supplied:** Inj 10, 20 mg/mL **Caution/Contra:** [B (D if prolonged or high doses at term), ?] Sulfite sensitivity **Notes/SE:** Causes CNS depression and drowsiness; caution in patients receiving opiates

Naloxone (Narcan) **Uses:** Reversal of narcotics **Action:** Competitive narcotic antagonist **Dose:** *Adults.* 0.4–2.0 mg IV, IM, or SC q5min; max total dose, 10 mg. *Peds.* 0.01–1.0 mg/kg/dose IV, IM, or SC; repeat IV q3min ×3 doses PRN **Caution/Contra:** [B, ?] May precipitate acute withdrawal in addicts **Supplied:** Inj 0.4, 1.0 mg/mL; neonatal inj

0.02 mg/mL **Notes/SE:** If no response after 10 mg, suspect nonnarcotic cause; hypotension, tachycardia, irritability, GI upset, pulmonary edema

Naltrexone (ReVia) Uses: Alcohol and narcotic addiction **Action:** Competitively binds to opioid receptors **Dose:** 50 mg/d PO; do not give until opioid-free for 7–10 d **Caution/Contra:** [C, M] Acute hepatitis, liver failure; opioid use **Supplied:** Tabs 50 mg **Notes/SE:** May cause hepatotoxicity; insomnia, GI upset, joint pain, HA, fatigue

Naphazoline and Antazoline (Albalon-A Ophthalmic, others) Naphazoline and Pheniramine Acetate (Naphcon A) Uses: Temporary relief from ocular redness and itching caused by allergy **Action:** Vasoconstrictor and antihistamine **Dose:** 1–2 gtt up to 4×/d **Caution/Contra:** [C, +] Contra in glaucoma, children <6 y, and with contact lens **Supplied:** Soln 15 mL **Notes/SE:** Cardiovascular stimulation, dizziness, local irritation

Naproxen (Aleve, Naprosyn, Anaprox) Uses: Arthritis and pain **Action:** NSAID; inhibits prostaglandin synthesis **Dose:** *Adults & Peds >12 y.* 200–500 mg bid–tid to a max of 1500 mg/d; ↓ dose in hepatic impairment **Caution/Contra:** [B (D 3rd trimester), +] NSAID sensitivity, peptic ulcer **Supplied:** Tabs 200, 250, 375, 500 mg; delayed-release (EC) tabs 375, 500 mg; susp 125 mg/5 mL **Notes/SE:** Dizziness, pruritus, GI upset, peptic ulcer, edema

Naratriptan (Amerge) Uses: Acute migraine attacks **Action:** Serotonin 5-HT$_1$ receptor antagonist **Dose:** 1–2.5 mg PO once; repeat PRN in 4 h; ↓ dose in mild renal/hepatic insufficiency **Caution/Contra:** [C, M] Contra in severe renal/hepatic impairment, avoid in angina, ischemic heart disease, uncontrolled HTN, and ergot use **Supplied:** Tabs 1, 2.5 mg **Notes/SE:** Dizziness, sedation, GI upset, paresthesias, ECG changes, coronary vasospasm, arrhythmias

Nateglinide (Starlix) Uses: Type 2 DM **Action:** ↑ Pancreatic release of insulin **Dose:** 120 mg PO tid 1–30 min pc; ↓ to 60 mg tid if near target HbA$_{1c}$ **Caution/Contra:** [C, –]. Caution with drugs metabolized by CYP2C9/3A4 **Supplied:** Tabs 60, 120 mg **Notes/SE:** Hypoglycemia, URI; salicylates, nonselective β-blockers may enhance hypoglycemia

Nedocromil (Tilade) Uses: Mild–moderate asthma **Action:** Antiinflammatory agent **Dose:** 2 inhal 4×/d **Caution/Contra:** [B, ?/–] **Supplied:** Met-dose inhaler **Notes/SE:** Chest pain, dizziness, dysphonia, rash, GI upset, infection

Nefazodone (Serzone) WARNING: Fatal hepatitis and liver failure possible; DC if LFT >3× ULN; do not re-treat **Uses:** Depression **Action:** Inhibits neuronal uptake of serotonin and norepinephrine **Dose:** Initially 100 mg PO bid; usual 300–600 mg/d in 2 ÷ doses **Caution/Contra:** [C, ?] MAOIs, pimozide **Supplied:** Tabs 100, 150, 200, 250 mg **Notes/SE:** Orthostatic hypotension and allergic reactions; HA, drowsiness, xerostomia, constipation, GI upset

Nelfinavir (Viracept) Uses: HIV infection **Action:** Protease inhibitor; results in formation of immature, noninfectious virion **Dose:** *Adults.* 750 mg PO tid or 1250 mg PO bid. *Peds.* 20–30 mg/kg PO tid; with food **Caution/Contra:** [B, ?] Phenylketonuria, or triazolam/midazolam use **Supplied:** Tabs 250 mg; oral powder **Notes/SE:** Food ↑ absorption; interacts with St. John's wort; dyslipidemia, lipodystrophy, diarrhea, rash

Neomycin, Bacitracin, and Polymyxin B (Neosporin Ointment) (See Bacitracin, Neomycin, and Polymyxin, page 515)

Neomycin, Colistin, and Hydrocortisone (Cortisporin-TC Otic Drops)

Neomycin, Colistin, Hydrocortisone, and Thonzonium (Cortisporin-TC Otic Suspension) Uses: External otitis, infections of mastoidectomy and fenestration cavities **Action:** Antibiotic and antiinflammatory **Dose:** *Adults.*4–5 gtt in ear(s) tid–qid. *Peds.* 3–4 gtt in ear(s) tid–qid **Caution/Contra:** [C, ?] **Supplied:** Otic gtt and susp **Notes/SE:** Local irritation

Neomycin and Dexamethasone (AK-Neo-Dex Ophthalmic, NeoDecadron Ophthalmic) Uses: Steroid-responsive inflammatory conditions of the cornea, conjunctiva, lid, and anterior segment **Action:** Antibiotic with antiinflammatory corticosteroid **Dose:** 1–2 gtt in eye(s) q3–4h or thin coat tid–qid until response , then ↓ to qd **Caution/Contra:** [C, ?] **Supplied:** Cream neomycin 0.5%/dexamethasone 0.1%; oint neomycin

0.35%/dexamethasone 0.05%; soln neomycin 0.35%/dexamethasone 0.1% **Notes/SE:** Use under supervision of ophthalmologist; local irritation

Neomycin and Polymyxin B (Neosporin Cream) **Uses:** Infection in minor cuts, scrapes, and burns **Action:** Bactericidal antibiotic **Dose:** Apply bid–qid **Caution/Contra:** [C, ?] **Supplied:** Cream neomycin 3.5 mg/polymyxin B 10,000 U/g **Notes/SE:** Different from Neosporin oint; local irritation

Neomycin, Polymyxin B, and Dexamethasone (Maxitrol) **Uses:** Steroid-responsive ocular conditions with bacterial infection **Action:** Antibiotic with antiinflammatory corticosteroid **Dose:** 1–2 gtt in eye(s) q4–6h; apply oint in eye(s) 3–4×/d **Caution/Contra:** [C, ?] **Supplied:** Oint neomycin sulfate 3.5 mg/polymyxin B sulfate 10,000 U/dexamethasone 0.1%/g; susp identical/5 mL **Notes/SE:** Use under supervision of ophthalmologist; local irritation

Neomycin-Polymyxin Bladder Irrigant [GU Irrigant] **Uses:** Continuous irrigant for prophylaxis against bacteriuria and gram– bacteremia associated with indwelling catheter use **Action:** Bactericidal antibiotic **Dose:** 1 mL irrigant added to 1 L of 0.9% NaCl; continuous bladder irrigation with 1–2 L of soln/24 h **Caution/Contra:** [C (D if GU irrigant), ?] **Supplied:** Amp 1, 20 mL **Notes/SE:** Potential for bacterial or fungal superinfection; slight possibility for neomycin-induced ototoxicity or nephrotoxicity

Neomycin, Polymyxin, and Hydrocortisone (Cortisporin Ophthalmic and Otic) **Uses:** Ocular and otic bacterial infections **Action:** Antibiotic and antiinflammatory **Dose:** *Otic:* 3–4 gtt in the ear(s) 3–4×/d. *Ophth:* Apply a thin layer to the eye(s) or 1 gtt 1–4×/d **Caution/Contra:** [C, ?] **Supplied:** Otic susp; ophth soln; ophth oint **Notes/SE:** Local irritation

Neomycin, Polymyxin-B, and Prednisolone (Poly-Pred Ophthalmic) **Uses:** Steroid-responsive ocular conditions with bacterial infection **Action:** Antibiotic and antiinflammatory **Dose:** 1–2 gtt in eye(s) q4–6h; apply oint in eye(s) 3–4×/d **Caution/Contra:** [C, ?] **Supplied:** Susp neomycin 0.35%/polymyxin B 10,000 U/prednisolone 0.5%/mL **Notes/SE:** Use under supervision of ophthalmologist

Neomycin Sulfate **Uses:** Hepatic coma and preoperative bowel preparation **Action:** Aminoglycoside, poorly absorbed orally; suppresses GI bacterial flora **Dose:** *Adults.* 3–12 g/24 h PO in 3–4 ÷ doses. *Peds.* 50–100 mg/kg/24 h PO in 3–4 ÷ doses **Caution/Contra:** [C, ?/–] Caution in renal failure, neuromuscular disorders, hearing impairment. Do not use parenterally. **Supplied:** Tabs 500 mg; oral soln 125 mg/5 mL **Notes/SE:** Part of the Condon bowel prep; hearing loss with long-term use; rash, N/V

Nesiritide (Natrecor) **Uses:** Acutely decompensated CHF **Action:** Human B-type natriuretic peptide **Dose:** 2-mcg/kg IV bolus, then 0.01 mcg/kg/min IV **Caution/Contra:** [C, ?/–] BP <90, cardiogenic shock; low cardiac filling pressures; patients in whom vasodilators are not appropriate **Supplied:** Vials 1.5 mg **Notes/SE:** Hypotension, requires continuous BP monitoring; HA, back pain, GI upset, arrhythmias, ↑ Cr

Nevirapine (Viramune) **WARNING:** Reports of fatal hepatotoxicity even after short-term use; severe life-threatening skin reactions (Stevens–Johnson syndrome, toxic epidermal necrolysis, and hypersensitivity reactions); monitor closely during 1st 8 wk of treatment **Uses:** HIV infection **Action:** Nonnucleoside reverse transcriptase inhibitor **Dose:** *Adults.* Initially 200 mg/d for 14 d, then 200 mg bid. *Peds.* <8 y: 4 mg/kg/d for 14 d, then 7 mg/kg bid. >8 y: 4 mg/kg/d for 14 d, then 4 mg/kg bid; give without regard to food **Caution/Contra:** [C, +/–] Oral contraceptive use **Supplied:** Tabs 200 mg; susp 50 mg/5 mL **Notes/SE:** May cause life-threatening rash; HA, fever, diarrhea, neutropenia, hepatitis

Niacin (Nicolar, Niaspan) **Uses:** Adjunctive therapy in patients with significant hyperlipidemia **Action:** Inhibits lipolysis; decreases esterification of triglycerides; increases lipoprotein lipase activity **Dose:** 1–6 g tid; max of 9 g/d **Caution/Contra:** [A (C if doses >RDA), +] Liver disease, peptic ulcer, arterial hemorrhage **Supplied:** SR caps 125, 250, 300, 400, 500 mg; tabs 25, 50, 100, 250, 500 mg; SR tabs 150, 250, 500, 750 mg; elixir 50 mg/5 mL **Notes/SE:** Upper body and facial flushing and warmth following dose; may cause GI upset; HA, flatulence, paresthesias, liver damage

Nicardipine (Cardene) **Uses:** Chronic stable angina and HTN; prophylaxis of migraine **Action:** Ca channel blocker **Dose:** *Oral:* 20–40 mg PO tid. *SR:* 30–60 mg PO bid.

IV: 5 mg/h IV cont inf; ↑ by 2.5 mg/h q15min to max 15 mg/h; take with food (not high fat); ↓ dose in renal/hepatic impairment **Caution/Contra:** [C, ?/–] Heart block, cardiogenic shock **Supplied:** Caps 20, 30 mg; SR caps 30, 45, 60 mg; inj 2.5 mg/mL **Notes/SE:** *Oral-to-IV conversion:* 20 mg tid = 0.5 mg/h, 30 mg tid = 1.2 mg/h, 40 mg tid = 2.2 mg/h; flushing, tachycardia, hypotension, edema, HA

Nicotine Gum (Nicorette, Nicorette DS) **Uses and Action:** See Nicotine Nasal Spray **Dose:** Chew 9–12 pieces/d PRN; max 30 pieces/d **Caution/Contra:** [C, ?] Life-threatening arrhythmias, unstable angina **Supplied:** 2 mg (96 pieces/box); Nicorette DS has 4 mg/piece **Notes/SE:** Patients must stop smoking and perform behavior modification for max effect; tachycardia, HA, GI upset

Nicotine Nasal Spray (Nicotrol NS) **Uses:** Aid to smoking cessation for the relief of nicotine withdrawal **Action:** Provides systemic delivery of nicotine **Dose:** 0.5 mg/actuation; 1–2 sprays/h, not to exceed 10 sprays/h **Caution/Contra:** [D, M] Life-threatening arrhythmias, unstable angina **Supplied:** Nasal inhaler 10 mg/mL **Notes/SE:** Patients must stop smoking and perform behavior modification for max effect; local irritation, tachycardia, HA, taste perversion

Nicotine Transdermal (Habitrol, Nicoderm, Nicotrol, ProStep) **Uses:** Aid to smoking cessation for the relief of nicotine withdrawal **Action:** Provides systemic delivery of nicotine **Dose:** Individualized to the patient's needs; apply 1 patch (14–22 mg/d), and taper over 6 wk **Caution/Contra:** [D, M] Life-threatening arrhythmias, unstable angina **Supplied:** Habitrol and Nicoderm 7, 14, 21 mg of nicotine/24 h; Nicotrol 5, 10, 15 mg/24 h; ProStep 11, 22 mg/24 h **Notes/SE:** Nicotrol to be worn for 16 h to mimic smoking patterns; others worn for 24 h; patients must stop smoking and perform behavior modification for max effect; insomnia, pruritus, erythema, local site reaction, tachycardia

Nifedipine (Procardia, Procardia XL, Adalat, Adalat CC) **Uses:** Vasospastic or chronic stable angina and HTN; tocolytic **Action:** Ca channel blocker **Dose:** *Adults.* SR tabs 30–90 mg/d. *Tocolysis:* 10–20 mg PO q4–6h. *Peds.* 0.6–0.9 mg/kg/24 h ÷ tid–qid **Caution/Contra:** [C, +] Heart block, aortic stenosis **Supplied:** Caps 10, 20 mg; SR tabs 30, 60, 90 mg **Notes/SE:** Adalat CC and Procardia XL not interchangeable; SL administration not recommended; HAs common on initial treatment; reflex tachycardia may occur with regular release dosage forms; edema, hypotension, flushing, dizziness

Nilutamide (Nilandron) WARNING: Interstitial pneumonitis possible; most cases in 1st 3 mon; follow CXR before Rx **Uses:** Combination with surgical castration for metastatic prostate CA **Action:** Nonsteroidal antiandrogen **Dose:** 300 mg/d in ÷ doses for 30 d, then 150 mg/d **Caution/Contra:** [N/A] Severe hepatic impairment or respiratory insufficiency **Supplied:** Tabs 50 (phased out), 150 mg **Notes/SE:** Hot flashes, loss of libido, impotence, N/V/D, gynecomastia, hepatic dysfunction (follow LFTs), interstitial pneumonitis

Nimodipine (Nimotop) **Uses:** Prevent vasospasm following subarachnoid hemorrhage **Action:** Ca channel blocker **Dose:** 60 mg PO q4h for 21 d; ↓ dose in hepatic failure **Caution/Contra:** [C, ?] **Supplied:** Caps 30 mg **Notes/SE:** Contents of caps may be administered via NG tube if caps cannot be swallowed whole; hypotension, HA, constipation

Nisoldipine (Sular) **Uses:** HTN **Action:** Ca channel blocker **Dose:** 10–60 mg/d PO; do not take with grapefruit juice or high-fat meal; ↓ starting doses in elderly or hepatic impairment **Caution/Contra:** [C, ?] **Supplied:** ER tabs 10, 20, 30, 40 mg **Notes/SE:** Edema, HA, flushing

Nitazoxanide (Alinia) **Uses:** *Cryptosporidium* or *Giardia*-induced diarrhea in patients 1–11 years **Action:** Antiprotozoal **Dose:** Peds. 12–47 months: 5 mL (100 mg) PO q 12h × 3 days. 4–11 years: 10 mL (200 mg) PO q 12h × 3 days; take with food **Caution/Contra:** [B, ?] **Supplied:** 100 mg/5 mL oral susp **Notes/SE:** suspension contains sucrose; likely to interact with highly protein-bound drugs; abdominal pain

Nitrofurantoin (Macrodantin, Furadantin, Macrobid) WARNING: Pulmonary reactions possible **Uses:** Prevention and Rx UTI **Action:** Bacteriostatic; interferes with carbohydrate metabolism **Dose:** *Adults.* *Suppression:* 50–100 mg/d PO. *Rx:* 50–100 mg PO qid. *Peds.* 5–7 mg/kg/24 h in 4 ÷ doses; take with food, milk, or antacid **Caution/Contra:** [B, +] Avoid if CrCl <50 mL/min, pregnant at term, infants <1 mon (hemolytic anemia risk) **Supplied:** Caps and tabs 50, 100 mg; SR caps 100 mg; susp 25 mg/5 mL **Notes/SE:** Macrocrystals (Macrodantin) cause less nausea than other forms of the drug;

GI side effects common; dyspnea and a variety of acute and chronic pulmonary reactions, peripheral neuropathy

Nitroglycerin (Nitrostat, Nitrolingual, Nitro-Bid Ointment, Nitro-Bid IV, Nitrodisc, Transderm-Nitro, others) **Uses:** Angina pectoris, acute and prophylactic therapy, CHF, BP control **Action:** Relaxation of vascular smooth muscle **Dose** *Adults.* *SL:* 1 tab q5min SL PRN for 3 doses. *Translingual:* 1–2 met-doses sprayed onto oral mucosa q3–5min, max 3 doses. *Oral:* 2.5–9 mg tid. *IV:* 5–20 mcg/min, titrated to effect. *Topical:* Apply 1–2 in. of oint to the chest wall tid, wipe off at night. *TD:* 5–20 cm patch qd. *Peds.* 1 mcg/kg/min IV, titrated to effect **Caution/Contra:** [B, ?] Pericardial tamponade, restrictive cardiomyopathy, constrictive pericarditis **Supplied:** SL tabs 0.3, 0.4, 0.6 mg; translingual spray 0.4 mg/dose; SR caps 2.5, 6.5, 9, 13 mg; SR tabs 2.6, 6.5, 9.0 mg; inj 0.5, 5, 10 mg/mL; oint 2%; TD patches 2.5, 5, 7.5, 10, 15 mg/24 h; buccal CR 1, 2, 3 mg **Notes/SE:** Tolerance to nitrates develops with chronic use after 1–2 wk; can be avoided by providing a nitrate-free period each day, using shorter-acting nitrates tid, and removing long-acting patches and oint before hs to prevent development of tolerance; HA, hypotension, lightheadedness, GI upset

Nitroprusside (Nipride, Nitropress) **Uses:** Hypertensive emergency, aortic dissection, pulmonary edema **Action:** ↓ SVR **Dose:** *Adults & Peds.* 0.5–10 mcg/kg/min IV inf, titrated to effect; usual dose 3 mcg/kg/min **Caution/Contra:** [C, ?] Decreased cerebral perfusion, compensatory HTN **Supplied:** Inj 10 mg/mL, 25 mg/mL **Notes/SE:** Thiocyanate, the metabolite, excreted by the kidney; thiocyanate toxicity at levels of 5–10 mg/dL; if used to treat aortic dissection, use β-blocker concomitantly; excessive hypotensive effects, palpitations, HA

Nizatidine (Axid) **Uses:** Duodenal ulcers, GERD, heartburn **Action:** H₂-receptor antagonist **Dose:** *Active ulcer:* 150 mg PO bid or 300 mg PO hs; maint 150 mg PO hs. *GERD:* 300 mg PO bid; maint PO bid. *Heartburn:* 75 mg PO bid; ↓?dose in renal impairment **Caution/Contra:** [B, +] H₂-antagonist sensitivity **Supplied:** Caps 75, 150, 300 mg **Notes/SE:** Dizziness, HA, constipation, diarrhea

Norepinephrine (Levophed) **Uses:** Acute hypotensive states **Action:** Peripheral vasoconstrictor acting on both the arterial and venous beds **Dose:** *Adults.* 8–12 mcg/min IV, titrate to effect. *Peds.* 0.05–0.1 mg/kg/min IV, titrate to effect **Caution/Contra:** [C, ?] **Supplied:** Inj 1 mg/mL **Notes/SE:** Correct blood volume depletion as much as possible prior to vasopressor therapy; interaction with TCAs leads to severe HTN; infuse into large vein to avoid extravasation; phentolamine 5–10 mg/10 mL NS injected locally for extravasation

Norfloxacin (Noroxin) **Uses:** Complicated and uncomplicated UTI due to gram– bacteria, prostatitis, and infectious diarrhea **Action:** Quinolone, inhibits DNA gyrase **Dose:** *Adults.* 400 mg PO bid. *Gonorrhea:* 800 mg single dose. *Conjunctivitis:* 1–2 gtt qid **Caution/Contra:** [X, –] Do not use in PRG; quinolone sensitivity **Supplied:** Tabs 400 mg; ophth soln 0.3%; ↓ in renal impairment **Notes/SE:** Photosensitivity; drug interactions with antacids, theophylline, and caffeine; good concs in the kidney and urine, poor blood levels; do not use for urosepsis

Norgestrel (Ovrette) **Uses:** Contraceptive **Action:** Prevent follicular maturation and ovulation **Dose:** 1 tab/d; begin day 1 of menses **Caution/Contra:** [X, ?] Thromboembolism, severe hepatic disease, breast CA **Supplied:** Tabs 0.075 mg **Notes/SE:** Progestin-only products have higher risk of failure in prevention of PRG; edema, breakthrough bleeding, thromboembolism

Nortriptyline (Aventyl, Pamelor) **Uses:** Endogenous depression **Action:** TCA; increases the synaptic CNS concs of serotonin and/or norepinephrine **Dose:** *Adults.* 25 mg PO tid–qid; doses >150 mg/d not recommended. *Elderly.* 10–25 mg hs. *Peds.* 6–7 y: 10 mg/d. 8–11 y: 10–20 mg/d. >11 y: 25–35 mg/d; ↓ dose with hepatic insufficiency **Caution/Contra:** [D, +/–] Narrow-angle glaucoma, TCA hypersensitivity **Supplied:** Caps 10, 25, 50, 75 mg; soln 10 mg/5 mL **Notes/SE:** Max effect seen after 2 wk of therapy. Many anticholinergic side effects (blurred vision, urinary retention, xerostomia)

Nystatin (Mycostatin) **Uses:** Mucocutaneous *Candida* infections (thrush, vaginitis) **Action:** Alters membrane permeability **Dose:** *Adults.* *Oral:* 400,000–600,000 U PO "swish and swallow" qid. *Vaginal:* 1 tab vaginally hs for 2 wk. *Topical:* Apply bid–tid to affected area. *Peds.* *Infants:* 200,000 U PO q6h. *Children:* See adult dosage **Caution/Contra:**

[B (C oral), +] **Supplied:** Oral susp 100,000 U/mL; oral tabs 500,000 U; troches 200,000 U; vaginal tabs 100,000 U; topical cream and oint 100,000 U/g **Notes/SE:** Not absorbed orally; not effective for systemic infections; GI upset, Stevens-Johnson syndrome

Octreotide (Sandostatin, Sandostatin LAR) **Uses:** Suppresses/inhibits severe diarrhea associated with carcinoid and neuroendocrine GI tumors (ie, VIPoma, ZE syndrome); bleeding esophageal varices **Action:** Long-acting peptide; mimics natural hormone somatostatin **Dose:** *Adults.* 100–600 mcg/d SC in 2–4 ÷ doses; initiate at 50 mcg qd–bid. *Sandostatin LAR (depot):* 10–30 mg IM q4wk *Peds.* 1–10 mcg/kg/24 h SC in 2–4 ÷ doses **Caution/Contra:** [B, +] **Supplied:** Inj 0.05, 0.1, 0.2, 0.5, 1 mg/mL; 10, 20, 30 mg/5 mL depot **Notes/SE:** N/V, abdominal discomfort, flushing, edema, fatigue, cholelithiasis, hyper/hypoglycemia, hepatitis

Ofloxacin (Floxin, Ocuflox Ophthalmic) **Uses:** Lower respiratory tract, skin and skin structure, and UTIs, prostatitis, uncomplicated gonorrhea, and *Chlamydia* infections; topical for bacterial conjunctivitis; acute otitis media in children >1 y with tympanostomy tubes; otitis externa in adults and children >1 y; if perforated ear drum >12 y **Action:** Bactericidal; inhibits DNA gyrase **Dose:** *Adults.* 200–400 mg PO bid or IV q12h. *Adults & Peds >1 y.* Ophth 1–2 gtt in eye(s) q2–4h for 2 d, then qid for ≥5 d. *Peds.* Do not administer systemically in children <18 y. *Peds 1–12 y.* Otic 5 gtt in ear(s) bid for 10 d. *Adults & Peds >12 y.* Otic 10 gtt in ear(s) bid for 10 d; ↓ dose in renal impairment; take on empty stomach **Caution/Contra:** [C, –] Quinolone sensitivity; drug interactions with antacids, sucralfate, and Al^{2+}-, Ca^{2+}-, Mg^{2+}-, Fe^{2+}-, or Zn^{2+}-containing products, which ↓ absorption **Supplied:** Tabs 200, 300, 400 mg; inj 20, 40 mg/mL; ophth and otic 0.3% **Notes/SE:** Ophth form can be used in ears; N/V/D, photosensitivity, insomnia, and HA

Olanzapine (Zyprexa) **Uses:** Psychotic disorders, acute mania **Action:** Dopamine and serotonin antagonist **Dose:** 5–10 mg/d, ↑ weekly PRN to 20 mg/d max **Caution/Contra:** [C, –] **Supplied:** Tabs 2.5, 5, 7.5, 10, 15, 20 mg; oral disintegrating tabs 5, 10, 15, 20 mg **Notes/SE:** Takes wks to titrate to therapeutic dose; cigarette smoking decreases levels; HA, somnolence, orthostatic hypotension, tachycardia, dystonia, xerostomia, constipation

Olmesartan (Benicar) **Uses:** HTN **Action:** Angiotensin II antagonist **Dose:** 20–40 mg PO qd **Caution/Contra:** [C (1st trimester), D (2nd and 3rd trimesters), ?/–] **Supplied:** Tabs 5, 20, 40 mg **Notes/SE:** Use lower dose with depleted intravascular volume

Olopatadine (Patanol) **Uses:** Allergic conjunctivitis **Action:** H$_1$-receptor antagonist **Dose:** 1–2 gtt in eye(s) bid q6–8h **Caution/Contra:** [C, ?] **Supplied:** Soln 0.1% 5 mL **Notes/SE:** Do not instill if wearing contact lenses; local irritation, HA, rhinitis

Olsalazine (Dipentum) **Uses:** Maint of remission of ulcerative colitis **Action:** Topical antiinflammatory activity **Dose:** 500 mg PO bid; take with food **Caution/Contra:** [C, M] Salicylate sensitivity **Supplied:** Caps 250 mg **Notes/SE:** May cause diarrhea, HA, blood dyscrasias, hepatitis

Omeprazole (Prilosec) **Uses:** Duodenal and gastric ulcers, Zollinger–Ellison syndrome, GERD, and *H. pylori* infections **Action:** Proton-pump inhibitor **Dose:** 20–40 mg PO qd–bid **Caution/Contra:** [C, –] **Supplied:** Caps 10, 20, 40 mg **Notes/SE:** Combination (ie, antibiotic) therapy necessary for *H. pylori* infection; HA, diarrhea

Ondansetron (Zofran) **Uses:** Prevent chemotherapy-associated and postop N/V **Action:** Serotonin receptor antagonist **Dose:** *Adults & Peds. Chemotherapy:* 0.15 mg/kg/dose IV prior to chemotherapy, then repeat 4 and 8 h after 1st dose or 4–8 mg PO tid; give 1st dose 30 min prior to chemotherapy. *Adults. Postop:* 4 mg IV immediately before induction of anesthesia or postop; ↓ dose with hepatic impairment; administer on a schedule, not PRN **Caution/Contra:** [B, +/–] **Supplied:** Tabs 4, 8 mg; inj 2 mg/mL **Notes/SE:** Diarrhea, HA, constipation, dizziness

Oprelvekin (Neumega) **Uses:** Prevent severe thrombocytopenia due to chemotherapy **Action:** Promotes proliferation and maturation of megakaryocytes (interleukin-11) **Dose:** *Adults.* 50 mcg/kg/d SC for 10–21 d. *Peds.* 75–100 mcg/kg/d SC for 10–21 d; *<12y:* Use only in clinical trials **Caution/Contra:** [C, ?/–] **Supplied:** Inj **Notes/SE:** Tachycardia, palpitations, arrhythmias, edema, HA, dizziness, insomnia, fatigue, fever, nausea, anemia, dyspnea

22 **Oral Contraceptives, Biphasic, Monophasic, Triphasic, Progestin Only (Table 7, page 617)** **Uses:** Birth control and regulation of anovulatory bleeding **Ac-**

tion: *Birth control:* Suppresses LH surge, prevents ovulation; progestins thicken cervical mucus; inhibits fallopian tubule cilia, ↓ endometrial thickness to ↓ chances of fertilization. *Anovulatory bleeding:* Cyclic hormones mimic body's natural cycle and help regulate endometrial lining, resulting in regular bleeding q28d; may also reduce uterine bleeding and dysmenorrhea **Dose:** 28-d cycle pills taken qd; 21-d cycle pills taken qd, no pills taken during the last 7 d of the cycle (during menses) **Caution/Contra:** [X, +] *Absolute contraindications:* Undiagnosed abnormal vaginal bleeding, PRG, estrogen-dependent malignancy, hypercoagulation disorders, liver disease, hemiplegic migraine, and smokers >35 y. *Relative caution/contra:* Migraine HAs, HTN, diabetes, sickle cell disease, and gallbladder disease **Supplied:** 28-d cycle pills (21 hormonally active pills + 7 placebo/Fe supplementation); 21-d cycle pills (21 hormonally active pills). Table 7, page 617 **Notes/SE:** Taken correctly, 99.9% effective for preventing PRG; not protective against STDs; encourage additional barrier contraceptive. Long term, can ↓ risk of ectopic pregnancy, benign breast disease, ovarian and uterine CA. *Rx for menstrual cycle control:* Start with a monophasic pill. Pill must be taken for 3 mon before switching to another brand. If abnormal bleeding continues, change to pill with higher estrogen dose. *Rx for birth control:* Choose pill with most beneficial side effect profile for particular patient. Side effects numerous and due to symptoms of estrogen excess or progesterone deficiency. Each pill's side effect profile is unique (found in package insert); tailor Rx to specific patient. *Common SE:* Intermenstrual bleeding, oligomenorrhea, amenorrhea, ↑ appetite/weight gain, loss of libido, fatigue, depression, mood swings, mastalgia, HAs, melasma, ↑ vaginal discharge, acne/greasy skin, corneal edema, nausea

Orphenadrine (Norflex) **Uses:** Muscle spasms **Action:** Central atropine-like effects cause indirect skeletal muscle relaxation, euphoria, and analgesia **Dose:** 100 mg PO bid, 60 mg IM/IV q12h **Caution/Contra:** [C, +] Glaucoma, GI obstruction, cardiospasm, MyG **Supplied:** Tabs 100 mg; SR tabs 100 mg; inj 30 mg/mL **Notes/SE:** Drowsiness, dizziness, blurred vision, flushing, tachycardia, constipation

Oseltamivir (Tamiflu) **Uses:** Prevention and Rx of influenza A and B **Action:** Inhibits viral neuraminidase **Dose:** *Adults.* Rx 75 mg bid for 5 d. *Peds.* PO bid dosing: <15 kg, 30 mg; 16–23 kg, 45 mg; 24–40 kg, 60 mg; >41 kg, as adult; ↓ dose in renal impairment **Caution/Contra:** [C, ?/–] **Supplied:** Caps 75 mg, powder 12 mg/mL **Notes/SE:** Initiate within 48 h of symptom onset or exposure; N/V, insomnia

Oxacillin (Bactocill, Prostaphlin) **Uses:** Infections caused by susceptible strains of *S. aureus* and *Streptococcus* **Action:** Bactericidal; inhibits cell wall synthesis **Dose:** *Adults.* 250–500 mg (1 g severe) IM/IV q4–6h. *Peds.* 150–200 mg/kg/d IV ÷ q4–6h; ↓ dose in significant renal disease **Caution/Contra:** [B, M] Penicillin sensitivity **Supplied:** Inj; caps 250, 500 mg; soln 250 mg/5 mL **Notes/SE:** GI upset, interstitial nephritis, blood dyscrasias

Oxaprozin (Daypro) **Uses:** Arthritis and pain **Action:** NSAID; inhibits prostaglandin synthesis **Dose:** 600–1200 mg/d; ↓ dose in renal/hepatic impairment **Caution/Contra:** [C (D in 3rd trimester or near term), ?] ASA/NSAID sensitivity, peptic ulcer, bleeding disorders **Supplied:** Caplets 600 mg **Notes/SE:** CNS inhibition, sleep disturbance, rash, GI upset, peptic ulcer, edema, renal failure

Oxazepam (Serax) [C-IV] **Uses:** Anxiety, acute alcohol withdrawal, anxiety with depressive symptoms **Action:** Benzodiazepine **Dose:** *Adults.* 10–15 mg PO tid–qid; severe anxiety and alcohol withdrawal may require up to 30 mg qid. *Peds.* 1 mg/kg/d in ÷ doses; avoid abrupt DC **Caution/Contra:** [D, ?] **Supplied:** Caps 10, 15, 30 mg; tabs 15 mg **Notes/SE:** One of the metabolites of diazepam (Valium); sedation, ataxia, dizziness, rash, blood dyscrasias, dependence

Oxcarbazepine (Trileptal) **Uses:** Partial seizures **Action:** Blocks voltage-sensitive Na^+ channels, resulting in stabilization of hyperexcited neural membranes **Dose:** *Adults.* 300 mg bid, ↑ dose weekly; usual dose of 1200–2400 mg/d. *Peds.* 8–10 mg/kg bid, 600 mg/d max; ↑ dose weekly to target maint dose; ↓ dose in renal insufficiency **Caution/Contra:** [C, –] Possible cross-sensitivity to carbamazepine **Supplied:** Tabs 150, 300, 600 mg **Notes/SE:** Hyponatremia; HA, dizziness, fatigue somnolence, GI upset, diplopia, mental conc difficulties; do not abruptly DC

Oxiconazole (Oxistat) **Uses:** Tinea pedis, tinea cruris, and tinea corporis **Action:** Antifungal antibiotic **Dose:** Apply bid **Caution/Contra:** [B, M] **Supplied:** Cream 1%; lotion **Notes/SE:** Local irritation

22

Oxybutynin (Ditropan, Ditropan XL) **Uses:** Symptomatic relief of urgency, nocturia, and incontinence associated with neurogenic or reflex neurogenic bladder **Action:** Direct smooth muscle antispasmodic; ↑ bladder capacity **Dose:** *Adults & Peds >5 y.* 5 mg PO tid–qid. *Adults.* XL 5 mg PO qd; ↑ to 30 mg/d PO (5 and 10 mg/tab). *Peds 1–5 y.* 0.02 mg/kg/dose bid–qid (syrup 5 mg/5 mL); ↓ dose in elderly; periodic drug holidays recommended **Caution/Contra:** [B, ? (use with caution)] Glaucoma, MyG, GI or GU obstruction, ulcerative colitis, megacolon **Supplied:** Tabs 5 mg; XL tabs 5, 10, 15 mg; syrup 5 mg/5 mL **Notes/SE:** Anticholinergic side effects; drowsiness, xerostomia, constipation, tachycardia

Oxycodone [Dihydrohydroxycodeinone] (OxyContin, OxyIR, Roxicodone) [C-II] WARNING: Swallow whole, do not crush. **Uses:** Moderate–severe pain, normally used in combination with nonnarcotic analgesics **Action:** Narcotic analgesic **Dose:** *Adults.* 5 mg PO q6h PRN. *Peds. 6–12 y:* 1.25 mg PO q6h PRN. *>12 y:* 2.5 mg q6h PRN; ↓ in severe liver disease **Caution/ Contra:** [B (D if prolonged use or near term), M] **Supplied:** Immediate release caps (OxyIR) 5 mg; tabs (Percolone) 5 mg; CR (OxyContin) 10, 20, 40, 80 mg; liq 5 mg/mL; soln conc 20 mg/mL **Notes/SE:** Usually prescribed in combination with APAP or ASA; OxyContin used for chronic CA pain; hypotension, sedation, dizziness, GI upset, constipation, risk of abuse

Oxycodone and Acetaminophen (Percocet, Tylox) [C-II] **Uses:** Moderate–severe pain **Action:** Narcotic analgesic **Dose:** *Adults.* 1–2 tabs/caps PO q4–6h PRN (acetaminophen max dose 4 g/d). *Peds.* Oxycodone 0.05–0.15 mg/kg/dose q4–6h PRN; up to 5 mg/dose **Caution/Contra:** [B (D if prolonged use or near term), M] **Supplied:** Percocet tabs, mg oxycodone/mg APAP: 2.5/325, 5/325, 7.5/325, 10/325, 7.5/500, 10/650; Tylox caps 5 mg of oxycodone, 500 mg of APAP; soln 5 mg of oxycodone and 325 mg of APAP/5 mL **Notes/SE:** Hypotension, sedation, dizziness, GI upset, constipation

Oxycodone and Aspirin (Percodan, Percodan-Demi) [C-II] **Uses:** Moderate–moderately severe pain **Action:** Narcotic analgesic with NSAID **Dose:** *Adults.* 1–2 tabs/caps PO q4–6h PRN. *Peds.* 0.05–0.15 mg/kg/dose q4–6h, max 5 mg/dose (based on oxycodone); ↓ dose in severe hepatic failure **Caution/Contra:** [B (D if prolonged use or near term), M] Peptic ulcer **Supplied:** Percodan 4.5 mg oxycodone HCl, 0.38 mg oxycodone terephthalate, 325 mg ASA; Percodan-Demi 2.25 mg oxycodone hydrochloride, 0.19 mg oxycodone terephthalate, 325 mg ASA **Notes/SE:** Sedation, dizziness, GI upset, constipation

Oxymorphone (Numorphan) [C-II] **Uses:** Moderate–severe pain, sedative **Action:** Narcotic analgesic **Dose:** 0.5 mg IM, SC, IV initially, 1–1.5 mg q4–6h PRN. *PR:* 5 mg q4–6h PRN **Caution/Contra:** [B, ?] **Supplied:** Inj 1, 1.5 mg/mL; supp 5 mg **Notes/SE:** Chemically related to hydromorphone; hypotension, sedation, GI upset, constipation, histamine release

Oxytocin (Pitocin) **Uses:** Induction of labor and control of postpartum hemorrhage; promote milk letdown in lactating woman **Action:** Stimulate muscular contractions of the uterus, stimulate milk flow during nursing **Dose:** 0.001–0.002 U/min IV inf; titrate to desired effect to a max of 0.02 U/min. *Breast-feeding:* 1 spray in both nostrils 2–3 min before feeding **Caution/Contra:** [Uncategorized, no anomalies expected, +/–] **Supplied:** Inj 10 U/mL; nasal soln 40 U/mL **Notes/SE:** Monitor vital signs closely; nasal form for breast-feeding only; can cause uterine rupture and fetal death; arrhythmias, anaphylaxis, water intoxication

Paclitaxel (Taxol) **Uses:** Ovarian and breast CA **Action:** Mitotic spindle poison promotes microtubule assembly and stabilization against depolymerization **Dose:** 135–250 mg/m^2 as a 3–24 h IV inf; glass or polyolefin containers using polyethylene-lined nitroglycerin tubing sets; PVC inf sets result in leaching of plasticizer; ↓ dose in hepatic failure; maintain adequate hydration **Caution/Contra:** [D, – (unknown excretion, but nursing must be stopped)] **Supplied:** Inj 6 mg/mL **Notes/SE:** Hypersensitivity reactions (dyspnea, hypotension, urticaria, rash) usually within 10 min of starting inf; minimize with corticosteroid, antihistamine (H$_1$- and H$_2$-antagonist) pretreatment. Myelosuppression, peripheral neuropathy, transient ileus, myalgia, bradycardia, hypotension, mucositis, N/V/D, fever, rash, HA, and phlebitis; hematologic toxicity schedule-dependent; leukopenia dose-limiting by 24-h inf; neurotoxicity dose-limiting by short (1–3 h) inf

Palivizumab (Synagis) **Uses:** Prevent RSV **Action:** RSV fusion protein monoclonal antibody **Dose:** *Peds.* 15 mg/kg IM monthly, typically Nov–Apr **Caution/Contra:** [C, ?]

22

Caution in renal or hepatic dysfunction **Supplied:** Vials 50, 100 mg **Notes/SE:** URI, rhinitis, cough, ↑ LFT, local irritation

Pamidronate (Aredia)   **Uses:** Hypercalcemia of malignancy and Paget's disease; palliation of symptomatic bone metastases **Action:** Inhibition of normal and abnormal bone resorption **Dose:** *Hypercalcemia:* 60 mg IV over 4 h or 90 mg IV over 24 h. *Paget's disease:* 30 mg/d IV for 3 d; slow inf rate necessary **Caution/ Contra:** [C, ?/–] **Supplied:** Powder for inj 30, 60, 90 mg **Notes/SE:** Fever, tissue irritation at inj site, uveitis, fluid overload, HTN, abdominal pain, N/V, constipation, UTI, bone pain, hypokalemia, hypocalcemia, hypomagnesemia, and hypophosphatemia

Pancrelipase (Pancrease, Cotazym, Creon, Ultrase)   **Uses:** Exocrine pancreatic secretion deficiency (CF, chronic pancreatitis, other pancreatic insufficiency) and for steatorrhea of malabsorption syndrome **Action:** Pancreatic enzyme supplementation **Dose:** *Adults & Peds.* 1–3 caps (tabs) with meals and snacks; dosage ↑ to 8 caps (tabs); do not crush or chew EC products; dosage is dependent on digestive requirements of patient; avoid antacids. **Caution/Contra:** [C, ?/–] **Supplied:** Caps, tabs **Notes/SE:** N/V, abdominal cramps

Pancuronium (Pavulon)   **Uses:** Rx of patients on mechanical ventilation **Action:** Nondepolarizing neuromuscular blocker **Dose:** *Adults.* 2–4 mg IV q2–4h PRN. *Peds.* 0.02–0.10 mg/kg/dose q2–4h PRN; ↓ dose for renal/hepatic impairment; intubate patient and keep on controlled ventilation; use an adequate amount of sedation or analgesia **Caution/Contra:** [C, ?/–] **Supplied:** Inj; 1, 2 mg/mL **Notes/SE:** Tachycardia, HTN, pruritus, other histamine reactions

Pantoprazole (Protonix)   **Uses:** GERD, PUD, erosive gastritis, ZE syndrome **Action:** Proton-pump inhibitor **Dose:** 40 mg/d PO; do not crush or chew tablets; 40 mg IV/d (not >3 mg/min and use Protonix filter) **Caution/Contra:** [B, ?/–] **Supplied:** Tabs 40 mg; inj **Notes/SE:** Chest pain, anxiety, GI upset, ↑ levels on LFTs

Paregoric (Camphorated Tincture of Opium) [C-III]   **Uses:** Diarrhea, pain, and neonatal opiate withdrawal syndrome **Action:** Narcotic **Dose:** *Adults.* 5–10 mL PO qd–qid PRN. *Peds.* 0.25–0.5 mL/kg qd–qid. *Neonatal withdrawal syndrome:* 3–6 gtt PO q3–6h PRN to relieve symptoms for 3–5 d, then taper over 2–4 wk **Caution/Contra:** [B (D if prolonged use or high dose near term, +] **Supplied:** Liq 2 mg morphine = 20 mg opium/ 5 mL **Notes/SE:** Contains anhydrous morphine from opium; short-term use only; hypotension, sedation, constipation

Paroxetine (Paxil, Paxil CR)   **Uses:** Depression, OCD, panic disorder, social anxiety disorder, PMDD **Action:** Serotonin reuptake inhibitor **Dose:** 10–60 mg PO single daily dose in AM; CR 25 mg/d PO; ↑ 12.5 mg/wk (max range 26–62.5 mg/d) **Caution/Contra:** [B, ?/–] DDI, MAOI **Supplied:** Tabs 10, 20, 30, 40 mg; susp 10 mg/5 mL; CR 12.5, 25 mg **Notes/SE:** Sexual dysfunction, HA, somnolence, dizziness, GI upset, diarrhea, xerostomia, tachycardia

Pegfilgrastim (Neulasta)   **Uses:** ↓ Frequency of infection in patients with non-myeloid malignancies receiving myelosuppressive anticancer drugs that cause febrile neutropenia **Actions:** Colony-stimulating factor **Dose:** *Adults:* 6 mg SC × 1/chemo cycle; Never give between 14 d before and 24 h after dose of cytotoxic chemotherapy **Contra/Caution:** [C, M] Contra in patients hypersensitive to drugs used to treat *E. coli* or to filgrastim, caution in sickle cell **Supplied:** Syringes: 6 mg/0.6 mL **Notes:** HA, fever weakness, fatigue, dizziness, insomnia, edema, N/V/D, stomatitis, anorexia, constipation, taste perversion, dyspepsia, abdominal pain, granulocytopenia, neutropenic fever, ↑ LFT, uric acid, arthralgia, myalgia, bone pain, ARDS, alopecia, splenic rupture, aggravation of sickle cell disease

Peg Interferon Alfa 2a (Pegasys)   **Uses:** Chronic hepatitis C with compensated liver disease **Action:** BRM **Dose:** 180 mcg (1 mL) SQ once weekly × 48 wk; ↓ dose in renal impairment **Caution/Contra:** [C, /?–] Autoimmune hepatitis, decompensated liver disease **Supplied:** 180 mcg/mL inj **Notes/SE:** May aggravate neuropsychiatric, autoimmune, ischemic, and infectious disorders

Peg Interferon Alfa 2b (PEG-Intron)   **Uses:** Rx hepatitis C **Action:** Immune modulation **Dose:** 1 mcg/kg/wk SC; 1.5 mcg/kg/wk combined with ribavirin **Caution/Contra:**

[C, ?/–] Contra in hemoglobinopathy; caution in patients with psychiatric Hx **Supplied:** Vials 50, 80, 120, 150 mcg/0.5 mL **Notes/SE:** ↓ Flu-like symptoms by giving hs or with APAP; neutropenia and thrombocytopenia may require DC; follow CBC and platelets; depression, insomnia, suicidal behavior, GI upset, alopecia, pruritus

Pemirolast (Alamast) Uses: Allergic conjunctivitis **Action:** Mast cell stabilizer **Dose:** 1–2 gtt in each eye qid **Caution/Contra:** [C, ?/–] **Supplied:** 1 mg/mL **Notes/SE:** HA, rhinitis, cold/flu symptoms, local irritation, wait 10 min after instilling before inserting contacts

Penbutolol (Levatol) Uses: HTN **Action:** Competitively blocks β-adrenergic receptors, β_1, β_2 **Dose:** 20–40 mg/d; ↓ dose in hepatic insufficiency **Caution/ Contra:** [C (1st trimester; D if 2nd or 3rd trimester), M] Asthma, cardiogenic shock, cardiac failure, heart block, bradycardia **Supplied:** Tabs 20 mg **Notes/SE:** Flushing, hypotension, fatigue, hyperglycemia, GI upset, sexual dysfunction, bronchospasm

Penciclovir (Denavir) Uses: Herpes simplex (herpes labialis/cold sores) **Action:** Competitive inhibitor of DNA polymerase **Dose:** Apply topically at 1st sign of lesions, then q2h for 4 d **Caution/Contra:** [B, ?/–] **Supplied:** Cream 1% **Notes/SE:** Erythema, HA

Penicillin G, Aqueous (Potassium or Sodium) (Pfizerpen, Pentids) Uses: Most gram+ infections (except staphylococci), including streptococci; *N. meningitidis,* syphilis, clostridia, and anaerobes (except *Bacteroides*) **Action:** Bactericidal; inhibits cell wall synthesis **Dose:** *Adults.* 400,000–800,000 U PO qid; IV doses vary greatly depending on indications; range 0.6–24 MU/d in ÷ doses q4h *Peds. Newborns <1 wk:* 25,000–50,000 U/kg/dose IV q12h. *Infants 1 wk–<1 mon:* 25,000–50,000 U/kg/dose IV q8h. *Children:* 100,000–300,000 U/kg/24 h IV ÷ q4h; ↓ in renal impairment **Caution/Contra:** [B, M] **Supplied:** Tabs 200,000, 250,000, 400,000, 800,000 U; susp 200,000, 400,000 U/5 mL; powder for inj **Notes/SE:** Beware of hypersensitivity reactions; interstitial nephritis, diarrhea, hypersensitivity, seizures

Penicillin G Benzathine (Bicillin) Uses: Useful as a single-dose treatment regimen for streptococcal pharyngitis, rheumatic fever, and glomerulonephritis prophylaxis, and syphilis **Action:** Bactericidal; inhibits cell wall synthesis **Dose:** *Adults.* 1.2–2.4 MU deep IM inj q2–4wk. *Peds.* 50,000 U/kg/dose to a max of 2.4 MU/dose deep IM inj q2–4wk **Caution/Contra:** [B, M] **Supplied:** Inj 300,000, 600,000 U/mL **Notes/SE:** Sustained action with detectable levels up to 4 wk; considered drug of choice for treatment of noncongenital syphilis; Bicillin L-A contains the benzathine salt only; Bicillin C-R contains a combination of benzathine and procaine (300,000 U procaine with 300,000 U benzathine/mL or 900,000 U benzathine with 300,000 U procaine/2 mL); pain at inj site, acute interstitial nephritis, anaphylaxis

Penicillin G Procaine (Wycillin, others) Uses: Moderately severe infections caused by penicillin G-sensitive organisms that respond to low, persistent serum levels **Action:** Bactericidal; inhibits cell wall synthesis **Dose:** *Adults.* 0.6–4.8 MU/d in ÷ doses q12–24h. *Peds.* 25,000–50,000 U/kg/d IM ÷ qd–bid; give probenecid at least 30 min prior to penicillin to prolong action. **Caution/Contra:** [B, M] **Supplied:** Inj 300,000, 500,000, 600,000 U/mL **Notes/SE:** Long-acting parenteral penicillin; blood levels up to 15 h; pain at inj site, interstitial nephritis, anaphylaxis

Penicillin V (Pen-Vee K, Veetids, others) Uses: Most gram+ infections, including streptococci **Action:** Bactericidal; inhibits cell wall synthesis **Dose:** *Adults.* 250–500 mg PO q6h, q8h, q12h. *Peds.* 25–50 mg/kg/24 h PO in 4 ÷ doses; ↓ in severe renal disease; take on empty stomach **Caution/Contra:** [B, M] **Supplied:** Tabs 125, 250, 500 mg; susp 125, 250 mg/5 mL **Notes/SE:** Well-tolerated oral penicillin; 250 mg = 400,000 U of penicillin G; GI upset, interstitial nephritis, anaphylaxis, convulsions

Pentamidine (Pentam 300, NebuPent) Uses: Rx and prevention of PCP **Action:** Inhibits DNA, RNA, phospholipid, and protein synthesis **Dose:** *Adults & Peds.* 4 mg/kg/24 h IV qd for 14–21 d. *Adults & Peds >5 y. Prevention:* 300 mg once q4wk, administered via Respiragard II neb; IV requires ↓ dose in renal impairment. **Caution/Contra:** [C, ?] **Supplied:** Inj 300 mg/vial; aerosol 300 mg **Notes/SE:** Follow CBC (leukopenia and thrombocytopenia); monitor glucose and pancreatic function monthly for the 1st 3 mon; monitor for hypotension following IV administration; associated with pancreatic islet cell necrosis leading to hyperglycemia; chest pain, fatigue, dizziness, rash, GI upset, pancreatitis, renal impairment, blood dyscrasias

Pentazocine (Talwin) [C-IV] Uses: Moderate–severe pain Action: Partial narcotic agonist–antagonist Dose: *Adults.* 30 mg IM or IV; 50–100 mg PO q3–4h PRN. *Peds. 5–8 y:* 15 mg IM q4h PRN. *8–14 y:* 30 mg IM q4h PRN; ↓ dose in renal/hepatic impairment Caution/Contra: [C (1st trimester), D if prolonged use or high doses near term), +/–] Supplied: Tabs 50 mg (+ naloxone 0.5 mg); inj 30 mg/mL Notes/SE: 30–60 mg IM equianalgesic to 10 mg of morphine IM; associated with considerable dysphoria; drowsiness, GI upset, xerostomia, seizures

Pentobarbital (Nembutal, others) [C-II] Uses: Insomnia, convulsions, and induced coma following severe head injury Action: Barbiturate Dose: *Adults. Sedative:* 20–40 mg PO or PR q6–12h. *Hypnotic:* 100–200 mg PO or PR hs PRN. *Induced coma:* Load 5–10 mg/kg IV, then maint 1–3 mg/kg/h IV cont inf to keep the serum level between 20 and 50 mg/mL. *Peds. Hypnotic:* 2–6 mg/kg/dose PO hs PRN. *Induced coma:* See adult dosage Caution/Contra: [D, +/–] Significant hepatic impairment Supplied: Caps 50, 100 mg; elixir 18.2 mg/5 mL (= 20 mg pentobarbital); supp 30, 60, 120, 200 mg; inj 50 mg/mL Notes/SE: Tolerance to sedative-hypnotic effect acquired within 1–2 wk; can cause respiratory depression, hypotension when used aggressively IV for cerebral edema; bradycardia, hypotension, sedation, lethargy, hangover, rash, Stevens–Johnson syndrome, blood dyscrasias, respiratory depression

Pentosan Polysulfate Sodium (Elmiron) Uses: Relief of pain/discomfort associated with interstitial cystitis Action: Acts as buffer on bladder wall Dose: 100 mg PO tid on empty stomach with water 1 h ac or 2 h pc Caution/Contra: [B, ?/–] Supplied: Caps 100 mg Notes/SE: Alopecia, diarrhea, nausea, HAs, ↑ LFTs, anticoagulant effects, thrombocytopenia

Pentostatin (Nipent) WARNING: Fatal, acute pulmonary toxicity with concomitant administration of other chemotherapeutic agents Uses: Hairy cell leukemia, CLL, mycosis fungoides, ALL, and adult T-cell leukemia Action: Irreversible inhibitor of adenosine deaminase Dose: 4–5 mg/m²/wk for 3 consecutive wk; ↓ dose in renal/hepatic impairment Caution/Contra: [D, ?/–] Leukopenia Supplied: Inj 10 mg Notes/SE: Renal dysfunction; myelosuppression (especially leukopenia), lymphocytopenia, fever, and infection possible; neurologic toxicity symptoms (lethargy and fatigue), dry skin, keratoconjunctivitis, N/V

Pentoxifylline (Trental) Uses: Symptomatic management of peripheral vascular disease Action: Lowers blood cell viscosity by restoring erythrocyte flexibility Dose: 400 mg PO tid pc; treat for at least 8 wk to see full effect; ↓ to bid if GI or CNS effects occur Caution/Contra: [C, +/–] Cerebral or retinal hemorrhage Supplied: Tabs 400 mg Notes/SE: Dizziness, HA, GI upset

Pergolide (Permax) Uses: Parkinson's disease Action: Centrally active dopamine receptor agonist Dose: Initially, 0.05 mg PO tid, titrated q2–3d to desired effect; usual maint 2–3 mg/d in ÷ doses Caution/Contra: [B, ?/–] Ergot sensitivity Supplied: Tabs 0.05, 0.25, 1.0 mg Notes/SE: May cause hypotension during initiation of therapy; dizziness, somnolence, confusion, nausea, constipation, dyskinesia, rhinitis, MI

Perindopril Erbumine (Aceon) Uses: HTN, CHF, DN, post-MI Action: ACE inhibitor Dose: 4–8 mg/d; avoid taking with food; ↓ dose in elderly/renal impairment Caution/Contra: [C (1st trimester), D (2nd and 3rd trimesters), ?/–] ACE-inhibitor-induced angioedema, bilateral renal artery stenosis, primary hyperaldosteronism Supplied: Tabs 2, 4, 8 mg Notes/SE: HA, hypotension, dizziness, GI upset, cough

Permethrin (Nix, Elimite) Uses: Eradication of lice and scabies Action: Pediculicide Dose: *Adults & Peds.* Saturate hair and scalp; allow 10 min before rinsing Caution/Contra: [B, ?/–] Supplied: Topical liq 1%; cream 5% Notes/SE: Local irritation

Perphenazine (Trilafon) Uses: Psychotic disorders, intractable hiccups, severe nausea Action: Phenothiazine; blocks dopaminergic receptors in the brain Dose: *Adults. Antipsychotic:* 4–16 mg PO tid; max 64 mg/d. *Hiccups:* 5 mg IM q6h PRN or 1 mg IV at intervals not <1–2 mg/min to a max of 5 mg. *Peds. 1–6 y:* 4–6 mg/d in ÷ doses. *6–12 y:* 6 mg/d in ÷ doses. *>12 y:* 4–16 mg 2–4×/d; ↓ dose in hepatic insufficiency Caution/Contra: [C, ?/–] Phenothiazine sensitivity, narrow-angle glaucoma, bone marrow depression, severe liver or cardiac disease; severe hyper-/hypotension Supplied: Tabs 2, 4, 8, 16 mg; oral conc 16 mg/5 mL; inj 5 mg/mL Notes/SE: Hypotension, tachycardia, bradycardia, extrapyramidal symptoms, drowsiness, seizures, photosensitivity, skin discoloration, blood dyscrasias, constipation

22

Phenazopyridine (Pyridium, others) Uses: Lower urinary tract irritation **Action:** Local anesthetic on urinary tract mucosa **Dose:** *Adults.* 100–200 mg PO tid. *Peds 6–12 y.* 12 mg/kg/24 h PO in 3 ÷ doses; ↓ in renal insufficiency **Caution/Contra:** [B, ?] Renal/hepatic disease **Supplied:** Tabs 100, 200 mg **Notes/SE:** GI disturbances; causes red-orange urine color, which can stain clothing; HA, dizziness, acute renal failure, methemoglobinemia

Phenelzine (Nardil) Uses: Depression **Action:** MAOI **Dose:** *Adults.* 15 mg tid. *Elderly:* 15–60 mg/d in ÷ doses; avoid tyramine-containing foods **Caution/Contra:** [C, –] Interactions with SSRI, ergots, tripans **Supplied:** Tabs 15 mg **Notes/SE:** May cause orthostatic hypotension; edema, dizziness, sedation, rash, sexual dysfunction, xerostomia, constipation, urinary retention; may take 2–4 wk to see therapeutic effect

Phenobarbital [C-IV] Uses: Seizure disorders, insomnia, and anxiety **Action:** Barbiturate **Dose:** *Adults. Sedative-hypnotic:* 30–120 mg/d PO or IM PRN. *Anticonvulsant:* Loading dose of 10–12 mg/kg in 3 ÷ doses, then 1–3 mg/kg/24 h PO, IM, or IV. *Peds. Sedative-hypnotic:* 2–3 mg/kg/24 h PO or IM hs PRN. *Anticonvulsant:* Loading dose of 15–20 mg/kg ÷ into 2 equal doses 4 h apart, then 3–5 mg/kg/24 h PO ÷ in 2–3 doses **Caution/Contra:** [D, M] Porphyria **Supplied:** Tabs 8, 15, 16, 30, 32, 60, 65, 100 mg; elixir 15, 20 mg/5 mL; inj 30, 60, 65, 130 mg/mL **Notes/SE:** Tolerance develops to sedation; paradoxic hyperactivity seen in pediatric patients; long half-life allows single daily dosing (Table 2, page 607); bradycardia, hypotension, hangover, Stevens–Johnson syndrome, blood dyscrasias, respiratory depression

Phenylephrine (Neo-Synephrine) Uses: Vascular failure in shock, hypersensitivity, or drug-induced hypotension; nasal congestion; mydriatic **Action:** α-Adrenergic agonist **Dose:** *Adults. Mild–moderate hypotension:* 2–5 mg IM or SC elevates BP for 2 h; 0.1–0.5 mg IV elevates BP for 15 min. *Severe hypotension/shock:* Initiate cont inf 100–180 mg/min; after BP is stabilized, maint rate of 40–60 mg/min. *Nasal congestion:* 1–2 sprays/nostril PRN. *Ophth:* 1 gt 15–30 min before exam. *Peds. Hypotension:* 5–20 mcg/kg/dose IV q10–15min or 0.1–0.5 mg/kg/min IV inf, titrated to desired effect. *Nasal congestion:* 1 spray/nostril q3–4h PRN **Caution/Contra:** [C, +/–] HTN, bradycardia, arrhythmias, acute pancreatitis, hepatitis, coronary disease, narrow-angle glaucoma **Supplied:** Inj 10 mg/mL; nasal soln 0.125, 0.16, 0.25, 0.5, 1%; ophth soln 0.12, 2.5, 10% **Notes/SE:** Promptly restore blood volume if loss has occurred; use large veins for inf to avoid extravasation; phentolamine 10 mg in 10–15 mL of NS for local inj as antidote for extravasation; arrhythmias, HTN, peripheral vasoconstriction activity potentiated by oxytocin, MAOIs, and TCAs; HA, weakness, necrosis, ↓ renal perfusion

Phenytoin (Dilantin) Uses: Seizure disorders **Action:** Inhibits seizure spread in the motor cortex **Dose:** *Adults & Peds. Load:* 15–20 mg/kg IV, max inf rate 25 mg/min or PO in 400-mg doses at 4-h intervals. *Adults. Maint:* Initially, 200 mg PO or IV bid or 300 mg hs; then follow serum conc. *Peds. Maint:* 4–7 mg/kg/24 h PO or IV ÷ qd–bid; avoid oral susp if possible due to erratic absorption **Caution/Contra:** [D, +] Heart block, sinus bradycardia **Supplied:** Caps 30, 100 mg; chew tabs 50 mg; oral susp 30, 125 mg/5 mL; inj 50 mg/mL **Notes/SE:** Follow levels (Table 2, page 607); note: Phenytoin is bound to albumin, and levels reflect both bound and free phenytoin; in the presence of ↓ albumin and azotemia, low phenytoin levels may be therapeutic (normal free levels); nystagmus and ataxia early signs of toxicity; gum hyperplasia with long-term use. *IV:* Hypotension, bradycardia, arrhythmias, phlebitis; peripheral neuropathy, rash, blood dyscrasias, Stevens–Johnson syndrome

Physostigmine (Antilirium) Uses: Antidote for TCA, atropine, and scopolamine overdose; glaucoma **Action:** Reversible cholinesterase inhibitor **Dose:** *Adults.* 2 mg IV or IM q20min. *Peds.* 0.01–0.03 mg/kg/dose IV q15–30min to total of 2 mg if necessary **Caution/Contra:** [C, ?] GI or GU obstruction **Supplied:** Inj 1 mg/mL; ophth oint 0.25% **Notes/SE:** Rapid IV administration associated with convulsions; cholinergic side effects; may cause asystole sweating, salivation, lacrimation, GI upset, changes in heart rate

Phytonadione [Vitamin K] (AquaMEPHYTON, others) Uses: Coagulation disorders caused by faulty formation of factors II, VII, IX, and X; hyperalimentation **Action:** Needed for the production of factors II, VII, IX, and X **Dose:** *Children and Adults. Anticoagulant-induced prothrombin deficiency:* 1.0–10.0 mg PO or IV slowly. *Hyperalimentation:* 10 mg IM or IV qwk. *Infants.* 0.5–1.0 mg/dose IM, SC, or PO **Caution/Contra:** [C, +] **Supplied:** Tabs 5 mg; inj 2, 10 mg/mL **Notes/SE:** With parenteral Rx, the 1st change in prothrombin usually seen in 12–24 h; anaphylaxis can result from IV dosage; administer IV slowly; GI upset (oral), inj site reactions

Pimecrolimus (Elidel) Uses: Atopic dermatitis **Action:** T-lymphocyte inhibition **Dose:** Apply bid for at least 1 wk following resolution; apply to dry skin only; wash hands after **Caution/Contra:** [C, ?/–] Caution with local infection, lymphadenopathy **Supplied:** Ointment 0.03%, 0.1%: 30-g, 60-g tubes **Notes/SE:** Phototoxicity, local irritation/burning, flu-like symptoms

Pindolol (Visken) Uses: HTN **Action:** Competitively blocks β-adrenergic receptors, β_1, β_2, ISA **Dose:** 5–10 mg bid, 60 mg/d max; ↓ dose in hepatic/renal failure **Caution/ Contra:** [B (1st trimester); D if 2nd or 3rd trimester), +/–] Uncompensated CHF, cardiogenic shock, bradycardia, heart block, asthma, COPD **Supplied:** Tabs 5, 10 mg **Notes/SE:** Insomnia, dizziness, fatigue, edema, GI upset, dyspnea, fluid retention may exacerbate CHF

Pioglitazone (Actos) Uses: Type 2 DM **Action:** Increases insulin sensitivity **Dose:** 15–45 mg/d **Caution/Contra:** [C, –] Contra in hepatic impairment **Supplied:** Tabs 15, 30, 45 mg **Notes/SE:** Weight gain, URI, HA, hypoglycemia, edema

Pipecuronium (Arduan) Uses: Adjunct to general anesthesia **Action:** Nondepolarizing neuromuscular blocker **Dose:** *Adults & Peds.* 0.05–0.085 mg/kg initially, then 0.5–2 mcg/kg/min (ICU); ↓ dose in renal failure **Supplied:** Inj 10 mg; **Caution/Contra:** [C, ?] **Notes/SE:** Hypotension, bradycardia

Piperacillin (Pipracil) Uses: Infections caused by gram– bacteria (including *Klebsiella, Proteus, E. coli, Enterobacter, P. aeruginosa,* and *Serratia*) of skin, bone, respiratory tract, urinary tract, and abdomen, and septicemia **Action:** Bactericidal; inhibits cell wall synthesis **Dose:** *Adults.* 3 g IV q4–6h. *Peds.* 200–300 mg/kg/d IV ÷ q4–6h; ↓ dose in renal failure **Caution/Contra:** [B, M] Penicillin sensitivity **Supplied:** Inj **Notes/SE:** Often used in combination with aminoglycoside; ↓ platelet aggregation, interstitial nephritis, renal failure, anaphylaxis, hemolytic anemia

Piperacillin-Tazobactam (Zosyn) Uses: Infections caused by gram– bacteria (including *Klebsiella, Proteus, E. coli, Enterobacter, P. aeruginosa,* and *Serratia*) involving skin, bone, respiratory tract, urinary tract, and abdomen, and septicemia **Action:** Bactericidal; inhibits cell wall synthesis **Dose:** *Adults.* 3.375–4.5 g IV q6h; ↓ dose in renal failure **Caution/Contra:** [B, M] Penicillin or β-lactam sensitivity **Supplied:** Inj **Notes/SE:** Often used in combination with aminoglycoside; diarrhea, HA, insomnia, GI upset, serum sickness-like reaction, pseudomembranous colitis

Pirbuterol (Maxair) Uses: Prevention and Rx of reversible bronchospasm **Action:** β_2-Adrenergic agonists **Dose:** *Adults & Peds >12 y.* 2 inhal q4–6h; max 12 inhal/d **Caution/Contra:** [C, ?/–] **Supplied:** Aerosol 0.2 mg/actuation; Autohaler dry powder 0.2 mg/actuation **Notes/SE:** Nervousness, restlessness, trembling, HA, taste changes, tachycardia

Piroxicam (Feldene) Uses: Arthritis and pain **Action:** NSAID; inhibits prostaglandin synthesis **Dose:** 10–20 mg/d **Caution/Contra:** [B (1st trimester); D if 3rd trimester or near term), +] GI bleeding, ASA or NSAID sensitivity **Supplied:** Caps 10, 20 mg **Notes/SE:** Dizziness, rash, GI upset, edema, acute renal failure, peptic ulcer

Plasma Protein Fraction (Plasmanate, others) Uses: Shock and hypotension **Action:** Plasma volume expansion **Dose:** *Adults.* Initially, 250–500 mL IV (not >10 mL/min); subsequent inf depends on clinical response. *Peds.* 10–15 mL/kg/dose IV; subsequent inf depend on clinical response **Caution/Contra:** [C, +] **Supplied:** Inj 5% **Notes/SE:** 130–160 mEq Na/L; not substitute for RBC; hypotension associated with rapid inf; hypocoagulability, metabolic acidosis, PE

Plicamycin (Mithracin) Uses: Hypercalcemia of malignancy; disseminated embryonal cell carcinoma or germ cell tumors of the testis **Action:** Antibiotic; binds to the outside of the DNA molecule, interrupting DNA-directed RNA synthesis, DNA intercalation **Dose:** *Hypercalcemia:* 25 mcg/kg/d IV qod for 3–8 doses. *CA:* 25–30 mcg/kg/d for 8–10 d; ↓ dose in renal failure **Caution/Contra:** [D, ?] Thrombocytopenia, coagulation disorders, bone marrow impairment **Supplied:** Inj **Notes/SE:** Thrombocytopenia; drug-induced deficiency of clotting factors II, V, VII, and X, resulting in bleeding and bruising

Pneumococcal Vaccine, Polyvalent (Pneumovax-23) Uses: Immunization against pneumococcal infections in patients predisposed to or at high risk **Action:** Active immunization **Dose:** *Adults & Peds >2 y.* 0.5 mL IM **Caution/Contra:** [C, M] Do not vaccinate during immunosuppressive therapy, active infection, Hodgkin's disease, children <5 y. **Supplied:** Inj 25 mg each of polysaccharide isolates/0.5-mL dose **Notes/SE:** Local reactions, arthralgia, fever, myalgia

Pneumococcal 7-Valent Conjugate Vaccine (Prevnar) **Uses:** Immunization against pneumococcal infections in infants and children **Action:** Active immunization **Dose:** 0.5 mL IM/dose; series of 3 doses; 1st dose at 2 mon of age with subsequent doses q2mon **Caution/Contra:** [C, +] Diphtheria toxoid sensitivity, febrile illness, thrombocytopenia **Supplied:** Inj **Notes/SE:** Local reactions, arthralgia, fever, myalgia

Podophyllin (Podocon-25, Condylox Gel 0.5%, Condylox) **Uses:** Topical therapy of benign growths (genital and perianal warts [condylomata acuminata], papillomas, fibroids) **Action:** Direct antimitotic effect; exact mechanism unknown **Dose:** Condylox gel and Condylox: apply 3 consecutive d/wk for 4 wk. Use Podocon-25 sparingly on the lesion, leave on for 1–4 h, then thoroughly wash off **Caution/Contra:** [C, ?] DM, bleeding lesions, immunocompromise **Supplied:** Podocon-25 (w/benzoin) 15-mL bottles; Condylox gel 0.5% 35 g clear gel; Condylox soln 0.5% 35 g clear **Notes/SE:** Podocon-25 applied only by the clinician; do not dispense; local reactions, significant absorption; anemias, tachycardia, paresthesias, GI upset, renal/hepatic damage

Polyethylene Glycol [PEG]-Electrolyte Solution (GoLYTELY, CoLyte) **Uses:** Bowel prep prior to examination or surgery **Action:** Osmotic cathartic **Dose:** *Adults.* Following 3–4-h fast, drink 240 mL of soln q10min until 4 L is consumed. *Peds.* 25–40 mL/kg/h for 4–10 h **Caution/Contra:** [C, ?] GI obstruction, bowel perforation, megacolon, ulcerative colitis **Notes/SE:** Powder for reconstitution to 4 L in container **Notes/SE:** 1st BM should occur in approximately 1 h; cramping or nausea, bloating

Polymyxin B and Hydrocortisone (Otobiotic Otic) **Uses:** Superficial bacterial infections of external ear canal **Action:** Antibiotic antiinflammatory combination **Dose:** 4 gtt in ear(s) tid–qid **Caution/Contra:** [B, ?] **Supplied:** Soln polymyxin B 10,000 U/hydrocortisone 0.5%/mL **Notes/SE:** Useful in neomycin allergy, local irritation

Potassium Citrate (Urocit-K) **Uses:** Alkalinize urine, prevention of urinary stones (uric acid, Ca stones if hypocitraturic) **Action:** Urinary alkalinizer **Caution/Contra:** [A, +] Severe renal impairment, dehydration, hyperkalemia, peptic ulcer; use of K-sparing diuretics or salt substitutes **Dose:** 10–20 mEq PO tid with meals, max 100 mEq/d **Notes/SE:** Tabs 540 mg = 5 mEq, 1080 mg = 10 mEq; GI upset, hypocalcemia, hyperkalemia, metabolic alkalosis

Potassium Citrate and Citric Acid (Polycitra-K) **Uses:** Alkalinize urine, prevention of urinary stones (uric acid, Ca stones if hypocitraturic) **Action:** Urinary alkalinizer **Dose:** 10–20 mEq PO tid with meals, max 100 mEq/d **Caution/Contra:** [A, +] Severe renal impairment, dehydration, hyperkalemia, peptic ulcer; use of K-sparing diuretics or salt substitutes **Notes/SE:** Soln 10 mEq/5 mL; powder 30 mEq/packet; GI upset, hypocalcemia, hyperkalemia, metabolic alkalosis

Potassium Iodide [Lugol's Solution] (SSKI, Thyro-Block) **Uses:** Thyroid storm, reduction of vascularity before thyroid surgery, block thyroid uptake of radioactive isotopes of iodine, thin bronchial secretions **Action:** Iodine supplement **Dose:** *Adults & Peds. Preop thyroidectomy:* 50–250 mg PO tid (2–6 gtt strong iodine soln); administer 10 d preop. *Peds 1 y: Thyroid crisis:* 300 mg (6 gtt SSKI q8h). *<1 y:* ½ adult dose **Caution/Contra:** [D, +] Iodine sensitivity, hyperkalemia, tuberculosis, PE, bronchitis, renal impairment **Supplied:** Tabs 130 mg; soln (SSKI) 1 g/mL; Lugol's soln, strong iodine 100 mg/mL; syrup 325 mg/5 mL **Notes/SE:** Fever, HA, urticaria, angioedema, goiter, GI upset, eosinophilia

Potassium Supplements (Kaon, Kaochlor, K-Lor, Slow-K, Micro-K, Klorvess, others) **Uses:** Prevention or Rx of hypokalemia (often related to diuretic use) **Action:** Supplementation of K **Dose:** *Adults.* 20–100 mEq/d PO ÷ qd–bid; IV 10–20 mEq/h, max 40 mEq/h and 150 mEq/d (monitor frequent K levels when using high-dose IV infs). *Peds.* Calculate K deficit; 1–3 mEq/kg/d PO ÷ qd–qid; IV max dose 0.5–1 mEq/kg/h **Caution/Contra:** [A, +] Use cautiously in renal insufficiency as well as with NSAIDs and ACE inhibitors **Supplied:** Oral forms (Table 8, page 620); injectable forms **Notes/SE:** Can cause GI irritation; mix powder and liq with beverage (unsalted tomato juice, etc); follow serum K⁺; Cl⁻ salt recommended in coexisting alkalosis; for coexisting acidosis use acetate, bicarbonate, citrate, or gluconate salt; bradycardia, hyperkalemia, heart block

Pramipexole (Mirapex) Uses: Parkinson's disease **Action:** Dopamine agonist **Dose:** 1.5–4.5 mg/d, beginning with 0.375 mg/d in 3 ÷ doses; titrate dosage slowly **Caution/Contra:** [C, ?/–] **Supplied:** Tabs 0.125, 0.25, 1, 1.5 mg **Notes/SE:** Orthostatic hypotension, asthenia, somnolence, abnormal dreams, GI upset, EPS

Pramoxine (Anusol Ointment, Proctofoam-NS, others) Uses: Relief of pain and itching from external and internal hemorrhoids and anorectal surgery; topical for burns and dermatosis **Action:** Topical anesthetic **Dose:** Apply cream, oint, gel, or spray freely to anal area q3h **Caution/Contra:** [C, ?] **Supplied:** [OTC] All 1%; foam (Proctofoam NS), cream, oint, lotion, gel, pads, spray **Notes/SE:** Contact dermatitis

Pramoxine + Hydrocortisone (Enzone, Proctofoam-HC) Uses: Relief of pain and itching from hemorrhoids **Action:** Topical anesthetic, antiinflammatory **Dose:** Apply freely to anal area tid–qid **Caution/Contra:** [C, ?/–] **Supplied:** Cream pramoxine 1% acetate 0.5/1%; foam pramoxine 1% hydrocortisone 1%; lotion pramoxine 1% hydrocortisone 0.25/1/2.5%, pramoxine 2.5% and hydrocortisone 1% **Notes/SE:** Contact dermatitis

Pravastatin (Pravachol) Uses: Reduction of ↑ cholesterol levels **Action:** HMG-CoA reductase inhibitor **Dose:** 10–40 mg PO hs; ↓ dose with significant renal/hepatic insufficiency **Caution/Contra:** [X, –] Liver disease or persistent LFT ↑ **Supplied:** Tabs 10, 20, 40 mg **Notes/SE:** Use caution with concurrent gemfibrozil; HA, GI upset, hepatitis, myopathy, renal failure

Prazosin (Minipress) Uses: HTN **Action:** Peripherally acting α-adrenergic blocker **Dose:** *Adults.* 1 mg PO tid; can ↑ to max daily dose of up to 20 mg/d. *Peds.* 5–25 mcg/kg/dose q6h, up to 25 mcg/kg/dose **Caution/Contra:** [C, ?] **Supplied:** Caps 1, 2, 5 mg **Notes/SE:** Can cause orthostatic hypotension, take the 1st dose hs; tolerance develops to this effect; tachyphylaxis may result; dizziness, edema, palpitations, fatigue, GI upset

Prednisolone See Steroids, systemic, page 612 and topical, page 613

Prednisone See Steroids, systemic, page 612 and topical, page 613

Probenecid (Benemid, others) Uses: Prevention of gout and hyperuricemia; prolongs serum levels of penicillins or cephalosporins **Action:** Renal tube blocking agent **Dose:** *Adults. Gout:* 250 mg bid for? 1 wk, then 0.5 g PO bid; can ↑ by 500 mg/mon up to 2–3 g/d. *Antibiotic effect:* 1–2 g PO 30 min before antibiotic dose. *Peds >2 y.* 25 mg/kg, then 40 mg/kg/d PO ÷ qid **Caution/Contra:** [B, ?] High-dose ASA, moderate/severe renal impairment, age <2 y **Supplied:** Tabs 500 mg **Notes/SE:** Do not use during acute gout attack; HA, GI upset, rash, pruritus, dizziness, blood dyscrasias

Procainamide (Pronestyl, Procan) Uses: Supraventricular and ventricular arrhythmias **Action:** Class 1A antiarrhythmic **Dose:** *Adults. Recurrent VF/VT:* 20 mg/min IV (max total 17 mg/kg). *Maint:* 1–4 mg/min. *Stable wide-complex tachycardia of unknown origin, AF with rapid rate in WPW syndrome:* 20 mg/min IV until arrhythmia suppression, hypotension, QRS widens >50%, then 1–4 mg/min. *Chronic dosing:* 50 mg/kg/d PO in ÷ doses q4–6h. *Peds. Chronic maint:* 15–50 mg/kg/24 h PO ÷ q3–6h; ↓ dose in renal/hepatic impairment **Caution/Contra:** [C, +] CHB, 2nd- or 3rd-degree heart block w/o pacemaker, torsades de pointes, SLE **Supplied:** Tabs and caps 250, 375, 500 mg; SR tabs 250, 500, 750, 1000 mg; inj 100, 500 mg/mL **Notes/SE:** Follow levels (Table 22–2, page 607); can cause hypotension and a lupus-like syndrome; GI upset, taste perversion, arrhythmias, tachycardia, heart block, angioneurotic edema

Procarbazine (Matulane) **WARNING: Highly toxic; handle with care** Uses: Hodgkin's disease, NHL, brain tumors **Action:** Alkylating agent; inhibits DNA and RNA synthesis **Dose:** 2–4 mg/kg/d ×7 d, then 4–6 mg/kg/d until response; maint 1–2 mg/kg/d/ in combination, 60–100 mg/m²/d ×10–14 d **Caution/Contra:** [D, ?] Alcohol ingestion **Supplied:** Caps 50 mg **Notes/SE:** Myelosuppression, hemolytic reactions (with G6PD deficiency), N/V/D; disulfiram-like reaction; cutaneous reactions; constitutional symptoms, myalgia, and arthralgia; CNS effects, azoospermia, and cessation of menses

22

Prochlorperazine (Compazine) Uses: N/V, agitation, and psychotic disorders **Action:** Phenothiazine; blocks postsynaptic dopaminergic CNS receptors **Dose:** *Adults. Antiemetic:* 5–10 mg PO tid–qid or 25 mg PR bid or 5–10 mg deep IM q4–6h. *Antipsychotic:* 10–20 mg IM acutely or 5–10 mg PO tid–qid for maint. *Peds.* 0.1–0.15 mg/kg/dose IM q4–6h or 0.4 mg/kg/24 h PO ÷ tid–qid; ↑ doses may be required for antipsychotic effect **Caution/Contra:** [C, +/–] Phenothiazine sensitivity, narrow-angle glaucoma, bone marrow suppression, severe liver/cardiac disease **Supplied:** Tabs 5, 10, 25 mg; SR caps 10, 15, 30 mg; syrup 5 mg/5 mL; supp 2.5, 5, 25 mg; inj 5 mg/mL **Notes/SE:** Extrapyramidal side effects common; treat with diphenhydramine

Procyclidine (Kemadrin) Uses: Parkinson's syndrome **Action:** Blocks excess acetylcholine **Dose:** 2.5 mg PO tid, up to 20 mg/d **Caution/Contra:** [C, ?] Contra in glaucoma **Supplied:** Tabs 5 mg **Notes/SE:** Anticholinergic side effects

Promethazine (Phenergan) Uses: N/V, motion sickness **Action:** Phenothiazine; blocks postsynaptic mesolimbic dopaminergic receptors in the brain **Dose:** *Adults.* 12.5–50 mg PO, PR, or IM bid–qid PRN. *Peds.* 0.1–0.5 mg/kg/dose PO or IM q12–6h PRN **Caution/Contra:** [C, +/–] **Supplied:** Tabs 12.5, 25, 50 mg; syrup 6.25 mg/5 mL, 25 mg/5 mL; supp 12.5, 25, 50 mg; inj 25, 50 mg/mL **Notes/SE:** Drowsiness, tardive dyskinesia, EPS, lowered seizure threshold, hypotension, GI upset, blood dyscrasias, photosensitivity

Propafenone (Rythmol) Uses: Life-threatening ventricular arrhythmias and AF **Action:** Class IC antiarrhythmic **Dose:** 150–300 mg PO q8h **Caution/Contra:** [C, ?] Uncontrolled CHF, bronchospasm, cardiogenic shock, conduction disorders, amprenavir or ritonavir use **Supplied:** Tabs 150, 225, 300 mg **Notes/SE:** Dizziness, unusual taste, 1st-degree heart block, arrhythmias, prolongation of QRS and QT intervals; fatigue, GI upset, blood dyscrasias

Propantheline (Pro-Banthine) Uses: Symptomatic treatment of small intestine hypermotility, spastic colon, ureteral spasm, bladder spasm, pylorospasm **Action:** Antimuscarinic agent **Dose:** *Adults.* 15 mg PO ac and 30 mg PO hs. *Peds.* 1–3 mg/kg/24 h PO ÷ tid–qid; ↓ dose in elderly **Caution/Contra:** [C, ?] Narrow-angle glaucoma, ulcerative colitis, toxic megacolon, GI or GU obstruction **Supplied:** Tabs 7.5, 15 mg **Notes/SE:** Anticholinergic side effects (xerostomia and blurred vision common)

Propofol (Diprivan) Uses: Induction or maint of anesthesia; continuous sedation in intubated patients **Action:** Sedative hypnotic; mechanism unknown **Dose:** *Adults. Anesthesia:* 2–2.5 mg/kg induction, then 0.1–0.2 mg/kg/min inf. *ICU sedation:* 5–50 mcg/kg/min cont inf. *Peds. Anesthesia:* 2.5–3.5 mg/kg induction, then 125–300 mcg/kg/min; ↓ dose in elderly, debilitated, or ASA II or IV patients **Caution/Contra:** [B, +] **Supplied:** Inj 10 mg/mL **Notes/SE:** 1 mL of propofol contains 0.1 g fat; may ↑ triglycerides with extended dosing; hypotension, pain at inj site, apnea, anaphylaxis

Propoxyphene (Darvon), Propoxyphene and Acetaminophen (Darvocet), and Propoxyphene and Aspirin (Darvon Compound-65, Darvon-N + Aspirin) [C-IV] Uses: Mild–moderate pain **Action:** Narcotic analgesic **Dose:** 1–2 PO q4h PRN; ↓ dose in hepatic impairment, elderly **Caution/Contra:** [C (D if prolonged use), M] Hepatic impairment (APAP), peptic ulcer (ASA); severe renal impairment **Supplied:** *Darvon:* Propoxyphene HCl caps 65 mg. *Darvon-N:* Propoxyphene napsylate 100-mg tabs. *Darvocet-N:* Propoxyphene napsylate 50 mg/APAP 325 mg. *Darvocet-N 100:* Propoxyphene napsylate 100 mg/APAP 650 mg. *Darvon Compound-65:* Propoxyphene HCl 65-mg/ASA 389-mg/caffeine 32-mg caps. *Darvon-N with ASA:* Propoxyphene napsylate 100 mg/ASA 325 mg **Notes/SE:** Overdose can be lethal; hypotension, dizziness, sedation, GI upset, ↑ levels on LFTs

Propranolol (Inderal) Uses: HTN, angina, MI, hyperthyroidism; prevents migraines and atrial arrhythmias **Action:** Competitively blocks β-adrenergic receptors, $β_1$, $β_2$; only β-blocker to block conversion of T_4 to T_3 **Dose:** *Adults. Angina:* 80–320 mg/d PO ÷ bid–qid or 80–160 mg/d SR. *Arrhythmia:* 10–80 mg PO tid–qid or 1 mg IV slowly, repeat q5min up to 5 mg. *HTN:* 40 mg PO bid or 60–80 mg/d SR, ↑ weekly to max 640 mg/d. *Hypertrophic subaortic stenosis:* 20–40 mg PO tid–qid. *MI:* 180–240 mg PO ÷ tid–qid. *Migraine prophylaxis:* 80 mg/d ÷ qid–tid, ↑ weekly to max 160–240 mg/d ÷ tid–qid; wean off if no response in 6 wk. *Pheochromocytoma:* 30–60 mg/d ÷ tid–qid. *Thyrotoxicosis:* 1–3 mg IV single dose; 10–40 mg PO q6h. *Tremor:* 40 mg PO bid, ↑ as needed to max 320 mg/d. *Peds. Arrhythmia:* 0.5–1.0 mg/kg/d ÷ tid–qid, ↑ as needed q3–7d to max 60 mg/d; 0.01–0.1 mg/kg IV over

10 min, max dose 1 mg. *HTN:* 0.5–1.0 mg/kg ÷ bid–qid, ↑ as needed q3–7d to 2 mg/kg/d max; ↓ dose in renal impairment **Caution/Contra:** [C (1st trimester, D if 2nd or 3rd trimester), +] Uncompensated CHF, cardiogenic shock, bradycardia, heart block, PE, severe respiratory disease **Supplied:** Tabs 10, 20, 40, 60, 80 mg; SR caps 60, 80, 120, 160 mg; oral soln 4, 8 mg/mL, 80 mg/mL; inj 1 mg/mL **Notes/SE:** Bradycardia, hypotension, fatigue, GI upset, erectile dysfunction, hypoglycemia

Propylthiouracil [PTU] Uses: Hyperthyroidism **Action:** Inhibits production of T_3 and T_4 and conversion of T_4 to T_3 **Dose:** *Adults. Initial:* 100 mg PO q8h (may need up to 1200 mg/d); after patient euthyroid (6–8 wk), taper dose by ½ q4–6wk to maint: 50–150 mg/24 h; can usually be DC in 2–3 y. *Peds. Initial:* 5–7 mg/kg/24 h PO ÷ q8h. *Maint:* 1/3–2/3 of initial dose; ↓ dose in elderly **Caution/Contra:** [D, –] **Supplied:** Tabs 50 mg **Notes/SE:** Monitor patient clinically; monitor TFT, fever, rash, leukopenia, dizziness, GI upset, taste perversion, SLE-like syndrome

Protamine (Generic) Uses: Reversal of heparin effect **Action:** Neutralizes heparin by forming a stable complex **Dose:** *Adults & Peds.* Based on amount of heparin reversal desired; give IV slowly; 1 mg reverses approximately 100 U of heparin given in the preceding 3–4 h, 50 mg max dose **Caution/Contra:** [C, ?] **Supplied:** Inj 10 mg/mL **Notes/SE:** Follow coagulation studies; may have anticoagulant effect if given without heparin; hypotension, bradycardia, dyspnea, hemorrhage

Pseudoephedrine (Sudafed, Novafed, Afrinol, others) Uses: Decongestant **Action:** Stimulates α-adrenergic receptors, resulting in vasoconstriction **Dose:** *Adults.* 30–60 mg PO q6–8h; SR caps 120 mg PO q12h. *Peds.* 4 mg/kg/24 h PO ÷ qid **Caution/Contra:** [C, +] Contra in poorly controlled HTN or CAD disease and in MAOIs **Supplied:** Tabs 30, 60 mg; caps 60 mg; SR tabs 120, 240 mg; SR caps 120 mg; liq 7.5 mg/0.8 mL, 15, 30 mg/5 mL; ↓ dose in renal insufficiency **Notes/SE:** Ingredient in many cough and cold preparations; HTN, insomnia, tachycardia, arrhythmias, nervousness, tremor

Psyllium (Metamucil, Serutan, Effer-Syllium) Uses: Constipation and diverticular disease of the colon **Action:** Bulk laxative **Dose:** 1 tsp (7 g) in a glass of water qd–tid **Caution/Contra:** [B, ?] Do not use if suspected bowel obstruction; psyllium in effervescent (Effer-Syllium) form usually contains K^+; use caution in patients with renal failure; phenylketonuria (in products with aspartame) **Supplied:** Granules 4, 25 g/tsp; powder 3.5 g/packet **Notes/SE:** Diarrhea, abdominal cramps, bowel obstruction, constipation, bronchospasm

Pyrazinamide (Generic) Uses: Active TB in combination with other agents **Action:** Bacteriostatic; mechanism unknown **Dose:** *Adults.* 15–30 mg/kg/24 h PO ÷ tid–qid; max 2 g/d. *Peds.* 15–30 mg/kg/d PO ÷ qd–bid; dosage regimen differs for directly observed therapy; ↓ dose for renal/hepatic impairment **Caution/ Contra:** [C, +/–] Severe hepatic damage, acute gout **Supplied:** Tabs 500 mg **Notes/SE:** Use in combination with other anti-TB drugs; consult *MMWR* for the latest TB recommendations; hepatotoxicity, malaise, GI upset, arthralgia, myalgia, gout, photosensitivity

Pyridoxine [Vitamin B_6] Uses: Rx and prevention of vitamin B_6 deficiency **Action:** Supplementation of vitamin B_6 **Dose:** *Adults. Deficiency:* 10–20 mg/d PO. *Drug-induced neuritis:* 100–200 mg/d; 25–100 mg/d prophylaxis. *Peds.* 5–25 mg/d ×3 wk **Caution/ Contra:** [A (C if doses exceed RDA), +] **Supplied:** Tabs 25, 50, 100 mg; inj 100 mg/mL **Notes/SE:** Allergic reactions, HA, nausea

Quazepam (Doral) [C-IV] Uses: Insomnia **Action:** Benzodiazepine **Dose:** 7.5–15 mg PO hs PRN; ↓ dose in the elderly, hepatic failure **Caution/Contra:** [X, ?/–] Narrow-angle glaucoma **Supplied:** Tabs 7.5, 15 mg **Notes/SE:** Do not DC abruptly; sedation, hangover, somnolence, respiratory depression

Quetiapine (Seroquel) Uses: Acute exacerbations of schizophrenia **Action:** Serotonin and dopamine antagonism **Dose:** 150–750 mg/d; initiate at 25–100 mg bid–tid; slowly ↑ dose; ↓ dose for hepatic and geriatric patients **Caution/Contra:** [C, –] **Supplied:** Tabs 25, 100, 200 mg **Notes/SE:** Multiple reports of confusion with Serzone (nefazodone); HA, somnolence, weight gain, orthostatic hypotension, dizziness, cataracts, neuroleptic malignant syndrome, tardive dyskinesia, QT prolongation

Quinapril (Accupril) Uses: HTN, CHF, DN, post-MI **Action:** ACE inhibitor **Dose:** 10–80 mg PO qd in a single dose; ↓ dose in renal impairment **Caution/Contra:** [D, +] ACE

22

inhibitor sensitivity or angioedema **Supplied:** Tabs 5, 10, 20, 40 mg **Notes/SE:** Dizziness, HA, hypotension, impaired renal function, angioedema, taste perversion, cough

Quinidine (Quinidex, Quinaglute) **Uses:** Prevention of tachydysrhythmias **Action:** Class 1A antiarrhythmic **Dose:** *Adults. Conversion of AF or flutter:* Use after digitalization, 200 mg q2–3h for 8 doses; then ↑ daily dose to a max of 3–4 g or until normal rhythm. *Peds.* 15–60 mg/kg/24 h PO in 4–5 ÷ doses; ↓ dose in renal impairment **Caution/Contra:** [C, +] Contra in digitalis toxicity and AV block; conduction disorders; sparfloxacin or ritonavir use **Supplied:** *Sulfate:* Tabs 200, 300 mg; SR tabs 300 mg. *Gluconate:* SR tabs 324 mg; inj 80 mg/mL **Notes/SE:** Follow serum levels (Table 2, page 607); extreme hypotension may be seen with IV administration. Sulfate salt is 83% quinidine; gluconate salt is 62% quinidine; syncope, QT prolongation, GI upset, arrhythmias, fatigue, cinchonism (tinnitus, hearing loss, delirium, visual changes), fever, hemolytic anemia, thrombocytopenia, rash

Quinupristin-Dalfopristin (Synercid) **Uses:** Infections caused by vancomycin-resistant *E. faecium* and other gram+ organisms **Action:** Inhibits both the early and late phases of protein synthesis at the ribosomes **Dose:** *Adults & Peds.* 7.5 mg/kg IV q8–12h (use central line if possible); not compatible with NS or heparin; therefore, flush IV lines with dextrose; ↓ in hepatic failure **Caution/Contra:** [B, M] **Supplied:** Inj 500 mg (150 mg quinupristin/350 mg dalfopristin) **Notes/SE:** Hyperbilirubinemia, inf site reactions and pain, arthralgia, myalgia

Rabeprazole (Aciphex) **Uses:** PUD, GERD, ZE **Action:** Proton-pump inhibitor **Dose:** 20 mg/d; may be ↑ to 60 mg/d; do not crush tabs **Caution/Contra:** [B, ?/–] **Supplied:** Tabs 60 mg **Notes/SE:** HA, fatigue, GI upset

Raloxifene (Evista) **Uses:** Prevention of osteoporosis **Action:** Partial antagonist of estrogen that behaves like estrogen **Dose:** 60 mg/d **Caution/Contra:** [X, –] Thromboembolism **Supplied:** Tabs 60 mg **Notes/SE:** Chest pain, insomnia, rash, hot flashes, GI upset, hepatic dysfunction

Ramipril (Altace) **WARNING:** ACE inhibitors used during the 2nd and 3rd trimesters of PRG can cause injury and even death to the developing fetus. **Uses:** HTN, CHF, DN, post-MI **Action:** ACE inhibitor **Dose:** 2.5–20 mg/d PO ÷ qd–bid; ↓ in renal failure **Caution/Contra:** [D, +] ACE-inhibitor-induced angioedema **Supplied:** Caps 1.25, 2.5, 5, 10 mg **Notes/SE:** May use in combination with diuretics; may cause cough; HA, dizziness, hypotension, renal impairment, angioedema

Ranitidine (Zantac) **Uses:** Duodenal ulcer, active benign ulcers, hypersecretory conditions, and GERD **Action:** H_2-receptor antagonist **Dose:** *Adults. Ulcer:* 150 mg PO bid, 300 mg PO hs, or 50 mg IV q6–8h; or 400 mg IV/d cont inf, then maint of 150 mg PO hs. *Hypersecretion:* 150 mg PO bid, up to 600 mg/d. *GERD:* 300 mg PO bid; maint 300 mg PO hs. *Peds.* 0.75–1.5 mg/kg/dose IV q6–8h or 1.25–2.5 mg/kg/dose PO q12h; ↓ dose in renal failure **Caution/Contra:** [B, +] **Supplied:** Tabs 75, 150, 300 mg; syrup 15 mg/mL; inj 25 mg/mL **Notes/SE:** Oral and parenteral doses are different; dizziness, sedation, rash, GI upset

Rasburicase (Elitek) **Uses:** ↑ Plasma uric acid due to tumor lysis (pediatrics) **Action:** Catalyzes uric acid **Dose:** *Peds.* 0.15 or 0.20 mg/kg IV over 30 min, qd × 5 **Caution/Contra:** [C, ?/–] Anaphylaxis, screen for G6PD deficiency to avoid hemolysis, methemoglobinemia; falsely ↓ uric acid values **Supplied:** 1.5 mg inj **Notes/SE:** Fever, neutropenia, GI upset, HA, rash

Repaglinide (Prandin) **Uses:** Type 2 DM **Action:** Stimulates insulin release from pancreas **Dose:** 0.5–4 mg ac, start 1–2 mg, ↑ to 16 mg/d max; take pc **Caution/Contra:** [C, ?/–] DKA, type 1 DM **Supplied:** Tabs 0.5, 1, 2 mg **Notes/SE:** HA, hyper-/hypoglycemia, GI upset

Reteplase (Retavase) **Uses:** Post-AMI **Action:** Thrombolytic agent **Dose:** 10 U IV over 2 min, 2nd dose in 30 min 10 U IV over 2 min **Caution/Contra:** [C, ?/–] Internal bleeding, spinal surgery or trauma, Hx CVA vascular malformations, uncontrolled hypotension, sensitivity to thrombolytics **Supplied:** Inj 10.8 U/2 mL **Notes/SE:** Bleeding, allergic reactions

Ribavirin (Virazole) **Uses:** RSV infection in infants and hepatitis C (in combination with interferon alfa-2b) **Action:** Unknown **Dose:** *RSV:* 6 g in 300 mL sterile water inhaled over 12–18 h. *Hep C:* 600 mg PO bid in combination with interferon alfa-2b (see Rebetron, page 554) **Caution/Contra:** [X, ?] Autoimmune hepatitis **Supplied:** Powder for aerosol 6 g; caps 200 mg **Notes/SE:** Aerosolized by a SPAG; may accumulate on soft contact lenses; monitor H/H frequently; PRG test monthly; fatigue, HA, GI upset, anemia, myalgia, alopecia, bronchospasm

Rifabutin (Mycobutin) **Uses:** Prevention of *M. avium* complex infection in AIDS patients with a CD4 count <100 **Action:** Inhibits DNA-dependent RNA polymerase activity **Dose:** 150–300 mg/d PO **Caution/Contra:** [B; ?/–] WBC <1000/mm^3 or platelets <50,000/mm^3; ritonavir **Supplied:** Caps 150 mg **Notes/SE:** Adverse effects/drug interactions similar to rifampin; discolored urine, rash, neutropenia, leukopenia, myalgia, ↑ LFTs

Rifampin (Rifadin) **Uses:** TB and Rx and prophylaxis of *N. meningitidis, H. influenzae,* or *S. aureus* carriers; adjunct for severe *S. aureus* **Action:** Inhibits DNA-dependent RNA polymerase activity **Dose:** *Adults. N. meningitidis and H. influenzae carrier:* 600 mg/d PO for 4 d. *TB:* 600 mg PO or IV qd or 2×/wk with combination therapy regimen. *Peds.* 10–20 mg/kg/dose PO or IV qd–bid; ↓ dose in hepatic failure **Caution/Contra:** [C, +] Amprenavir, multiple drug interactions **Supplied:** Caps 150, 300 mg; inj 600 mg **Notes/SE:** Never use as single agent for active TB; orange-red discoloration of bodily secretions; rash, GI upset, ↑ LFTs, flushing, HA; multiple drug interactions

Rifapentine (Priftin) **Uses:** TB **Action:** Inhibits DNA-dependent RNA polymerase activity **Dose:** *Intensive phase:* 600 mg PO 2 ×/wk for 2 mon; separate doses by 3 or more days. *Continuation phase:* 600 mg/wk **Caution/Contra:**[C, ?/–] **Supplied:** Tabs 150 mg **Notes/SE:** Adverse effects/drug interactions similar to rifampin; hyperuricemia, HTN, HA, dizziness, rash, GI upset, blood dyscrasias, ↑ LFTs, hematuria, discolored secretions

Rimantadine (Flumadine) **Uses:** Prophylaxis and Rx of influenza A virus infections **Action:** Antiviral agent **Dose:** *Adults.* 100 mg PO bid. *Peds.* 5 mg/kg/d PO, 150 mg/d max; ↓ dose in severe renal/hepatic impairment, elderly; initiate within 48 h of symptom onset **Caution/Contra:** [C, –] **Supplied:** Tabs 100 mg; syrup 50 mg/5 mL **Notes/SE:** Orthostatic hypotension, edema, dizziness, GI upset, lowered seizure threshold

Rimexolone (Vexol Ophthalmic) **Uses:** Postop inflammation and uveitis **Action:** Steroid **Dose:** *Adults & Peds >2 y. Uveitis:* 1–2 gtt/h daytime and q2h at night, taper to 1 gtt q4h; postop 1–2 gtt qid up to 2 wk **Caution/Contra:**[C, ?/–] Ocular infections **Supplied:** Susp 1% **Notes/SE:** Taper dose to zero; blurred vision, local irritation

Risedronate (Actonel) **Uses:** Prevention and Rx of postmenopausal osteoporosis; Paget's disease **Action:** Bisphosphonate; inhibits osteoclast-mediated bone resorption **Dose:** 5 mg/d PO with 6–8 oz water; 30 mg/d for 2 mon for Paget's; take 30 min before 1st food/drink of the day; maintain upright position for at least 30 min after administration **Caution/Contra:** [C, ?/–] Not recommended in moderate–severe renal impairment; esophageal structural abnormality, inability to stand or sit upright; interaction with Ca supplements **Supplied:** Tabs 5, 30 mg **Notes/SE:** GI distress, arthralgia; rash, abdominal pain, esophagitis, arthralgia, diarrhea, bone pain

Risperidone (Risperdal) **Uses:** Psychotic disorders **Action:** Benzisoxazole antipsychotic agent **Dose:** 1–6 mg PO bid; ↓ starting doses in elderly, renal/hepatic impairment **Caution/Contra:** [C, –] **Supplied:** Tabs 1, 2, 3, 4 mg **Notes/SE:** Orthostatic hypotension, extrapyramidal reactions with higher doses, tachycardia, arrhythmias, sedation, dystonias, neuroleptic malignant syndrome, sexual dysfunction, constipation, xerostomia, blood dyscrasias, cholestatic jaundice, weight gain

Ritonavir (Norvir) **Uses:** HIV infection **Actions:** Protease inhibitor; inhibits maturation of immature noninfectious virions to mature infectious virus **Dose:** 600 mg PO bid or 400 mg PO bid in combination with saquinavir; titrate over 1 wk to ↓ GI complications; take with food **Caution/Contra:** [B, +] Ergotamine, amiodarone, bepridil, flecainide, propafenone, quinidine, pimozide, midazolam, triazolam **Supplied:** Caps 100 mg; soln 80 mg/mL **Notes/SE:** Many drug interactions; store in refrigerator; perioral and peripheral paresthesias; dyslipidemia, lipodystrophy, hyperglycemia, GI upset, ↑ LFTs, decreased mentation, rash, blood dyscrasias

Rivastigmine (Exelon) **Uses:** Mild–moderate dementia associated with Alzheimer's disease **Action:** Enhances cholinergic activity **Dose:** 1.5 mg bid; ↑ to 6 mg bid, with increases at 2-wk intervals **Caution/Contra:** [B, ?] **Supplied:** Caps 1.5, 3, 4.5, 6 mg; soln 2 mg/mL **Notes/SE:** Dose-related GI adverse effects; dizziness, somnolence, tremor, diaphoresis

Rizatriptan (Maxalt) Uses: Acute migraine Action: Serotonin 5-HT$_1$ receptor antagonist Dose: 5–10 mg PO; may repeat once in 2 h Caution/Contra: [C, M] Ischemic heart disease, Prinzmetal's angina, uncontrolled HTN, within 2 wk of MAOI use, ergots Supplied: Tabs 5, 10 mg; disintegrating tabs 5, 10 mg Notes/SE: GI adverse effects (dose-related); ↑ BP, chest pain, dizziness, drowsiness, fatigue, flushing, dyspnea, coronary vasospasm

Rofecoxib (Vioxx) Uses: Osteoarthritis, RA, acute pain, and primary dysmenorrhea Action: NSAID; COX-2 inhibitor Dose: 12.5–50 mg/d; ↓ dose in severe renal/hepatic impairment, elderly Caution/Contra: [C, ?/–] ASA or NSAID sensitivity Supplied: Tabs 12.5, 25 mg; susp 12.5, 25 mg/5 mL Notes/SE: Alert patients about GI ulceration or bleeding; dizziness, edema, HTN, HA, renal failure; no effect on bleeding parameters, may ↑ thromboembolism risk

Rosiglitazone (Avandia) Uses: Type 2 DM Action: ↑ Insulin sensitivity Dose: 4–8 mg/d PO or in 2 ÷ doses without regard to meals Caution/Contra: [C, –] Contra in active liver disease Supplied: Tabs 2, 4, 8 mg Notes/SE: Weight gain, hyperlipidemia, HA, edema, fluid retention, exacerbate CHF, hyper-/hypoglycemia, hepatic damage

Salmeterol (Serevent) Uses: Asthma, exercise-induced bronchospasm, COPD Action: Sympathomimetic bronchodilator Dose: 2 inhal bid Caution/ Contra: [C, ?/–] Do not use within 14 d of MAOI use Supplied: Met-dose inhaler Notes/SE: Not for acute attacks; HA, pharyngitis, tachycardia, arrhythmias, nervousness, GI upset, tremors

Saquinavir (Fortovase) Uses: HIV infection Action: HIV protease inhibitor Dose: 1200 mg PO tid within 2 h pc Caution/Contra: [B, +] Triazolam, midazolam, ergots Supplied: Caps 200 mg Notes/SE: Dyslipidemia, lipodystrophy, rash, hyperglycemia, GI upset, weakness, hepatic dysfunction

Sargramostim [GM-CSF] (Prokine, Leukine) Uses: Myeloid recovery following BMT or CA chemotherapy Action: Activates mature granulocytes and macrophages Dose: *Adults & Peds.* 250 mg/m^2/d IV for 21 d (BMT) Caution/Contra: [C, ?/–] > (10% blasts) Supplied: Inj 250, 500 mg Notes/SE: Bone pain, fever, hypotension, tachycardia, flushing, GI upset, myalgia

Scopolamine, Scopolamine Transdermal (Scopace, Transderm-Scop) Uses: Prevention of N/V associated with motion sickness, anesthesia, and opiates; mydriatic, cycloplegic, Rx iridocilitis Action: Anticholinergic, antiemetic Dose: Apply 1 TD patch behind the ear q3d; 0.4–0.8 PO, repeat PRN q4–6h; apply at least 4 h before exposure; ↓ dose in elderly Caution/ Contra: [C, +] Narrow-angle glaucoma, GI or GU obstruction, thyrotoxicosis, paralytic ileus Supplied: Patch 1.5 mg; tabs 0.4 mg, ophthalmic 0.25% Notes/SE: Xerostomia, drowsiness, blurred vision, tachycardia, constipation

Secobarbital (Seconal) [C-II] Uses: Insomnia Action: Rapid-acting barbiturate Dose: *Adults.* 100–200 mg. *Peds.* 3–5 mg/kg/dose, up to 100 mg; ↓ dose in elderly Caution/Contra: [D, +] Porphyria Supplied: Caps 100 mg Notes/SE: Tolerance acquired in 1–2 wk; respiratory depression, CNS depression, porphyria, photosensitivity

Selegiline (Eldepryl) Uses: Parkinson's disease Action: Inhibits MAO activity Dose: 5 mg PO bid; ↓ dose in elderly Caution/Contra: [C, ?] Meperidine, SSRI, and TCAs Supplied: Tabs 5 mg Notes/SE: Nausea, dizziness, orthostatic hypotension, arrhythmias, tachycardia, edema, confusion, xerostomia

Selenium Sulfide (Exsel Shampoo, Selsun Blue Shampoo, Selsun Shampoo) Uses: Scalp seborrheic dermatitis, itching and flaking of the scalp due to dandruff; treatment of tinea versicolor Action: Antiseborrheic Dose: *Dandruff, seborrhea:* Massage 5–10 mL into wet scalp, leave on 2–3 min, rinse, and repeat; use 2×/wk, then once q1–4wk PRN. *Tinea versicolor:* Apply 2.5% qd for 7 d on area and lather with small amounts of water; leave on skin for 10 min, then rinse Caution/Contra: [C, ?] Supplied: Shampoo 1, 2.5% Notes/SE: Dry or oily scalp, lethargy, hair discoloration, local irritation

Serotonin 5-HT$_1$ Receptor Agonists (See Table 11, page 623) Uses: Migraine w/wo aura Action: Serotonin receptor antagonism results in vasoconstriction Dose: See Table 11, page 623 Caution/Contra: [C, ?, sumatriptan –] Contra in sumatriptan sensitivity, ischemic CAD, MI Notes/SE: Flushing, dizziness, pressure/heaviness

Sertraline (Zoloft) **Uses:** Depression, panic disorders, obsessive–compulsive disorder, posttraumatic stress disorders (PTSD), social anxiety disorder **Action:** Inhibits neuronal uptake of serotonin **Dose:** *Depression:* 50–200 mg/d PO. *PTSD:* 25 mg PO qd ×1 wk, then 50 mg PO qd, max 200 mg/d **Caution/Contra:** [C, ?/–] MAOI use within 14 d; caution in hepatic impairment, concomitant pimozide **Supplied:** Tabs 25, 50, 100 mg **Notes/SE:** Can activate manic/hypomanic state; has caused weight loss in clinical trials; insomnia, somnolence, fatigue, tremor, xerostomia, nausea, dyspepsia, diarrhea, ejaculatory dysfunction, ↓ libido, hepatotoxicity

Sibutramine (Meridia) **Uses:** Obesity **Action:** Blocks uptake of norepinephrine, serotonin, and dopamine **Dose:** 10 mg/d, may ↓ to 5 mg after 4 wk **Caution/Contra:** [C, –] MAOI use within 14 d, uncontrolled HTN, arrhythmias **Supplied:** Caps 5, 10, 15 mg **Notes/SE:** Use with low-calorie diet, monitor BP and HR; HA, insomnia, xerostomia, constipation, rhinitis, tachycardia, HTN

Sildenafil (Viagra) **Uses:** Erectile dysfunction **Action:** Smooth muscle relaxation and ↑ inflow of blood to the corpus cavernosum; inhibits phosphodiesterase type 5 responsible for cGMP breakdown; ↑ cGMP activity **Dose:** 25–100 mg 1 h before sexual activity, max dosing is once daily; ↓ dose if >65 y; avoid fatty foods with dose **Caution/Contra:** [B, ?] Contra with nitrates of any form; retinitis pigmentosa; potent CYP3A4 inhibitors (ie, protease inhibitors); hepatic/severe renal impairment **Supplied:** Tabs 25, 50, 100 mg **Notes/SE:** HA, flushing, dizziness, blue haze visual disturbance, usually reversible; cardiac events in absence of nitrates debatable

Silver Nitrate (Dey-Drop, others) **Uses:** Prevent ophthalmia neonatorium due to GC; remove granulation tissue and warts and cauterize wounds **Action:** Caustic antiseptic and astringent **Dose:** *Adults & Peds.* Apply to moist surface 2–3×/wk for several wks or until effect. *Peds. Newborns:* Apply 2 gtt into conjunctival sac immediately after birth **Caution/Contra:** [C, ?] Do not use on broken skin **Supplied:** Topical impregnated applicator sticks, oint 10%, soln 10, 25, 50%; ophth 1% amp **Notes/SE:** May stain tissue black, usually resolves; local irritation, methemoglobinemia

Silver Sulfadiazine (Silvadene) **Uses:** Prevention of sepsis in 2nd- and 3rd-degree burns **Action:** Bactericidal **Dose:** *Adults & Peds.* Aseptically cover the affected area with $^1/_{16}$-in. coating bid **Caution/Contra:** [B, ?/–] Age <2 mon **Supplied:** Cream 1% **Notes/SE:** Can have systemic absorption with extensive application; itching, rash, skin discoloration, blood dyscrasias, hepatitis, allergy

Simethicone (Mylicon) **Uses:** Flatulence **Action:** Defoaming action **Dose:** *Adults & Peds.* 40–125 mg PO pc and hs PRN **Caution/Contra:** [C, ?] Intestinal perforation or obstruction **Supplied:** Tabs 80, 125 mg; caps 125 mg; gtt 40 mg/0.6 mL **Notes/SE:** Diarrhea, nausea

Simvastatin (Zocor) **Uses:** ↓ of elevated cholesterol levels **Action:** HMG-CoA reductase inhibitor **Dose:** 5–80 mg PO; with meals; ↓ dose in renal insufficiency **Caution/Contra:** [X, –] Avoid concurrent use of gemfibrozil; liver disease **Supplied:** Tabs 5, 10, 20, 40 mg **Notes/SE:** Use caution with concurrent use of gemfibrozil; HA, GI upset, myalgia, myopathy, hepatitis

Sirolimus [Rapamycin] (Rapamune) WARNING: Can cause immunosuppression and infections **Uses:** Prophylaxis of organ rejection **Action:** Inhibits T-lymphocyte activation **Dose:** 2 mg/d PO; dilute in water or orange juice; do not drink grapefruit juice while on sirolimus; take 4 h after cyclosporin; ↓ dose in hepatic impairment **Caution/Contra:** [C, ?/–] Grapefruit juice, ketoconazole **Supplied:** Soln 1 mg/mL **Notes/SE:** Routine blood levels not needed except in peds or liver failure (trough 9–17 ng/mL); HTN, edema, chest pain, fever, HA, insomnia, acne, rash, hypercholesterolemia, hyper-/hypokalemia, GI upset, infections, blood dyscrasias, arthralgia, tachycardia, renal impairment, hepatic artery thrombosis, graft loss and death in de novo liver transplant

Smallpox Vaccine (Dryvax) **Uses:** Immunization against smallpox (variola virus) **Actions:** Active immunization (live attenuated vaccinia virus) **Dose:** *Adults* (routine nonemergency) or all ages (emergency): 2–3 punctures of bifurcated needle dipped in vaccine into deltoid, posterior triceps muscle; check site for reaction in 6–8 d; if major reaction, the site will scab, and heal, leaving a scar; if mild–equivocal reaction, repeat using 15 punctures

Contra/Caution: [X, –] in nonemergency use, contra in children < 18 y, in febrile illness, immunosuppression, Hx of eczema and their household contacts; in emergency situations, no absolute contraindications. **Supplied:** Vial for reconstitution: ≅100 million pock-forming units/mL **Notes/SE:** Malaise, fever, regional lymphadenopathy, encephalopathy, rashes, spread of inoculation to other sites administered; Stevens–Johnson syndrome, eczema vaccinatum with severe disability

Sodium Bicarbonate (NaHCO₃) **Uses:** Alkalinization of urine, RTA, metabolic acidosis **Dose:** *Adults. ECC:* Initiate adequate ventilation, 1 mEq/kg/dose IV; can repeat 0.5 mEq/kg in 10 min once or based on acid–base status. *Metabolic acidosis:* 2–5 mEq/kg IV over 8 h and PRN based on acid–base status. *Alkalinize urine:* 4 g (48 mEq) PO, then 1–2 g q4h; adjust based on urine pH; 2 amp in 1 L D₅W @100–250 mL/h IV, monitor urine pH and serum bicarbonate. *Chronic renal failure:* 1–3 mEq/kg/d. *Distal RTA:* 1 mEq/kg/d PO. *Peds >1 y: ECC:* See Adults. *Peds <1 y: ECC:* Initiate adequate ventilation, 1:1 dilution 1 mEq/mL dosed 1 mEq/kg IV; can repeat with 0.5 mEq/kg in 10 min once or based on acid–base status. *Chronic renal failure:* See Adults. *Distal RTA:* 2–3 mEq/kg/d PO. *Proximal RTA:* 5–10 mEq/kg/d titrate based on serum bicarbonate levels. *Urine alkalinization:* 84–840 mg/kg/d (1–10 mEq/kg/d) ÷ doses; adjust based on urine pH **Caution/Contra:** [C, ?] **Supplied:** IV inf, powder, and tabs; 300 mg = 3.6 mEq; 325 mg = 3.8 mEq; 520 mg = 6.3 mEq; 600 mg = 7.3 mEq; 650 mg = 7.6 mEq **Notes/SE:** 1 g neutralizes 12 mEq of acid; in infants, do not exceed 10 mEq/min inf; belching, edema, flatulence, hypernatremia, metabolic alkalosis

Sodium Citrate (Bicitra) **Uses:** Alkalinize urine; dissolve uric acid and cysteine stones **Action:** Urinary alkalinizer **Dose:** *Adults.* 2–6 tsp (10–30 mL) diluted in 1–3 oz water pc and hs. *Peds.* 1–3 tsp (5–15 mL) diluted in 1–3 oz water pc and hs; best after meals **Caution/Contra:** [C, +] Do not give to patients on aluminum-based antacids. Contra in severe renal impairment or Na-restricted diets **Supplied:** 15- or 30-mL unit dose: 16 (473 mL) or 4 (118 mL) fl oz **Notes/SE:** Tetany, metabolic alkalosis, hyperkalemia, GI upset; avoid use of multiple 50-mL amps; can cause hypernatremia/hyperosmolality

Sodium Oxybate (Xyrem) [C-III] **Uses:** Narcolepsy-associated cataplexy **Action:** Inhibitory neurotransmitter **Dose:** 2.25 g PO qhs, second dose 2.5–4 h later; may increase to max of 9 g/d **Caution/Contra:** [B, ?/–] May lead to dependence; significant vomiting, respiratory depression, psychiatric symptoms; contra in succinic semialdehyde dehydrogenase deficiency; potentiates ethanol **Supplied:** 500 mg/mL 180 mL oral soln **Notes/SE:** Synonym for γ-hydroxybutyrate (GHB), a substance abused recreationally and as a "date rape drug;" controlled distribution requires prescriber and patient registration; must be administered when patient in bed; confusion, depression, diminished level of consciousness, incontinence

Sodium Polystyrene Sulfonate (Kayexalate) **Uses:** Hyperkalemia **Action:** Na and K ion-exchange resin **Dose:** *Adults.* 15–60 g PO or 30–60 g PR q6h based on serum K⁺. *Peds.* 1 g/kg/dose PO or PR q6h based on serum K⁺; given with an agent, eg, sorbitol, to promote movement through the bowel **Caution/Contra:** [C, M] Hypernatremia **Supplied:** Powder; susp 15 g/60 mL sorbitol **Notes/SE:** Can cause hypernatremia, hypokalemia, Na⁺ retention, GI upset, fecal impaction; enema acts more quickly than PO

Sorbitol (generic) **Uses:** Constipation **Action:** Laxative **Dose:** 30–60 mL of a 20–70% soln PRN **Caution/Contra:** [B, +] Anuria **Supplied:** Liq 70% **Notes/SE:** Edema, electrolyte losses, lactic acidosis, GI upset, xerostomia

Sotalol (Betapace) **WARNING:** Monitor patients for 1st 3 d of therapy to reduce risks of induced arrhythmia **Uses:** Ventricular arrhythmias, AF **Action:** β-Adrenergic-blocking agent **Dose:** 80 mg PO bid; may be ↑ to 240–320 mg/d; ↓ dose in renal failure **Caution/Contra:** [B (1st trimester) (D if 2nd or 3rd trimester), +] Asthma, bradycardia, prolonged QT interval, 2nd- or 3rd-degree heart block w/o pacemaker, cardiogenic shock, uncontrolled CHF, CrCl <40 mL/min **Supplied:** Tabs 80, 120, 160, 240 mg **Notes/SE:** Betapace should not be substituted for Betapace AF because of significant differences in labeling; bradycardia, chest pain, palpitations, fatigue, dizziness, weakness, dyspnea

Sotalol (Betapace AF) **WARNING:** To minimize risk of induced arrhythmia, patients initiated/reinitiated on Betapace AF should be placed for a minimum of 3 d (on their maint dose) in a facility that can provide cardiac resuscitation, continuous ECG monitoring, and calculations of CrCl; Betapace should not be substituted for Betapace AF because of differences in labeling. **Uses:** Maintain sinus rhythm for symptomatic AF/flutter

Action: β-Adrenergic-blocking agent **Dose:** *Initial CrCl >60 mL/min:* 80 mg PO q12h. *ClCr 40–60 mL/min:* 80 mg PO q2h; ↑ to 120 mg during hospitalization; monitor QT interval 2–4 h after each dose, with dose reduction or discontinuation if QT interval >500 ms **Caution/Contra:** [B (1st trimester; D if 2nd or 3rd trimester), +] Asthma, bradycardia, prolonged QT interval, 2nd- or 3rd -degree heart block w/o pacemaker, cardiogenic shock, uncontrolled CHF, CrCl <40 mL/min; caution if converting from previous antiarrhythmic therapy **Supplied:** Tabs 80, 120, 160 mg **Notes/SE:** Bradycardia, chest pain, palpitations, fatigue, dizziness, weakness, dyspnea; routinely evaluate renal function and QT interval

Sparfloxacin (Zagam)   **Uses:** Community-acquired pneumonia, acute exacerbations of chronic bronchitis **Action:** Quinolone antibiotic; Inhibits DNA gyrase **Dose:** 400 mg PO on day 1, then 200 mg q24h for 10 days; ↓ dose in renal dysfunction **Caution/Contra:** [C, ?/–] Significant phototoxicity (even from sunlight through windows); QT prolongation; do not administer with drugs that prolong QT interval **Supplied:** Tabs 200 mg **Notes/SE:** Interactions with theophylline, caffeine, sucralfate, warfarin, and antacids; restlessness, N/V/D, rash, ruptured tendons, ↑ LFTs, sleep disorders, confusion, convulsions; must protect from sunlight up to 5 days after last dose

Spironolactone (Aldactone)   **Uses:** Hyperaldosteronism, ascites from CHF or cirrhosis **Action:** Aldosterone antagonist; K⁺-sparing diuretic **Dose:** *Adults.* 25–100 mg PO qid; CHF (NYHA class III–IV) 25–50 mg/d. *Peds.* 1–3.3 mg/kg/24 h PO ÷ bid–qid. *Neonates* 0.5–1 mg/kg/dose q8h; take with food **Caution/Contra:** [D, +] Hyperkalemia, renal failure, anuria **Supplied:** Tabs 25, 50, 100 mg **Notes/SE:** Hyperkalemia and gynecomastia, arrhythmia, sexual dysfunction, confusion, dizziness

Stavudine (Zerit)   **WARNING:** Lactic acidosis and severe hepatomegaly with steatosis and pancreatitis reported **Uses:** Advanced HIV disease **Action:** Reverse-transcriptase inhibitor **Dose:** *Adults.* *>60 kg:* 40 mg bid. *<60 kg:* 30 mg bid; **Peds.** Birth–13 d:0.5 mg/kg q12h;>14 d and < 30 kg: 1 mg/kg q12h; ≥ 30 kg adult dose; ↓ dose in renal failure **Caution/Contra:** [C, +] **Supplied:** Caps 15, 20, 30, 40 mg; soln 1 mg/mL **Notes/SE:** May cause peripheral neuropathy, HA, chills, fever, malaise, rash, GI upset, anemias, lactic acidosis, ↑ levels on LFTs, pancreatitis

Steroids, Systemic (Table 4, page 612)   The following relates only to the commonly used systemic glucocorticoids **Uses:** Endocrine disorders (adrenal insufficiency), rheumatoid disorders, collagen-vascular diseases, dermatologic diseases, allergic states, cerebral edema, nephritis, nephrotic syndrome, immunosuppression for transplantation, hypercalcemia, malignancies (breast, lymphomas), preoperatively (in any patient who has been on steroids in the previous year, known hypoadrenalism, preop for adrenalectomy); inj into joints/tissue **Action:** Glucocorticoid **Dose:** Varies with use and institutional protocols. *Adrenal insufficiency, acute:* **Adults.** *Hydrocortisone:* 100 mg IV; then 300 mg/d ÷ q6h; convert to 50 mg PO q8h ×6 doses, taper to 30–50 mg/d ÷ bid. **Peds.** *Hydrocortisone:* 1–2 mg/kg IV; then 150–250 mg/d ÷ tid. *Adrenal insufficiency, chronic (physiologic replacement):* May need mineralocorticoid supplementation such as Florinef. **Adults.** Hydrocortisone 20 mg PO qAM, 10 mg PO qPM; cortisone 0.5–0.75 mg/kg/d ÷ bid; cortisone 0.25–0.35 mg/kg/d IM; dexamethasone 0.03–0.15 mg/kg/d or 0.6–0.75 mg/m²/d ÷ q6–12h PO, IM, IV. **Peds.** Hydrocortisone 0.5–0.75 mg/kg/d PO tid; hydrocortisone succinate 0.25–0.35 mg/kg/d IM. *Asthma, acute:* **Adults.** Methylprednisolone 60 mg q6h, **Peds.** Prednisolone 1–2 mg/kg/d or prednisone 1–2 mg/kg/d ÷ qd–bid for up to 5 d; prednisolone 2–4 mg/kg/d IV ÷ tid. *Congenital adrenal hyperplasia:* **Peds.** Initially hydrocortisone 30–36 mg/m²/d PO ÷ 1/3 dose qAM, ⅔ dose qPM; maint 20–25 mg/m²/d ÷ bid. *Extubation/airway edema:* Dexamethasone 0.5–1 mg/kg/d IM/IV ÷ q6h, start beginning 24 h prior to extubation; continue for 4 additional doses. *Immunosuppressive/antiinflammatory:* **Adults & Older Peds.** Hydrocortisone 15–240 mg PO, IM, IV q12h; methylprednisolone: 4–48 mg/d PO, taper to lowest effective dose; methylprednisolone Na succinate 10–80 mg/d IM. **Adults.** Prednisone or prednisolone 5–60 mg/d PO ÷ qd–qid. *Infants & Younger Children.* Hydrocortisone 2.5–10 mg/kg/d PO ÷ q6–8h; 1–5 mg/kg/d IM/IV ÷ bid. *Nephrotic syndrome:* **Peds.** Prednisolone or prednisone 2 mg/kg/d PO ÷ tid–qid until urine is protein-free for 5 d, use up to 28 d; for persistent proteinuria, 4 mg/kg/d PO qod max 120 mg/d for an additional 28 d; maint 2 mg/kg/dose qod for 28 d; taper over 4–6 wk (max 80 mg/d). *Septic shock* (controversial): **Adults.** Hydrocortisone 500 mg–1 g IM/IV q2–6h. **Peds.** Hydrocortisone 50 mg/kg IM/IV, repeat q4–24 h PRN. *Status asthmaticus: Adults & Peds.* Hydrocortisone 1–

2 mg/kg/dose IV q6h; then decrease by 0.5–1 mg/kg q6h. *Rheumatic disease: Adults.* Intraarticular: Hydrocortisone acetate 25–37.5 mg large joint, 10–25 mg small joint; methylprednisolone acetate 20–80 mg large joint, 4–10 mg small joint. *Intrabursal:* Hydrocortisone acetate 25–37.5 mg. *Intraganglial:* Hydrocortisone acetate 25–37.5 mg. *Tendon sheath:* Hydrocortisone acetate 5–12.5 mg. *Perioperative steroid coverage:* Hydrocortisone 100 mg IV night before surgery, 1 h preop, intraop, and 4, 8, and 12 h postop; pod #1 100 mg IV q6h; pod #2 100 mg IV q8h; pod #3 100 mg IV q12h; pod #4 50 mg IV q12h; pod #5 25 mg IV q12h; then resume prior oral dosing if chronic use or DC if only perioperative coverage required. *Cerebral edema:* Dexamethasone 10 mg IV; then 4 mg IV q4–6h **Caution/Contra:** [C, ?/–] **Supplied:** Table 4, page 612 **Notes/SE:** Hydrocortisone succinate administered systemically, acetate form intraarticular; all can cause ↑ appetite, hyperglycemia, hypokalemia, osteoporosis, nervousness, insomnia, "steroid psychosis," adrenal suppression; never abruptly stop steroids, especially in chronic treatment; taper dose

Steroids, Topical (See also Table 5, page 613)   **Uses:** Relief of inflammatory and pruritic manifestations of corticosteroid-responsive dermatoses **Action:** Corticosteroid, antiinflammatory **Dose:** Varies widely with indication and formulation. Table 5 (page 613) for frequency of application of various agents **Caution/Contra:** [?, ?] Contra in viral, fungal, or tubercular skin lesions **Supplied:** Table 5, page 613 **Notes/SE:** Topical use should be short term

Streptokinase (Streptase, Kabikinase)   **Uses:** Coronary artery thrombosis, acute massive PE, DVT, and some occluded vascular grafts **Action:** Activates plasminogen to plasmin that degrades fibrin **Dose:** *Adults. PE:* Loading dose of 250,000 IU IV through a peripheral vein over 30 min, then 100,000 IU/h IV for 24–72 h. *Coronary artery thrombosis:* 1.5 MU IV over 60 min. *DVT or arterial embolism:* Load as with PE, then 100,000 IU/h for 72 h. *Peds.* 3500–4000 U/kg over 30 min, followed by 1000–1500 U/kg/h **Caution/Contra:** [C, +] Streptococcal infection or streptokinase use in last 6 mon, active bleeding, CVA, TIA, spinal surgery, or trauma in last month, vascular anomalies, severe hepatic or renal disease, endocarditis, pericarditis, severe uncontrolled HTN **Supplied:** Powder for inj 250,000, 600,000, 750,000, 1,500,000 IU **Notes/SE:** If maint inf inadequate to maintain thrombin clotting time 2–5× control, refer to the package insert, *PDR,* or the AHFS Drug Information service for adjustments. Antibodies remain 3–6 mon following dose; bleeding, hypotension, fever, bruising, rash, GI upset, hemorrhage, anaphylaxis

Streptomycin   **Uses:** TB **Action:** Aminoglycoside; interferes with protein synthesis **Dose:** 1–4 g/d IM in 1–2 ÷ doses (endocarditis); TB 15 mg/kg/d; ↓ dose in renal failure **Caution/Contra:** [D, +] **Supplied:** Inj 400 mg/mL **Notes/SE:** ↑ incidence of vestibular and auditory toxicity, neurotoxicity, nephrotoxicity

Streptozocin (Zanosar)   **Uses:** Pancreatic islet cell tumors and carcinoid tumors **Action:** DNA–DNA (interstrand) cross-linking; DNA, RNA, and protein synthesis inhibitor **Dose:** 1–1.5 g/m² q4wk (single agent); 500 mg/m²/d for 5 d or 100 mg/m²/wk for 1st 2 wk q6wk (combination regimens); ↓ dose in renal failure **Caution/Contra:** [D, ?/–] Caution in renal failure. **Supplied:** Inj 1 g **Notes/SE:** N/V, duodenal ulcers; myelosuppression rare (20%) and mild; nephrotoxicity (proteinuria and azotemia often heralded by hypophosphatemia) dose limiting. Hypo-/hyperglycemia may occur; phlebitis and pain at the site of inj

Succimer (Chemet)   **Uses:** Lead poisoning **Action:** Heavy-metal-chelating agent **Dose:** *Adults & Peds.* *8–15 kg:* 100 mg PO. *16–23 kg:* 200 mg PO. *24–34 kg:* 300 mg PO. *35–44 kg:* 400 mg PO. *>45 kg:* 500 mg PO; give dose noted q8h for 5 d, q12h for 14 d; drink fluids liberally **Caution/Contra:** [C, ?] **Supplied:** Caps 100 mg **Notes/SE:** Rash, fever, GI upset, hemorrhoids, metallic taste, drowsiness, ↑ LFTs

Succinylcholine (Anectine, Quelicin, Sucostrin)   **Uses:** Adjunct to general anesthesia to facilitate ET intubation and to induce skeletal muscle relaxation during surgery or mechanically supported ventilation **Action:** Depolarizing neuromuscular blocking agent **Dose:** *Adults.* 0.6 mg/kg IV over 10–30 s, followed by 0.04–0.07 mg/kg as needed to maintain muscle relaxation. *Peds.* 1–2 mg/kg/dose IV, followed by 0.3–0.6 mg/kg/dose at intervals of 10–20 min; ↓ in severe liver disease **Caution/Contra:** [C, M] At risk for malignant hyperthermia; myopathy; recent major burn, multiple trauma, extensive skeletal muscle denervation **Supplied:** Inj 20, 50, 100 mg/mL; powder for inj 100, 500 mg, 1 g/vial **Notes/SE:** May precipitate malignant hyperthermia, respiratory depression, or prolonged apnea; many drug interactions potentiate succinylcholine; observe for cardiovascular effects (arrhythmias, hypotension, brady/tachycardia); ↑ intraocular pressure, postoperative stiffness, salivation, myoglobinuria; in children, acute rhabdomyolysis, hyperkalemia, arrhythmia, and death

Sucralfate (Carafate) **Uses:** Duodenal and gastric ulcers **Action:** Forms ulcer-adherent complex that protects against acid, pepsin, and bile acid **Dose:** *Adults.* 1 g PO qid, 1 h prior to meals and hs. *Peds.* 40–80 mg/kg/d ÷ q6h; continue 4–8 wk unless healing demonstrated by x-ray or endoscopy; separate from other drugs by 2 h (can inhibit absorption); take on empty stomach (before meals acceptable) **Caution/Contra:** [B, +] **Supplied:** Tabs 1 g; susp 1 g/10 mL **Notes/SE:** Constipation frequent; diarrhea, dizziness, xerostomia; aluminum may accumulate in renal failure.

Sufentanil (Sufenta) [C-II] **Uses:** Analgesic adjunct to maintain balanced general anesthesia **Action:** Potent synthetic opioid **Dose:** *Adjunctive:* 1–8 mcg/kg with nitrous oxide/oxygen; maint of 10–50 mcg PRN. *General anesthesia:* 8–30 mcg/kg with oxygen and a skeletal muscle relaxant. *Maint:* 25–50 mcg PRN. Give over 3–5 min **Caution/Contra:** [C, ?] **Supplied:** Inj 50 mcg/mL **Notes/SE:** Respiratory depressant effects last longer than analgesia; bradycardia, hypotension, drowsiness, GI upset, arrhythmias, biliary tract spasm, blurred vision, pruritus

Sulfacetamide (Bleph-10, Cetamide, Sodium Sulamyd) **Uses:** Conjunctival infections **Action:** Sulfonamide antibiotic **Dose:** 10% Oint apply qid and hs; soln for keratitis apply q2–3h depending on severity **Caution/Contra:** [C, M] Sulfonamide sensitivity; age <2 mon **Supplied:** Oint 10%; soln 10, 15, 30% **Notes/SE:** Irritation, burning; blurred vision, brow ache, Stevens–Johnson syndrome, photosensitivity

Sulfacetamide and Prednisolone (Blephamide, others) **Uses:** Steroid-responsive inflammatory ocular conditions with infection or a risk of infection **Action:** Antibiotic and antiinflammatory **Dose:** *Adult and Peds* >2 y. Apply oint to lower conjunctival sac qd–qid; soln 1–3 gtt 2–3 h while awake **Caution/Contra:** [C, ?/–] Sulfonamide sensitivity; age <2 mon **Supplied:** Oint sulfacetamide 10%/prednisolone 0.5%, sulfacetamide 10%/prednisolone 0.2%, sulfacetamide 10%/prednisolone 0.25%; susp sulfacetamide 10%/prednisolone 0.25%, sulfacetamide 10%/prednisolone 0.5%, sulfacetamide 10%/prednisolone 0.2%. **Notes/SE:** Ophth susp can be used as an otic agent; irritation, burning, blurred vision, brow ache, Stevens–Johnson syndrome, photosensitivity

Sulfasalazine (Azulfidine, Azulfidine EN) **Uses:** Ulcerative colitis, active Crohn's, juvenile RA **Action:** Sulfonamide; actions not clear **Dose:** *Adults.* Initially, 1 g tid–qid; ↑ to a max of 8 g/d in 3–4 ÷ doses; maint 500 mg PO qid. *Peds.* Initially, 40–60 mg/kg/24 h PO ÷ q4–6h; maint 20–30 mg/ kg/24 h PO ÷ q6h; RA >6 y 30–50 mg/kg/d (%) in 2 doses, start with 1/4–1/3 described maint dose, ↑ weekly until dose reached at 1 mon, 2 g/d max; ↓ dose in renal failure **Caution/Contra:** [B (D if near term), M] Sulfonamide or salicylate sensitivity, porphyria, GI or GU obstruction; avoid in hepatic impairment **Supplied:** Tabs 500 mg; EC tabs 500 mg; oral susp 250 mg/5 mL **Notes/SE:** Can cause severe GI upset; discolors urine; dizziness, HA, photosensitivity, oligospermia, anemias, Stevens–Johnson syndrome

Sulfinpyrazone (Anturane) **Uses:** Acute and chronic gout **Action:** Inhibits renal tubular absorption of uric acid **Dose:** 100–200 mg PO bid for 1 wk, then ↑ as needed to maint of 200–400 mg bid; take with food or antacids, take with plenty of fluids; avoid salicylates **Caution/Contra:** [C (per manufacturer), D (per expert analysis if near term), ?/–] Avoid in renal impairment, avoid salicylates; peptic ulcer; blood dyscrasias **Supplied:** Tabs 100 mg; caps 200 mg **Notes/SE:** N/V, stomach pain, urolithiasis, leukopenia

Sulindac (Clinoril) **Uses:** Arthritis and pain **Action:** NSAID; inhibits prostaglandin synthesis **Dose:** 150–200 mg bid with food **Caution/Contra:** [B (D if 3rd trimester or near term), ?] NSAID or ASA sensitivity, peptic ulcer, GI bleeding **Supplied:** Tabs 150, 200 mg **Notes/SE:** Dizziness, rash, GI upset, pruritus, edema, ↓ renal blood flow, renal failure (may have fewer renal effects than other NSAIDs), peptic ulcer, GI bleeding

22

Sumatriptan (Imitrex) Uses: Acute treatment of migraine attacks Action: Vascular serotonin receptor agonist Dose: *SC:* 6 mg SC as a single dose PRN; can repeat in 1 h to a max of 12 mg/24 h. *Oral:* 25 mg, repeat in 2 h, PRN, 100 mg/d max oral dose; max 300 mg/d. *Nasal spray:* 1 single spray into 1 nostril, may repeat in 2 h to a max of 40 mg/24 h Caution/Contra: [C, M] Avoid in patients with angina, ischemic heart disease, uncontrolled HTN, ergot use, MAOI use within 14 d Supplied: Inj 6 mg/mL; tabs 25, 50 mg; nasal spray 5, 20 mg Notes/SE: Pain and bruising at the inj site; dizziness, hot flashes, paresthesias, chest pain, weakness, numbness, coronary vasospasm, HTN

Tacrine (Cognex) Uses: Mild–moderate dementia Action: Cholinesterase inhibitor Dose: 10–40 mg PO qid to 160 mg/d; separate doses from food Caution/Contra: [C, ?] Supplied: Caps 10, 20, 30, 40 mg Notes/SE: May ↑ LFT, HA, dizziness, GI upset, flushing, confusion, ataxia, myalgia, bradycardia

Tacrolimus [FK 506] (Prograf, Protopic) Uses: Prophylaxis of organ rejection, eczema Action: Macrolide immunosuppressant Dose: *IV:* 0.05–0.1 mg/ kg/d as cont inf. *PO:* 0.15–0.3 mg/kg/d ÷ into 2 doses. *Eczema:* Apply bid, continue 1 wk after clearing; ↓ dose in hepatic/renal impairment Caution/Contra: [C, –] Do not use with cyclosporine Supplied: Caps 1, 5 mg; inj 5 mg/mL; ointment 0.03, 0.1% Notes/SE: Neurotoxicity and nephrotoxicity, HTN, edema, HA, insomnia, fever, pruritus, hypo-/hyperkalemia, hyperglycemia, GI upset, anemia, leukocytosis, tremors, paresthesias, pleural effusion, seizures, lymphoma

Tamoxifen (Nolvadex) Uses: Breast CA (postmenopausal, estrogen receptor positive), endometrial CA, melanoma, reduction of breast CA in high-risk women Action: Nonsteroidal antiestrogen; mixed agonist–antagonist effect Dose: 20–40 mg/d (typically 10 mg bid or 20 mg/d) Caution/Contra: [D, –] Caution in leukopenia, thrombocytopenia, hyperlipidemia Supplied: Tabs 10, 20 mg Notes/SE: Uterine malignancy and thrombotic events notes when administered to reduce risk of breast CA; menopausal symptoms (hot flashes, N/V) in premenopausal patients; vaginal bleeding and menstrual irregularities; skin rash, pruritus vulvae, dizziness, HA, peripheral edema; acute flare of bone metastasis pain and hypercalcemia; retinopathy reported (high dose); ↑ risk of pregnancy in premenopausal women by inducing ovulation

Tamsulosin (Flomax) Uses: BPH Action: Antagonist of prostatic α-receptors Dose: 0.4 mg/d; do not crush, chew, or open caps Caution/Contra: [NA/NA (not for use in women)] Supplied: Caps 0.4, 0.8 mg Notes/SE: HA, dizziness, syncope, somnolence, decreased libido, GI upset, retrograde ejaculation, rhinitis, rash, angioedema

Tazarotene (Tazorac) Uses: Facial acne vulgaris; stable plaque psoriasis up to 20% body surface area Action: Keratolytic Dose: *Adults & Peds >12 y. Acne:* Cleanse face, dry, and apply thin film qd hs on acne lesions. *Psoriasis:* Apply hs Caution/Contra: [X, ?/–] Retinoid sensitivity Supplied: Gel 0.05, 0.1% Notes/SE: Burning, erythema, irritation, rash, photosensitivity, desquamation, bleeding, skin discoloration

Tegaserod maleate (Zelnorm) Uses: Short-term treatment of constipation-predominant IBS in women Action: 5HT$_4$ serotonin agonist Dose: 6 mg PO bid pc for 4–6 wk; may continue for 2nd course Caution/Contra: [B, ?/–] Contra in severe renal, moderate-severe hepatic impairment, Hx of bowel obstruction, gallbladder disease, sphincter of Oddi dysfunction, abdominal adhesions Supplied: Tabs 2, 6 mg Notes/SE: Do not administer if diarrhea present, as ↑ GI motility; D/C if abdominal pain worsens

Telmisartan (Micardis) Uses: HTN, CHF, DN Action: Angiotensin II receptor antagonist Dose: 40–80 mg/d Caution/Contra: [C (1st trimester; D 2nd and 3rd trimesters), ?/–] Angiotensin II receptor antagonist sensitivity Supplied: Tabs 40, 80 mg Notes/SE: Edema, GI upset, HA, angioedema, renal impairment, orthostatic hypotension

Temazepam (Restoril) [C-IV] Uses: Insomnia Action: Benzodiazepine Dose: 15–30 mg PO hs PRN; ↓ dose in elderly Caution/Contra: [X; ?/–] Narrow-angle glaucoma Supplied: Caps 7.5, 15, 30 mg Notes/SE: Confusion, dizziness, drowsiness, hangover

Tenecteplase (TNKase) Uses: Reduction of mortality associated with AMI Action: Thrombolytic; TPA Dose: 30–50 mg; see following table: Caution/Contra: [C, ?]

Bleeding, CVA, major surgery (intracranial, intraspinal) or trauma within 2 mon **Supplied:** Inj 50 mg, reconstitute with 10 mL sterile water **Notes/SE:** Bleeding, hypersensitivity

Weight (kg)	TNKase (mg)	TNKase[a] Volume (mL)
<60	30	6
≥60–70	35	7
≥70–80	40	8
≥80–90	45	9
≥90	50	10

[a]From one vial of reconstituted TNKase.

Tenofovir (Viread) **Uses:** HIV infection **Action:** Nucleotide reverse transcriptase inhibitor **Dose:** 300 mg PO qd with a meal **Caution/Contra:** [B, ?/–] CrCl <60 mL/min; caution with known risk factors for liver disease **Supplied:** Tabs 300 mg **Notes/SE:** GI upset, metabolic syndrome, hepatotoxicity; separate didanosine doses by 2 h

Terazosin (Hytrin) **Uses:** BPH and HTN **Action:** α_1-Blocker (blood vessel and bladder neck/prostate) **Dose:** Initially, 1 mg PO hs; ↑ 20 mg/d max **Caution/Contra:** [C, ?] α-Antagonist sensitivity **Supplied:** Tabs 1, 2, 5, 10 mg; caps 1, 2, 5, 10 mg **Notes/SE:** Hypotension and syncope following 1st dose; dizziness, weakness, nasal congestion, peripheral edema common, palpitations, GI upset

Terbinafine (Lamisil) **Uses:** Onychomycosis, athlete's foot **Action:** Inhibits squalene epoxidase resulting in fungal death **Dose:** *Oral:* 250 mg/d PO for 6–12 wk. *Topical:* Apply to affected area; ↓ dose in renal/hepatic impairment **Caution/Contra:** [B, –] Liver disease or kidney impairment **Supplied:** Tabs 250 mg; cream 1% **Notes/SE:** Effect may take months due to need for new nail growth; do not use occlusive dressings; HA, dizziness, rash, pruritus, alopecia, GI upset, taste perversion, neutropenia, retinal damage, Stevens–Johnson syndrome

Terbutaline (Brethine, Bricanyl) **Uses:** Reversible bronchospasm (asthma, COPD); inhibition of labor **Action:** Sympathomimetic **Dose:** *Adults. Bronchodilator:* 2.5–5 mg PO qid or 0.25 mg SC; may repeat in 15 min (max 0.5 mg in 4 h). *Met-dose inhaler:* 2 inhal q4–6h. *Premature labor:* Acutely 2.5–10 mg/min/IV, gradually ↑ as tolerated q10–20min; maint 2.5–5 mg PO q4–6h until term. *Peds. Oral:* 0.05–0.15 mg/kg/dose PO tid; max 5 mg/24 h; ↓ dose in renal failure **Caution/Contra:** [B, +] Caution with diabetes, HTN, hyperthyroidism; tachycardia **Supplied:** Tabs 2.5, 5 mg; inj 1 mg/mL; met-dose inhaler **Notes/SE:** Caution with diabetes, HTN, hyperthyroidism; high doses may precipitate β_1-adrenergic effects; nervousness, trembling, tachycardia, HTN, dizziness

Terconazole (Terazol 7) **Uses:** Vaginal fungal infections **Action:** Topical antifungal **Dose:** 1 applicatorful or 1 supp intravaginally hs for 7 d **Caution/Contra:** [C, ?] **Supplied:** Vaginal cream 0.4%, vaginal supp 80 mg **Notes/SE:** Vulvar or vaginal burning

Teriparatide (Forteo) **Uses:** Severe/refractory osteoporosis **Action:** PTH (recombinant) **Dose:** 20 μg/d SQ in thigh or abdomen **Caution/Contra:** [C, ?/–) Osteosarcoma in animals—do not administer if Paget's disease, pediatric, prior radiation, bone metastases, hypercalcemia; caution in urolithiasis **Supplied:** 3 mL prefilled device (discard after 28 d) **Notes/SE:** Symptomatic orthostatic hypotension on administration, N/D, ↑ Ca, leg cramps; not recommended for use > 2 y

Tetanus Immune Globulin **Uses:** Passive immunization against tetanus for a suspected contaminated wound and unknown immunization status **Action:** Passive immunization **Dose:** *Adults & Peds.* 250–500 U IM (higher doses if delayed therapy); Table 9, page 621 **Caution/Contra:** [C, ?] Thimerosal sensitivity **Supplied:** Inj 250-U vial or syringe **Notes/SE:** May begin active immunization series at different inj site if required; pain, tenderness, erythema at inj site; fever, angioedema, muscle stiffness, anaphylaxis

Tetanus Toxoid **Uses:** Protection against tetanus **Action:** Active immunization **Dose:** Based on previous immunization status; Table 9 (page 621). **Caution/Contra:** [C, ?] Chloramphenicol use, neurologic symptoms with previous use, active infection (for routine primary immunization) **Supplied:** Inj tetanus toxoid, fluid, measured in limes flocculation (Lf) units of toxoid: 4–5 Lf units/0.5 mL; tetanus toxoid, adsorbed, 5, 10 Lf units/0.5 mL **Notes/SE:** Local erythema, induration, sterile abscess; chills, fever, neurologic disturbances

Tetracycline (Achromycin V, Sumycin) **Uses:** Broad-spectrum antibiotic treatment against *Staphylococcus, Streptococcus, Chlamydia, Rickettsia,* and *Mycoplasma* **Action:** Bacteriostatic; inhibits protein synthesis **Dose:** *Adults.* 250–500 mg PO bid–qid. *Peds >8 y.* 25–50 mg/kg/24 h PO q6–12h; ↓ dose in renal/hepatic impairment **Caution/Contra:** [D, +] Do not use with antacids; children ≤8 y **Supplied:** Caps 100, 250, 500 mg; tabs 250, 500 mg; oral susp 250 mg/5 mL **Notes/SE:** Can stain tooth enamel and depress bone formation in children; photosensitivity, GI upset, renal failure, pseudotumor cerebri, hepatic impairment

Theophylline (Theolair, Somophyllin, others) **Uses:** Asthma, bronchospasm **Action:** Relaxes smooth muscle of the bronchi and pulmonary blood vessels **Dose:** *Adults.* 900 mg PO ÷ q6h; SR products may be ÷ q8–12h × (maint). *Peds.* 16–22 mg/kg/24 h PO ÷ q6h; SR products may be ÷ q8–12h × (maint); ↓ dose in hepatic failure **Caution/Contra:** [C, +] Arrhythmia, hyperthyroidism, uncontrolled seizures **Supplied:** Elixir 80, 150 mg/15 mL; liq 80, 160 mg/15 mL; caps 100, 200, 250 mg; tabs 100, 125, 200, 225, 250, 300 mg; SR caps 50, 75, 100, 125, 200, 250, 260, 300 mg; SR tabs 100, 200, 250, 300, 400, 450, 500 mg **Notes/SE:** See drug levels in Table 2 (page 607); many drug interactions; N/V, tachycardia, and seizures; nervousness, arrhythmias

Thiamine [Vitamin B₁] **Uses:** Thiamine deficiency (beriberi), alcoholic neuritis, Wernicke's encephalopathy **Action:** Dietary supplementation **Dose:** *Adults. Deficiency:* 100 mg/d IM for 2 wk, then 5–10 mg/d PO for 1 mon. *Wernicke's encephalopathy:* 100 mg IV in single dose, then 100 mg/d IM for 2 wk. *Peds.* 10–25 mg/d IM for 2 wk, then 5–10 mg/24 h PO for 1 mon **Caution/Contra:** [A (C if doses exceed RDA), +] **Supplied:** Tabs 5, 10, 25, 50, 100, 500 mg; inj 100, 200 mg/mL **Notes/SE:** IV thiamine use associated with anaphylactic reaction; give IV slowly; angioedema, paresthesias, rash

Thiethylperazine (Torecan) **Uses:** N/V **Action:** Antidopaminergic antiemetic **Dose:** 10 mg PO, PR, or IM qd–tid; ↓ dose in hepatic failure **Caution/Contra:** [X, ?] Phenothiazine and sulfite sensitivity **Supplied:** Tabs 10 mg; supp 10 mg; inj 5 mg/mL **Notes/SE:** Extrapyramidal reactions may occur; xerostomia, drowsiness, orthostatic hypotension, tachycardia, confusion

6-Thioguanine [6-TG] (Tabloid) **Uses:** AML, ALL, CML **Action:** Purine-based antimetabolite (substitutes for natural purines interfering with nucleotide synthesis) **Dose:** 2–3 mg/kg/d; ↓ dose in severe renal/hepatic impairment **Caution/Contra:** [D, –] Resistance to mercaptopurine **Supplied:** Tabs 40 mg **Notes/SE:** Myelosuppression (especially leukopenia and thrombocytopenia), N/V/D, anorexia, stomatitis, rash, hyperuricemia; hepatotoxicity occurs rarely

Thioridazine (Mellaril) WARNING: Dose-related QT prolongation **Uses:** Psychotic disorders; short-term treatment of depression, agitation, organic brain syndrome **Action:** Phenothiazine antipsychotic **Dose:** *Adults.* Initially, 50–100 mg PO tid; maint 200–800 mg/24 h PO in 2–4 ÷ doses. *Peds >2 y.* 0.5–3 mg/kg/24 h PO in 2–3 ÷ doses **Caution/Contra:** [C, ?] Phenothiazine sensitivity **Supplied:** Tabs 10, 15, 25, 50, 100, 150, 200 mg; oral conc 30, 100 mg/mL; oral susp 25, 100 mg/5 mL **Notes/SE:** Low incidence of extrapyramidal effects; ventricular arrhythmias; hypotension, dizziness, drowsiness, neuroleptic malignant syndrome, seizures, skin discoloration, photosensitivity, constipation, sexual dysfunction, blood dyscrasias, pigmentary retinopathy, hepatic impairment

Thiothixene (Navane) **Uses:** Psychotic disorders **Action:** Antipsychotic **Dose:** *Adults & Peds >12 y. Mild–moderate psychosis:* 2 mg PO tid, up to 20–30 mg/d. *Severe psychosis:* 5 mg PO bid; ↑ to a max of 60 mg/24 h PRN. *IM use:* 16–20 mg/24 h ÷ bid–qid; max 30 mg/d. *Peds <12 y.* 0.25 mg/kg/24 h PO ÷ q6–12h **Caution/Contra:** [C, ?] Phenothiazine sensitivity **Supplied:** Caps 1, 2, 5, 10, 20 mg; oral conc 5 mg/mL; inj 2, 5 mg/mL **Notes/SE:** Drowsiness and extrapyramidal side effects most common; hypotension, dizziness, drowsiness, neuroleptic malignant syndrome, seizures, skin discoloration, photosensi-

22

tivity, constipation, sexual dysfunction, blood dyscrasias, pigmentary retinopathy, hepatic impairment

Tiagabine (Gabitril) **Uses:** Adjunctive therapy in treatment of partial seizures **Action:** Inhibition of GABA **Dose:** Initial 4 mg/d, ↑ by 4 mg during 2nd wk; ↑ PRN by 4–8 mg/d based on response, 56 mg/d/max **Caution/Contra:** [C, M] **Supplied:** Tabs 4, 12, 16, 20 mg **Notes/SE:** Use gradual withdrawal; used in combination with other anticonvulsants; dizziness, HA, somnolence, memory impairment, tremors

Ticarcillin (Ticar) **Uses:** Infections due to gram– bacteria (*Klebsiella, Proteus, E. coli, Enterobacter, P. aeruginosa,* and *Serratia*) involving the skin, bone, respiratory tract, urinary tract, and abdomen, and septicemia **Action:** Bactericidal; inhibits cell wall synthesis **Dose:** *Adults.* 3 g IV q4–6h. *Peds.* 200–300 mg/kg/d IV ÷ q4–6h; ↓ dose in renal failure **Caution/Contra:** [B, +] Penicillin sensitivity **Supplied:** Inj **Notes/SE:** Often used in combination with aminoglycosides; interstitial nephritis, anaphylaxis, bleeding, rash, hemolytic anemia

Ticarcillin/Potassium Clavulanate (Timentin) **Uses:** Infections caused by gram– bacteria (*Klebsiella, Proteus, E. coli, Enterobacter, P. aeruginosa,* and *Serratia*) involving the skin, bone, respiratory tract, urinary tract, and abdomen, and septicemia **Action:** Bactericidal; inhibits cell wall synthesis; clavulanic acid blocks β-lactamase activity **Dose:** *Adults.* 3.1 g IV q4–6h. *Peds.* 200–300 mg/kg/d IV ÷ q4–6h; ; ↓ dose in renal failure **Caution/Contra:** [B, +/–] Penicillin sensitivity **Supplied:** Inj **Notes/SE:** Often used in combination with aminoglycosides; hemolytic anemia

Ticlopidine (Ticlid) **WARNING:** Neutropenia/agranulocytosis, TTP, and aplastic anemia reported; monitor hematologic status 1st 3 mon **Uses:** ↓ risk of thrombotic stroke **Action:** Platelet aggregation inhibitor **Dose:** 250 mg PO bid with food **Caution/Contra:** [B, ?/–] Bleeding, hepatic impairment, neutropenia, thrombocytopenia **Supplied:** Tabs 250 mg **Notes/SE:** Bleeding, GI upset, rash, ↑ on LFTs

Timolol (Blocadren) **WARNING:** Exacerbation of ischemic heart disease following abrupt withdrawal **Uses:** HTN and MI **Action:** Competitively blocks β-adrenergic receptors, β_1, β_2 **Dose:** *HTN:* 10–20 mg bid, up to 60 mg/d. *MI:* 10 mg bid **Caution/Contra:** [C (1st trimester) (D if 2nd or 3rd trimester), +] Uncomplicated CHF, cardiogenic shock, bradycardia, heart block, COPD, asthma **Supplied:** Tabs 5, 10, 20 mg **Notes/SE:** Sexual dysfunction, arrhythmia, dizziness, fatigue, CHF

Timolol, Ophthalmic (Timoptic) **Uses:** Glaucoma **Action:** β-Blocker **Dose:** 0.25% 1 gt bid; ↓ to qd when controlled; use 0.5% if needed; 1 gtt/d gel **Caution/Contra:** [C (1st trimester, D 2nd or 3rd), ?/+] **Supplied:** Soln 0.25/0.5%; Timoptic XE (0.25, 0.5%) gel-forming soln **Notes/SE:** Local irritation

Tinzaparin (Innohep) **Uses:** Rx of DVT with or without PE **Action:** LMW heparin **Dose:** 175 units/kg SC qd at least 6 d until warfarin dose stabilized **Caution/Contra:** [B, ?] Pork hypersensitivity, sulfites, HIT, active bleeding; caution in mild–moderate renal dysfunction **Supplied:** Multidose vials 20,000 U/mL in 2 mL **Notes/SE:** Anti-Xa levels monitoring tool; no effect on bleeding time, platelet function, PT, or aPTT; bleeding, bruising, thrombocytopenia, pain at inj site, ↑ LFTs

Tioconazole (Vagistat-1) **Uses:** Vaginal fungal infections **Action:** Topical antifungal **Dose:** 1 applicatorful intravaginally hs (single dose) **Caution/Contra:** [C, ?] **Supplied:** Vaginal oint 6.5% **Notes/SE:** Local burning, itching, soreness, polyuria

Tirofiban (Aggrastat) **Uses:** Acute coronary syndrome **Action:** Glycoprotein IIB/IIIa inhibitor **Dose:** Initial 0.4 mcg/kg/min for 30 min, followed by 0.1 mcg/kg/min; use in combination with heparin; ↓ dose in renal insufficiency **Caution/Contra:** [B, ?/–] Bleeding, intracranial neoplasm, vascular malformation, stroke/surgery/trauma within last 30 d, severe HTN **Supplied:** Inj 50, 250 mcg/mL **Notes/SE:** Bleeding, bradycardia, coronary dissection, pelvic pain, rash

Tobramycin (Nebcin) **Uses:** Serious gram– infections, especially *Pseudomonas* **Action:** Aminoglycoside; inhibits protein synthesis **Dose:** *Adults.* 1–2.5 mg/kg/dose IV q8–24h **Peds.** 2.5 mg/kg/dose IV q8h; ↓ with renal insufficiency **Caution/Contra:** [C, M] Aminoglycoside sensitivity **Supplied:** Inj 10, 40 mg/mL **Notes/SE:** Nephrotoxic and ototoxic; monitor CrCl and serum concs for dosage adjustments (Table 2, page 607)

22

Tobramycin Ophthalmic (AKTob, Tobrex) Uses: Ocular bacterial infections **Action:** Aminoglycoside **Dose:** 1–2 gtt q4h; oint bid–tid; if severe infections, use oint q3–4h, or 2 gtt q30–60min, then less frequently **Caution/Contra:** [C, M] Aminoglycoside sensitivity **Supplied:** Oint and soln tobramycin 0.3% **Notes/SE:** Ocular irritation

Tobramycin and Dexamethasone Ophthalmic (TobraDex) Uses: Ocular bacterial infections associated with significant inflammation **Action:** Antibiotic with antiinflammatory **Dose:** 0.3% oint apply q3–8h or soln 0.3% apply 1–2 gtt q1–4h **Caution/Contra:** [C, M] Aminoglycoside sensitivity **Supplied:** Oint and soln tobramycin 0.3% and dexamethasone 0.1% **Notes/SE:** Local irritation or edema; use under ophthalmologist's direction

Tocainide (Tonocard) WARNING: Blood dyscrasias reported, follow hematologic parameters; pulmonary fibrosis reported, follow Sx and CXR **Uses:** Suppression of ventricular arrhythmias, including PVCs, and ventricular tachycardia **Action:** Class IB antiarrhythmic **Dose:** 400–600 mg PO q8h, up to 2400 mg/d; ↓ dose in renal failure **Caution/Contra:** [C, +/–] Heart block w/o pacemaker, amide-type anesthetic sensitivity **Supplied:** Tabs 400, 600 mg **Notes/SE:** SE similar to those for lidocaine; CNS and GI SE common; dizziness, tachycardia, hypotension, arrhythmias, HA, rash, hepatitis

Tolazamide (Tolinase) Uses: Type 2 DM **Action:** Sulfonylurea; stimulates the release of insulin from the pancreas; increases insulin sensitivity at peripheral sites; ↓ hepatic glucose output **Dose:** 100–500 mg/d (no benefit >1 g/d) **Caution/Contra:** [C, +/–] Caution in elderly or in hepatic or renal impairment **Supplied:** Tabs 100, 250, 500 mg **Notes/SE:** HA, dizziness, GI upset, rash, hyperglycemia, photosensitivity, blood dyscrasias

Tolazoline (Priscoline) Uses: Persistent pulmonary vasoconstriction and HTN of the newborn, peripheral vasospastic disorders **Action:** Competitively blocks α-adrenergic receptors **Dose:** *Adults.* 10–50 mg IM/IV/SC qid. *Neonates.* 1–2 mg/kg IV over 10–15 min, then 1–2 mg/kg/h **Caution/Contra:** [C, ?] CAD **Supplied:** Inj 25 mg/mL **Notes/SE:** Hypotension, peripheral vasodilation, tachycardia, arrhythmias, GI upset, blood dyscrasias, renal failure, GI bleeding

Tolbutamide (Orinase) Uses: Type 2 DM **Action:** Sulfonylurea; stimulates the release of insulin from the pancreas; increases insulin sensitivity at peripheral sites; ↓ hepatic glucose output **Dose:** 500–1000 mg bid; ↓ dose in hepatic failure **Caution/Contra:** [C, +] Sulfonylurea sensitivity **Supplied:** Tabs 500 mg **Notes/SE:** HA, dizziness, GI upset, rash, photosensitivity, blood dyscrasias, hypoglycemia

Tolmetin (Tolectin) Uses: Arthritis and pain **Action:** NSAID; inhibits prostaglandin synthesis **Dose:** 200–600 mg tid 2000; mg/d max **Caution/Contra:** [C (D in 3rd trimester or near term), +] NSAID or ASA sensitivity **Supplied:** Tabs 200, 600 mg; caps 400 mg **Notes/SE:** Dizziness, rash, GI upset, edema, GI bleeding, renal failure

Tolnaftate (Tinactin) Uses: Tinea pedis, tinea cruris, tinea corporis, tinea manus, tinea versicolor **Action:** Topical antifungal **Dose:** Apply to area bid for 2–4 wk **Caution/Contra:** [C, ?] **Supplied:** OTC 1% liq; gel; powder; cream; soln **Notes/SE:** Local irritation

Tolterodine (Detrol, Detrol LA) Uses: Overactive bladder (frequency, urgency, urge incontinence) **Action:** Anticholinergic **Dose:** Detrol 1–2 mg PO bid; Detrol LA 2–4 mg/d **Caution/Contra:** [C, ?/–] Urinary retention, gastric retention, or uncontrolled narrow-angle glaucoma; significant drug interactions with CYP2D6, CYP3A3/4 substrates **Supplied:** Tabs 1, 2 mg; Detrol LA tabs 2, 4 mg **Notes/SE:** Xerostomia common side effect

Topiramate (Topamax) Uses: Partial-onset seizures **Action:** Anticonvulsant **Dose:** Total dose 400 mg/d. See product information for 8-wk titration schedule; ↓ dose in renal failure **Caution/Contra:** [C, ?/–] **Supplied:** Tabs 25, 100, 200 mg; caps sprinkles 15, 25, 50 mg **Notes/SE:** May precipitate kidney stones; fatigue, dizziness, psychomotor slowing, memory impairment, GI upset, tremor, nystagmus

Topotecan (Hycamtin) WARNING: Chemotherapy precautions, myelosuppression possible **Uses:** Ovarian CA (cisplatin-refractory), small-cell lung CA, and NHL **Action:** Topoisomerase I inhibitor; interferes with DNA synthesis **Dose:** 1.5 mg/m^2/d as a 1-h IV inf for 5 consecutive days, repeated q3wk; ↓ dose in renal failure **Caution/Contra:** [D, –] Sup-

plied: Vials containing 4 mg lyophilized drug reconstituted in sterile water and diluted in NS or 5% dextrose **Notes/SE:** Myelosuppression, N/V/D, drug fever, skin rash

Torsemide (Demadex) **Uses:** Edema, HTN, CHF, and hepatic cirrhosis **Action:** Loop diuretic; inhibits reabsorption of Na and Cl in ascending loop of Henle and distal tubule **Dose:** 5–20 mg/d PO or IV **Caution/Contra:** [B, ?] Sulfonylurea sensitivity **Supplied:** Tabs 5, 10, 20, 100 mg; inj 10 mg/mL **Notes/ SE:** Orthostatic hypotension, HA, dizziness, photosensitivity, electrolyte imbalance, blurred vision, renal impairment

Tramadol (Ultram) **Uses:** Moderate–severe pain **Action:** Centrally acting analgesic **Dose:** 50–100 mg PO q4–6h PRN, not to exceed 400 mg/d **Caution/Contra:** [C, ?/–] Opioid dependency; MAOIs **Supplied:** Tabs 50 mg **Notes/SE:** Lowers seizure threshold, tolerance or dependence may develop; dizziness, HA, somnolence, GI upset, respiratory depression, anaphylaxis (sensitivity to codeine)

Tramadol/Acetaminophen (Ultracet) **Uses:** Short-term management of acute pain (<5 d) **Action:** Centrally acting analgesic; nonnarcotic analgesic **Dose:** 2 tab PO q4–6h PRN; 8 tab/d max; *Elderly/renal impairment:* Use lowest possible dose; 2 tab q12h max if CrCl <30 **Caution/Contra:** [C, –] Contra in allergy to either drug, in acutely intoxicated patients; caution in seizures, hepatic/renal impairment, or Hx addictive tendencies **Supplied:** Tab 37.5 mg tramadol/325 mg APAP **Notes/SE:** Avoid alcohol use; SSRIs, TCAs, opioids, MAOIs increase risk of seizures; dizziness, somnolence, tremor, HA, risk of seizures, N/V/D, constipation, xerostomia, liver toxicity, rash, pruritus, ↑ sweating, physical dependence

Trandolapril (Mavik) WARNING: Use in PRG in 2nd/3rd trimester can result in fetal death. **Uses:** HTN, CHF, LVD, post-AMI **Action:** ACE inhibitor **Dose:** *HTN:* 2–4 mg/d. *CHF/LVD:* 4 mg/d; ↓ dose in severe renal/hepatic impairment **Caution/Contra:** [D, +] ACE inhibitor sensitivity, angioedema with ACE inhibitors **Supplied:** Tabs 1, 2, 4 mg **Notes/SE:** Hypotension, bradycardia, dizziness, hyperkalemia, GI upset, renal impairment, cough, angioedema

Trazodone (Desyrel) **Uses:** Depression and insomnia associated with anxiety and depression **Action:** Antidepressant; inhibits reuptake of serotonin and norepinephrine **Dose:** *Adults & Adolescents.* 50–150 mg PO qd–qid; max 600 mg/d. *Sleep:* 50 mg PO, qhs, PRN **Caution/Contra:** [C, ?/–] **Supplied:** Tabs 50, 100, 150, 300 mg **Notes/SE:** May take 1–2 wk for symptomatic improvement; anticholinergic side effects; dizziness, HA, sedation, nausea, xerostomia, syncope, confusion, tremor, hepatitis, extrapyramidal reactions

Treprostinil Sodium (Remodulin) **Uses:** NYHA Class II–IV pulmonary arterial hypertension **Action:** Vasodilation, inhibition of platelet aggregation **Dose:** 0.625–1.25 ng/kg/min cont inf **Caution/Contra:** [B, ?/–] Initiate in monitored setting; do not DC or reduce dose abruptly **Supplied:** 1, 2.5, 5, 10 mg/mL inj **Notes/SE:** Additive effects with anticoagulants, antihypertensives; inf site reactions

Tretinoin, Systemic [Retinoic Acid] (Vesanoid) **Uses:** APL induction therapy **Action:** Differentiating agent; all *trans* retinoic acid **Dose:** 45 mg/m^2/d in ÷ doses for approximately 40 d; with food **Caution/Contra:** [D, ?] Retinoid sensitivity **Supplied:** Caps 10 mg **Notes/SE:** Cutaneous (dryness, chafing), neurologic (HA), hypertriglyceridemia, and treatment-related leukocytosis reported in APL, as well as "retinoic acid syndrome"

Tretinoin, Topical [Retinoic Acid] (Retin-A, Avita, Renova) **Uses:** Acne vulgaris, sun-damaged skin, wrinkles (aka photo aging), some skin CAs **Action:** Exfoliant retinoic acid derivative **Dose:** Adults & Peds >12 y. Apply qd hs; if irritation develops, ↓ frequency; photoaging, start 0.025%, increase to 0.1% over several months; apply only every 3 d if on neck area; dark skin may require bid application **Caution/Contra:** [C, ?] Retinoid sensitivity **Supplied:** Cream 0.025, 0.05, 0.1%; gel 0.01, 0.025, 0.1%; microformulation gel 0.1%;liq 0.05% **Notes/SE:** Avoid sunlight; edema; skin dryness, erythema, scaling, changes in pigmentation, stinging, photosensitivity

Triamcinolone and Nystatin (Mycolog-II) **Uses:** Cutaneous candidiasis **Action:** Antifungal and antiinflammatory **Dose:** Apply lightly to area bid; max 25 d **Caution/Contra:** [C, ?] Varicella; systemic fungal infections **Supplied:** Cream and oint 15, 30, 60, 120 mg **Notes/SE:** Local irritation, hypertrichosis, changes in pigmentation

Triamterene (Dyrenium) **Uses:** Edema associated with CHF, cirrhosis **Action:** K$^+$-sparing diuretic **Dose:** *Adults.* 100–300 mg/24 h PO ÷ qd–bid. *Peds.* 2–4 mg/kg/d in 1–2

÷ doses; ↓ dose in renal/hepatic impairment **Caution/Contra:** [B (manufacturer; D expert opinion), ?/–] Hyperkalemia, renal impairment, diabetes; caution with other K+-sparing diuretics **Supplied:** Caps 50, 100 mg **Notes/SE:** Hyperkalemia, blood dyscrasias, liver damage, and other reactions

Triazolam (Halcion) [C-IV]　**Uses:** Short-term management of insomnia **Action:** Benzodiazepine **Dose:** 0.125–0.25 mg/d PO hs PRN; additive CNS depression with alcohol and other CNS depressants; ↓ dose in elderly **Caution/Contra:** [X, ?/–] Narrow-angle glaucoma; cirrhosis, amprenavir, ritonavir, nelfinavir **Supplied:** Tabs 0.125, 0.25 mg **Notes/SE:** Tachycardia, chest pain, drowsiness, fatigue, memory impairment, GI upset

Triethanolamine (Cerumenex)　**Uses:** Cerumen removal **Action:** Ceruminolytic agent **Dose:** Fill the ear canal and insert the cotton plug; irrigate with water after 15 min; repeat PRN **Caution/Contra:** [C, ?] Perforated tympanic membrane, otitis media **Supplied:** Soln 6, 12 mL **Notes/SE:** Local dermatitis, pain, erythema, pruritus

Triethylene-Triphosphamide (Thio-Tepa, Tespa, TSPA)　**Uses:** Hodgkin's and NHLs; leukemia; breast, ovarian, and bladder CAs (IV and intravesical therapy), preparative regimens for allogeneic and autologous BMT in high doses **Action:** Polyfunctional alkylating agent **Dose:** 0.5 mg/kg q1–4wk, 6 mg/m^2 IM or IV ×4 d q2–4wk, 15–35 mg/m^2 by cont IV inf over 48 h; 60 mg into the bladder and retained 2 h q1–4wk; 900–125 mg/m^2 in ABMT regimens (the highest dose that can be administered without ABMT is 180 mg/m^2); 1–10 mg/m^2 (typically 15 mg) IT once or twice a wk; 0.8 mg/kg in 1–2 L of soln may be instilled intraperitoneally; ↓ dose in renal failure **Caution/Contra:** [D, –] **Supplied:** Inj 15 mg **Notes/SE:** Myelosuppression, N/V, dizziness, HA, allergy, paresthesias, alopecia

Trifluoperazine (Stelazine)　**Uses:** Psychotic disorders **Action:** Phenothiazine; blocks postsynaptic CNS dopaminergic receptors in the brain **Dose:** *Adults.* 2–10 mg PO bid. *Peds 6–12 y.* 1 mg PO qd–bid initially, gradually ↑ to 15 mg/d; ↓ dose in elderly/debilitated patients **Caution/Contra:** [C, ?/–] Hx blood dyscrasias; phenothiazine sensitivity **Supplied:** Tabs 1, 2, 5, 10 mg; oral conc 10 mg/mL; inj 2 mg/mL **Notes/SE:** Oral conc must be diluted to 60 mL or more prior to administration; requires several wks for onset of effects; orthostatic hypotension, EPS, dizziness, neuroleptic malignant syndrome, skin discoloration, lowered seizure threshold, photosensitivity, blood dyscrasias

Trifluridine (Viroptic)　**Uses:** Herpes simplex keratitis and conjunctivitis **Action:** Antiviral **Dose:** 1 gtt q2h (max 9 gtt/d); ↓ to 1 gtt q4h after healing begins; treat up to 14 d **Caution/Contra:** [C, M] **Supplied:** Soln 1% **Notes/SE:** Local burning, stinging

Trihexyphenidyl (Artane)　**Uses:** Parkinson's disease **Action:** Blocks excess acetylcholine at cerebral synapses **Dose:** 2–5 mg PO qd–qid **Caution/Contra:** [C, +] Narrow-angle glaucoma, GI obstruction, MyG, bladder obstructions **Supplied:** Tabs 2, 5 mg; SR caps 5 mg; elixir 2 mg/5 mL **Notes/SE:** Dry skin, constipation, xerostomia, photosensitivity, tachycardia, arrhythmias

Trimethobenzamide (Tigan)　**Uses:** N/V **Action:** Inhibits medullary chemoreceptor trigger zone **Dose:** *Adults.* 250 mg PO or 200 mg PR or IM tid–qid PRN. *Peds.* 20 mg/kg/24 h PO or 15 mg/kg/24 h PR or IM in 3–4 ÷ doses (not recommended for infants) **Caution/Contra:** [C, ?] Benzocaine sensitivity; inj in children; suppositories in premature infants or neonates **Supplied:** Caps 100, 250 mg; supp 100, 200 mg; inj 100 mg/mL **Notes/SE:** In the presence of viral infections, may mask emesis or mimic CNS effects of Reye's syndrome; may cause parkinsonian-like syndrome; drowsiness, hypotension, dizziness; hepatic impairment, blood dyscrasias, seizures

Trimethoprim (Trimpex, Proloprim)　**Uses:** UTI due to susceptible gram+ and gram– organisms; suppression of UTI **Action:** Inhibits dihydrofolate reductase **Dose:** *Adults.* 100 mg/d PO bid or 200 mg/d PO. *Peds.* 4 mg/kg/d in 2 ÷ doses; ↓ dose in renal failure **Caution/Contra:** [C, +] Megaloblastic anemia due to folate deficiency **Supplied:** Tabs 100, 200 mg; oral soln 50 mg/5 mL **Notes/SE:** Rash, pruritus, megaloblastic anemia, hepatic impairment, blood dyscrasias

Trimethoprim-Sulfamethoxazole [Co-Trimoxazole] (Bactrim, Septra)　**Uses:** UTI treatment and prophylaxis, otitis media, sinusitis, bronchitis, and *Shigella, P. carinii,* and *Nocardia* infections **Action:** SMX-inhibiting synthesis of dihydrofolic acid; TMP-inhibiting dihydrofolate reductase to impair protein synthesis **Dose:** *Adults.* 1 DS tab PO bid or 5–20 mg/kg/24 h (based on TMP) IV in 3–4 ÷ doses. *P. carinii:* 15–20 mg/kg/d

22

IV or PO (TMP) in 4 ÷ doses. *Nocardia:* 10–15 mg/kg/d IV or PO (TMP) in 4 ÷ doses. *UTI prophylaxis:* 1 PO qd. **Peds.** 8–10 mg/kg/24 h (TMP) PO ÷ into 2 doses or 3–4 doses IV; do not use in newborns; ↓ dose in renal failure; maintain hydration **Caution/Contra:** [B (D if near term), +] Sulfonamide sensitivity, porphyria, megaloblastic anemia with folate deficiency, significant hepatic impairment, age <2 mon, interacts with warfarin **Supplied:** Regular tabs 80 mg TMP/400 mg SMX; DS tabs 160 mg TMP/800 mg SMX; oral susp 40 mg TMP/200 mg SMX/5 mL; inj 80 mg TMP/ 400 mg SMX/5 mL **Notes/SE:** Synergistic combination; allergic skin reactions, photosensitivity, GI upset, Stevens-Johnson syndrome, blood dyscrasias, hepatitis

Trimetrexate (Neutrexin) WARNING: Must be used with leucovorin to avoid toxicity **Uses:** Moderate–severe PCP **Action:** Inhibits dihydrofolate reductase **Dose:** 45 mg/m^2 IV q24h for 21 d; ↓ in hepatic impairment **Caution/Contra:** [D, ?/–] Methotrexate sensitivity **Supplied:** Inj **Notes/SE:** Administer with leucovorin 20 mg/m^2 IV q6h for 24 d; use cytotoxic cautions; infuse over 60 min; seizure, fever, rash, GI upset, anemias, and ↑ LFTs, peripheral neuropathy, renal impairment

Trimipramine (Surmontil) **Uses:** Depression **Action:** TCA; increases synaptic conc of serotonin and/or norepinephrine in CNS **Dose:** 50–300 mg/d PO hs; avoid grapefruit juice **Caution/Contra:** [C, ?] Narrow-angle glaucoma **Supplied:** Caps 25, 50, 100 mg **Notes/SE:** Arrhythmias, hypotension, tachycardia, confusion, photosensitivity, sexual dysfunction, xerostomia, constipation, urinary retention, EPS, hepatic damage, blood dyscrasias; do not DC abruptly in hyperthyroid patients

Triptorelin (Trelstar Depot, Trelstar LA) **Uses:** Palliation of advanced prostate CA **Action:** ↓ Gonadotropin secretion when given continuously; following 1st administration, there is a transient surge in LH, FSH, testosterone, and estradiol. After chronic/continuous administration (usually 2–4 wk), a sustained decrease in LH and FSH secretion and marked reduction of testicular and ovarian steroidogenesis is observed. A reduction of serum testosterone similar to surgical castration. **Dose:** 3.75 mg IM monthly or 11.25 mg IM q3mon **Caution/Contra:** [X, NA] Not indicated in females **Supplied:** Inj depot 3.75 mg; LA 11.25 mg **Notes/SE:** Dizziness, emotional lability, fatigue, HA, insomnia HTN, diarrhea, vomiting, impotence, urinary retention, UTI, pruritus, anemia, inj site pain, musculoskeletal pain, allergic reactions

Urokinase (Abbokinase) **Uses:** PE, DVT, restore patency to IV catheters **Action:** Converts plasminogen to plasmin that causes clot lysis **Dose:** *Adults & Peds. Systemic effect:* 4400 IU/kg IV over 10 min, followed by 4400–6000 IU/kg/h for 12 h. *Restore catheter patency:* Inject 5000 IU into catheter and gently aspirate **Caution/Contra:** [B, +] Do not use within 10 d of surgery, delivery, or organ biopsy; bleeding, CVA, vascular malformation **Supplied:** Powder for inj 5000 IU/mL, 250,000 IU vial **Notes/SE:** Bleeding , hypotension, dyspnea, bronchospasm, anaphylaxis, cholesterol embolism

Valacyclovir (Valtrex) **Uses:** Herpes zoster; genital herpes **Action:** Prodrug of acyclovir, inhibits viral DNA replication **Dose:** 1 g PO tid. *Genital herpes:* 500 mg bid ×7 d. *Herpes prophylaxis:* 500–1000 mg/d; ↓ dose in renal failure **Caution/Contra:** [B, +] **Supplied:** Caplets 500 mg **Notes/SE:** HA, GI upset, dizziness, pruritus, photophobia

Valdecoxib (Bextra) **Uses:** RA, osteoarthritis, primary dysmenorrhea **Action:** COX-II inhibition **Dose:** *Arthritis:* 10 mg PO qd. *Dysmenorrhea:* 20 mg PO bid, PRN **Caution/Contra:** [C, ?] Asthma, urticaria, allergic-type reactions after ASA or NSAIDs, sulfonamide hypersensitivity **Supplied:** Tabs 10, 20 mg **Notes/SE:** ↑ LFT, GI ulceration or bleeding; dizziness, edema, HTN, HA, peptic ulcer, renal failure; serious hypersensitivity reactions have occurred, including Stevens–Johnson syndrome

Valganciclovir (Valcyte) **Uses:** Treatment of CMV **Action:** Ganciclovir prodrug, inhibits viral DNA synthesis **Dose:** Induction, 900 mg PO bid with food ×21 days, then 900 mg/d PO **Caution/Contra:** Caution in renal impairment [C, ?/–] **Supplied:** Tabs 450 mg **Notes/SE:** Dose adjustment in renal dysfunction; bone marrow suppression, requires frequent CBCs; renal function monitoring required; caution with imipenem/cilastatin, nephrotoxic drugs

Valproic Acid (Depakene, Depakote) **Uses:** Rx epilepsy, mania; prophylaxis of migraines **Action:** Anticonvulsant; increases the availability of GABA **Dose:** *Adults & Peds. Seizures:* 30–60 mg/kg/24 h PO ÷ tid (after initiation of 10–15 mg/kg/24 h). *Mania:* 750 mg in 3 ÷ doses, ↑ 60 mg/kg/d max. *Migraines:* 250 mg bid, ↑ 1000 mg/d max; ↓ dose in hepatic impairment **Caution/Contra:** [D, +] Hepatic impairment **Supplied:** Caps 250 mg; syrup 250 mg/5 mL **Notes/SE:** Monitor LFTs and serum levels (Table 2, page 607); phenobarbital and phenytoin may alter levels; somnolence, dizziness, GI upset, diplopia, ataxia, rash, thrombocytopenia, hepatitis, pancreatitis, prolonged bleeding times, alopecia, weight gain, hyperammonemic encephalopathy reported in patients with urea cycle disorders

Valsartan (Diovan) WARNING: Use during 2nd/3rd trimester of PRG can cause fetal harm. **Uses:** HTN, CHF, DN **Action:** Angiotensin II receptor antagonist **Dose:** 80–160 mg/d; caution with K⁺-sparing diuretics or K⁺ supplements **Caution/Contra:** [C (1st trimester), D (2nd and 3rd trimesters), ?/–] Severe hepatic impairment, biliary cirrhosis, biliary obstruction, primary hyperaldosteronism, bilateral renal artery stenosis **Supplied:** Caps 80, 160 mg **Notes/SE:** Hypotension, dizziness

Vancomycin (Vancocin, Vancoled) **Uses:** Serious MRSA infections; enterococcal infections; oral Rx of *C. difficile* pseudomembranous colitis **Action:** Inhibits cell wall synthesis **Dose:** *Adults.* 1 g IV q12h; for colitis 125–500 mg PO q6h. *Peds (NOT neonates).* 40 mg/kg/24 h IV in ÷ doses q6–12h; ↓ in renal insufficiency **Caution/Contra:** [C, M] **Supplied:** Caps 125, 250 mg; powder for oral soln; powder for inj 500 mg, 1000 mg, 10 g/vial **Notes/SE:** Not absorbed PO, local effect in gut only; give IV dose slowly (over 1 h) to prevent "red-neck syndrome"; ↓ in renal insufficiency (for drug levels, Table 2, page 607). Ototoxic and nephrotoxic; GI upset (oral), neutropenia

Varicella Virus Vaccine (Varivax) **Uses:** Prevention of varicella (chickenpox) infection **Action:** Active immunization **Dose:** *Adults & Peds.* 0.5 mL SC, repeated in 4–8 wk **Caution/Contra:** [C, M] Contra in immunocompromised patients; neomycin-anaphylactoid reaction, blood dyscrasias; immunosuppressive drugs; avoid pregnancy for 3 mon after inj **Supplied:** Powder for inj **Notes/SE:** Live attenuated virus; may cause mild varicella infection; fever, local reactions, irritability, GI upset

Vasopressin [Antidiuretic Hormone, ADH] (Pitressin) **Uses:** Diabetes insipidus; relieve gaseous GI tract distention; severe GI bleeding **Action:** Posterior pituitary hormone, potent GI vasoconstrictor **Dose:** *Adults & Peds. Diabetes insipidus:* 2.5–10 U SC or IM tid–qid or 1.5–5.0 U IM q1–3d of the tannate; *GI hemorrhage:* 0.2–0.4 U/min; ↓ dose in cirrhosis; caution in vascular disease **Caution/Contra:** [B, +] **Supplied:** Inj 20 U/mL **Notes/SE:** HTN, arrhythmias, fever, vertigo, GI upset, tremor

Vecuronium (Norcuron) **Uses:** Skeletal muscle relaxation during surgery or mechanical ventilation **Action:** Nondepolarizing neuromuscular blocker **Dose:** *Adults & Peds.* 0.08–0.1 mg/kg IV bolus; maint 0.010–0.015 mg/kg after 25–40 min; additional doses q12–15min PRN; ↓ dose in severe renal/hepatic impairment **Caution/Contra:** [C, ?] **Supplied:** Powder for inj 10 mg **Notes/SE:** Drug interactions causing ↑ effect of vecuronium (eg, aminoglycosides, tetracycline, succinylcholine); fewer cardiac effects than with pancuronium; bradycardia, hypotension, rash

Venlafaxine (Effexor) **Uses:** Depression, generalized anxiety, social anxiety disorder **Action:** Potentiation of CNS neurotransmitter activity **Dose:** 75–375 mg/d ÷ into 2–3 equal doses; ↓ dose in renal/hepatic impairment **Caution/Contra:** [C, ?/–] MAOIs **Supplied:** Tabs 25, 37.5, 50, 75, 100 mg; ER caps 37.5, 75, 150 mg **Notes/SE:** HTN, HA, somnolence, GI upset, sexual dysfunction; actuates mania or seizures

Verapamil (Calan, Isoptin) **Uses:** Angina, essential HTN, arrhythmias; migraine prophylaxis **Action:** Ca²⁺ channel blocker **Dose:** *Adults. Arrhythmias:* 2nd line for PSVT with narrow QRS complex and adequate BP 2.5–5.0 mg IV over 1–2 min; repeat 5–10 mg in 15–30 min PRN (30 mg max). *Angina:* 80–120 mg PO tid, ↑ 480 mg/24 h max. *HTN:* 80–180 mg PO tid or SR tabs 120–240 mg PO qd to 240 mg bid. *Peds. <1 y:* 0.1–0.2 mg/kg IV over 2 min (may repeat in 30 min). *1–16 y:* 0.1–0.3 mg/kg IV over 2 min (may repeat in 30 min); 5 mg max. *Oral: 1–5 y:* 4–8 mg/kg/d in 3 ÷ doses. *>5 y:* 80 mg q6–8h; ↓ dose in renal/hepatic impairment **Caution/Contra:** [C, +] Conduction disorders, cardiogenic shock; caution with elderly patients **Supplied:** Tabs 40, 80, 120 mg; SR tabs 120, 180, 240 mg; SR caps 120, 180, 240, 360 mg; inj 5 mg/2 mL **Notes/SE:** Gingival hyperplasia, constipation, hypotension, bronchospasm, heart rate or conduction disturbances

Vinblastine (Velban, Velbe) WARNING: Chemotherapeutic agent; handle with caution **Uses:** Hodgkin's and NHLs, mycosis fungoides, CAs (testis, renal cell, breast, non-small-cell lung, AIDS-related Kaposi's sarcoma, choriocarcinoma), histiocytosis X **Action:** Inhibits microtubule assembly through binding to tubulin **Dose:** 0.1–0.5 mg/kg/wk (4–20 mg/m^2); ↓ dose in hepatic failure **Caution/ Contra:** [D, ?] IT use **Supplied:** Inj 1 mg/mL **Notes/SE:** Myelosuppression (especially leukopenia), N/V (rare), constipation, neurotoxicity (like vincristine but less frequent), alopecia, rash; myalgia tumor pain

Vincristine (Oncovin, Vincasar PFS) WARNING: Chemotherapeutic agent; handle with caution **Uses:** ALL, breast and small-cell lung carcinoma, sarcoma (eg, Ewing's, rhabdomyosarcoma), Wilms' tumor, Hodgkin's and NHLs, neuroblastoma, multiple myeloma **Action:** Promotes disassembly of mitotic spindle, causing metaphase arrest **Dose:** 0.4–1.4 mg/m^2 (single doses 2 mg/max); ↓ dose in hepatic failure **Caution/Contra:** [D, ?] IT use **Supplied:** Inj 1 mg/mL **Notes/SE:** Neurotoxicity commonly dose limiting, jaw pain (trigeminal neuralgia), fever, fatigue, anorexia, constipation and paralytic ileus, bladder atony; no significant myelosuppression with standard doses; soft tissue necrosis possible with extravasation

Vinorelbine (Navelbine) WARNING: Chemotherapeutic agent; handle with caution **Uses:** Breast and non-small-cell lung CA (alone or with cisplatin) **Action:** Inhibits polymerization of microtubules, impairing mitotic spindle formation; semisynthetic vinca alkaloid **Dose:** 30 mg/m^2/wk; ↓ dose in hepatic failure **Caution/Contra:** [D, ?] IT use **Supplied:** Inj 10 mg **Notes/SE:** Myelosuppression (especially leukopenia), mild GI effects, and infrequent neurotoxicity (6–29%); constipation and paresthesias (rare); tissue damage can result from extravasation

Vitamin B₁ See Thiamine (page 596)

Vitamin B₆ See Pyridoxine (page 585)

Vitamin B₁₂ See Cyanocobalamin (page 528)

Vitamin K See Phytonadione (page 580)

Voriconazole (VFEND) **Uses:** Invasive aspergillosis, serious infections caused by *Scedosporium* or *Fusarium* spp. **Action:** Inhibits ergosterol synthesis **Dose:** IV: 6 mg/kg q12h × 2, then 4 mg/kg bid; may reduce to 3 mg/kg/dose. PO: <40 kg–100 mg q 12h, up to 150 mg; >40 kg–200 mg q 12 h, up to 300 mg. ↓ dose in mild/moderate hepatic impairment **Caution/Contra:** [D,?/–] Severe hepatic impairment **Supplied:** Tabs 50, 200 mg; 200 mg inj **Notes/SE:** Must screen for multiple drug interactions (eg, increase dose when given with phenytoin); administer oral doses on empty stomach; visual changes, fever, rash, GI upset, ↑ LFTs

Warfarin (Coumadin) **Uses:** Prophylaxis and Rx of PE and DVT, AF with embolization, other postoperative indications **Action:** Inhibits vitamin K-dependent production of clotting factors in the order VII-IX-X-II **Dose:** Table 10 (page 622) for anticoagulation guidelines. *Adults.* Adjust to keep INR 2.0–3.0 for most; mechanical valves INR is 2.5–3.5. *ACCP guidelines:* 5 mg initially, (unless rapid therapeutic INR needed) use 7.5–10 mg or patient elderly or has other bleeding risk factors ↓. *Alternative:* 10–15 mg PO, IM, or IV qd for 1–3 d; maint 2–10 mg/d PO, IV, or IM; follow daily INR initially to adjust dosage. *Peds.* 0.05–0.34 mg/kg/24 h PO, IM, or IV; follow PT/INR to adjust dosage; monitor vitamin K intake; consider ↓ doses in hepatic impairment or elderly **Caution/Contra:** [X, +] Severe hepatic or renal disease, bleeding, peptic ulcer **Supplied:** Tabs 1, 2, 2.5, 3, 4, 5, 6, 7.5, 10 mg; inj **Notes/SE:** INR preferred test rather than PT; follow INR; bleeding caused by excessive anticoagulation (PT >3× control or INR >5.0–6.0); to rapidly correct excessive anticoagulation, use vitamin K, FFP or both; highly teratogenic; do not use in PRG. Caution patient on taking warfarin with other meds, especially ASA. *Common warfarin interactions:* Potentiated by APAP, alcohol (with liver disease), amiodarone, cimetidine, ciprofloxacin, co-trimoxazole, erythromycin, fluconazole, flu vaccine, isoniazid, itraconazole, metronidazole, omeprazole, phenytoin, propranolol, quinidine, tetracycline. Inhibited by barbiturates, carbamazepine, chlordiazepoxide, cholestyramine, dicloxacillin, nafcillin, rifampin, sucralfate, high vitamin K foods; bleeding, alopecia, skin necrosis, purple toe syndrome

Witch Hazel (Tucks Pads, others) **Uses:** After bowel movement cleansing to decrease local irritation or relieve hemorrhoids; after anorectal surgery, episiotomy **Dose:** Apply PRN **Caution/Contra:** [?, ?] **Supplied:** Presoaked pads, liq **Notes/SE:** Mild itching or burning

Zafirlukast (Accolate) **Uses:** Prophylaxis and chronic Rx of asthma **Action:** Selective and competitive inhibitor of leukotrienes **Dose:** 20 mg bid; empty stomach

22

Caution/Contra: [B,–] Interacts with warfarin, can ↑ PT **Supplied:** Tabs 20 mg **Notes/SE:** Not for acute asthma; hepatic dysfunction, usually reversible on discontinuation; HA, dizziness, GI upset; Churg–Strauss syndrome

Zalcitabine (Hivid) WARNING: Use with caution in patients with neuropathy, pancreatitis, lactic acidosis, hepatitis **Uses:** HIV **Action:** Antiretroviral agent **Dose:** 0.75 mg PO tid; ↓ dose in renal failure **Caution/Contra:** [C, +] **Supplied:** Tabs 0.375, 0.75 mg **Notes/SE:** May be used in combination with zidovudine; peripheral neuropathy, pancreatitis, fever, malaise, anemia, hypo-/hyperglycemia, hepatic impairment

Zaleplon (Sonata) **Uses:** Insomnia **Action:** A nonbenzodiazepine sedative hypnotic, a pyrazolopyrimidine **Dose:** 5–20 mg hs PRN; ↓ dose in renal/hepatic insufficiency, elderly **Caution/Contra:** [C, ?/–] Caution in mental/psychologic conditions **Supplied:** Caps 5, 10 mg **Notes/SE:** HA, edema, amnesia, somnolence, photosensitivity

Zanamivir (Relenza) **Uses:** Influenza A and B **Action:** Inhibits viral neuraminidase **Dose:** *Adults & Peds >7 y.* 2 inhal (10 mg) bid for 5 d; initiate within 48 h of symptoms **Caution/Contra:** [C, M] Pulmonary disease **Supplied:** Powder for inhal 5 mg **Notes/SE:** Uses a Diskhaler for administration; bronchospasm, HA, GI upset

Zidovudine (Retrovir) WARNING: Neutropenia, anemia, lactic acidosis, and hepatomegaly with steatosis **Uses:** HIV infection **Action:** Inhibits reverse transcriptase **Dose:** *Adults.* 200 mg PO tid or 300 mg PO bid or 1–2 mg/kg/dose IV q4h. *Pregnancy:* 100 mg PO 5×/d until the start of labor, then during labor 2 mg/kg over 1 h followed by 1 mg/kg/h until clamping of the umbilical cord. *Peds.* 160 mg/m^2/dose q8h; ↓ dose in renal failure **Caution/Contra:** [C, ?/–] **Supplied:** Caps 100 mg; tabs 300 mg; syrup 50 mg/5 mL; inj 10 mg/mL **Notes/SE:** Hematologic toxicity, HA, fever, rash, GI upset, malaise

Zidovudine and Lamivudine (Combivir) WARNING: Neutropenia, anemia, lactic acidosis, and hepatomegaly with steatosis **Uses:** HIV infections **Action:** Combination inhibitors of reverse transcriptase **Dose:** *Adults & Peds >12 y.* 1 tab bid; ↓?dose in renal failure **Caution/Contra:** [C, ?/–] **Supplied:** Caps zidovudine 300 mg/lamivudine 150 mg **Notes/SE:** An alternative to ↓ number of caps for combination therapy with the two agents; hematologic toxicity, HA, fever, rash, GI upset, malaise, pancreatitis

Zileuton (Zyflo) **Uses:** Prophylaxis and chronic treatment of asthma **Action:** Inhibitor of 5-lipoxygenase **Dose:** 600 mg qid **Caution/Contra:** [C, ?/–] Hepatic impairment **Supplied:** Tabs 600 mg **Notes/SE:** Must take on a regular basis; not for acute asthma; hepatic damage, HA, GI upset, leukopenia

Ziprasidone (Geodon) **Uses:** Schizophrenia, acute agitation **Action:** Atypical antipsychotic **Dose:** 20 mg PO bid with food, may increase in 2-day intervals up to 80 mg bid; agitation 10–20 mg IM PRN up to 40 mg/d. Separate 10 mg doses by 2h and 20 mg doses by 4 h **Caution/Contra:** [C, –] QT prolongation, recent MI, uncompensated heart failure, meds that prolong QT interval **Supplied:** Caps 20, 40, 60, 80 mg; Inj 20 mg/mL **Notes/SE:** Caution in hypokalemia/hypomagnesemia, bradycardia; monitor electrolytes; rash, somnolence, respiratory disorder, EPS, weight gain, orthostatic hypotension

Zoledronic acid (Zometa) **Uses:** Hypercalcemia of malignancy (HCM), ↓ skeletal-related events in prostate CA, multiple myeloma, and metastatic bone lesions **Action:** Bisphosphonate; inhibits osteoclastic bone resorption **Dose:** *HCM:* 4 mg IV over at least 15 min; may retreat in 7 days if adequate renal function. *Bone lesions/myeloma:* 4 mg IV over at least 15 min repeat q3–4wk PRN; prolonged with Cr ↑ **Caution/Contra:** [C, ?/–] Contra if bisphosphonate hypersensitive; caution with loop diuretics and aminoglycosides; adverse effects ↑ with renal dysfunction; caution in ASA-sensitive asthmatics **Supplied:** Vial 4 mg **Notes/SE:** Requires vigorous prehydration; do not exceed recommended doses/inf duration to minimize dose-related renal dysfunction; follow Cr; fever, flu-like syndrome, GI upset, insomnia, anemia; electrolyte abnormalities

Zolmitriptan (Zomig) **Uses:** Acute Rx migraine **Action:** Selective serotonin agonist; causes vasoconstriction **Dose:** Initial 2.5 mg, may repeat after 2 h to 10 mg max in 24 h **Caution/Contra:** [C, ?/–] Ischemic heart disease, Prinzmetal's angina, uncontrolled HTN, accessory conduction pathway disorders, ergots, MAOIs **Supplied:** Tabs 2.5, 5 mg **Notes/SE:** Dizziness, hot flashes, paresthesias, chest tightness, myalgia, diaphoresis

Zolpidem (Ambien) **Uses:** Short-term treatment of insomnia **Action:** Hypnotic agent **Dose:** 5–10 mg PO hs PRN; ↓ dose in elderly, hepatic insufficiency **Caution/Contra:** [B, +] **Supplied:** Tabs 5, 10 mg **Notes/SE:** HA, dizziness, drowsiness, nausea, myalgia

Zonisamide (Zonegran) **Uses:** Partial seizures **Action:** Anticonvulsant **Dose:** Initial 100 mg/d; may ↑ to 400 mg/d **Caution/Contra:** [C, –] Hypersensitivity to sulfonamides, oligohidrosis and hypothermia in peds **Supplied:** Caps 100 mg **Notes/SE:** Dizziness, drowsiness, confusion, ataxia, memory impairment, paresthesias, psychosis, nystagmus, diplopia, tremor; anemia, leukopenia; GI upset, nephrolithiasis, Stevens–Johnson syndrome; monitor for ↓ sweating and ↑ body temperature

TABLE 22-1
Quick Guide to Dosing of Acetaminophen Based on the Tylenol Product Line

	Suspension[a] Drops and Original Drops 80 mg/0.8 mL Dropperful	Chewable[a] Tablets 80-mg tabs	Suspension[a] Liquid and Original Elixir 160 mg/5 ml	Junior[a] Strength 160-mg Caplets/ Chewables	Regular[b] Strength 325-mg Caplets/ Tablets	Extra Strength[b] 500-mg Caplets/ Gelcaps
Birth–3 mo/6–11 lb/2.5–5.4 kg	½ dppr[c] (0.4 ml)					
4–11 mo/12–17 lb/5.5–7.9 kg	1 dppr[c] (0.8 ml)		½ tsp			
12–23 mo/18–23 lb/8.0–10.9 kg	1½ dppr[c] (1.2 ml)		¾ tsp			
2–3 y/24–35 lb/11.0–15.9 kg	2 dppr[c] (1.6 ml)	2 tab	1 tsp			
4–5 y/36–47 lb/16.0–21.9 kg		3 tab	1½ tsp			
6–8 y/48–59 lb/22.0–26.9 kg		4 tab	2 tsp	2 cap/tab		
9–10 y/60–71 lb/27.0–31.9 kg		5 tab	2½ tsp	2½ cap/tab		
11 y/72–95 lb/32.0–43.9 kg		6 tab	4 tsp	3 cap/tab		
Adults & children 12 y and over/96 lb and over/44.0 kg and over				4 cap/tab	1 or 2 caps/tabs	2 caps/gel

[a]Doses should be administered 4 or 5 times daily. Do not exceed 5 doses in 24 h.
[b]No more than 8 dosage units in any 24-h period. Not to be taken for pain for more than 10 days or for fever for more than 3 days unless directed by a physician.
[c]Dropperful.

TABLE 22-2
Common Drug Levels[a]

Drug	When to Sample	Therapeutic Levels	Usual Half-life	Potentially Toxic Levels
ANTIBIOTICS				
Gentamicin	Peak: 30 min after 30-min infusion (peak level not necessary if extended-interval dosing: 6 mg/kg/dose)	Peak: 5–8 mcg/mL Trough <2 mg/mL <1.0 µg/mL for extended intervals (6 mg/kg/dose) (peak levels not needed with extended-interval dosing)	2 h	Peak: >12 mcg/mL
	Trough: <0.5 h before next dose			
Tobramycin	Same as above	Same as above	Same as above	Same as above
Amikacin	Same as above	Peak: 20–30 mcg/mL	2 h	Peak: >35 mcg/mL
Vancomycin	Peak: 1 h after 1-h infusion	Peak: 30–40 mcg/mL	6–8 h	Peak: >50 mcg/mL
	Trough: <0.5 h before next dose			Trough: >15 mcg/mL
ANTICONVULSANTS				
Carbamazepine	Trough: just before next oral dose	8–12 mcg/mL (monotherapy) 4–8 mcg/mL (polytherapy)	15–20 h	Trough: >12 mcg/mL
Ethosuximide	Trough: just before next oral dose	40–100 mcg/mL	30–60 h	Trough: >100 mcg/mL

(continued)

TABLE 22–2
(Continued)

Drug	When to Sample	Therapeutic Levels	Usual Half-life	Potentially Toxic Levels
Phenobarbital	Trough: just before next dose	15–40 mcg/mL	40–120 h	Trough: >40 mcg/mL
Phenytoin	May use free phenytoin to monitor[b]	10–20 mcg/mL	Concentration-dependent	>20 mcg/mL
Primidone	Trough: just before next dose	5–12 mcg/mL	10–12 h	>12 mcg/mL
	Trough just before next dose (primidone is metabolized to phenobarb; order levels separately)			
Valproic acid	Trough: just before next dose	50–100 mcg/mL	5–20 h	>100 mcg/mL
BRONCHODILATORS				
Caffeine	Trough: just before next dose	Adults 5–15 mcg/mL Neonate 6–11 mg/mL	Adults 3–4 h Neonates 30–140 h	20 mcg/mL
Theophylline (IV)	IV: 12–24 h after infusion started	5–15 mcg/mL	Nonsmoking adult-8 h Children and smoking adults 4 h	>20 mcg/mL

(continued)

TABLE 22–2
(Continued)

Drug	When to Sample	Therapeutic Levels	Usual Half-life	Potentially Toxic Levels
Theophylline (PO)	Peak levels: not recommended Trough level: just before next dose	5–15 mcg/mL		
CARDIOVASCULAR AGENTS				
Amiodarone	Trough: just before next dose	1–2.5 mcg/mL	30–100 days	>2.5 mcg/mL
Digoxin	Trough: just before next dose (levels drawn earlier than 6 h after a dose will be artificially elevated)	0.8–2.0 ng/mL	36 h	>2 ng/mL
Disopyramide	Trough: just before next dose	2–5 mcg/mL	4–10 h	>5 mcg/mL
Flecainide	Trough: just before next dose	0.2–1.0 mcg/mL	11–14 h	>1.0 mcg/mL
Lidocaine	Steady-state levels are usually achieved after 6–12 h	1.2–5.0 mcg/mL	1.5 h	>6 mcg/mL
Procainamide	Trough: just before next oral dose	4–10 mcg/mL NAPA + Procaine: 5–30 mcg/mL	Procaine: 3–5 h NAPA: 6–10 h	>10 mcg/mL >30 mcg/mL (NAPA + Procaine)
Quinidine	Trough: just before next oral dose	2–5 mcg/mL	6 h	0.5 mcg/mL

(continued)

TABLE 22–2
(Continued)

Drug	When to Sample	Therapeutic Levels	Usual Half-life	Potentially Toxic Levels
OTHER AGENTS				
Amitriptyline plus nortriptyline	Trough: just before next dose	120–250 ng/mL		
Nortriptyline	Trough: just before next dose	50–140 ng/mL		
Lithium	Trough: just before next dose	0.5–1.5 mEq/mL	18–20 h	>1.5 mEq/mL
Imipramine plus desipramine	Trough: just before next dose	150–300 ng/mL		
Desipramine	Trough: just before next dose	50–300 ng/mL		
Methotrexate	By protocol	<0.5 μmol/L after 48 h		
Cyclosporine	Trough: just before next dose	Highly variable Renal: 150–300 ng/mL (RIA) Hepatic: 150–300 ng/mL	Highly variable	
Doxepin	Trough: just before next dose	100–300 ng/mL		
Trazodone	Trough: just before next dose	900–2100 ng/mL		

aResults of therapeutic drug monitoring *must* be interpreted in light of the complete clinical situation. For information on dosing or interpretation of drug levels contact the pharmacist or an order for a pharmacokinetic consult may be written in the patient's chart. Modified and reproduced with permission from the *Pharmacy and Therapeutics Committee Formulary*, 41st ed., Thomas Jefferson University Hospital, Philadelphia, PA.
bMore reliable in cases of uremia and hypoalbuminemia.

TABLE 22-3
Local Anesthetic Comparison Chart for Commonly Used Injectable Agents

Agent	Proprietary Names	Onset	Duration	Maximum Dose mg/kg	Maximum Dose Volume in 70-kg Adult[a]
Bupivacaine	Marcaine Sensoricaine	7–30 min	5–7 h	3	70 mL of 0.25% solution
Lidocaine	Xylocaine Anestacon	5–30 min	2 h	4	28 mL of 1% solution
Lidocaine with epinephrine (1:200,000)		5–30 min	2–3 h	7	50 mL of 1% solution
Mepivacaine	Carbocaine	5–30 min	2–3 h	7	50 mL of 1% solution
Procaine	Novocaine	Rapid	30 min–1 h	10–15	70–105 mL of 1% solution

[a]To calculate the maximum dose if not a 70-kg adult, use the fact that a 1% solution has 10 mg of drug per milliliter.

TABLE 22–4
Comparison of Systemic Steroids

Drug	Relative Equivalent Dose (mg)	Mineralo-corticoid Activity	Duration (h)	Route
Betamethasone	0.75	0	36–72	PO, IM
Cortisone (Cortone)	25.00	2	8–12	PO, IM
Dexamethasone (Decadron)	0.75	0	36–72	PO, IV
Hydrocortisone (Solu-Cortef, Hydrocortone)	20.00	2	8–12	PO, IM, IV
Methylprednisolone acetate (Depo-Medrol)	4.00	0	36–72	PO, IM, IV
Methylprednisolone succinate (Solu-Medrol)	4.00	0	8–12	PO, IM, IV
Prednisone (Deltasone)	5.00	1	12–36	PO
Prednisolone (Delta-Cortef)	5.00	1	12–36	PO, IM, IV

TABLE 22-5
Topical Steroid Preparations

Agent	Common Trade Names	Potency	Apply
Aclometasone dipropionate	Aclovate, cream, oint 0.05%	Low	bid/tid
Amcinonide	Cyclocort, cream, lotion, oint 0.1%	High	bid/tid
Betamethasone			
Betamethasone valerate	Valisone cream, lotion 0.01%	Low	qd/bid
Betamethasone valerate	Valisone cream, 0.01, 0.1%, oint, lotion 0.1%	Intermediate	qd/bid
Betamethasone dipropionate	Diprosone cream (0.05%)	High	qd/bid
	Diprosone aerosol (0.1%)		
Betamethasone dipropionate augmented	Diprolene oint, gel 0.05%	Ultrahigh	qd/bid
Clobetasol propionate	Temovate cream, gel, oint, scalp, soln 0.05%	Ultrahigh	bid (2 wk max)
Clocortolone pivalate	Cloderm cream 0.1%	Intermediate	qd-qid
Desonide	DesOwen, cream, oint, lotion 0.05%	Low	bid-qid
Desoximetasone			
Desoximetasone 0.05%	Topicort LP cream, gel 0.05%	Intermediate	
Desoximetasone 0.25%	Topicort cream, oint	High	
Dexamethasone base	Aeroseb-Dex aerosol 0.01%	Low	bid-qid
	Decadron cream 0.1%		
Diflorasone diacetate	Psorcon cream, oint 0.05%	Ultrahigh	bid/qid

(continued)

613

22

TABLE 22-5
(Continued)

Agent	Common Trade Names	Potency	Apply
Fluocinolone			
Fluocinolone acetonide 0.01%	Synalar cream, soln 0.01%	Low	bid/tid
Fluocinolone acetonide 0.025%	Synalar oint, cream 0.025%	Intermediate	bid/tid
Fluocinolone acetonide 0.2%	Synalar-HP cream 0.2%	High	bid/tid
Fluocinonide 0.05%	Lidex, anhydrous cream, gel, soln 0.05%	High	bid/tid oint
	Lidex-E aqueous cream 0.05%		
Flurandrenolide	Cordran cream, oint 0.025%	Intermediate	bid/tid
	cream, lotion, oint 0.05%	Intermediate	bid/tid
	tape, 4 µg/cm²	Intermediate	qd
Fluticasone propionate	Cultivate cream 0.05%, oint 0.005%	Intermediate	bid
Halobetasol	Ultravate cream, oint 0.05%	Very High	bid
Halcinonide	Halog cream 0.025%, emollient base 0.1% cream, oint, solution 0.1%	High	qd/tid
Hydrocortisone			
Hydrocortisone	Cortisone, Caldecort, Hycort, Hytone, etc.	Low	tid/qid
	aerosol 1%, cream: 0.5, 1, 2.5%, gel 0.5% oint 0.5, 1, 2.5%, lotion 0.5, 1, 2.5%, paste 0.5% soln 1%		

(continued)

TABLE 22–5
(Continued)

Agent	Common Trade Names	Potency	Apply
Hydrocortisone acetate	Corticaine cream, oint 0.5, 1%	Low	tid/qid
Hydrocortisone butyrate	Locoid oint, soln 0.1%	Intermediate	bid/tid
Hydrocortisone valerate	Westcort cream, oint 0.2%	Intermediate	bid/tid
Mometasone furoate	Elocon 0.1% cream, oint, lotion	Intermediate	qd
Prednicarbate	Dermatop 0.1% cream	Intermediate	bid
Triamcinolone			
Triamcinolone acetonide 0.025%	Aristocort, Kenalog cream, oint, lotion 0.025%	Low	tid/qid
Triamcinolone acetonide 0.1%	Aristocort, Kenalog cream, oint, lotion 0.1%	Intermediate	tid/qid
	Aerosol 0.2 mg/2-sec spray		
Triamcinolone acetonide 0.5%	Aristocort, Kenalog cream, oint 0.5%	High	tid/qid

TABLE 22–6
Comparison of Insulins

Type of Insulin	Onset (h)	Peak (h)	Duration (h)
ULTRA RAPID			
Humalog (lispro)	Immediate	0.5–1.5	3–5
NovoLog (insulin aspart)	Immediate	0.5–1.5	3–5
RAPID			
Regular Iletin II	0.25–0.5	2.0–4.0	5–7
Humulin R	0.5	2.5–4.0	6–8
Novolin R	0.5	2.0–5.0	5–8
Velosulin	0.5	2.0–5.0	6–8
INTERMEDIATE			
NPH Iletin II	1.0–2.0	6–12	18–24
Lente Iletin II	1.0–2.0	6–12	18–24
Humulin N	1.0–2.0	6–12	14–24
Novolin L	2.5–5.0	7–15	18–24
Novolin 70/30	0.5	7–12	24
PROLONGED			
Ultralente	4.0–6.0	14–24	28–36
Humulin U	4.0–6.0	8–20	24–28
Lantus (insulin glargine)	4.0–6.0	No peak	24
COMBINATION INSULINS			
Humalog Mix (lispro protamine/ lispro)	0.25–0.5	1–4	24

TABLE 22-7
Some Oral Contraceptives

Drug (Manufacturer)	Estrogen (mcg)[a]	Progestin (mg)[b]
MONOPHASICS		
Alesse 21, 28 (Wyeth)	Ethinyl estradiol (20)	Desogestrel (0.15)
Brevicon 21, 28 (Watson)[c]	Ethinyl estradiol (35)	Norethindrone (0.5)
Demulen 1/35 21 (Searle)[c]	Ethinyl estradiol (35)	Ethynodiol diacetate (1)
Demulen 1/50 21 (Searle)[c]	Ethinyl estradiol (50)	Ethynodiol diacetate (1)
Desogen (Organon)	Ethinyl estradiol (30)	Desogestrel (0.15)
Genora 1/50 28 (Physicians total care)	Mestranol (50)	Norethindrone (1)
Genora 1/35 21, 28 (Physicians total care)	Ethinyl estradiol (35)	Norethindrone (1)
Levlen 21, 28 (Berlex)	Ethinyl estradiol (30)	Levonorgestrel (0.15)
Levlite 21, 28 (Berlex)	Ethinyl estradiol (20)	Levonorgestrel (0.1)
Levora 21, 28 (Watson)	Ethinyl estradiol (30)	Levonorgestrel (0.15)
Loestrin 1.5/30 21, 28 (Parke-Davis)	Ethinyl estradiol (30)	Norethindrone acetate (1.5)
Loestrin 1/20 21, 28 (Parke-Davis)	Ethinyl estradiol (20)	Norethindrone acetate (1)
Lo/Ovral (Wyeth)[c]	Ethinyl estradiol (30)	Norgestrel (0.3)
Low-Ogestrel (Watson)	Ethinyl estradiol (30)	Norgestrel (0.3)
Modicon 28 (Ortho-McNeil)	Ethinyl estradiol (35)	Norethindrone (0.5)
Necon 1/50 21, 28 (Watson)	Mestranol (50)	Norethindrone (1)
Necon 0.5/35E 21, 28 (Watson)	Ethinyl estradiol (35)	Norethindrone (0.5)
Necon 1/35 21, 28 (Watson)	Ethinyl estradiol (35)	Norethindrone (1)
Nelova 0.5/35E 21 (Warner-Chilcott)[c]	Ethinyl estradiol (35)	Norethindrone (0.5)

(continued)

617

22

TABLE 22–7
(Continued)

Drug	Estrogen (mcg)[a]	Progestin (mg)[b]
Nelova 1/35 21 (Warner-Chilcott)	Ethinyl estradiol (35)	Norethindrone (1)
Nelova 1/50 21 (Warner-Chilcott)[c]	Mestranol (50)	Norethindrone (1)
Nordette-21 (Wyeth)[c]	Ethinyl estradiol (30)	Levonorgestrel (0.15)
Norinyl 1/35 21, 28 (Watson)	Ethinyl estradiol (35)	Norethindrone (1)
Norinyl 1/50 21, 28 (Watson)	Mestranol (50)	Norethindrone (1)
Ogestrel-28 (Watson)	Ethinyl estradiol (50)	Norgestrel (0.5)
Ortho-Cept 21 (Ortho-McNeil)[c]	Ethinyl estradiol (30)	Desogestrel (0.15)
Ortho-Cyclen 21 (Ortho-McNeil)[c]	Ethinyl estradiol (35)	Norgestimate (0.25)
Ortho-Novum 1/35 21 (Ortho-McNeil)[c]	Ethinyl estradiol (35)	Norethindrone (1)
Ortho-Novum 1/50 21 (Ortho-McNeil)[c]	Mestranol (50)	Norethindrone (1)
Ovcon 35 21, 28 (Warner-Chilcott)	Ethinyl estradiol (35)	Norethindrone (0.4)
Ovcon 50 21, 28 (Warner-Chilcott)	Ethinyl estradiol (50)	Norethindrone (1)
Ovral (Wyeth-Ayerst)[c]	Ethinyl estradiol (50)	Norgestrel (0.5)
Zovia 1/50E 21, 28 (Watson)	Ethinyl estradiol (50)	Ethynodiol diacetate (1)
Zovia 1/35E 21, 28 (Watson)	Ethinyl estradiol (35)	Ethynodiol diacetate (1)
BIPHASICS		
Jenest-28 (Organon)	Ethinyl estradiol (35)	Norethindrone (0.5, 1)
Necon 10/11 21, 28 (Watson)[c]	Ethinyl estradiol (35)	Norethindrone (0.5, 1)
Nelova 10/11 21 (Warner-Chilcott-McNeil)	Ethinyl estradiol (35)	Norethindrone (0.5, 1)
Ortho-Novum 10/11 21 (Ortho-McNeil)[c]	Ethinyl estradiol (35, 35)	Norethindrone (0.5, 1.0)

(continued)

TABLE 22-7
(Continued)

Drug	Estrogen (mcg)[a]	Progestin (mg)[b]
TRIPHASICS[d]		
Estrostep 28 (Parke-Davis)	Ethinyl estradiol (20, 30, 35)	Norethindrone acetate (1)
Mircette 28 (Organon)	Ethinyl estradiol (20, 0, 10)	Desogestrel (0.15)
Ortho Tri-Cyclen (Ortho-McNeil)[c]	Ethinyl estradiol (35, 35, 35)	Norgestimate (0.18, 0.215, 0.25)
Ortho-Novum 7/7/7 21 (Ortho-McNeil)[c]	Ethinyl estradiol (35, 35, 35)	Norethindrone (0.5, 0.75, 1.0)
Tri-Levlen 21, 28 (Berlex)	Ethinyl estradiol (30, 40, 30)	Levonorgestrel (0.05, 0.075, 0.125)
Tri-Norinyl 21, 28 (Watson)	Ethinyl estradiol (35, 35, 35)	Norethindrone (0.5, 1.0, 0.5)
Triphasil-21 (Wyeth)[c]	Ethinyl estradiol (30, 40, 30)	Levonorgestrel (0.05, 0.075, 0.125)
Trivora-28 (Watson)	Ethinyl estradiol (30, 40, 30)	Levonorgestrel (0.05, 0.075, 0.125)
PROGESTIN ONLY		
Micronor (Ortho-McNeil)	None	Norethindrone (0.35)
Nor-QD (Watson)	None	Norethindrone (0.35)
Ovrette (Wyeth-Ayerst)	None	Norgestrel (0.075)

[a]Ethinyl estradiol and mestranol are not equivalent milligram for milligram; the results of some studies indicate that 35 µg of ethinyl estradiol is equivalent to 50 mg of mestranol.
[b]Different progestins are not equivalent milligram for milligram.
[c]Also available in a 28-day regimen at slightly different cost.
[d]Estrogen/progesterone dose varies based on the time of the cycle (ie, days 1–7, 8–14, 15–21).

22

619

TABLE 22-8
Some Common Oral Potassium Supplements

Brand Name	Salt	Form	mEq Potassium/ Dosing Unit
Glu-K	Gluconate	Tablet	2 mEq/tablet
Kaochlor 10%	KCl	Liquid	20 mEq/15 mL
Kaochlor S-F 10% (sugar-free)	KCl	Liquid	20 mEq/15 mL
Kaochlor Eff	Bicarbonate/ KCl/citrate	Effervescent tablet	20 mEq/tablet
Kaon elixir	Gluconate	Liquid	20 mEq/15 mL
Kaon	Gluconate	Tablets	5 mEq/tablet
Kaon-Cl	KCl	Tablet, SR	6.67 mEq/tablet
Kaon-Cl 20%	KCl	Liquid	40 mEq/15 mL
KayCiel	KCl	Liquid	20 mEq/15 mL
K-Lor	KCl	Powder	15 or 20 mEq/packet
Klorvess	Bicarbonate/KCl	Liquid	20 mEq/15 mL
Klotrix	KCl	Tablet, SR	10 mEq/tablet
K-Lyte	Bicarbonate/ citrate	Effervescent tablet	25 mEq/tablet
K-Tab	KCl	Tablet, SR	10 mEq/tablet
Micro-K	KCl	Capsules, SR	8 mEq/capsule
Slow-K	KCl	Tablet, SR	8 mEq/tablet
Tri-K	Acetate/bicar- bonate and citrate	Liquid	45 mEq/15 mL
Twin-K	Citrate/gluconate	Liquid	20 mEq/5 mL

SR = sustained release.

22

TABLE 22–9
Tetanus Prophylaxis

History of Absorbed Tetanus Toxoid Immunization	Clean, Minor Wounds		All Other Wounds[a]	
	Td[b]	TIG[c]	Td[d]	TIG[c]
Unknown or <3 doses	Yes	No	Yes	No
<3 doses	No[e]	No	No[f]	No

[a]Such as, but not limited to, wounds contaminated with dirt, feces, soil, saliva, etc.; puncture wounds; avulsions; and wounds resulting from missiles, crushing, burns, and frostbite.
[b]Td = tetanus-diptheria toxoid (adult type), 0.5 mL IM.
  • For children < 7 y, DPT (DT, if pertussis vaccine is contraindicated) is preferred to tetanus toxoid alone.
  • For persons > 7 y, Td is preferred to tetanus toxoid alone.
  • DT = Diptheria-tetanus toxoid (pediatric), used for those who cannot receive pertussis.
[c]TIG = tetanus immune globulin, 250 U IM.
[d]If only 3 doses of fluid toxoid have been received, then a fourth dose of toxoid, preferably an absorbed toxoid, should be given.
[e]Yes, if > 10 y since last dose.
[f]Yes, if > 5 y since last dose.
Source: Based on guidelines from the Centers for Disease Control and Prevention and reported in *MMWR*.

TABLE 22–10
Oral Anticoagulant Standards of Practice

Thromboembolic Disorder	INR	Duration
DEEP VENOUS THROMBOSIS		
Prophylaxis (High-Risk Surgery)	10 mg night before surgery 5 mg night of surgery	Short term only
Treatment single episode	2–3	3–6 mon
Recurrent	2–3	Indefinite
PREVENTION OF SYSTEMIC EMBOLISM		
Atrial fibrillation (AF)[a]	2–3	Indefinite
AF: cardioversion	2–3	3 wk prior; 4 wk post sinus rhythm
Valvular heart disease	2–3	Indefinite
Cardiomyopathy	2–3	Indefinite
ACUTE MYOCARDIAL INFARCTION		
Prevention of systemic embolization	2–3	<3 mon
Prevention of recurrence	2.5–3.5	Indefinite
PROSTHETIC VALVES		
Tissue heart valves	2–3	3 mon
Bileaflet mechanical valve in aortic position	2–3	2–3 mon Indefinite
Other mechanical prosthetic valves[b]	2.5–3.5	Indefinite

[a]With high-risk factors or multiple moderate risk factors.
[b]May add aspirin 81 mg to warfarin in patients with ball–cage valves or with additional risk factors.
INR = international normalized ratio.
Source: Based on data published in *Chest* 2001;119 Supplement 1S–307S.

TABLE 22–11
Serotonin 5-HT₁ Receptor Agonists

Drug	Initial Dose	Repeat Dose	Max Dose/24h	Supplied
Almotriptan (Axert)	6.25 or 12.5 mg PO	× 1 in 2 h	25 mg	Tabs 6.25, 12.5 mg
Frovatriptan (Frova)	2.5 mg PO	in 2 h	7.5 mg	Tabs 2.5 mg
Naratriptan (Amerge)	1 or 2.5 mg PO^a	in 4h	5 mg	Tabs 1, 2.5 mg
Rizatriptan (Maxalt)	5 or 10 mg PO^b	in 2 h	30 mg	Tabs 5, 10 mg
				Disintegrating tabs, 5, 10 mg
Sumatriptan (Imitrex)	25, 50, or 100 mg PO	in 2 h	200 mg	Tabs 25, 50 mg
	5–20 mg intranasally	in 2 h	40 mg	Nasal spray 5, 20 mg
	6 mg SC	in 1 h	12 mg	Inj 12 mg/mL
Zolmitriptan (Zomig)	2.5 or 5 mg PO	in 2 h	10 mg	Tabs 2.5, 5 mg

Precautions/contraindications: (C, M) ischemic heart disease, coronary artery vasospasm, Prinzmetal's angina, uncontrolled HTN, hemiplegic or basilar migraine, ergots, use of another serotonin agonist within 24 h, use with MAOI. Side effects: dizziness, somnolence, paresthesias, nausea, flushing, dry mouth, coronary vasospasm, chest tightness, HTN, GI upset.
^aReduce dose in mild renal and hepatic insufficiency (2.5 mg/d MAX); contraindicated with severe renal (CrCl < 15 mL/min) or hepatic impairment.
^bInitiate therapy at 5 mg PO (15 mg/d max) in patients receiving propanolol.

APPENDIX

APGAR SCORES

Apgar scores (Table A-1, page 262) are a numerical expression of a newborn infant's physical condition. Usually determined 1 min after birth and again at 5 min, the score is the sum of points gained on assessment of color, heart rate, reflex irritability, muscle tone, and respirations.

BODY SURFACE AREA FOR ADULTS AND CHILDREN

Figure A-1 is a nomogram for determining the body surface area of an adult. Figure A-2 is a nomogram for determining the body surface area of children.

BODY MASS INDEX

Table A-2 gives BMI useful in the determination of obesity and other health-related risks. It also provides useful information for counseling patients on target body weights. Underweight = < 18.5 ; normal weight = 18.5–24.9; overweight = 25–29.9; obesity = BMI of 30 or greater. (From the National Heart Lung and Blood Institute (NIH) Bethesda MD 2003 http://www.nhlbisupport.com/bmi)

EPIDEMIOLOGY BASICS

$$\text{Prevalance} = \frac{\text{Number of persons who have a disease at one point in time}}{\text{Number of persons at risk at that point}}$$

$$\text{Incidence} = \frac{\text{Number of new cases of a disease over a period of time}}{\text{Number of persons at risk during that period}}$$

Sensitivity = Proportion of subjects with the disease who have a positive test
$$= (a / a = c)$$

Specificity = Proportion of subjects without the disease who have a negative test
$$= (d / b + d)$$

Predictive value = Positive: likelihood of a positive test indicates disease
$$= (a / a + b)$$
    = Negative: likelihood of a negative test indicates lack of disease
$$= (d / c + d)$$

Disease is
* (Present) – (Absent)

	Present	Absent
+	A	b
–	C	d

GLASGOW COMA SCALE

The Glasgow Coma Scale (*EMV* Scale) gives a fairly reliable, objective way to monitor changes in levels of consciousness. It is based on *E*ye opening, *M*otor responses, and *V*erbal responses. A person's EMV score is based on the total of the three responses. The score ranges from 3 (lowest) to 15 (highest) (Table A-3, page 630).

IMMUNIZATION GUIDELINES

Figure A-3, page 631 indicates the currently recommended childhood and adolescent immunization schedule in the United States for 2003. For additional details, see the CDC Website   http://www.cdc.gov/mmwr/preview/mmwrhtml/mm5204-immunizational.htm

MEASUREMENT EQUIVALENTS (APPROXIMATE)

Length

1 centimeter (cm) = 0.4 in.
1 meter (m) = 39.4 in.

Household

1 teaspoon (tsp) = 5 mL
1 tablespoon (tbsp) = 15 mL
1 ounce (oz) = 30 mL
8 ounces (oz) = 1 cup = 240 mL
1 quart (qt) = 946 mL

TABLE A-1
Apgar Scores

	Score		
Sign	0	1	2
Appearance (color)	Blue or pale	Pink body with blue extremities	Completely pink
Pulse (heart rate)	Absent	Slow (< 100/min)	> 100/min
Grimace (reflex irritability	No response	Grimace	Cough or sneeze
Activity (muscle tone)	Limp	Some flexion	Active movement
Respirations	Absent	Slow, irregular	Good, crying

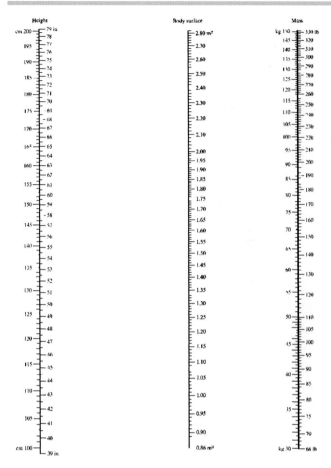

FIGURE A-1. Body surface area: Adult. Use a straight edge to connect the height and mass. The point of intersection on the body surface line gives the body surface area (in m²). (Reprinted, with permission, from: Lentner C [ed]: *Geigy Scientific Tables,* 8th ed. Ciba-Geigy, San Francisco, CA, 1981, Vol. 1, p. 226.)

Apothecary

1 grain (gr) = 60 mg
30 g = 1 oz
1 g = 15 gr

MEASUREMENT PREFIXES AND SYMBOLS

Factor	Prefix	Symbol
10^9	giga	G
10^6	mega	M

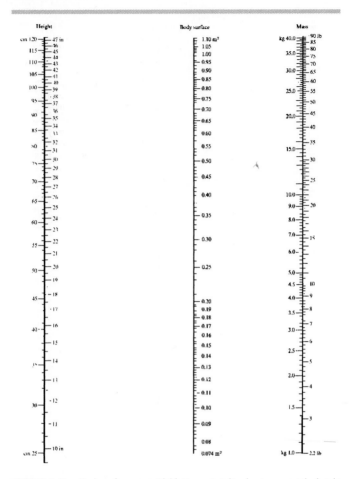

FIGURE A–2. Body surface area: Child. Use a straight edge to connect the height and mass. The point of intersection on the body surface line gives the body surface area (in m²). (Reprinted, with permission, from: Lentner C [ed]: *Geigy Scientific Tables,* 8th ed. Ciba-Geigy, San Francisco, CA, 1981, Vol. 1, p. 226.)

Factor	Prefix	Symbol
10^3	kilo	k
10^2	hecto	h
10^1	deka	da
10^{-1}	deci	d
10^{-2}	centi	c
10^{-3}	milli	m
10^{-6}	micro	m
10^{-9}	nano	n
10^{-12}	pico	p
10^{-15}	femto	f

TABLE A–2
Body Mass Index

Height ↓ / Weight →	120	130	140	150	160	170	180	190	200	210	220	230	240	250
4'6"	29	31	34	36	39	41	43	46	48	51	53	56	58	60
4'8"	27	29	31	34	36	38	40	43	45	47	49	52	54	56
4'10"	25	27	29	31	34	36	38	40	42	44	46	48	50	52
5'0"	23	25	27	29	31	33	35	37	39	41	43	45	47	49
5'2"	22	24	26	27	29	31	33	35	37	38	40	42	44	46
5'4"	21	22	24	26	28	29	31	33	34	36	38	40	41	43
5'6"	19	21	23	24	26	27	29	31	32	34	36	37	39	40
5'8"	18	20	21	23	24	26	27	29	30	32	34	35	37	38
5'10"	17	19	20	22	23	24	26	27	29	30	32	33	35	36
6'0"	16	18	19	20	22	23	24	26	27	28	30	31	33	34
6'2"	15	17	18	19	21	22	23	24	26	27	28	30	31	32
6'4"	15	16	17	18	20	21	22	23	24	26	27	28	29	30
6'6"	14	15	16	17	19	20	21	22	23	24	25	27	28	29
6'8"	13	14	15	17	18	19	20	21	22	23	24	25	26	28

TABLE A–3
Glasgow Coma Scale

Parameter	Response		Score
Eyes	Open: Spontaneously		4
		To verbal command	3
		To pain	2
		No response	1
Best motor response	To verbal command To painful stimulus	Obeys	6
		Localized pain	5
		Flexion-withdrawal	4
		Decorticate (flex)	3
		Decerebrate (extend)	2
		No response	1
Best verbal response		Oriented, converses	5
		Disoriented, converses	4
		Inappropriate responses	3
		Incomprehensible sounds	2
		No response	1

PERFORMANCE STATUS SCALES

Table A-4, page 634 lists the most common performance scales used clinically.

RADIATION TERMINOLOGY

Measure	Old Term	SI Unit
Activity	curie	becquerel (Bq)
Absorbed dose	rad	gray (Gy)

TEMPERATURE CONVERSION

Table A-5 gives information for converting temperature from the Fahrenheit (F) scale to the centigrade, or Celsius (C), scale and vice versa.

TNM AND OTHER SYSTEMS OF CLASSIFICATION FOR COMMON TUMORS

TNM stands for "tumor, nodes, metastasis" and is a universally accepted classification system for malignancy staging. The UICC (Union Internationale Contre le Cancer) and the AJCC (American Joint Committee on Cancer) have adopted this system and have published the most recent update of this system in *TNM Classification of Malignant Tumours,* 6th ed published by Springer, New York, 2002. The following is a highly selected listing of commonly encountered solid tumors (breast, bladder, cervix, colon and rectum, kidney, lung, melanoma, ovary, stomach, thyroid, uterus, and prostate) as well as the classification for lymphomas. Where appropriate, other common staging systems are noted (ie, Duke's classification of colon cancer) (see p. 634).

FIGURE A–3. Abbreviations: Diptheria and tetanus toxoids and acellular pertussis vaccine (DTaP); *Haemophilus influenza type b* vaccine (HiB); inactivated poliovirus (IPV); measles, mumos, and rubella vaccine (MMR); pneumococcal conjugate vaccine (PCV); tetanus and dipheria toxoids vaccine (Td). (Reprinted, with permission, from Centers for Disease Control and Prevention Website: http://www.cdc.gov/mmwr/preview/mmwrhtml/mm5204-Immunizational.htm)

TABLE A-4
Performance Status Scales

Karnofsky			ECOG		AJCC	
Functional Status	% Normal Status	Activity Level	Grade	Activity Level	Grade	Activity
Able to carry on normal activity; no special care needed	100	Normal; no complaints; no evidence of disease	0	Normal activity	H0	Normal activity
	90	Able to carry on normal activity; minor sign or symptoms of disease				
	80	Normal activity with effort; some signs or symptoms of disease	1	Symptoms but ambulatory	H1	Symptomatic and ambulatory; cares for self
Unable to work; able to live at home; cares for most personal needs, varying amount of assistance needed	70	Cares for self; unable to carry on normal activity or progressing rapidly to active work				
	60	Requires occasional assistance but able to care for self	2	In bed 50% of time	H2	Ambulatory 50% of time; occasionally needs assistance

(continued)

TABLE A–4
(Continued)

Functional Status	Karnofsky		ECOG		AJCC	
	% Normal Status	Activity Level	Grade	Activity Level	Grade	Activity
	50	Requires considerable assistance and frequent medical care				
Unable to care for self; requires equivalent of needed institutional or hospital care; may be progressing rapidly	40	Disabled; requires special care and assistance	3	In bed 50% of time	H3	Ambulatory 50% of time; nursing care
	30	Severely disabled; hospitalization indicated through death not imminent				
	20	Very sick; hospitalization necessary	4	100% bedridden	H4	Bedridden; may need hospitalization
	10	Moribund; fatal processes				
	0	Dead				

ECOG = Eastern Cooperative Oncology Group; AJCC = American Joint Committee on Cancer.
Source: Reprinted, with permission, from Cameron R (ed): *Practical Oncology.* Originally published by Appleton & Lange. Copyright © 1993. McGraw-Hill Companies, Inc.

TABLE A–5
Temperature Conversion Table

F	C	C	F
0	–17.7	0	32.0
95.0	35.0	35.0	95.0
96.0	35.5	35.5	95.9
97.0	36.1	36.0	96.8
98.0	36.6	36.5	97.7
98.6	37.0	37.0	98.6
99.0	37.2	37.5	99.5
100.0	37.7	38.0	100.4
101.0	38.3	38.5	101.3
102.0	38.8	39.0	102.2
103.0	39.4	39.5	103.1
104.0	40.0	40.0	104.0
105.0	40.5	40.5	104.9
106.0	41.1	41.0	105.8
$C = (F - 32) \times 5/9$		$F = (C \times 9/5) + 32$	

F = degrees Fahrenheit; C = degrees Celsius.

(TNM—Continued from p. 630.)

(TNM—Continued from p. 630.)

Breast

Primary Tumor (T)

TX   Primary tumor cannot be assessed

T0   No evidence of primary tumor

Tis Carcinoma in situ: Intraductal carcinoma, lobular carcinoma in situ, or Paget's disease of the nipple with no tumor. *Note:* Paget disease associated with a tumor is classified according to the size of the tumor.

T1   Tumor 2 cm or less in greatest dimension

    T1mic Microinvasion 0.1 cm or less in greatest dimension

    T1a   More than 0.1 cm but not more than 0.5 cm in greatest dimension

    T1b   More than 0.5 cm but not more than 1 cm in greatest dimension

    T1c   More than 1 cm but not more than 2 cm in greatest dimension

T2   Tumor more than 2 cm but not more than 5 cm in greatest dimension

T3   Tumor more than 5 cm in greatest dimension

T4   Tumor of any size with direct extension to chest wall or skin

    T4a   Extension of the chest wall. not including pectoralis muscle

    T4b   Edema (including peau d'orange) or ulceration of the skin of breast or satellite skin nodules confined to same breast

    T4c   Both T4a and T4b

    T4d   Inflammatory carcinoma

Lymph Node (N)

NX   Regional lymph nodes cannot be assessed

N0   No regional lymph node metastasis

N1   Metastasis to movable ipsilateral axillary lymph nodes(s)

N2a Metastasis to ipsilateral axillary lymph node(s) fixed, or matted, to one another or to other structures

N2b Metastasis only in clinically apparent (by imaging or clinical exam) ipsilateral internal mammary nodes in the absence of clinically evident axillary nodes

N3a Metastasis in ipsilateral infraclavicular and axillary nodes

N3b Metastasis in ipsilateral internal mammary and axillary nodes

N3c Metastasis in ipsilateral supraclavicular nodes

Pathologic Classification (pTNM)

(pT) Primary Tumor

The pT categories correspond to the T categories.

(pN) Regional Lymph Nodes

pNX Regional lymph nodes cannot be assessed

pN0 No regional lymph node metastasis

     (i–/i+) with negative/positive immunohistochemistry)

     (mo1–/mo1+) with negative/positive molecular (RT-PCR) findings

    pN1mi Micrometastasis (0.2–2.0 mm)

    pN1a Metastasis in 1–3 axillary nodes

    pN1b Metastasis in internal mammary nodes with microscopic disease detected by sentinel lymph node dissection but not clinically apparent (by imaging or clinical exam)

    pN1c Metastasis in 1–3 axillary nodes and internal mammary nodes with microscopic disease detected by sentinel lymph node dissection but not clinically apparent (by imaging or clinical exam)

    pN2a Metastasis in 4–9 axillary nodes (at least one > 2.0 mm)

    pN2b Metastasis in clinically apparent (by imaging or clinical exam) internal mammary nodes in the absence of axillary nodes

    pN3a Metastasis in $\geq$ 10 axillary nodes (at least one > 2.0 mm) or metastasis in infraclavicular nodes

    pN3b Metastasis in clinically apparent (by imaging or clinical exam) ipsilateral internal mammary nodes with $\geq$ 1 positive axillary node or > 3 axillary nodes and internal mammary nodes with microscopic disease detected in sentinel lymph node but not clinically apparent

    pN3c Metastasis in ipsilateral and supraclavicular nodes

pM Distant Metastasis (M)

MX Presence of distant metastasis cannot be assessed

M0 No distant metastasis

M1 Distant metastasis

Bladder

Primary Tumor (T)

TX Primary tumor cannot be assessed

T0 No evidence of primary tumor

    Tis Carcinoma in situ: "flat tumor"

    Ta Noninvasive papillary carcinoma

T1 Tumor invades subepithelial connective tissue

T2 Tumor invades muscle

    T2a Tumor invades superficial muscle (inner half)

    T2b Tumor invades deep muscle (outer half)

T3 Tumor invades perivesical tissue

    T3a Microscopically

    T3b Macroscopically (extravesical mass)

T4   Tumor invades any of the following: prostate, uterus, vagina, pelvic wall, abdominal wall

     T4a   Tumor invades prostate or uterus or vagina

     T4b   Tumor invades pelvic wall or abdominal wall

Lymph Node (N)

NX   Regional lymph nodes cannot be assessed

N0   No regional lymph node metastasis

N1   Metastasis in a single lymph node, 2 cm or less in greatest dimension

N2   Metastasis in a single lymph node, more than 2 cm but not more than 5 cm in greatest dimension, or multiple lymph nodes, none more than 5 cm in greatest dimension

N3   Metastasis in a lymph node more than 5 cm in greatest dimension

Distant Metastasis (M)

MX   Presence of distant metastasis cannot be assessed

M0   No distant metastasis

M1   Distant metastasis

Pathologic Classification (pTNM)

The pT, pN, and pM categories correspond to the T, N , and M categories.

Cervix

Primary Tumor (T)

TX   Primary tumor cannot be assessed

T0   No evidence of primary tumor

Tis   Carcinoma in situ

T1   Cervical carcinoma confined to uterus

     T1a   Preclinical invasive carcinoma diagnosed by microscopy only

     T1b   Preclinical visible lesion confined to the cervix ormicroscopic lesion greater than T1a2

         T1a1   Stromal invasion ≤ 3.0 mm in depth and ≤ 7.0 mm in horizontal spread

         T1a2   Stromal invasion > 3.0 mm but ≤ 5.0 mm with a horizontal spread ≤ 7.0

     T1b   Clinically visible lesion confined to the cervix or microscopic lesion greater than T1a2

         T1b1   Clinically visible lesion ≤ 4 cm in greatest dimension

         T1b2   Clinically visible lesion > 4 cm in greatest dimension

T2   Cervical carcinoma invades beyond uterus but not to pelvic wall or to the lower third of vagina

     T2a   Tumor without parametrial invasion

     T2b   Tumor with parametrial invasion

T3   Cervical carcinoma extends to pelvic wall and/or involves lower third of vagina and/or causes hydronephrosis or nonfunctioning kidney

     T3a   Tumor involves lower third of the vagina, no extension to pelvic wall

     T3b   Tumor extends to pelvic wall and/or causes hydronephrosis or nonfunctioning kidney

T4   Tumor invades mucosa of bladder or rectum and/or extends beyond the true pelvis. *Note:* The presence of bullous edema is not sufficient to classify a tumor as T4.

Lymph Node (N)

NX   Regional lymph nodes cannot be assessed

N0   No regional lymph node metastasis

N1   Regional lymph node metastasis

Distant Metastasis (M)

MX Presence of distant metastasis cannot be assessed
M0 No distant metastasis
M1 Distant metastasis

Pathologic Classification (pTNM)

The pT, pN and pM categories correspond to the T, N , and M categories.

Colon and Rectum

Primary Tumor (T)

TX   Primary tumor cannot be assessed
T0   No evidence of primary tumor
Tis Carcinoma in situ: intraepithelial or invasion of lamina propria. *Note:* Tis includes cancer cells confined within a glandular basement membrane (intraepithelial) or lamina propria (intramucosal) with no extension through muscularis mucosa into submusosa
T1   Tumor invades submucosa
T2   Tumor invades muscularis propria
T3   Tumor invades through muscularis propria into subserosa, or into nonperitonealized pericolic or perirectal tissues
T4   Tumor perforates visceral peritoneum and/or directly invades other organs or structures

Lymph Node (N)

NX   Regional lymph nodes cannot be assessed
N0   No regional lymph node metastasis
N1   Metastasis in 1–3 or more pericolic or perirectal lymph nodes
N2   Metastasis in 4 or more pericolic or perirectal lymph nodes

Distant Metastasis (M)

MX   Presence of distant metastasis cannot be assessed
M0   No distant metastasis
M1   Distant metastasis

Pathologic Classification (pTNM)

The pT, pN and pM categories correspond to the TNM categories.

DUKES' CLASSIFICATION (ASTER–COLLER MODIFICATION) OF COLON CANCER

STAGE A:	Limited to the mucosa
STAGE B1:	Into muscularis propria, nodes negative
STAGE B2:	Extends through entire wall, nodes negative
STAGE C1:	Extends into muscularis propria, nodes positive
STAGE C2:	Extends through entire wall, nodes positive
STAGE D:	Metastatic disease

Kidney

Primary Tumor (T)

TX   Primary tumor cannot be assessed
T0   No evidence of primary tumor
T1a Tumor ≤ 4.0 cm in greatest dimension, limited to the kidney
T1b Tumor 4.0–7.0 cm in greatest dimension, limited to the kidney
T2   Tumor > 7 cm in greatest dimension, limited to the kidney

T3   Tumor extends into major veins or invades adrenal gland or perinephric tissues but not beyond Gerota's fascia

    T3a   Tumor invades adrenal gland or perirenal and/or renal sinus fat but not beyond Gerota's fascia

    T3b   Tumor grossly extends into renal vein(s) or vena cava below diaphragm

    T3c   Tumor grossly extends into vena cava above diaphragm or invades wall of vena cava

T4   Tumor invades beyond Gerota's fascia

Lymph Node (N)

NX   Regional lymph nodes cannot be assessed

N0   No regional lymph node metastasis

N1   Metastasis in a single regional lymph node

N2   Metastasis in more than one regional lymph node

Distant Metastasis (M)

MX   Presence of distant metastasis cannot be assessed

M0   No distant metastasis

M1   Distant metastasis

Pathologic Classification (pTNM)

The pT, pN and pM categories correspond to the T, N , and M categories.

Lung

Primary Tumor (T)

TX   Primary tumor cannot be assessed, or tumor proven by presence of malignant cells in sputum or bronchial washings but not visualized by imaging or bronchoscopy

T0   No evidence of primary tumor

Tis   Carcinoma in situ

T1   Tumor ≤ 3 cm in greatest dimension, surrounded by lung or visceral pleura, without bronchoscopic evidence of invasion more proximal than the lobar bronchus

T2   Tumor with *any* of the following features of size or extent:

    > 3 cm in greatest dimension

    Involves main bronchus, ≥ 2 cm distal to the carina

    Invades the visceral pleura

    Associated with atelectasis or obstructive pneumonitis that extends to the hilar region but does not involve the entire lung

T3   Tumor of any size that directly invades any of the following: chest wall (including superior sulcus tumors), diaphragm, mediastinal pleura, parietal pericardium; or tumor in the main bronchus < 2 cm distal to the carina but without involvement of the carina; or associated atelectasis or obstructive pneumonitis of the entire lung

T4   Tumor of any size that invades any of the following: mediastinum, heart, great vessels, trachea, esophagus, vertebral body, carina; or separate tumor nodules in the same lobe, or tumor with a malignant pleural effusion

Lymph Node (N)

NX   Regional lymph nodes cannot be assessed

N0   No regional lymph node metastasis

N1   Metastasis in ipsilateral peribronchial and/or ipsilateral hilar lymph nodes, and intrapulmonary nodes, including direct extension

N2   Metastasis in ipsilateral mediastinal and/or subcarinal lymph node(s)

N3   Metastasis in contralateral mediastinal, contralateral hilar, ipsilateral or contralateral scalene or supraclavicular lymph node(s)

Distant Metastasis (M)

MX   Presence of distant metastasis cannot be assessed

M0   No distant metastasis

M1   Distant metastasis (includes separate tumor nodule(s) in a different lobe, ipsilateral or contralateral)

Pathologic Classification (pTNM)

The pT, pN and pM categories correspond to the T, N , and M categories.

ANN ARBOR STAGING CLASSIFICATION

Lymphoid Neoplasms

Stage	Definition
I	Limited to one area
II	Involvement in two or more areas on the same side of the diaphragm
III	Involvement in two or more areas on both sides of the diaphragm
III_E	Adjacent lymph node involvement: Upper abdomen, spleen, splenic and hilar nodes
III_S	Involvement of the spleen
$III_{E,S}$	Both of the above
IV	Diffuse or disseminated involvement of one or more extralymphatic organs, with or without associated lymph node involvement

Melanoma of the Skin (Excluding Eyelid)

Primary Tumor (pT)

pTX   Primary tumor cannot be assessed

pT0   No evidence of tumor

pTis   Melanoma in situ (atypical melanotic hyperplasia, severe melanotic dysplasia), not an invasive lesion (Clark's level I)

pT1a   Tumor ≤ 1.0 mm and Clark's level II or III, no ulceration

pT1b   Tumor ≤ 1.0 mm and Clark's level IV or V, with ulceration

pT2a   Melanoma 1.01–2.0 mm, no ulceration

pT2b   Melanoma 1.01–2.0 mm, with ulceration

pT3a   Melanoma 2.01–4.0 mm, no ulceration

pT3b   Melanoma 2.01–4.0 mm, with ulceration

pT2a   Melanoma > 4.0 mm, no ulceration

pT2b   Melanoma > 4.0 mm, with ulceration

Lymph Node (N)

NX   Regional lymph nodes cannot be assessed

N0   No regional lymph node metastasis

N1   Metastasis in one lymph node

N1a   Microscopic metastasis

N1b   Clinically apparent (macroscopic) metastasis

N2   Metastasis in 2–3 regional nodes or intralymphatic regional metastasis without nodal metastasis

N2a   Microscopic metastasis

N2b   Clinically apparent (macroscopic) metastasis

N2c Satellite or in-transit metastasis without nodal metastasis
N3   Metastasis in ≥ 4 regional nodes, or matted metastatic nodes, or in-transit metastasis or satellite(s) with metastasis in regional node(s)

Distant Metastasis (M)
MX   Presence of distant metastasis cannot be assessed
M0   No distant metastasis
M1   Distant metastasis
    M1a Metastasis in skin or subcutaneous tissue or lymph node(s) beyond the regional lymph nodes
    M1b Metastasis to lung
    M1c Metastasis to all other visceral sites or distant metastasis at any site associated with an elevated serum LDH

Ovary

Primary Tumor (T)

TNM	FIGO	Definition
TX		Primary tumor cannot be assessed
T0		No evidence of primary tumor
T1	1	Tumor limited to ovaries
T1a	1a	Tumor limited to one ovary; capsule intact, no tumor on ovarian surface, no malignant cells in ascites or peritoneal washings
T1b	1b	Tumor limited to both ovaries; capsules intact, no tumor on ovarian surface, no malignant cells in ascites or peritoneal washings
T1c	1c	Tumor limited to one or both ovaries with any of the following: capsule ruptured, tumor on ovarian surface, malignant cells in ascites or peritoneal washings
T2	11	Tumor involves one or both ovaries with pelvic extension
T2a	11a	Extension and/or implants on uterus and/or tubes
T2b	11b	Extension and/or implants to other pelvic tissues
T2c	11c	Pelvic extension and/or implants (2a or 2b) with malignant cells in ascites or peritoneal washing
T3*	111	Tumor involves one or both ovaries with microscopically confirmed peritoneal metastasis outside the pelvis
T3a	111a	Microscopic peritoneal metastasis beyond pelvis
T3b	111b	Microscopic peritoneal metastasis beyond pelvis ≤ 2 cm in greatest dimension
T3c	111c	Peritoneal metastasis beyond pelvis ≥ 2 cm in greatest dimension and/or regional lymph node metastasis

*Liver capsule metastasis is T3/stage III, liver parenchymal metastasis M1/stage IV. Pleural effusion must have positive cytology for M1/stage IV.
FIGO = Fédération Internationale de Gynécologie et d' Obstétrique.

Lymph Node (N)

NX Regional lymph nodes cannot be assessed
N0 No regional lymph node metastasis
N1 IIIC Regional lymph node metastasis

Distant Metastasis (M)

TNM	FIGO	Definition
MX		Presence of distant metastasis cannot be assessed
M0		No distant metastasis
M1	IV	Distant metastasis (excludes peritoneal metastasis)

FIGO = Fédération Internationale de Gynécologie et d' Obstétrique.

Stomach

Primary Tumor (T)

TX Primary tumor cannot be assessed
T0 No evidence of primary tumor
Tis Carcinoma in situ: Intraepithelial tumor without invasion of lamina propria
T1 Tumor invades lamina propria or submucosa
T2a Tumor invades muscularis propria
T2a Tumor invades subserosa
T3 Tumor penetrates serosa (visceral peritoneum) without invasion of adjacent structures
T4 Tumor invades adjacent structures

Lymph Node (N)

NX Regional lymph node(s) cannot be assessed
N0 No regional lymph node metastasis
N1 Metastasis in 1–6 regional lymph node(s)
N2 Metastasis in 7–15 regional lymph nodes(s)
N3 Metastasis in > 15 regional lymph nodes(s)

Distant Metastasis (M)

MX Presence of distant metastasis cannot be assessed
M0 No distant metastasis
M1 Distant metastasis

Pathologic Classification (pTNM)

The pT, pN and pM categories correspond to the T, N, and M categories.

Thyroid Gland

Primary Tumor (T)

All categories may be subdivided: (a) solitary; (b) multifocal—measure the largest for classification
TX Primary tumor cannot be assessed
T0 No evidence of primary tumor
T1 Tumor ≤ 2.0 cm in greatest dimension, limited to the thyroid
T2 Tumor 2.01–4.0 cm in greatest dimension, limited to the thyroid
T3 Tumor > 4.0 cm in greatest dimension, limited to the thyroid, or any tumor with extrathyroid extension

T4   Tumor of any size extending beyond the thyroid capsule

Lymph Node (N)

Regional nodes are the central compartment, lateral and cervical, and upper mediastinal lymph nodes

NX   Regional lymph nodes cannot be assessed

N0   No regional lymph node metastasis

N1   Regional lymph node metastasis

  N1a Metastasis to level VI nodes (pretracheal, paratracheal, and prelaryngeal nodes)

  N1b Metastasis in unilateral, bilateral, or contralateral cervical or superior, mediastinal lymph nodes

Distant Metastasis (M)

MX   Presence of distant metastasis cannot be assessed

M0   No distant metastasis

M1   Distant metastasis

Pathologic Classification (pTNM)

The pT, pN, and pM categories correspond to the T, N, and M categories.

Uterus

Primary Tumor (T)

TNM	FIGO	Definition
TX		Primary tumor cannot be assessed
T0		No evidence of primary tumor
Tis	0	Carcinoma in situ
T1	1	Tumor confined to corpus
T1a	1A	Tumor limited to endometrium
T1b	1B	Tumor invades less than one half of myometrium
T1c	1C	Tumor invades one half, or more, of myometrium
T2	11	Tumor invades cervix but does not extend beyond uterus
T2a	IIA	Endocervical glandular endothelial involvement only
T2b	IIB	Cervical stomal invasion
T3	111	Local and/or regional spread as defined below:
T3a	IIIA	Tumor involves serosa and/or adnexa (direct extension or metastasis) and/or cancer cells in ascites or peritoneal washings
T3b	IIIB	Vaginal involvement (direct extension or metastasis)
T4*	IVA	Tumor involves bladder mucosa and/or bowel mucosa

*The presence of bullous edema is not sufficient evidence to classify a tumor T4.

Lymph Node (N)

NX   Regional lymph nodes cannot be assessed

N0   No regional lymph node metastasis

N1   IIIC Regional lymph node metastasis to pelvis and/or paraaortic lymph nodes

Distant Metastasis (M)

TNM	FIGO	Definition
MX		Presence of distant metastasis cannot be assessed
M0		No distant metastasis
M1	IVB	Distant metastasis includes metastasis to intraabdominal lymph nodes other than paraaortic and/or inguinal lymph nodes, excludes metastasis to vagina, pelvic serosa, or adnexa

FIGO = Fédération Internationale de Gynécologie et d' Obstétrique.

Pathologic Classification (pTNM)

The pT, pN, and pM categories correspond to the T, N, and M categories.

Prostate

TX   Primary tumor cannot be assessed

T0   No evidence of primary tumor

T1   Nonpalpable disease *Note:* There is no pT1 category because there is insufficient tissue to assess the highest pT category.

    T1a   Tumor incidentally found in ≤ 5% of resected tissue

    T1b   Tumor incidentally found in > 5% of resected tissue

    T1c   No palpable tumor, diagnosed by biopsy for elevated PSA, for clinical staining *only!*

T2   Tumor present clinically or grossly, limited to the gland

    T2a   Tumor unilateral in ≤ ½ of lobe

    T2b   Tumor unilateral in > ½ of lobe

    T2c   Tumor involves both lobes

T3   Tumor extends through the prostatic capsule

    T3a   Extracapsular extension (unilateral or bilateral)

    T3b   Tumor invades seminal vesical(s)

T4   Tumor is fixed or invades adjacent structures other than seminal vesicles: bladder neck, external sphincter, rectum, levator muscles, and/or pelvic wall.

Lymph Nodes (N)

NX   Regional lymph nodes cannot be assessed

N0   No regional lymph node metastasis

N1   Regional lymph node metastasis

Distant Metastasis (M)

MX   Distant metastasis cannot be assessed

M0   No distant metastasis

M1   Distant metastasis

M1a   Nonregional lymph node(s)

M1b   Bone(s)

M1c   Other site(s)

Pathologic Classification (pTNM)

The pT, pN and pM categories correspond to the T, N, and M categories.

TABLE A–6
Weight Conversion Table

lb	kg	kg	lb
1	0.5	1	2.2
2	0.9	2	4.4
4	1.8	3	6.6
6	2.7	4	8.8
8	3.6	5	11.0
10	4.5	6	13.2
20	9.1	8	17.6
30	13.6	10	22.0
40	18.2	20	44.0
50	22.7	30	66.0
60	27.3	40	88.0
70	31.8	50	110.0
80	36.4	60	132.0
90	40.9	70	154.0
100	45.4	80	176.0
150	68.2	90	198.0
200	90.8	100	220.9

$kg = lb \times 0.454$ $lb = kg \times 2.2$

WEIGHT CONVERSION

Table A-6 (above) gives information for converting weight in pounds (lb) to weight in kilograms (kg) and vice versa.

INDEX

Note: Page numbers followed by f *indicate figures; those followed by* t *indicate tables.*